Handbook of Self-Management and the Lived Experience of Healthcare

This edited book focuses on the role of self-management in healthcare and how it may enhance the medical treatment, management, and rehabilitation of service users. It offers expert perspectives on topics covering tools and techniques and how they are being incorporated into healthcare, but also critically appraising forthcoming implementation.

Handbook of Self-Management and the Lived Experience of Healthcare begins by introducing the importance of self-management with contemporary and innovative approaches. The book focuses on the impact of self-management and how it affects interpersonal and client-based perspectives. The chapters examine how these strategies can help and/or hinder patient/service user outcomes. Each chapter explores the multifaceted use and application of each self-management strategy within its respective specialty and its impacts on diagnosis, treatment, and future management of individuals. It encompasses an array of examples of self-management strategies that will remain pertinent to caregivers, families, practitioners, service users, and policymakers. This is not a text on self-management alone but on the societal implications, accompanied by ethical, altruistic and moral examples for such advances within the healthcare field. The book offers original discussions surrounding the interconnectivity of technology and medicine, rehabilitation and patient care.

This book will be useful for healthcare practitioners, researchers, and academics as it provides insight into both contemporary and innovative approaches within the medical field, and it can be used as a text to enrich scholarly learning, teaching, and assessment to healthcare programs nationally and internationally.

Christopher M. Hayre is Associate Professor at Monash University. He has published several textbooks, which are widely implemented into academic curriculum worldwide, with translations into other languages. His research impact is evidenced on an international scale, not only influencing policy and practice, but engagement as respected PhD supervisor to students in the UK, UAE, Australia, and South Africa. His areas of expertise are medical imaging, health research, emerging technology, and ethnography.

Dave J. Muller is currently a Co-Editor of the *Rehabilitation in Practice Series*, published by CRC Press. He is the Editor-in-Chief of *Disability and Rehabilitation* and has been involved in the publication of over 50 books and has published over 40 referred papers. He is a visiting Professor at the University of Suffolk, United Kingdom.

Marcia Scherer is a rehabilitation psychologist and founding President of the Institute for Matching Person & Technology. She is Editor in Chief to *Disability and Rehabilitation* and also Professor of Physical Medicine and Rehabilitation, University of Rochester Medical Center where she received both her PhD and MPH degrees. She is Co-Editor of the book series for CRC Press, *Rehabilitation Science in Practice Series*.

Paul M.W. Hackett has wide experience in social science and humanities research and is the originator of the declarative mapping approach to qualitative research. His research interests span many aspects of behavior and experience focusing upon the investigation of ontologies and epistemologies that have originated in the African continent. He has around 300 publications including more than 30 books. He is a visiting research professor in the department of philosophy at Nnamdi Azikiwe University, Nigeria, an honorary fellow in the philosophy department at University of Wales Trinity St David and a PhD supervisor at the same university, and a visiting professor in health research methods at the University of Suffolk. He holds a PhD in psychology and a PhD in fine art. He has held appointments at universities, including Oxford, Cambridge, Tufts, Harvard, Cardiff, and Durham.

Ava Gordley-Smith is a lecturer at Emerson College and a PhD research student at the University of Wales Trinity Saint David. Her research aims to develop a multidimensional psychological framework for understanding the relationship and intersection of attitudes toward environmental and social justice issues. Outside of her PhD research, her work focuses more broadly on both theoretical and applied methodologies in health and rehabilitation, the social sciences, and communication studies.

Rehabilitation Science in Practice Series

Series Editors:
Marcia J. Scherer
Institute for Matching Person & Technology, Webster, New York, USA

Dave Muller
University of Suffolk, UK

Everyday Technologies in Healthcare
Christopher M. Hayre, Dave Muller, Marcia Scherer

Enhancing Healthcare and Rehabilitation: The Impact of Qualitative Research
Christopher M. Hayre and Dave Muller

Neurological Rehabilitation: Spasticity and Contractures in Clinical Practice and Research
Anand D. Pandyan, Hermie J. Hermens, Bernard A. Conway

Quality of Life Technology Handbook
Richard Schulz

Computer Systems Experiences of Users with and Without Disabilities: An Evaluation Guide for Professionals
Simone Borsci, Masaaki Kurosu, Stefano Federici, Maria Laura Mele

Assistive Technology Assessment Handbook - 2nd Edition
Stefano Federici, Marcia Scherer

Ambient Assisted Living
Nuno M. Garcia, Joel Jose P.C. Rodrigues

Rehabilitation Engineering: Principles and Practice
Alex Mihailidis, Roger Smith

Emerging Technologies in Healthcare: Interpersonal and Client Based Perspectives
Christopher M. Hayre, Dave Muller, Marcia Scherer, Paul M. W Hackett, Ava Gordley-Smith

Handbook of Self-Management and the Lived Experience of Healthcare
Edited by Christopher M. Hayre, Dave J. Muller, Marcia Scherer, Paul M.W. Hackett, and Ava Gordley-Smith

Principles and Practice For more information about this series, please visit: https://www.crcpress.com/Rehabilitation-Science-in-Practice-Series/book-series/CRCPRESERIN

Handbook of Self-Management and the Lived Experience of Healthcare

Edited by
Christopher M. Hayre, Dave J. Muller,
Marcia Scherer, Paul M.W. Hackett,
and Ava Gordley-Smith

CRC Press
Taylor & Francis Group
Boca Raton London New York

CRC Press is an imprint of the
Taylor & Francis Group, an **informa** business

Designed cover image: © Shutterstock

First edition published 2027
by CRC Press
2385 NW Executive Center Drive, Suite 320, Boca Raton FL 33431

and by CRC Press
4 Park Square, Milton Park, Abingdon, Oxon, OX14 4RN

CRC Press is an imprint of Taylor & Francis Group, LLC

ISBN: 978-1-032-98516-9 (hbk)
ISBN: 978-1-032-98515-2 (pbk)
ISBN: 978-1-003-59907-4 (ebk)

DOI: 10.1201/9781003599074

Typeset in Times
by KnowledgeWorks Global Ltd.

Christopher M. Hayre would like to dedicate this book to his family, in particular his wife Charlotte for her unwavering support and to his daughters Ayva and Ellena. This book is also dedicated to the memory of Evelynn.

Dave J. Muller would like to dedicate this book to his grandchildren Edie, Freya, Toby and Kaya in hope of a better future.

Collectively the editors congratulate one another for completing a worthwhile and enjoyable collaborative project.

Contents

Preface

This book presents the collaborative work of experienced researchers worldwide. It brings together practitioners and researchers who are either utilizing or critically evaluating self-management in a range of health and rehabilitation settings. The chapters presented here delve into the use of self-management for a number of health and rehabilitation conditions; this is coupled with lived experiences and also perspectives from internationally recognized peers working in this field. This book presents a range of topics and contexts pertinent to health disciplines worldwide, but it will naturally present researchers and scholars with methodological insights which are translatable to other disciplines. The examination of this topic among our experts seeks to provide greater impact to an array of readers internationally.

This book offers a multitude of perspectives in a range of contexts for self-management. Here, we appreciate the wide acceptance and impact of self-management as a topic and how it looks to enhance not only service users, but perhaps ourselves. In short, this book will offer value to undergraduate and postgraduate students given the magnitude of references signposting them to key materials. In addition, this book aims to remain pivotal for practitioners and prospective researchers in this important field providing methodological and empirical insights in advancing evidence-based practice, while supporting the development of novelty in their respective field.

Christopher M. Hayre

Dave J. Muller

Marcia Scherer

Paul M.W. Hackett

Ava Gordley-Smith

List of Contributors

Israel Ikechukwu Adandom
Department of Kinesiology
College of Education
University of Alabama
USA

Carole Anglade
École d'Orthophonie et d'audiologie, Université de Montréal
Centre for Interdisciplinary Research in Rehabilitation of Greater Montreal
Canada

Ebuka Miracle Anieto
School of Health, Sciences and Society
University of Suffolk
UK

Ijeoma Blessing Anieto
Pure Physiotherapy
UK

Ganette Apeadu-Baah
College of Health and Public Service
University of North Texas
USA

Elijah Areli
Centre for Health, Activity and Rehabilitation Research
School of Physiotherapy
University of Otago
New Zealand

Jerome Atutornu
School of Health, Sciences and Society
University of Suffolk
UK
and
Kavli Centre for Ethics, Science and the Public
University of Cambridge
England

Vasiliki B Darsaklis
Shriners Hospital for Children
Canada

Liesbet De Baets
Musculoskeletal Rehabilitation Research Group
Department of Rehabilitation Sciences
Faculty of Movement and Rehabilitation Sciences
The Leuven Centre for Algology and Pain Management
Division of Physical Medicine and Rehabilitation, University Hospitals Leuven, and
Pain in Motion (PAIN) Research Group, Vrije Universiteit Brussel
Belgium

Clíodhna Ní Bhroin
School of Postgraduate Studies
RCSI
University of Medicine and Health Sciences
Ireland

Cecilia (Nowak) Bushby
retired

Christopher P. Bushby
retired

Sarah-Jane Byrne
School of Postgraduate Studies
RCSI
University of Medicine and Health Sciences
Ireland

Sarah Cachecho
Shriners Hospital for Children
Canada

Olaf Kraus de Camargo
CanChild Centre for Childhood-Onset Disability Research
McMaster University
Canada

Lizz Carrington
Centre for Health, Activity and Rehabilitation Research
School of Physiotherapy
University of Otago
New Zealand

Elizabeth Chambers
CanChild Centre for Childhood-Onset Disability Research
McMaster University
Canada

Chungyi Chiu
Department of Health and Kinesiology
University of Illinois Urbana-Champaign
USA

Stephanie R. Cimino
Lawson Research Institute
St. Joseph's Health Care
Canada
and
School of Health Studies
The University of Western Ontario
Canada

Shane Clifton
Centre for Disability Research and Policy
Disability Studies and Ethics
School of Health Sciences
Faculty of Medicine
University of Sydney
Australia

Olivia Crozier
School of Occupational Therapy
The University of Western Ontario
Canada
and
Lawson Research Institute
St. Joseph's Health Care
Canada

Genevieve Currie
Mount Royal University
Canada

Noémi Dahan-Oliel
Shriners Hospital for Children
Canada
and
School of Occupational and Physical Therapy
Faculty of Medicine and Health Sciences
McGill University
Canada

Astrid Jensen Damgaard
Centre for Expertise in Rheumatology
Danish Hospital for Rheumatic Diseases
University Hospital of Southern Denmark
Denmark
and
Department of Regional Health Research
University of Southern Denmark
Denmark

Henrik Danielsson
Department of Behavioural Sciences and Learning
Linköping University
Sweden

Claudia Didyk
Caring Futures Institute
College of Nursing and Health Sciences
Flinders University
Australia
and
School of Allied Health Science and Practice
The University of Adelaide (Adelaide University)
Australia

Klaus Dieterich
Centre Hospitalier Universitaire Grenoble Alpes
France
and
Medical Genetics
Université Grenoble Alpes
France

Nicola Diviani
Person-Centered Healthcare and Health Communication Group
Swiss Paraplegic Research
Switzerland
and
Faculty of Health Sciences and Medicine
University of Lucerne
Switzerland

Kristen Donlevie
NAPA Center
USA

Maureen Donohoe
Nemours Children's Hospital
USA

Jacobi Elliott
Lawson Research Institute
St. Joseph's Health Care
Canada
and
School of Health Studies
The University of Western Ontario
Canada

Alicja Fąfara
Institute of Physiotherapy
Jagiellonian University Medical College
Poland

B.R. Kristoffersen-Fait
Department of Psychology
University of Oslo
Norway
and
Fredrikstad Community Mental Health Centre
General Outpatient Clinic
Norway

Emna Fakhfakh
École d'Orthophonie et d'audiologie
Université de Montréal
Canada
and
Centre for Interdisciplinary Research in Rehabilitation of Greater Montreal
Canada

Daniela Figueiredo
RISE-Health
School of Health Sciences
University of Aveiro
Aveiro, Portugal

Hermann Fricke-Comellas
CTS 1110: Understanding Movement and Self in health from Science (UMSS) Research Group
Departamento de Fisioterapia
Facultad de Enfermería, Fisioterapia y Podología
Universidad de Sevilla
Spain
and
Instituto de Biomedicina de Sevilla-IBiS (Hospitales Universitarios Virgen del Rocío y Macarena/CSIC/Universidad de Sevilla)
Spain

Mats Granlund
CHILD Research Group
School of Health Sciences
Jönköping University
Sweden
and
Centre for Augmentative and Alternative Communication
University of Pretoria
South Africa

Paul M.W. Hackett
Department of Philosophy
Nnamdi Azikiwe University
Nigeria
Health and Wellbeing Research Institute
University of Suffolk
England
Doctoral College
Prifysgol Cymru Y Drindod Dewi Sant (University of Wales Trinity Saint David)
Wales
School of Communication
Emerson College
USA
Patricia Hall
School of Public Health, Physiotherapy and Sports Science
Health Science Centre
University College Dublin
Ireland

Leigh Hale
Centre for Health, Activity and Rehabilitation Research
School of Physiotherapy
University of Otago
New Zealand

Buxin Han
State Key Laboratory of Cognitive Science and Mental Health
Institute of Psychology
Chinese Academy of Sciences (Department of Psychology
University of Chinese Academy of Sciences
China

S.L. Hauger
Department of Psychology
University of Oslo
and
Department of Research and Innovation
Sunnaas Rehabilitation Hospital
Norway

Jiali He
Feinberg School of Medicine
Northwestern University
Center for Rehabilitation Outcomes Research
Shirley Ryan AbilityLab
USA

Alberto Marcos Heredia-Rizo
CTS 1110: Understanding Movement and Self in health from Science (UMSS) Research Group
Departamento de Fisioterapia
Facultad de Enfermería, Fisioterapia y Podología
Universidad de Sevilla
and
Instituto de Biomedicina de Sevilla-IBiS
(Hospitales Universitarios Virgen del Rocío y Macarena/CSIC/Universidad de Sevilla)
Spain

Ann Marie Hestetun-Mandrup
Faculty of Health Sciences
Department of Rehabilitation Science and Health Technology
Interaction, Development and Innovation
Oslo Metropolitan University
and
Sunnaas Rehabilitation Hospital
Norway

Anne Hickey
Department of Health Psychology
School of Population Health
RCSI University of Medicine and Health Sciences
Ireland

Frances Horgan
School of Physiotherapy
RCSI University of Medicine and Health Sciences
Ireland

Mona Hoy
Centre Hospitalier Universitaire Grenoble Alpes
France

Claire Huzar
Centre Hospitalier Universitaire Grenoble Alpes
France

Christine Imms
Healthy Trajectories Child and Youth Disability Research Hub
Department of Paediatrics
The University of Melbourne
Australia

Tristram Ingham
Ngāti Kahungunu ki Heretaunga, Ngāti Porou (iwi tribal affiliation)
Department of Medicine
University of Otago
New Zealand

Magnus Ivarsson
Department of Behavioural Sciences and Learning
Linköping University
Sweden

Bernadette Jones
Ngā Wairiki, Ngāti Apa (iwi tribal affiliation)
Department of Medicine
University of Otago
New Zealand

Mojtaba Khaliji
Department of Health and Kinesiology
University of Illinois Urbana-Champaign
USA

Kirsten Lykke Knak
Centre for Expertise in Rheumatology
Danish Hospital for Rheumatic Diseases
University Hospital of Southern Denmark
Denmark
and
Department of Regional Health Research
University of Southern Denmark
Denmark

Francis Lacombe
Centre de réadaptation Lucie-Bruneau
Canada

Lena Wekre Lande
TRS National Resource Centre for Rare Disorders
Sunnaas Rehabilitation Hospital
Norway

Belinda Lange
Caring Futures Institute
College of Nursing and Health Sciences
Flinders University
Australia

Brason Lee
California Department of Public Health
Sacramento, California, USA

Olive Lennon
School of Public Health, Physiotherapy and Sports Science
Health Science Centre
University College Dublin
Ireland

Lucy Kate Lewis
Caring Futures Institute
College of Nursing and Health Sciences
Flinders University
Australia

Ziwei Li
Feinberg School of Medicine
Northwestern University
USA

Kristin Schewe Loxley
TRS National Resource Centre for Rare Disorders
Sunnaas Rehabilitation Hospital
Norway

Anne Lund
Faculty of Health Sciences
Department of Rehabilitation Science and Health Technology
Interaction, Development and Innovation
Oslo Metropolitan University
Norway
and
Sunnaas Rehabilitation Hospital
Norway

Christina Merete Tvede Madsen
Centre for Expertise in Rheumatology
Danish Hospital for Rheumatic Diseases
University Hospital of Southern Denmark
Sønderborg, Denmark
and
User Perspectives and Community-based Interventions
Department of Public Health
University of Southern Denmark
Odense, Denmark

Valentina Maestri
Azienda Ospedaliero Universitaria Ancona
Italy

Molly Manning
School of Allied Health, and Health Research Institute
University of Limerick
Ireland

Anne Catrine Trægde Martinsen
Faculty of Health Sciences
Department of Rehabilitation Science and Health Technology
Interaction, Development and Innovation
Oslo Metropolitan University
Norway
and
Sunnaas Rehabilitation Hospital
Norway

Thomas Matheve
Spine, Head and Pain Research Unit Ghent
Department of Rehabilitation Sciences
Ghent University
Belgium
and
Hasselt University
REVAL Rehabilitation Research Center
Belgium

Elias Mpofu
College of Health and Public Service
University of North Texas
USA
and
School of Health Sciences
University of Sydney
Australia

Carolina Navalòn
Asociación Artrogriposis Múltiple Congénita España
Spain

John Naylor
Physiotherapy Department
Hull University Teaching Hospitals NHS Trust (HUTH)
NHS Humber Health Partnership (HHP)
England

Eugene Nizeyimana
Division of Physiotherapy
Department of Health and Rehabilitation Sciences
Stellenbosch University
South Africa

Geraldine O'Callaghan
School of Physiotherapy
RCSI University of Medicine and Health Sciences
Ireland
and
Health Service Executive (HSE)
Longford/Westmeath Community Healthcare Services
Ireland

Mary O'Neill
Codesigning a Life After Stroke (CLASP) Project
RCSI University of Medicine and Health Sciences
Ireland

Hanne Pallesen
Hammel Neurorehabilitation Centre and University Research Clinic
Department of Clinical Medicine
University of Aarhus
Denmark

Sedsel Kristine Stage Pedersen
Hammel Neurorehabilitation Centre and University Research Clinic
Department of Clinical Medicine
University of Aarhus
Denmark

Jacinta Pennacchia
Healthy Trajectories Child and Youth Disability Research Hub
Department of Paediatrics
The University of Melbourne
Australia

Meredith Perry
Centre for Health, Activity and Rehabilitation Research
School of Physiotherapy
University of Otago
New Zealand

Minna Pikkarainen
Faculty of Health Sciences
Department of Rehabilitation Science and Health Technology
Postgraduate Studies, Faculty of Technology, Art and Design
Department of Product Design
Oslo Metropolitan University
Norway

Kinga Pozniak
CanChild Centre for Childhood-Onset Disability Research
McMaster University
Canada

Jette Primdahl
Centre for Expertise in Rheumatology
Danish Hospital for Rheumatic Diseases
Department of Public Health
Department of Regional Health Research
University of Southern Denmark
Denmark
and
Hospital Sønderjylland
University Hospital of Southern Denmark
Denmark

Enxhi Qama
Person-Centered Healthcare and Health Communication Group
Swiss Paraplegic Research
Switzerland
and
Faculty of Health Sciences and Medicine
University of Lucerne
Switzerland

Oscar Ribeiro
RISE-Health
Department of Education and Psychology
University of Aveiro
Aveiro, Portugal

Pablo Rodríguez-Sánchez-Laulhé
Departamento Ciencias de la Salud y Biomédicas
Universidad Loyola Andalucía
Spain
and
CTS 1110: Understanding Movement and Self in Health from Science (UMSS) Research Group
Spain

Sheeba Rosewilliam
School of Sport, Exercise and Rehabilitation Sciences
College of Life and Environmental Sciences
University of Birmingham
UK

Ahman Sahely
Department of Physical Therapy
College of Nursing and Health Sciences
Jazan University
Saudi Arabia
and
School of Sport, Exercise and Rehabilitation Sciences
College of Life and Environmental Sciences
University of Birmingham
UK

Md Refat Uz Zaman Sajib
Department of Health and Kinesiology
University of Illinois Urbana-Champaign
USA

Jesús Salas-González
CTS 1110: Understanding Movement and Self in health from Science (UMSS) Research Group
Spain
and
Instituto de Biomedicina de Sevilla-IBiS
Spain

Ani Samargian
Arthrogryposis Multiplex Congenita Support Inc
USA

Jessica B. Schwarzenbach
Independent Scholar

Megan Jaclyn Sions
Department of Physical Therapy
University of Delaware
USA

Susanne Lillelund Sørensen
Hammel Neurorehabilitation Centre and University Research Clinic
Department of Clinical Medicine
University of Aarhus
Denmark

Helena Sousa
RISE-Health
Department of Education and Psychology
University of Aveiro
Portugal

Ferhan Tanrıöğer Soyuer
Antalya Bilim University
Turkey

Yiling Tang
School of Kinesiology
University of British Columbia
Canada

Véronique Thellier
Centre Hospitalier Universitaire Grenoble Alpes
France

Michał T. Tomczak
Faculty of Management and Economics
Gdańsk University of Technology
Poland

Janelle Unger
Lawson Research Institute
St. Joseph's Health Care
Canada
and
School of Physical Therapy
The University of Western Ontario
Canada

K.T.A. Ustrimova
Department of Psychology
University of Oslo
Norway
and
Department of Functional Assessment
Sunnaas Rehabilitation Hospital
Norway

Lisa Wagner
Senior Occupational Therapist
Shriners Hospitals for Children
USA

Misha Walker
The Dream Walker Project
Peru

Lauren Winterbottom
Instructor in Clinical Rehabilitation & Regenerative Medicine (Occupational Therapy)
Research Occupational Therapist
Department of Rehabilitation & Regenerative Medicine
Columbia University Irving Medical Center
USA

Dalton L. Wolfe
Lawson Research Institute
St. Joseph's Health Care
Canada
and
School of Health Studies
The University of Western Ontario
Canada

Yong Yang
State Key Laboratory of Cognitive Science & Mental Health
Institute of Psychology
Chinese Academy of Sciences
Department of Psychology
University of Chinese Academy of Sciences
China

Acknowledgments

The editors would like to thank all contributing authors for sharing their innovative work in the field of self-management. This is a growing area of interest for practitioners and researchers which is demonstrated by the quality of chapters in this Handbook. The authors commitment to this book reflects the ongoing importance of this topic. On behalf of the editors, it has been a great pleasure working with you all in bringing together this collection. The work demonstrates not only the existing virtues of self-management for health and rehabilitation conditions, but we also observe important reflections of lived-experiences and lastly perspectives in the field from experts working in this space. This has been a thoroughly enjoyable project as we have been able to collaborate with colleagues from various parts of the world. Thank you.

Contributing Authors stated that they've used Chat GPT Versions 4 and 5.2, Open AI SIKT, Deep L, Grammarly, and Claude to assist with language improvement and refinement, and to improve readability. None of the text or images were generated using AI. All text was generated by the authors and edited using the AI programs listed above.

Section I

Health and Rehabilitation Conditions

1 Self-Management for Traumatic Injuries in Rehabilitation Settings

From Theory to Clinical Practice

K.T.A. Ustrimova, B.R. Kristoffersen-Fait, and S.L. Hauger

INTRODUCTION

Significant advancements in acute medical care have increased survival rates for patients with severe traumatic injuries. Nonetheless, these conditions often result in secondary complications, psychosocial issues, and disability (Haagsma et al., 2012; Lo et al., 2021). Consequently, the survivors frequently require an extended and intensive period of inpatient rehabilitation. Patients most commonly seen in rehabilitation settings often include those with traumatic brain injuries (TBIs), traumatic spinal cord injuries (SCIs), major or multitrauma, and burn injuries.

Traumatic Injuries: Types, Prevalence, and Consequences

Traumatic injuries usually encompass physical damage to the head and/or the body with an abrupt onset and a severity warranting urgent medical attention (Bonatti and Calland, 2008). Traumatic brain injury (TBI) is defined as an "alteration in brain function, or other evidence of brain pathology, caused by an external force" (Menon et al., 2010). As with other traumatic injuries, it is often caused by motor vehicle accidents, falls, and sports injuries (Ponsford, 2013). Each year, between 27 and 69 million individuals worldwide sustain TBI (Dewan et al., 2019; GBD 2016 Neurology Collaborators, 2019; "Traumatic Brain Injury (TBI) | National Institute of Neurological Disorders and Stroke," n.d.), and about 20% of patients are admitted to hospitals with moderate to severe brain injuries (Bruns Jr. and Hauser, 2003). Most TBI survivors are males in their early adulthood, which often compromises their future educational and occupational prospects, as well as their family and community roles (Ponsford, 2013). Regardless of the age of onset, individuals with TBI report long-term physical, cognitive, and emotional challenges that affect their daily lives, work, and community reintegration, leading to decreased health-related quality of life (HRQoL) decades after the injury (Andelic et al., 2018, 2015, 2009; Hammond et al., 2021; Soberg et al., 2013).

Traumatic spinal cord injuries (SCIs) constitute damage to the spinal cord due to trauma, resulting in loss of function and long-term impairments across multiple domains (Ahuja et al., 2017). The global incidence of SCI ranges from 250,000 to 500,000 cases annually, with younger adults being affected more frequently (Bickenbach et al., 2013). SCI usually results in both significant motor sequelae and secondary complications, such as chronic pain and pressure ulcers (Aaby et al., 2020; Adriaansen et al., 2016; Carrard et al., 2021; Jensen et al., 2012). Furthermore, it is often followed by challenges within the family, growing social isolation, employment issues, a reduced quality of life, and psychological distress that may persist decades after the injury (Pollard and Kennedy, 2007; Post and van Leeuwen, 2012).

Major trauma involves significant injuries across two or more body regions, such as complex fractures, peripheral nerve damage, internal organ injuries, and amputations (Alberdi et al., 2014;

DOI: 10.1201/9781003599074-2

Thompson et al., 2021). It is the sixth leading cause of death and the fifth most common cause of moderate to severe disability, greatly impacting health-related quality of life (World Health Organization, n.d.a). Survivors often experience decreased functional capacity, psychological issues, chronic pain, employment difficulties, and reduced social participation (de Munter et al., 2020; Gabbe et al., 2017; Haagsma et al., 2012; Soberg et al., 2012; Vincent et al., 2015). Burn injuries, the fourth most frequent civilian trauma, are injuries to skin or other tissues caused by heat, radiation, electricity, or chemicals (World Health Organization, n.d.b). These injuries frequently result in long-lasting skin alterations and an increased risk of secondary problems such as chronic pain, scar contractures, and scar hypertrophy (Allahham et al., 2024; Cariello et al., 2021; Jeschke et al., 2020; Smolle et al., 2017). Burn survivors typically face challenges with body image, sexual health, psychological well-being, as well as social participation and employment (Enblom et al., 2022; Moi et al., 2016; Spronk et al., 2018).

The complex and long-term consequences of traumatic injuries highlight the need for ongoing lifestyle changes that affected individuals must make to manage their everyday lives. Furthermore, survivors also experience increased healthcare needs that must be handled on a day-to-day basis, which influences both the quality of life, educational and occupational opportunities, and community participation (Andelic et al., 2018; Corrigan and Hammond, 2013; Gabbe et al., 2017; Wilson et al., 2017). In addition, ageing with traumatic injuries presents considerable challenges for patients, their caregivers, healthcare providers, and communities (Rabinowitz et al., 2021; Sabariego et al., 2023; Sullivan et al., 2018). There is also evidence that the psychosocial consequences of traumatic injuries may have more impact on an individual's identity than the mechanism or location of the injury, shifting rehabilitation focus from working with specific deficits to a broader approach that targets both strengths and challenges, helping individuals to negotiate a new identity and meaningful life roles in the process of adjustment to persistent injury-related consequences (Beadle et al., 2016).

However, despite the complexity surrounding both the nature of traumatic injuries and their multifactorial consequences, rehabilitation services for survivors often remain under-prioritised, and many patients experience unmet healthcare needs years after injury (Andelic et al., 2021; Cieza et al., 2020; Kamenov et al., 2019; Moksnes et al., 2023). This occurs against a backdrop of a generally increasing demand for healthcare, driven by a rising prevalence of chronic diseases and an ageing population (Choi et al., 2024; Holman, 2020). Self-management (SM) interventions have recently emerged as a promising approach to address the healthcare needs of people with traumatic injuries, aiming to enhance patients' confidence in managing their health, improve health literacy, and promote adaptive health behaviours (Jones et al., 2016; Jones and Demain, 2020). Self-management interventions are inherently complex due to the numerous issues they aim to address. Earlier studies on self-management have demonstrated its efficacy in managing chronic conditions, such as diabetes, arthritis, and asthma (Barlow et al., 2002; Lorig et al., 2001, 2016; Lorig and Holman, 2003). The long-term effects of traumatic injuries allow us to view them as chronic conditions (Corrigan and Hammond, 2013). In this context, self-management can help address the daily challenges faced by survivors and their caregivers. Indeed, emerging evidence suggests that self-management interventions could be beneficial in the rehabilitation of stroke, TBI, and SCI, thereby offering a means to alleviate the long-term healthcare burden. Several systematic reviews of self-management interventions for stroke and SCI patients highlight a modest impact on independence, quality of life, and self-efficacy, as well as an increase in physical activity, improvement in activities of daily living (ADL), and improved psychosocial well-being in caregivers (Baron et al., 2018a, 2018b; Cheng et al., 2014; Foster et al., 2007; Fryer et al., 2016; Jones et al., 2015; Parke et al., 2015; Prados-Román et al., 2024). Unfortunately, the evidence was often deemed inconclusive due to the insufficient quality of research, the risk of bias, and poor reporting. However, despite this, the growing literature and knowledge point out that self-management has the potential to support patients with traumatic injuries in managing injury-related consequences. Additionally, many of the ongoing symptoms and challenges that follow serious traumatic injuries overlap with the issues faced by patients with other chronic conditions (e.g. fatigue, chronic pain, and emotional difficulties)

(Lorig and Holman, 2003). Hence, with necessary adjustments, evidence and knowledge gained from existing interventions for chronic conditions such as diabetes and arthritis can also inform self-management support (SMS) approaches for patients with traumatic injuries in rehabilitation settings (Barlow et al., 2002; Lorig et al., 2001).

SELF-MANAGEMENT: THEORETICAL CONCEPTS IMPORTANT IN REHABILITATION

Self-management programs are complex interventions that require a solid theoretical foundation relevant to their intended outcomes to effectively cater to the specific needs of their target populations (Skivington et al., 2021). For self-management interventions, this foundation should identify the underlying mechanisms of behaviour change for a given patient population, informing the selection and efficient delivery of intervention ingredients (Bandura, 2004a; Lorig and Holman, 2003; Wilson, 2009). The literature on self-management often mentions social cognitive theory (SCT), the health belief model (HBM), and the transtheoretical model (TTM) as the frequently used theoretical frameworks (Bandura, 2004b; Glanz et al., 2008; Taylor, 2018).

The SCT, proposed by Albert Bandura, explains behaviour change through the dynamic interaction of personal factors, behaviour, and the environment (Bandura, 1997). A central construct is self-efficacy, defined as "belief in one's capabilities to organise and execute the courses of action required to produce given attainments" (Bandura, 1997, p. 3). Self-efficacy is influenced by four primary sources: enactive mastery, experiences, vicarious experiences (e.g. through peer involvement), external persuasion, and physiological and affective states (Bandura, 1997). In the context of rehabilitation, self-efficacy is thus a key concept, denoting the belief that one can achieve a successful recovery following a traumatic injury and foster effective rehabilitation through experiences of mastery. Enhancing self-efficacy is therefore a primary goal in self-management interventions.

The HBM posits that an individual's engagement in health-protective actions is determined by their appraisal of several factors: perceived susceptibility to a condition, its perceived severity, the perceived benefits of taking action, and the perceived barriers or costs associated with that action (Hochbaum, 1958; Rosenstock, 1974). For example, the HBM can be used to model adherence to preventative care engagement, such as mobilisation to prevent skin ulceration and increasing physical activity. Good compliance is theorised to correlate with a belief in susceptibility to the issues perceived as a severe enough threat, and the benefits of the preventive action outweigh the barriers (such as time investment or physical disability).

The TTM conceptualises behaviour change as a process that occurs in five stages for each potential change: precontemplation (not yet acknowledging the problem), contemplation (acknowledging the problem, but not yet ready to make a change), preparation (getting ready to change), action (actively changing behaviour), and maintenance (sustaining the behaviour change). However, it is essential to note that the progression between stages is not always linear (Prochaska and DiClemente, 1982, 1983). For example, a person might be in the "action" stage for their physical rehabilitation goals but in the "precontemplation" stage for managing the social anxiety related to their injury.

These theories provide models that can inform the design of self-management interventions aimed at supporting individuals in rebuilding their lives after injury by restoring a sense of control, confidence, and managing injury-related consequences. This could involve supporting a TBI survivor in managing their memory issues by using memory apps and to-do lists or providing training to an SCI survivor on how to self-monitor early signs of pressure ulcers, along with educating patients on when, how, and whom to contact in case of symptom worsening.

Despite existing theoretical frameworks supporting key elements of self-management, there is no universal consensus on the definition of "self-management," and terms such as "self-care" or "disease management" are often used interchangeably (Barlow et al., 2002; Jones and Demain, 2020;

Ustrimova et al., 2025). Furthermore, literature reviews repeatedly show that a substantial portion of studies on self-management interventions fail to explicitly state a guiding theoretical framework (Jaarsma et al., 2020; Painter et al., 2008; Prestwich et al., 2014; Ustrimova et al., 2025).

The lack of definitional consensus extends to the core elements of the concept. Some authors view self-management as patient compliance, which involves taking active responsibility for one's health through informed decisions (Ellis et al., 2017). Others define it as the capacity to manage symptoms, treatment, and the broader physical and psychological impacts of chronic illness (Barlow et al., 2002). Lorig and Holman outline the concept using three domains: medical, role, and emotional management (Lorig and Holman, 2003). In contrast, Jonkman et al. defined self-management interventions as those that equip persons with skills through knowledge acquisition and training in at least two other areas, such as problem-solving or changing health behaviours (Jonkman et al., 2016a).

While various theoretical models support the key notions of self-management, other issues, such as a lack of consensus on the definition of self-management and methodological issues surrounding implementation and evaluation, make it challenging to compare the effects of interventions on patient outcomes. In this regard, a stronger commitment to operationalisation and the proactive use of theory would help build more robust, replicable, and effective interventions that can be implemented in rehabilitation settings.

SELF-MANAGEMENT IN REHABILITATION SETTINGS: CURRENT EVIDENCE

The evidence for self-management in many chronic conditions is widely available, but less is known about it in traumatic injuries (Foster et al., 2007; Taylor et al., 2014). There are a few systematic and scoping reviews focused on specific conditions seen in rehabilitation settings, such as stroke and SCI (Baron et al., 2018a, 2018b; Cheng et al., 2014; Fryer et al., 2016). However, at the time of writing, few comprehensive reviews have examined self-management interventions across various traumatic injuries, except for one scoping review conducted by the authors of this chapter (Ustrimova et al., 2025). Based on this review, a summary of the findings on existing self-management interventions for individuals with traumatic injuries is provided in the following section to offer relevant perspectives for clinical applications in these populations.

Among different aetiologies of traumatic injuries, most existing interventions target survivors of SCI. The interest in self-management for this group may reflect profound and well-documented impacts of the condition, as well as the complex comorbidities that these individuals experience daily (Aaby et al., 2020; Adriaansen et al., 2016; Carrard et al., 2021; Jensen et al., 2012). The review findings showed that the volume of literature on self-management in the TBI population was larger than anticipated, potentially indicating a growing interest in this topic and an increasing understanding of brain injury as a chronic condition (Corrigan and Hammond, 2013). However, the literature on self-management interventions for major trauma and burn injuries is alarmingly limited, despite both conditions having a significant impact on the lives of the survivors.

Existing studies of self-management interventions for SCI survivors typically included 7 to 12 sessions, primarily delivered at home and/or outpatient settings by healthcare providers face-to-face and/or via phone. The delivery settings may reflect the mobility issues that persons with SCI face, thereby removing this significant barrier. Most interventions employed psychoeducation about the injury and its secondary complications, as well as training in stress management, problem-solving, action planning, and the provision of social support through peer and community involvement. Some interventions offered education on maintaining an active lifestyle and proactive coping. However, surprisingly, information on pain management, nutrition, and training in activities of daily living was often absent, despite these persisting issues experienced by patients with traumatic injuries. The outcomes of interventions varied, with some studies not finding significant effects (Guihan et al., 2014; Kooijmans et al., 2017), while others demonstrated significant improvements in quality of life and health symptoms in the intervention group (Goyaghaj et al., 2019; Schulz et al., 2009).

The profile of self-management interventions for patients with TBI was somewhat different. The intervention dose in reviewed studies ranged from five to 22 sessions, and the interventions were primarily delivered in hospitals and/or outpatient settings. Interventions were most commonly provided face-to-face by healthcare professionals. The patients were likely to be given psychoeducation on brain injury and its emotional and behavioural consequences, as well as receive training in problem-solving and goal setting. Some interventions also offered help with stress management and communication with healthcare providers. Surprisingly, mood management and cognitive training were rarely given, despite evidence of deficits in these domains. The results of the interventions varied as well, with McShan et al. (2023) reporting no significant differences between groups post-intervention, while other authors described substantial improvements in various areas, such as anger and self-efficacy (Backhaus et al., 2016; Hart et al., 2017; Niemeier et al., 2019).

Only two studies were found to investigate self-management interventions in patients with major trauma. One of these (Bérubé et al., 2018) described the development of an intervention aimed at preventing chronic pain in patients with major lower extremity trauma, and the other was an RCT conducted across six Level I Trauma Centres (Consortium [METRC], 2019). The latter study assessed the effects of early intervention delivered face-to-face and via telehealth by both healthcare professionals and peers. The program included psychoeducation, a personalised recovery plan, and guidance on managing depression and post-traumatic stress symptoms. Patients received assistance with seeking social support and were provided with advice on healthy living. The results showed a small positive effect in the intervention group for pain, depression, and PTSD, along with greater self-efficacy in returning to work and managing finances.

Similarly, only two studies examined self-management interventions for burn survivors. Gonçalves et al. (2016) offered participants six to eight sessions, delivered both in hospital and at home, by healthcare providers, face-to-face and via phone. The intervention included psychoeducation, education on skin function, practical burn care, and training in communication with their families and social interactions. The results indicated a significant decrease in anxiety and post-traumatic stress during rehabilitation in the intervention group. Notably, no effect on health status, self-efficacy, or depression was observed at six months post-discharge. Shokre et al. (2024) investigated the impact of an empowerment program on early adjustment among 80 burn survivors in hospital and outpatient settings. Healthcare providers delivered eight sessions focused on psychoeducation, training in practical skills, stress management, and the development of problem-solving and decision-making strategies. Participants also received training in emotional regulation and non-pharmacological pain management. The results showed significant improvements in body image satisfaction, coping abilities, and a reduction in post-traumatic symptoms.

In summary, the review findings suggest a high degree of similarity in the self-management ingredients used in the interventions for these traumatic injuries. Psychoeducation, problem-solving, stress management, goal setting, and communication training were frequently used in the interventions, possibly reflecting their benefits in promoting self-management in other chronic health conditions (De Silva, 2011). However, the rationale behind the choice of specific intervention ingredients and their role in alleviating condition-specific issues was rarely explained in the studies. For example, goal setting is frequently mentioned in the literature as a key ingredient for successful self-management, and yet, many studies did not include it (Silvester et al., 2024). Unfortunately, this is a known issue in the self-management literature (Coster et al., 2020; De Silva, 2011; Hoffmann et al., 2015; Van Hecke et al., 2017).

Overall, very few ingredients were used specifically within a particular patient group, and few studies explicitly described tailoring of self-management interventions for traumatic injuries. However, individuals with traumatic injuries can often encounter specific barriers to the implementation of self-management, e.g. cognitive and mobility issues, fatigue, and emotional symptoms (Jeschke et al., 2020; Martino et al., 2020; Rahman et al., 2023). Van Wyk et al. (2015) highlighted the need to adapt self-management programs for SCI survivors by explicitly addressing both physical and psychological barriers, thus proposing a focus on education and individualised planning. Sander et al. (2024) found a lack of reported adaptations of self-management interventions for patients with TBI, especially concerning challenges with planning, self-monitoring, and goal setting. The absence of such adjustments is puzzling, as cognitive deficits, reported in both TBI and SCI populations, are often quite debilitating (Andelic et al., 2018; Jensen et al., 2012). Neither was there evidence for the carryover or adoption of specific ingredients across different aetiologies. For example, education on extensive skin care and sexual health was primarily used in the interventions targeting SCI. However, skin damage is also frequent across other injuries (e.g. burns, major trauma), and sexual issues are often reported by TBI survivors (Jeschke et al., 2020; Ponsford et al., 2017). The knowledge and experience gained by applying these ingredients in some groups can potentially be extrapolated to other groups, ensuring a shared approach across rehabilitation settings and among different therapists.

Most of the interventions were carried out in the chronic phase, with only a fraction of studies conducted in the subacute phase (Consortium (METRC), 2019; Mäkelä et al., 2014). It reflects the nature of the original self-management programs, which targeted patients who had lived with their chronic conditions for some time (Lorig et al., 2001). However, the newer literature suggests the potential of implementing self-management interventions at earlier stages following the injury. There are reports on interventions for patients with acquired brain injury (ABI) that start during inpatient care or immediately after discharge (Eliassen et al., 2023). There is also evidence that early interventions might reduce caregiver burden by providing skills and knowledge required for caring for an injured family member (Adelman et al., 2014). Research on the benefits and disadvantages of implementing self-management at different phases is still in its early stages. Nevertheless, it seems essential that the intervention first and foremost aligns with the goals and needs of the injured individual and their family.

Despite being implemented in the chronic phase, many interventions were still often conducted face-to-face by healthcare providers in hospital settings. It is surprising, considering that self-management, at its core, focuses on health management outside of these contexts. Peers were also seldom included or mentioned in connection with the vaguely defined concept of "peer support." The rare inclusion of peers is discussed in the literature, which points out that self-management programs are often delivered by nurses (Coster et al., 2020; Ruksakulpiwat and Zhou, 2021). There is also evidence that self-management programs delivered by peers may be less effective (Jonkman et al., 2016b). In addition, we found that caregivers were rarely included, despite evidence supporting the importance of family participation in implementing self-management in everyday life.

It is worth noting that many studies provided only limited information and presented inconsistent or ambiguous descriptions of dose, delivery mode, provider, setting, and ingredients (Ustrimova et al., 2025). This is a known issue in the field, highlighting the fact that, despite the existence of guidelines for design, clinical trial reporting, evaluation, and review of self-management programs, no consensus exists on the recommended key ingredients that should comprise a self-management intervention (Jonkman et al., 2016b; Pearce et al., 2016; Taylor et al., 2014). The use of theory varied as well, despite explicit recommendations for the use of a theoretical framework for designing complex interventions (Moreels et al., 2023; Skivington et al., 2021; Taylor et al., 2014). The RCTs and controlled studies were more likely to have a theoretical framework, whereas 30% of all included studies did not specify any theoretical background (Ustrimova et al., 2025).

Finally, regarding the effects of the interventions, the evidence also varies. A large proportion of reviewed RCTs report significant improvements in perceived self-efficacy, increased physical and psychological well-being, as well as reduced caregiver burden and increased quality of life across different aetiologies (Ustrimova et al., 2025). Nevertheless, it should be noted that the literature often cites insufficient evidence to support the conclusive findings on self-management interventions (Coster et al., 2020; Wessol et al., 2017; Wray et al., 2018). For example, previous reviews of self-management interventions for SCI survivors failed to demonstrate effects on preventing pressure ulcers or managing secondary complications (Baron et al., 2018a; Cadel et al., 2020; Cogan et al., 2017). Sander et al. (2024) attempted to conduct an umbrella review of self-management interventions targeting TBI survivors but were unsuccessful due to the lack of such reviews. Reviews reporting the effects of self-management in multitrauma and burn injuries are also lacking. The current situation is likely multifactorial, involving limited information in studies, heterogeneity of outcomes, and structural issues such as insufficient funding and recruitment challenges. However, the current literature suggests that the field is in its development, with the first attempts to implement self-management interventions in rehabilitation settings and a potential for wider and interchangeable use of certain ingredients that prove especially valuable for patients with traumatic injuries.

CLINICAL RECOMMENDATIONS FOR SELF-MANAGEMENT INTERVENTIONS

SMS in Rehabilitation

Fostering SMS in patients with traumatic injuries requires interventions to be built around person-centred care, where the individual's needs, preferences, and values are prioritised. This approach emphasises the active role of patients and views them as partners in the rehabilitation process (Health Foundation (Great Britain), 2016) by employing SMS to enhance patient involvement, promote shared decision-making, and uphold respect and dignity throughout recovery (Ahmad et al., 2014). Existing insights from self-management interventions for other chronic conditions and emerging literature on SMS for traumatic injuries can inform clinical strategies tailored to address the unique needs of patients facing injury-related challenges. The evidence presented in this chapter also indicates the feasibility of SMS interventions for various traumatic injuries, including TBI, SCI, major trauma, and burns.

Supporting Self-Management Skills in Patients with Traumatic Injuries

Self-management programs aim to increase self-efficacy by developing skills in decision-making, goal setting, action planning and utilising available resources (Van de Velde et al., 2019). To promote self-management in rehabilitation settings, clinicians should focus on fostering the following seven key self-management skills (Bandura, 1977; Jones and Demain, 2020; Lorig and Holman, 2003):

- Problem-solving: developing flexible thinking and using adaptive strategies to overcome current and potential difficulties.
- Reflection: encouraging awareness of the impact of personal coping efforts on progress and change.
- Goal setting: establishing personally meaningful goals.
- Accessing resources: utilising available support, technology, and healthcare resources.
- Self-discovery: recognising one's strengths, finding new ways of coping and exploring new activities.
- Taking action: pursuing goals, engaging in daily activities, and seeking meaningful endeavours.
- Knowledge: understanding injury-related symptoms and adaptive health behaviours, such as compensatory strategies for cognitive deficits following TBI or non-pharmacological pain management in SCI.

By targeting these skills and ensuring that self-management is a fundamental part of all clinical interactions, clinicians can help patients increase self-efficacy and encourage positive health behaviours. In this context, a clinical assessment of individual self-management competencies is essential to pinpoint areas needing support and to create an environment that fosters shared decision-making, respecting the patient's expertise, goals, and values.

Core SMS Ingredients in Clinical Settings

SMS for patients with traumatic injuries remains a relatively unexplored area, but arguably, there are key components that should be integrated into clinical practice to begin the process. Here is a brief overview of these ingredients.

Psychoeducation

Psychoeducation should be given to provide insights into injury management and personalise information relevant to the patient's current situation.

SMART Goals

Goal-oriented rehabilitation with active patient involvement is considered a key approach to rehabilitation (Rose et al., 2017; Wilson, 2009). One recommended approach is the SMART goal method, which helps patients set Specific, Measurable, Achievable, Relevant, and Time-bound goals that are personally meaningful (Bovend'Eerdt et al., 2009).

Action Planning

Action planning involves assisting patients in tracking their progress towards the goals and encouraging reflection on coping strategies (Borgen et al., 2022; Jones and Demain, 2020). Figure 1.1 "Self-management goal and action plan" presents an example of action planning for SMART goal formulation.

Flexible Problem Solving

This component helps patients find creative solutions to dealing with challenging situations, practical difficulties, and emotional issues by selecting effective strategies and breaking tasks into manageable steps (D'Zurilla and Goldfried, 1971; Jones and Demain, 2020).

Positive Prompting

Positive prompting employs motivational interviewing techniques and open-ended questions to explore patients' perspectives and encourage adaptive behavioural changes. Clinicians should create an environment that fosters curiosity about the patient's experiences and provide feedback that acknowledges progress and personal strengths (Jones and Demain, 2020).

Supporting Emotional Coping and Identity Issues Post-Trauma

Sharing experiences with peers is essential, as it brings a sense of community and mutual understanding (De Silva, 2011). Peer modelling through encouragement, social support, and belonging to beneficial social networks can facilitate emotional coping and adaptive health behavioural change (Lorig and Holman, 2003; Reeves et al., 2014; Vassilev et al., 2014). Incorporating vignettes of coping experiences from peers with lived experiences with traumatic injuries can also provide essential support and build knowledge on managing common issues and emotional resilience (Bridges Self-Management, n.d.).

Tailoring SMS in Rehabilitation Settings

Effective SMS requires tailoring interventions to specific diagnostic groups and addressing individual needs. For instance, individuals with TBI may need support for their cognitive deficits,

Self-management goal and action plan

Personal goal

I. What specific goal do you want to work on? (something that is important for you)

Goal:

Steps for a SMART goal (Specific, Measurable, Achievable, Relevant, and Timed):

- How:
- Where:
- When:
- Frequency:

II. Barriers and supports

- What barriers could get in the way, and how would you overcome them?
- What kind of support do you need?
- What strategies can you use to achieve this goal?

III. Confidence level

How confident do you feel about this action plan (circle the number below)

1 2 3 4 5 6 7 8 9 10

No confidence ... Full confidence

IV. Goal achievement

How would you rate your achievement of this goal, once completed? (circle the number below)

1 2 3 4 5 6 7 8 9 10

Not achieved ... Fully achieved

Evaluation note (obtained experiences) **Date: / /**

____

____

____

____

FIGURE 1.1 Self-management goal and action plan.

fatigue, and challenges with emotional functioning and social roles. In an attempt to help a group of TBI survivors manage their anger issues, Hart et al. developed a tailored intervention which employed psychoeducation on anger, development, and practice of relevant skills, as well as training in self-monitoring (Hart et al., 2017).

For individuals with SCI, a key focus of the intervention may be on achieving independence, such as enhancing mobility and acquiring skills to function more effectively in their daily lives. It may also include skills to manage secondary complications, including pain and pressure ulcers.

Kooijmans et al. (2017) attempted to address physical inactivity and designed an intervention that specifically aimed to promote an active lifestyle in individuals with long-term SCI. The program included peer support and trained participants in action planning to promote healthy and active living, while also teaching them how to monitor their activities. It also provided a self-help workbook and a booklet titled "How to Stay Fit With SCI."

Survivors of major trauma may benefit from tailored support in managing physical limitations, pain, mental well-being, and participation in everyday life. For instance, the Trauma Collaborative Care Program was specifically developed to support management of trauma recovery at an individual level, starting from the early inpatient phase through transition to community, with a strong emphasis on assessment and a recovery plan tailored to particular challenges, such as depression, post-traumatic symptoms, pain, or substance abuse (Consortium (METRC), 2019).

Individuals with severe burn injuries may need help with managing skin care and working with challenges related to stigma and body image. To address these issues, Gonçalves et al. (2016) designed and implemented a self-management intervention focused on education on skin function and practical training in burn care. The program also included skills related to communication with family and social interaction, as well as advice on leisure activities, targeting specific difficulties that burn injury survivors may face.

Additionally, interventions should be tailored to different phases of recovery. SMS in the acute phase of injury must address the individual needs related to the injury's complexity, its nature, and the necessary treatment (Hollinshead et al., 2019). While transitioning to the chronic phase, patients with traumatic injuries often face many overlapping consequences and ongoing life changes that must be navigated daily (Ustrimova et al., 2025). In this phase, SMS in a group-based format can be valuable in facilitating the exchange of coping experiences and social encouragement (Lorig and Holman, 2003).

Facilitators and Barriers

The successful implementation of SMS can face many facilitators and barriers. Organisational support, clinician training, and cultural adaptations are essential for effective delivery (Hollinshead et al., 2019). Additionally, understanding patients' readiness, motivation, level of health literacy, and cultural background is critical for assessing individual engagement in self-management practices (Jones and Demain, 2020). Patients often present with various levels of self-efficacy. Some individuals can lack confidence and adaptive strategies, while others are highly motivated and employ effective health behaviours. Thus, SMS needs to be tailored to the individual level of confidence in self-management and personal resources (Jones and Demain, 2020). It is essential to remember that every person is engaged in managing their health situation to some extent, and as Lorig has described it, "one cannot not manage" (Lorig and Holman, 2003). Therefore, the vital question is how, exactly, one manages, and how clinicians can meet each patient and promote support for adaptive health behaviours that strengthen patients' self-management.

Recommendations for the Development of SMS Interventions in Rehabilitation Settings

The complexity of SMS and the inclusion of multiple target ingredients require interventions to be theory-driven and incorporate a solid understanding of the proposed behavioural change mechanisms (Skivington et al., 2021). The development of manuals facilitates clinician training and ensures the fidelity of the intervention across different settings, thereby maintaining the quality of the intervention. Furthermore, involving patients in co-design processes and incorporating stakeholders' feedback are crucial for developing relevant and effective self-management programs that meet patients' needs (Jones and Demain., 2020). For example, Mäkelä et al. (2019)

invited individuals with lived experiences of TBI to co-design a self-management intervention tailored for patients with brain injuries in a rehabilitation setting. The intervention included co-designed resources, such as a three-stage training workshop for multidisciplinary teams and leaders, as well as books for patients and their families. These books incorporated vignettes describing coping strategies and the experiences of individuals with TBI and their loved ones.

CONCLUSION

Seen through the lenses of various theories, such as SCT and the HBM, building self-efficacy and addressing barriers to health management are essential to fostering positive health behaviours. By focusing on existing knowledge from the SMS interventions for traumatic injuries and the clinical recommendations outlined in this chapter, healthcare providers can utilise self-management as a framework to empower patients to take an active role in their recovery, enhance their self-efficacy, promote symptom management, and help increase health-related quality of life.

While the potential of self-management interventions for the trauma population is promising, the evidence base remains in its early stages, with significant gaps in research, particularly across different traumatic aetiologies. To bridge these gaps, future efforts should aim to establish clear recommendations for the design, implementation, and evaluation of interventions, thereby enhancing the quality of studies and creating opportunities for high-quality systematic reviews. Involving individuals with lived experiences of traumatic injuries in the development of interventions is essential to ensure patient engagement and intervention use.

REFERENCES

Aaby, A., Ravn, S.L., Kasch, H. and Andersen, T.E. (2020) 'The associations of acceptance with quality of life and mental health following spinal cord injury: A systematic review', *Spinal Cord*, 58, pp. 130–148. doi:10.1038/s41393-019-0379-9.

Adelman, R.D., Tmanova, L.L., Delgado, D., Dion, S. and Lachs, M.S. (2014) 'Caregiver burden: A clinical review', *JAMA*, 311(10), pp. 1052–1060. doi:10.1001/jama.2014.304.

Adriaansen, J., Ruijs, L., Koppenhagen, C., van Asbeck, F., Snoek, G., van Kuppevelt, D., Visser-Meily, J. and Post, M. (2016) 'Secondary health conditions and quality of life in persons living with spinal cord injury for at least ten years', *Journal of Rehabilitation Medicine*, 48, pp. 853–860. doi:10.2340/16501977-2166.

Ahmad, N., Ellins, J., Krelle, H. and Lawrie, M. (2014) *Person-centred care: From ideas to action. Bringing together the evidence on shared decision making and self-management support.* London: The Health Foundation.

Ahuja, C., Wilson, J., Nori, S., Kotter, M.R.N., Druschel, C., Curt, A. and Fehlings, M.G. (2017) 'Traumatic spinal cord injury', *Nature Reviews Disease Primers*, 3, p. 17018. doi:10.1038/nrdp.2017.18.

Alberdi, F., García, I., Atutxa, L. and Zabarte, M. (2014) 'Epidemiology of severe trauma', *Medicina Intensiva (English Edition)*, 38, pp. 580–588. doi:10.1016/j.medine.2014.06.002.

Allahham, A., Rowe, G., Stevenson, A., Fear, M.W., Vallence, A.-M. and Wood, F.M. (2024) 'The impact of burn injury on the central nervous system', *Burns & Trauma*, 12, tkad037. doi:10.1093/burnst/tkad037.

Andelic, N., Hammergren, N., Bautz-Holter, E., Sveen, U., Brunborg, C. and Røe, C. (2009) 'Functional outcome and health-related quality of life 10 years after moderate-to-severe traumatic brain injury', *Acta Neurologica Scandinavica*, 120, pp. 16–23. doi:10.1111/j.1600-0404.2008.01116.x.

Andelic, N., Howe, E.I., Hellstrøm, T., Sanchez, M.F., Lu, J., Løvstad, M. and Røe, C. (2018) 'Disability and quality of life 20 years after traumatic brain injury', *Brain and Behavior*, 8, p. e01018. doi:10.1002/brb3.1018.

Andelic, N., Perrin, P.B., Forslund, M.V., Soberg, H.L., Sigurdardottir, S., Sveen, U., Jerstad, T. and Røe, C. (2015) 'Trajectories of physical health in the first 5 years after traumatic brain injury', *Journal of Neurology*, 262, pp. 523–531. doi:10.1007/s00415-014-7595-1.

Andelic, N., Røe, C., Tenovuo, O., van der Naalt, J., Helseth, E., Azouvi, P., Dawes, H., van Heugten, C., Majdan, M. and Wilson, L. (2021) 'Unmet rehabilitation needs after traumatic brain injury across Europe: Results from the CENTER-TBI study', *Journal of Clinical Medicine*, 10(5), p. 1035. doi:10.3390/jcm10051035.

Backhaus, S., Ibarra, S., Parrott, D., and Malec, J. (2016). 'Comparison of a cognitive-behavioural coping skills group to a peer support group in a brain injury population', *Archives of Physical Medicine and Rehabilitation*, 97(2), pp. 281–291. doi:10.1016/j.apmr.2015.10.097.

Bandura, A. (1977) 'Self-efficacy: Toward a unifying theory of behavioral change', *Psychological Review*, 84, pp. 191–215. doi:10.1037/0033-295X.84.2.191.

Bandura, A. (1997) *Self-efficacy: The exercise of control*. New York: Freeman.

Bandura, A. (2004a) 'Health promotion by social cognitive means', *Health Education & Behavior*, 31, pp. 143–164. doi:10.1177/1090198104263660.

Bandura, A. (2004b) 'Swimming against the mainstream: The early years from chilly tributary to transformative mainstream', *Behaviour Research and Therapy*, 42, pp. 613–630. doi:10.1016/j.brat.2004.02.001.

Barlow, J., Wright, C., Sheasby, J., Turner, A. and Hainsworth, J. (2002) 'Self-management approaches for people with chronic conditions: A review', *Patient Education and Counseling*, 48, pp. 177–187. doi:10.1016/S0738-3991(02)00032-0.

Baron, J.S., Sullivan, K.J., Swaine, J.M., Jaglal, S., McCormick, A., Teasell, R., Mortenson, W.B. and Wolfe, D.L. (2018a) 'Self-management interventions for skin care in people with A spinal cord injury: Part 1 – A systematic review of intervention content and effectiveness', *Spinal Cord*, 56(9), pp. 823–836. doi:10.1038/s41393-018-0138-3.

Baron, J.S., Sullivan, K.J., Swaine, J.M., Jaglal, S., McCormick, A., Teasell, R., Mortenson, W.B. and Wolfe, D.L. (2018b) 'Self-management interventions for skin care in people with A spinal cord injury: Part 2 – A systematic review of use of theory and quality of intervention reporting', *Spinal Cord*, 56(9), pp. 837–846. doi:10.1038/s41393-018-0136-5.

Beadle, E.J., Ownsworth, T., Fleming, J., Shum, D. and Togher, L. (2016) 'The impact of traumatic brain injury on self-identity: A systematic review of the evidence for self-concept changes', *Journal of Head Trauma Rehabilitation*, 31(2), pp. E12–E25. doi:10.1097/HTR.0000000000000158.

Bérubé, M., Gélinas, C., Martorella, G., Michaud, C., Houle, F., Bérubé, S. and Choinière, M. (2018) 'Development and acceptability assessment of a self-management intervention to prevent acute to chronic pain transition after major lower extremity trauma', *Pain Management Nursing*, 19(6), pp. 671–692. doi:10.1016/j.pmn.2018.04.010.

Bickenbach, J., Officer, A., Shakespeare, T. and von Groote, P. (2013) *International perspectives on spinal cord injury*. Geneva: World Health Organization.

Bonatti, H. and Calland, J.F. (2008) 'Trauma', *Emergency Medicine Clinics of North America*, 26, pp. 625–648. doi:10.1016/j.emc.2008.05.001.

Borgen, I.M.H., Hauger, S.L., Forslund, M.V., Kleffelgård, I., Brunborg, C., Andelic, N., Sveen, U., Søberg, H.L., Sigurdardottir, S., Røe, C. and Løvstad, M. (2022) 'Goal attainment in an individually tailored and home-based intervention in the chronic phase after traumatic brain injury', *Journal of Clinical Medicine*, 11, p. 958. doi:10.3390/jcm11040958.

Bovend'Eerdt, T.J., Botell, R.E. and Wade, D.T. (2009) 'Writing SMART rehabilitation goals and achieving goal attainment scaling: A practical guide', *Clinical Rehabilitation*, 23, pp. 352–361. doi:10.1177/0269215508101741.

Bridges Self-Management (n.d.) *Bridges self-management website*. Available at: https://www.bridgesselfmanagement.org.uk/ (Accessed: 28 August 2025).

Bruns, J. Jr. and Hauser, W.A. (2003) 'The epidemiology of traumatic brain injury: A review', *Epilepsia*, 44(s10), pp. 2–10. doi:10.1046/j.1528-1157.44.s10.3.x.

Cadel, L., DeLuca, C., Hitzig, S. L., Packer, T. L., Lofters, A. K., Patel, T., and Guilcher, S. J. T. (2020). 'Self-management of pain and depression in adults with spinal cord injury: A scoping review', *The Journal of Spinal Cord Medicine*, 43(3), pp. 280–297. doi:10.1080/10790268.2018.1523776.

Cariello, A.N., Perrin, P.B., Tyler, C.M., Pierce, B.S., Maher, K.E., Librandi, H., Sutter, M.E. and Feldman, M.J. (2021) 'Mediational models of pain, mental health, and functioning in individuals with burn injury', *Rehabilitation Psychology*, 66, pp. 1–9. doi:10.1037/rep0000359.

Carrard, V., Kunz, S. and Peter, C. (2021) 'Mental health, quality of life, self-efficacy, and social support of individuals living with spinal cord injury in Switzerland compared to that of the general population', *Spinal Cord*, 59, pp. 398–409. doi:10.1038/s41393-020-00582-5.

Cheng, H.Y., Chair, S.Y. and Chau, J.P. (2014) 'The effectiveness of psychosocial interventions for stroke family caregivers and stroke survivors: A systematic review and meta-analysis', *Patient Education and Counseling*, 95(1), pp. 30–44. doi:10.1016/j.pec.2014.01.005.

Choi, M., Sempungu, J.K., Lee, E.H., Yu, C., Kim, D. and Kim, H. (2024) 'Living longer but in poor health: Healthcare system responses to ageing populations in industrialised countries based on the findings from the Global Burden of Disease Study 2019', *BMC Public Health*, 24(1), p. 576. doi:10.1186/s12889-024-18049-0.

Cieza, A., Causey, K., Kamenov, K., Hanson, S.W., Chatterji, S. and Vos, T. (2020) 'Global estimates of the need for rehabilitation based on the Global Burden of Disease Study 2019: A systematic analysis for the Global Burden of Disease Study 2019', *The Lancet*, 396(10267), pp. 2006–2017. doi:10.1016/S0140-6736(20)32340-0.

Cogan, A. M., Blanchard, J., Garber, S. L., Vigen, C. L. P., Carlson, M., and Clark, F. A. (2017). 'Systematic review of behavioral and educational interventions to prevent pressure ulcers in adults with spinal cord injury,' *Clinical Rehabilitation*, 31(7), pp. 871–880. doi:10.1177/0269215516660855.

Consortium (METRC), The Major Extremity Trauma Research Consortium. (2019) 'Early effects of the trauma collaborative care intervention: Results from a prospective multicenter cluster clinical trial', *Journal of Orthopaedic Trauma*, 33, p. 538. doi:10.1097/BOT.0000000000001581.

Corrigan, J.D. and Hammond, F.M. (2013) 'Traumatic brain injury as a chronic health condition', *Archives of Physical Medicine and Rehabilitation*, 94, pp. 1199–1201. doi:10.1016/j.apmr.2013.01.023.

Coster, S., Li, Y. and Norman, I.J. (2020) 'Cochrane reviews of educational and self-management interventions to guide nursing practice: A review', *International Journal of Nursing Studies*, 110, p. 103698. doi:10.1016/j.ijnurstu.2020.103698.

D'Zurilla, T.J. and Goldfried, M.R. (1971) 'Problem solving and behavior modification', *Journal of Abnormal Psychology*, 78, pp. 107–126. doi:10.1037/h0031360.

de Munter, L., Polinder, S., Haagsma, J.A., Kruithof, N., van de Ree, C.L., Steyerberg, E.W. and de Jongh, M. (2020) 'Prevalence and prognostic factors for psychological distress after trauma', *Archives of Physical Medicine and Rehabilitation*, 101, pp. 877–884. doi:10.1016/j.apmr.2019.12.002.

De Silva, D. (2011) *Evidence: Helping people help themselves. A review of the evidence considering whether it is worthwhile to support self-management.* London: The Health Foundation.

Dewan, M.C., Rattani, A., Gupta, S., Baticulon, R.E., Hung, Y.-C., Punchak, M., Agrawal, A., Adeleye, A.O., Shrime, M.G., Rubiano, A.M., Rosenfeld, J.V. and Park, K.B. (2019) 'Estimating the global incidence of traumatic brain injury', *Journal of Neurosurgery*, 130, pp. 1080–1097. doi:10.3171/2017.10.JNS17352.

Eliassen, M., Arntzen, C., Nikolaisen, M., Haugland, H., Rydning, J. and Johansen, T. (2023) 'Rehabilitation models that support transitions from hospital to home for people with acquired brain injury (ABI): A scoping review', *BMC Health Services Research*, 23(1), p. 814. doi:10.1186/s12913-023-09793-x.

Ellis, J., Boger, E., Latter, S., Kennedy, A., Jones, F., Foster, C. and Demain, S. (2017) 'Conceptualisation of the "good" self-manager: A qualitative investigation of stakeholder views on the self-management of long-term health conditions', *Social Science & Medicine*, 176, pp. 25–33. doi:10.1016/j.socscimed.2017.01.018.

Enblom, S., Sundin, E., Guné, G.E., Aspling, N. and Huss, F. (2022) 'The relationship between health-related quality of life, subjective scar estimation, and activity performance in adult burn patients 6 and 12 months after injury', *European Burn Journal*, 3, pp. 486–492. doi:10.3390/ebj3040042.

Foster, G., Taylor, S.J.C., Eldridge, S., Ramsay, J. and Griffiths, C.J. (2007) 'Self-management education programmes by lay leaders for people with chronic conditions', *Cochrane Database of Systematic Reviews*, (4), p. CD005108. doi:10.1002/14651858.CD005108.pub2.

Fryer, C.E., Luker, J.A., McDonnell, M.N. and Hillier, S. (2016) 'Self-management programmes for quality of life in people with stroke', *Cochrane Database of Systematic Reviews*, 2016(8), p. CD010442. doi:10.1002/14651858.CD010442.pub2.

Gabbe, B.J., Simpson, P.M., Cameron, P.A., Ponsford, J., Lyons, R.A., Collie, A., Fitzgerald, M., Judson, R., Teague, W.J., Braaf, S., Nunn, A., Ameratunga, S. and Harrison, J.E. (2017) 'Long-term health status and trajectories of seriously injured patients: A population-based longitudinal study', *PLoS Medicine*, 14, p. e1002322. doi:10.1371/journal.pmed.1002322.

GBD 2016 Neurology Collaborators. (2019) 'Global, regional, and national burden of neurological disorders, 1990–2016: A systematic analysis for the Global Burden of Disease Study 2016', *The Lancet Neurology*, 18, pp. 459–480. doi:10.1016/S1474-4422(18)30499-X.

Glanz, K., Rimer, B.K. and Viswanath, K. (2008) *Health behavior and health education: Theory, research, and practice.* 4th edn. San Francisco: Jossey-Bass.

Gonçalves, N., Ciol, M.A., Dantas, R.A.S., Almeida, A., Santana, R., Furtado, L., Oliveira, C., Silva, A. and Nogueira, L. (2016) 'A randomized controlled trial of an educational programme with telephone reinforcement to improve perceived health status of Brazilian burn victims at 6-month post-discharge', *Journal of Advanced Nursing*, 72(10), pp. 2508–2523. doi:10.1111/jan.13003.

Goyaghaj, N., Pishgooie, A.H., Aliyari, S., Hosseini, S.H. and Ahmadi, Z. (2019) 'The effect of self-care program training on self-efficacy in veterans with spinal cord injury: A randomized clinical trial study', *Archives of Neuroscience*, 6(3), p. e89001. doi:10.5812/ans.89001.

Guihan, M., Bombardier, C.H., Ehde, D.M., Burns, S.P., Gater, D.R., Holmes, S.A., Kraft, G.H., Weitzenkamp, D.A., Ford, C., Crane, D.A. and Chan, A. (2014) 'Comparing multicomponent interventions to improve skin care behaviors and prevent recurrence in veterans hospitalized for severe pressure ulcers', *Archives of Physical Medicine and Rehabilitation*, 95(7), pp. 1246–1253.e3. doi:10.1016/j.apmr.2014.01.012.

Haagsma, J.A., Polinder, S., Olff, M., Toet, H., Bonsel, G.J. and van Beeck, E.F. (2012) 'Posttraumatic stress symptoms and health-related quality of life: A two-year follow-up study of injury treated at the emergency department', *BMC Psychiatry*, 12, p. 1. doi:10.1186/1471-244X-12-1.

Hammond, F.M., Perkins, S.M., Corrigan, J.D., Nakase-Richardson, R., Brown, A.W., O'Neil-Pirozzi, T.M., Zasler, N.D. and Greenwald, B.D. (2021) 'Functional change from five to fifteen years after traumatic brain injury', *Journal of Neurotrauma*, 38, pp. 858–869. doi:10.1089/neu.2020.7287.

Hart, T., Brockway, J.A., Maiuro, R.D., Vaccaro, M., Fann, J.R., Mellick, D., Harrison-Felix, C., Barber, J. and Temkin, N. (2017) 'Anger self-management training for chronic moderate to severe traumatic brain injury: Results of a randomized controlled trial', *Journal of Head Trauma Rehabilitation*, 32, pp. 319–331. doi:10.1097/HTR.0000000000000316.

Health Foundation (Great Britain). (2016) *Person-centred care made simple: What everyone should know about person-centred care*. London: The Health Foundation.

Hochbaum, G.M. (1958) *Public participation in medical screening programs: A socio-psychological study*. Washington, DC: US Department of Health, Education, and Welfare, Public Health Service.

Hoffmann, T., Ownsworth, T., Eames, S., Sinclair, E., Walker, N., O'Connor, C. and Cameron, A. (2015) 'Evaluation of brief interventions for managing depression and anxiety symptoms during early discharge period after stroke: A pilot randomized controlled trial', *Topics in Stroke Rehabilitation*, 22(2), pp. 116–126. doi:10.1179/1074935714Z.0000000030.

Hollinshead, L., Jones, F. and Silvester, L. (2019) 'Implementing an integrated approach to self-management support in an acute major trauma therapy team: An improvement project', *BMJ Open Quality*, 8, p. e000415. doi:10.1136/bmjoq-2018-000415.

Holman, H.R. (2020) 'The relation of the chronic disease epidemic to the health care crisis', *ACR Open Rheumatology*, 2(3), pp. 167–173. doi:10.1002/acr2.11114.

Jaarsma, T., Strömberg, A., Dunbar, S.B., Fitzsimons, D., Lee, C., Middleton, S., Vellone, E., Freedland, K.E. and Riegel, B. (2020) 'Self-care research: How to grow the evidence base?, *International Journal of Nursing Studies*, 105, p. 103555. doi:10.1016/j.ijnurstu.2020.103555.

Jensen, M.P., Molton, I.R., Groah, S.L., Campbell, M.L., Charlifue, S., Chiodo, A., Forchheimer, M., Krause, J.S. and Tate, D. (2012) 'Secondary health conditions in individuals aging with SCI: Terminology, concepts and analytic approaches', *Spinal Cord*, 50, pp. 373–378. doi:10.1038/sc.2011.150.

Jeschke, M.G., Van Baar, M.E., Choudhry, M.A., Chung, K.K., Gibran, N.S. and Logsetty, S. (2020) 'Burn injury', *Nature Reviews Disease Primers*, 6, p. 11. doi:10.1038/s41572-020-0145-5.

Jones, F. and Demain, S. (2020) 'Self-management strategies in neurorehabilitation', in Dietz, V., Ward, N.S. and Kennard, C. (eds.) *Oxford textbook of neurorehabilitation*. Oxford: Oxford University Press, pp. 387–400. doi:10.1093/med/9780198824954.003.0028.

Jones, F., Gage, H., Drummond, A., Bhalla, A., Grant, R., Lennon, S., Watkins, C., Leathley, M., McKevitt, C. and Riazi, A. (2016) 'Feasibility study of an integrated stroke self-management programme: A cluster-randomised controlled trial', *BMJ Open*, 6(1), p. e008900. doi:10.1136/bmjopen-2015-008900.

Jones, T.M., Dean, C.M., Hush, J.M., Dear, B.F., Titov, N., Pedro, F., Longley, W.A. and Wootton, B.M. (2015) 'A systematic review of the efficacy of self-management programs for increasing physical activity in community-dwelling adults with acquired brain injury (ABI)', *Systematic Reviews*, 4(1), p. 51. doi:10.1186/s13643-015-0039-x.

Jonkman, N.H., Schuurmans, M.J., Groenwold, R.H.H., Hoes, A.W. and Trappenburg, J.C.A. (2016b) 'Identifying components of self-management interventions that improve health-related quality of life in chronically ill patients: Systematic review and meta-regression analysis', *Patient Education and Counseling*, 99(7), pp. 1087–1098. doi:10.1016/j.pec.2016.01.022.

Jonkman, N.H., Schuurmans, M.J., Jaarsma, T., Shortridge-Baggett, L.M., Hoes, A.W. and Trappenburg, J.C.A. (2016a) 'Self-management interventions: Proposal and validation of a new operational definition', *Journal of Clinical Epidemiology*, 80, pp. 34–42. doi:10.1016/j.jclinepi.2016.08.001.

Kamenov, K., Mills, J.-A., Chatterji, S. and Cieza, A. (2019) 'Needs and unmet needs for rehabilitation services: A scoping review', *Disability and Rehabilitation*, 41(10), pp. 1227–1237. doi:10.1080/09638288.2017.1422036.

Kooijmans, H., Post, M.W.M., Stam, H.J., van der Woude, L.H.V., Spijkerman, D.C.M., Snoek, G.J., Bongers-Janssen, H.M.H., van Koppenhagen, C.F., Twisk, J.W. and Bussmann, J.B.J. (2017) 'Effectiveness of a self-management intervention to promote an active lifestyle in persons with long-term spinal cord injury: The HABITS randomized clinical trial', *Neurorehabilitation and Neural Repair*, 31, pp. 991–1004. doi:10.1177/1545968317736819.

Lo, J., Chan, L. and Flynn, S. (2021) 'A systematic review of the incidence, prevalence, costs, and activity and work limitations of amputation, osteoarthritis, rheumatoid arthritis, back pain, multiple sclerosis, spinal cord injury, stroke, and traumatic brain injury in the United States: A 2019 update', *Archives of Physical Medicine and Rehabilitation*, 102, pp. 115–131. doi:10.1016/j.apmr.2020.04.001.

Lorig, K.R. and Holman, H.R. (2003) 'Self-management education: History, definition, outcomes, and mechanisms', *Annals of Behavioral Medicine*, 26, pp. 1–7. doi:10.1207/S15324796ABM2601_01.

Lorig, K.R., Ritter, P.L., Turner, R.M., English, K. and Laurent, D.D. (2016) 'Benefits of diabetes self-management for health plan members: A 6-month translation study', *Journal of Medical Internet Research*, 18(6), p. e164. doi:10.2196/jmir.5568.

Lorig, K.R., Sobel, D.S., Ritter, P.L., Laurent, D. and Hobbs, M. (2001) 'Effect of a self-management program on patients with chronic disease', *Effective Clinical Practice*, 4(6), pp. 256–262.

Mäkelä, P., Gawned, S. and Jones, F. (2014) 'Starting early: Integration of self-management support into an acute stroke service', *BMJ Quality Improvement Reports*, 3(1), p. u202037.w1759. doi:10.1136/bmjquality.u202037.w1759.

Mäkelä, P., Jones, F., De Sousa De Abreu, M.I., Hollinshead, L. and Ling, J. (2019) 'Supporting self-management after traumatic brain injury: Codesign and evaluation of a new intervention across a trauma pathway', *Health Expectations*, 22, pp. 632–642. doi:10.1111/hex.12898.

Martino, C., Russo, E., Santonastaso, D.P., Colella, F., Garofalo, G. and Servadei, F. (2020) 'Long-term outcomes in major trauma patients and correlations with the acute phase', *World Journal of Emergency Surgery*, 15(1), p. 6. doi:10.1186/s13017-020-0289-3.

McShan, E. E., Juengst, S., Douglas, M. E., Noorbakhsh, D., Calhoun, S., Bennett, M., Suhalka, A., Dubiel, R., and Driver, S. (2023). 'Efficacy of a group-based education intervention for people with traumatic brain injury: supplementary results from a 12-month randomized controlled trial', *Brain Injury*, 37(10), pp. 1205–1214.doi:10.1080/02699052.2023.2225874.

Menon, D.K., Schwab, K., Wright, D.W. and Maas, A.I.R.; Demographics and Clinical Assessment Working Group of the International and Interagency Initiative toward Common Data Elements for Research on Traumatic Brain Injury and Psychological Health. (2010) 'Position statement: Definition of traumatic brain injury', *Archives of Physical Medicine and Rehabilitation*, 91(11), pp. 1637–1640. doi:10.1016/j.apmr.2010.05.017.

Moi, A.L., Haugsmyr, E. and Heisterkamp, H. (2016) 'Long-term study of health and quality of life after burn injury', *Annals of Burns and Fire Disasters*, 29, pp. 295–299.

Moksnes, H., Schäfer, C., Rasmussen, M.S., et al. (2023) 'Functional outcomes at 6 and 12 months post-injury in a trauma centre population with moderate-to-severe traumatic injuries', *Journal of Clinical Medicine*, 12(16), p. 5300. doi:10.3390/jcm12165300.

Moreels, T., Cruyt, E., De Baets, S., Andries, L., Arts-Tielemans, M., Rodriguez-Bailon, M., Bergström, A., Boete, K., Bormans, I., Costa, U., Declercq, H., Dekelver, S., Dekyvere, V., Delooz, E., Engels, C., Helderweirt, S., Jarrey, M., Lenaerts, A., Leyman, A., … Van de Velde, D. (2023). 'Self-Management Analysis in Chronic Conditions (SMACC) checklist: an international consensus-based tool to develop, compare and evaluate self-management support programmes', *BMJ Open*, 13(12), p. e075676. doi:10.1136/bmjopen-2023-075676.

Niemeier, J.P., Kreutzer, J.S., Marwitz, J.H., Wilson, C.S., Deluca, T.M., Sander, A.M. and Zasler, N.D. (2019) 'A randomized controlled pilot study of a manualized intervention for caregivers of patients with traumatic brain injury in inpatient rehabilitation', *Archives of Physical Medicine and Rehabilitation*, 100(4S), pp. S65–S75. doi:10.1016/j.apmr.2018.07.422.

Painter, J.E., Borba, C.P.C., Hynes, M., Mays, D. and Glanz, K. (2008) 'The use of theory in health behavior research from 2000 to 2005: A systematic review', *Annals of Behavioral Medicine*, 35, pp. 358–362. doi:10.1007/s12160-008-9042-y.

Parke, H.L., Epiphaniou, E., Pearce, G., Taylor, S.J.C., Sheikh, A. and Pinnock, H. (2015) 'Self-management support interventions for stroke survivors: A systematic meta-review', *PLoS ONE*, 10(7), p. e0131448. doi:10.1371/journal.pone.0131448.

Pearce, G., Parke, H.L., Pinnock, H., Epiphaniou, E., Bourne, C.L., Sheikh, A. and Taylor, S.J.C. (2016) 'The PRISMS taxonomy of self-management support: Derivation of a novel taxonomy and initial testing of its utility', *Journal of Health Services Research & Policy*, 21(2), pp. 73–82. doi:10.1177/1355819615602725.

Pollard, C. and Kennedy, P. (2007) 'A longitudinal analysis of emotional impact, coping strategies and post-traumatic psychological growth following spinal cord injury: A 10-year review', *British Journal of Health Psychology*, 12, pp. 347–362. doi:10.1348/135910707X197046.

Ponsford, J. (2013) 'Mechanisms, recovery and sequelae of traumatic brain injury: A foundation for the REAL approach', in Ponsford, J., Sloan, S. and Snow, P. (eds.) *Traumatic brain injury: Rehabilitation for every-day adaptive living*. New York: Taylor & Francis, pp. 1–33.

Ponsford, J., Draper, K. and Schönberger, M. (2008) 'Functional outcome 10 years after traumatic brain injury: Its relationship with demographic, injury severity, and cognitive and emotional status', *Journal of the International Neuropsychological Society*, 14, pp. 233–242. doi:10.1017/S1355617708080272.

Ponsford, J. L., Downing, M., and Stolwyk, R. (2017). 'Sexuality and rehabilitation following acquired brain injury', in Wilson B. A., Winegardner, J. van Heugten, C. M., and Ownsworth, T. (eds.) *Neuropsychological rehabilitation: The international handbook*. London: Routledge, pp. 403–413.

Post, M.W.M. and van Leeuwen, C.M. (2012) 'Psychosocial issues in spinal cord injury: A review', *Spinal Cord*, 50, pp. 382–389. doi:10.1038/sc.2011.182.

Prados-Román, E., Cabrera-Martos, I., Martín-Nuñez, J., Díaz-Pelegrina, A., Valenza-Demet, G., Arroyo-Morales, M. and Valenza, M.C. (2024) 'Effectiveness of self-management interventions during the peri-hospitalization period in patients with stroke: A systematic review and meta-analysis', *Clinical Rehabilitation*, 38(1), pp. 34–46. doi:10.1177/02692155231193563.

Prestwich, A., Sniehotta, F.F., Whittington, C., Dombrowski, S.U., Rogers, L. and Michie, S. (2014) 'Does theory influence the effectiveness of health behavior interventions? Meta-analysis', *Health Psychology*, 33, pp. 465–474. doi:10.1037/a0032853.

Prochaska, J.O. and DiClemente, C.C. (1982) 'Transtheoretical therapy: Toward a more integrative model of change', *Psychotherapy: Theory, Research & Practice*, 19, pp. 276–288. doi:10.1037/h0088437.

Prochaska, J.O. and DiClemente, C.C. (1983) 'Stages and processes of self-change of smoking: Toward an integrative model of change', *Journal of Consulting and Clinical Psychology*, 51, pp. 390–395. doi:10.1037/0022-006X.51.3.390.

Rabinowitz, A.R., Kumar, R.G., Sima, A., Venkatesan, U.M., Juengst, S.B., O'Neil-Pirozzi, T.M., Watanabe, T.K., Goldin, Y., Hammond, F.M. and Dreer, L.E. (2021) 'Aging with traumatic brain injury: Deleterious effects of injury chronicity are most pronounced in later life', *Journal of Neurotrauma*, 38(19), pp. 2706–2713. doi:10.1089/neu.2021.0038.

Rahman, M.S., Peng, W., Adams, J., Hamilton-Bruce, M.A., Hughes, R., Redfern, J. and Middleton, S. (2023) 'The use of self-management strategies for stroke rehabilitation: A scoping review', *Topics in Stroke Rehabilitation*, 30(6), pp. 552–567. doi:10.1080/10749357.2022.2127651.

Reeves, D., Blickem, C., Vassilev, I., Brooks, H., Kennedy, A. and Richardson, G. (2014) 'The contribution of social networks to the health and self-management of patients with long-term conditions: A longitudinal study', *PLoS ONE*, 9, p. e98340. doi:10.1371/journal.pone.0098340.

Rose, A., Rosewilliam, S. and Soundy, A. (2017) 'Shared decision making within goal setting in rehabilitation settings: A systematic review', *Patient Education and Counseling*, 100, pp. 65–75. doi:10.1016/j.pec.2016.07.030.

Rosenstock, I.M. (1974) 'Historical origins of the health belief model', *Health Education Monographs*, 2, pp. 328–335. doi:10.1177/109019817400200403.

Ruksakulpiwat, S., and Zhou, W. (2021). 'Self-management interventions for adults with stroke: A scoping review', *Chronic Diseases and Translational Medicine*, 7(3), pp. 139–148. doi:10.1016/j.cdtm.2021.03.001.

Sabariego, C., Ehrmann, C., Bickenbach, J., Pacheco Barzallo, D., Schedin Leiulfsrud, A., Strøm, V., Osterthun, R., Tederko, P., Seijas, V., Eriks-Hoogland, I., Le Fort, M., Gonzalez Viejo, M.A., Bökel, A., Popa, D., Dionyssiotis, Y., Baricich, A., Juocevicius, A., Amico, P. and Stucki, G. (2023) 'Ageing, functioning patterns and their environmental determinants in the spinal cord injury (SCI) population: A comparative analysis across eleven European countries implementing the international spinal cord injury community survey', *PLoS ONE*, 18(4), p. e0284420. doi:10.1371/journal.pone.0284420.

Sander, A.M., Pappadis, M.R., Bushnik, T., Dreer, L.E., Hammond, F.M., Kreutzer, J.S., Juengst, S.B., Ketchum, J.M., Felix, E.R. and Hanks, R.A. (2024) 'An umbrella review of self-management interventions for health conditions with symptom overlap with traumatic brain injury', *Journal of Head Trauma Rehabilitation*, 39(2), pp. 140–151. doi:10.1097/HTR.0000000000000863.

Schulz, R., Czaja, S.J., Lustig, A., Zdaniuk, B., Martire, L.M. and Perdomo, D. (2009) 'Improving the quality of life of caregivers of persons with spinal cord injury: A randomized controlled trial', *Rehabilitation Psychology*, 54(1), pp. 1–15. doi:10.1037/a0014932.

Shokre, E.S., Mohammed, S.E.M., Elhapashy, H.M.M., Mostafa, N.E. and Eladham, A.M. (2024) 'The effectiveness of the psychosocial empowerment program in early adjustment among adult burn survivors', *BMC Nursing*, 23(1), p. 45. doi:10.1186/s12912-024-01700-x.

Silvester, L., Higo, A., Kearney, R.S., McDaid, C., O'Connor, C., Costa, M.L. and Willett, K. (2024) 'Key components of rehabilitation programmes for adults with complex fractures following traumatic injury: A scoping review', *Injury*, 55(10), p. 111801. doi:10.1016/j.injury.2024.111801.

Skivington, K., Matthews, L., Simpson, S.A., Craig, P., Baird, J., Blazeby, J.M., Boyd, K.A., Craig, N., French, D.P., McIntosh, E., Petticrew, M., Rycroft-Malone, J., White, M. and Moore, L. (2021) 'A new framework for developing and evaluating complex interventions: Update of Medical Research Council guidance', *BMJ*, n2061. doi:10.1136/bmj.n2061.

Smolle, C., Cambiaso-Daniel, J., Forbes, A.A., Wurzer, P., Hundeshagen, G., Branski, L.K., Huss, F. and Kamolz, L.-P. (2017) 'Recent trends in burn epidemiology worldwide: A systematic review', *Burns*, 43, pp. 249–257. doi:10.1016/j.burns.2016.08.013.

Soberg, H., Roe, C., Anke, A., Arango-Lasprilla, J., Skandsen, T., Sveen, U., Steinbüchel, N. and Andelic, N. (2013) 'Health-related quality of life 12 months after severe traumatic brain injury: A prospective nationwide cohort study', *Journal of Rehabilitation Medicine*, 45, pp. 785–791. doi:10.2340/16501977-1158.

Soberg, H.L., Finset, A., Roise, O. and Bautz-Holter, E. (2012) 'The trajectory of physical and mental health from injury to 5 years after multiple trauma: A prospective, longitudinal cohort study', *Archives of Physical Medicine and Rehabilitation*, 93, pp. 765–774. doi:10.1016/j.apmr.2011.08.050.

Spronk, I., Legemate, C., Oen, I., Van Loey, N., Polinder, S. and Van Baar, M. (2018) 'Health related quality of life in adults after burn injuries: A systematic review', *PLoS ONE*, 13, p. e0197507. doi:10.1371/journal.pone.0197507.

Sullivan, J., Mirbahai, L. and Lord, J.M. (2018) 'Major trauma and acceleration of the ageing process', *Ageing Research Reviews*, 48, pp. 32–39. doi:10.1016/j.arr.2018.10.001.

Taylor, S.E. (2018) *Health psychology*. 10th edn., international edition. New York: McGraw-Hill Education.

Taylor, S.J., Pinnock, H., Epiphaniou, E., Pearce, G., Parke, H.L., Schwappach, A., Purushotham, N., Jacob, S., Griffiths, C.J., Greenhalgh, T. and Sheikh, A. (2014) 'A rapid synthesis of the evidence on interventions supporting self-management for people with long-term conditions: PRISMS – practical systematic review of self-management support for long-term conditions', *Health Services and Delivery Research*, 2(53), pp. 1–580. doi:10.3310/hsdr02530.

Thompson, L., Hill, M., Lecky, F. and Shaw, G. (2021) 'Defining major trauma: A Delphi study', *Scandinavian Journal of Trauma, Resuscitation and Emergency Medicine*, 29, p. 63. doi:10.1186/s13049-021-00884-0.

Traumatic Brain Injury (TBI) | National Institute of Neurological Disorders and Stroke. (n.d.) *Traumatic brain injury (TBI)*. Available at: https://www.ninds.nih.gov/health-information/disorders/traumatic-brain-injury-tbi (Accessed: 20 April 2024).

Ustrimova, K.T.A., Fait, B.R., Reme, S.E., Rasmussen, M.S. and Hauger, S.L. (2025) 'Existing evidence of self-management interventions in acquired brain injuries and traumatic injuries: A scoping review', *Disability and Rehabilitation*, pp. 1–38. doi:10.1080/09638288.2025.2530159.

Van de Velde, D., De Zutter, F., Satink, T., Costa, U., Janquart, S., Senn, D. and De Vriendt, P. (2019) 'Delineating the concept of self-management in chronic conditions: A concept analysis', *BMJ Open*, 9, p. e027775. doi:10.1136/bmjopen-2018-027775.

Van Hecke, A., Heinen, M., Fernández-Ortega, P., Graue, M., Hendriks, J. M. L., Høy, B., Köpke, S., Lithner, M., and Van Gaal, B. G. I. (2017). 'Systematic literature review on effectiveness of self-management support interventions in patients with chronic conditions and low socio-economic status,' *Journal of Advanced Nursing*, 73(4), pp. 775–793. doi:10.1111/jan.13159.

Vassilev, I., Rogers, A. and Kennedy, A. (2014) 'The influence of social networks on self-management support: A metasynthesis', *BMC Public Health*, 14, p. 719. doi:10.1186/1471-2458-14-719.

Van Wyk, K., Backwell, A., and Townson, A. (2015). 'A narrative literature review to direct spinal cord injury patient education programming', *Topics in Spinal Cord Injury Rehabilitation*, 21(1), pp. 49–60. doi:10.1310/sci2101-49.

Vincent, H.K., Horodyski, M., Vincent, K.R., Brisbane, S.T. and Sadasivan, K.K. (2015) 'Psychological distress after orthopedic trauma: Prevalence in patients and implications for rehabilitation', *PM&R*, 7, pp. 978–989. doi:10.1016/j.pmrj.2015.03.007.

Wessol, J.L., Russell, C.L. and Cheng, A.L. (2017) 'A systematic review of randomized controlled trials of medication adherence interventions in adult stroke survivors', *Journal of Neuroscience Nursing*, 49(2), pp. 120–133. doi:10.1097/JNN.0000000000000266.

Wilson, B.A. (2009) *Neuropsychological rehabilitation: Theory, models, therapy and outcome*. Cambridge: Cambridge University Press.

Wilson, L., Stewart, W., Dams, -, O'Connor, K., Diaz-Arrastia, R., Horton, L., Menon, D.K. and Polinder, S. (2017) 'The chronic and evolving neurological consequences of traumatic brain injury', *The Lancet Neurology*, 16, pp. 813–825. doi:10.1016/S1474-4422(17)30279-X.

World Health Organization. (n.d.a) *Burns*. Available at: https://www.who.int/news-room/fact-sheets/detail/burns (Accessed: 29 August 2025).

World Health Organization. (n.d.b) *Injuries and violence*. Available at: https://www.who.int/news-room/fact-sheets/detail/injuries-and-violence (Accessed: 29 August 2025).

Wray, F., Clarke, D. and Forster, A. (2018) 'Post-stroke self-management interventions: A systematic review of effectiveness and investigation of the inclusion of stroke survivors with aphasia', *Disability and Rehabilitation*, 40(11), pp. 1237–1251.

2 Self-Management Support for Older Adults in Stroke Rehabilitation

Implications for Rehabilitation Practice

Sedsel Kristine Stage Pedersen, Susanne Lillelund Sørensen, and Hanne Pallesen

STROKE, AGEING, AND EVERYDAY LIFE: SETTING THE SCENE

Stroke is one of the leading causes of disability worldwide, and the number of people living with its long-term sequels is growing (Feigin et al., 2024; World Health Organisation, 2014). In Denmark with a population of approximately 6 million people, most people who have a stroke are over the age of 65, and around 60,000 people are currently living with stroke-related impairments. Each year, approximately 12,000 people in Denmark experience a stroke, and more than two-thirds of them are older adults (Danish Health Authority, 2024; Flachs, 2015). In Denmark, individuals become eligible for the old-age state pension at around the age of 65, although the official retirement age is gradually increasing (Danish Agency for Labour Market and Recruitment (STAR), 2025; Danish legal information (Retsinformation), 2021). Most older adults are no longer part of the labour market, which may increase vulnerability to loneliness due to the loss of social connections from the workplace (DaneAge Association (Ældre Sagen), 2025; Grøn and Andersen, 2014). The effects of stroke can make it even harder for older adults to reconnect socially, as physical or cognitive difficulties may limit their ability to reengage in usual activities or join new activities (Danish Health Authority, 2011; Grøn and Andersen, 2014). Older adults living with stroke may therefore need extra support to rebuild or form new social relationships. Reintegration often relies on family support, but the responsibility frequently falls on spouses, who take on the role of informal caregiver (, Danish Health Authority, 2011; Turner et al., 2007).

SELF-MANAGEMENT SUPPORT AND THE ROLE OF SELF-EFFICACY IN STROKE REHABILITATION

Self-management has become a central concept in the care of long-term conditions, referring to individuals' efforts to manage the medical, emotional, and social consequences of illness (Bodenheimer et al., 2005; de Silva, 2011; Lorig and Holman, 2003). According to de Silva (2011), this extends beyond symptom control to include behavioural and lifestyle adjustments and is increasingly seen as a collaborative process supported by health systems. In the present context, self-management support refers to assistance provided by health professionals to older adults with stroke and their informal caregivers, aiming to sustain former lifestyles or foster new, meaningful life perspectives (Bodenheimer et al., 2005; de Silva, 2011). Importantly, self-management and self-efficacy are closely interconnected concepts, with self-efficacy often regarded as a foundational mechanism enabling effective self-management (de Silva, 2011). This relationship is grounded in Bandura's

DOI: 10.1201/9781003599074-3

(1977) social cognitive theory, which posits that individuals are more likely to initiate and maintain health behaviours when they believe they are capable of doing so (Bandura, 1977). Consequently, self-efficacy is not only an outcome of self-management programmes but a central mechanism through which older adults recovering from stroke and their informal caregivers improve health behaviours, quality of life, and healthcare utilisation (de Silva, 2011; Ryan and Sawin, 2009).

FROM INDIVIDUAL TO DYAD: STRENGTHENING SELF-MANAGEMENT THROUGH CAREGIVER SUPPORT

The authors of this chapter carried out a review of research studies to find out how well self-management programmes work for older adults who have had a stroke, especially in terms of mental and social wellbeing (Pedersen et al., 2020). Self-management programmes were defined as structured ways of helping people change habits and improve their emotional health or social life. These programmes were run by healthcare professionals, sometimes with the help of technology, and were offered either one-to-one or in group sessions. The studies looked at a range of outcomes, including quality of life, self-efficacy, emotional wellbeing, ability to manage daily tasks, and progress toward a more active lifestyle. These outcomes were measured either as the key outcomes or as additional outcomes. Only studies where people were randomly placed into different types of care – called randomised controlled trials – were included. The first search for studies was done in May 2019 and updated in April 2020. Eleven studies were included in total. The review grouped the results into seven categories: (i) self-management skills, (ii) self-efficacy, (iii) quality of life, (iv) depression, (v) daily activities, (vi) active lifestyle, and (vii) other related outcomes. The review found that self-management programmes may help older adults gain skills and confidence in managing life after stroke, improve quality of life, support daily activities, and boost emotional wellbeing. However, the overall strength of the findings was limited because the studies differed in quality, programme design, follow-up time, and how the results were measured.

A follow-up search in May 2025 found five new studies, including one by the authors of this chapter (Amiri et al., 2022; Bragstad et al., 2020; Minshall et al., 2020; Pallesen et al., 2025; Vluggen et al., 2021). These new studies did not change the overall conclusions, but three of them showed that caregivers also benefited when the older adult with stroke and their informal caregiver were supported as a pair, rather than separately (Minshall et al., 2020; Pallesen et al., 2025; Vluggen et al., 2021). This suggests that future programmes should also include support for caregivers, recognising that the older adult with stroke and their informal caregiver often experience stroke recovery together, as a shared process, while still having their own individual needs.

WHAT MATTERS IN STROKE RECOVERY? LESSONS FROM A SELF-MANAGEMENT PROGRAMME FOR OLDER ADULTS AND THEIR INFORMAL CAREGIVERS

In a Danish clinical setting, a self-management programme that focused on social and emotional aspects of recovery – based on self-management principles – was integrated into local physiotherapy and occupational therapy services (Pallesen et al., 2025). The programme was designed for older adults recovering from stroke and their informal caregivers. The aim was to broaden the goals of rehabilitation – which have often focused on physical problems and daily tasks – to also include helping people take part in meaningful activities and stay connected with others. This approach, aligns with the International Classification of Functioning, Disability and Health (ICF) (Maribo, 2022; World Health Organisation, 2002). The programme was delivered during the subacute phase after stroke, starting two weeks before discharge from specialised inpatient neurorehabilitation centres, continuing through municipal rehabilitation, and extending up to nine months after discharge.

It was delivered by two mentors – a physiotherapist and an occupational therapist – both with strong experience in stroke rehabilitation. The mentors also had prior training in coaching techniques. The programme was offered alongside usual care and consisted of three to nine sessions, each lasting 40 to 60 minutes, over a nine-month period.

Key elements of the programme included using a person-centred approach, building trusting relationships, fostering open dialogue, engaging informal caregivers, transferring relearned or new activities and practising active reflection carried out in social settings that involved informal caregivers and broader social contacts such as friends, peers, or community groups. These elements supported older adults with stroke and their informal caregivers reflecting on their situation, taking initiative, and gaining a sense of control. The goal was to support personal change and learning, helping people rebuild a sense of self, manage their health, and return to a more active life (Sørensen et al., 2019). In some cases, the programme also strengthened cooperation and communication between the older adults and their informal caregiver. An overview of the programme and its main components is provided in Figure 2.1 with practical applications described in more detail later in this chapter.

To understand the potential impact of the programme, it was tested in a research study with 69 participants, who were randomly assigned to either usual care or the new self-management programme added to usual care. Overall, the results showed no clear improvements in self-efficacy, quality of life, participation, or autonomy compared with usual care. However, further analysis showed that the informal caregivers in the programme group reported feeling less burdened at both three and nine months. This suggests the programme may have had an early positive effect on informal caregiver wellbeing (Pallesen et al., 2025).

What Did the Programme Mean to Participants?

In follow-up interviews, many older adults who took part in the self-management programme said that support from their mentor was important in helping them make a plan and find ways to resume daily

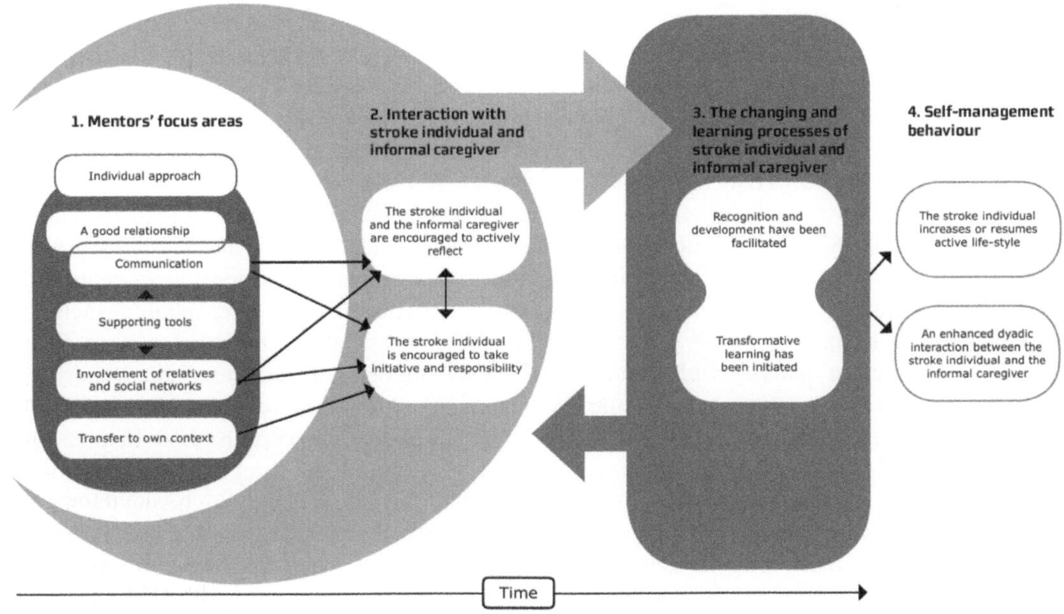

FIGURE 2.1 Overview of the main components in a Danish stroke self-management program (Sørensen et al., 2019). (Licensed under CC BY 4.0. Colour changed to black and white.)

life – emotionally, physically, and practically. They also felt that the mentor played a helpful role in supporting their informal caregivers. However, a few said they could probably have managed without the mentor's help. This suggests that older adults recovering from stroke have different support needs, and that a one-size-fits-all approach may not be suitable for everyone. Several older adults also said it was important to regain a sense of control over their lives after returning home. This included having time and space to think, reflect, and explore their new situation – without feeling constantly watched or evaluated. For the interviewed older adults and their informal caregivers, the combination of shared knowledge and practical application in daily life seemed to make a real difference.

The programme was evaluated in two ways: through questionnaires and through follow-up interviews. Interestingly, the findings from these two methods did not completely match. While the questionnaires offered structured ways of measuring change, the interviews provided more personal and detailed stories about how participants experienced the programme. This difference suggests that standard questionnaires may not fully capture the complexity or personal meaning of taking part in a self-management programme. It raises important questions about whether these tools are sufficient to reflect the full impact of such interventions – a point also raised by Bragstad et al. (2020).

CAPTURING COMPLEXITY: CHALLENGES IN MEASURING SELF-MANAGEMENT IN STROKE REHABILITATION

Measuring self-management in stroke rehabilitation is not straightforward. Current approaches – for example those that use self-efficacy as a proxy – may not fully reflect the complexity of the recovery process. The Stroke Self-Efficacy Questionnaire, developed by Jones et al. (2008), is widely used for this purpose. It builds on the idea that self-efficacy is an important mechanism to trigger self-management (Jones et al., 2008; Riazi et al., 2014). While self-efficacy is certainly important, we – the authors of this chapter – are concerned that focusing mainly on this concept may miss other essential parts of stroke recovery. For example, the emotional, social, and relational aspects are often overlooked in standard self-efficacy measures (Pallesen et al., 2025; Sørensen et al., 2019).

Self-management is often linked to social cognitive theory, which emphasises individual decision-making, knowledge, and behavioural skills (Knapp, 2000; Macgillivray et al., 2012). Accordingly, many self-management measures across rehabilitation and chronic disease care focus mainly on the individual's ability to control their own behaviour and carry out specific tasks. Examples include the Patient Activation Measure (Hibbard et al., 2004) and the Self-Management Ability Scales (Cramm et al., 2012). Within stroke rehabilitation, comparable task- and behaviour-oriented tools include the Southampton Stroke Self-Management Questionnaire (Boger et al., 2015). While these instruments provide useful insights, their narrow focus means that current measures often fail to capture the broader complexity and varied consequences of stroke – particularly for older adults – including emotional changes, shifts in family roles, and dependence on social and practical support. These aspects are difficult to quantify with standardised questionnaires. For this reason, we believe it is time to rethink how we define and measure self-management in stroke rehabilitation. Evaluation tools should go beyond measuring a person's confidence in performing certain tasks. Instead, they should aim to reflect the real-life experiences of older adults and their caregivers – including the emotional, social, and relational aspects of life after stroke. This also means recognising the mutual dependency within caregiving relationships, and the fact that self-management does not happen in isolation, but in the context of everyday life. Recent guidance from NHS England also emphasises the importance of selecting appropriate approaches for measuring supported self-management, recommending a structured process for planning how outcome measures are used in practice (National Health Service England, 2021). This underlines the need for tools that are both theoretically sound and contextually meaningful.

UNDERSTANDING THE LIMITS OF GENERALISED EVIDENCE: WHY OLDER ADULTS MAY NEED MORE

A Cochrane review – a comprehensive summary of high-quality research – looked at self-management programmes for adults recovering from stroke. The review, published in 2016, found that these programmes could improve quality of life. People reported feeling more in control, more able to do what mattered to them, and less dependent on others (Fryer et al., 2016). Importantly, the review found no evidence that the programmes caused harm. However, the review included adults of all ages, which makes it difficult to know whether the same positive results apply to older adults specifically. Older adults may have different needs, health challenges, and social circumstances that require more tailored support.

The review was based on 14 studies published up to April 2016, involving a total of about 1,800 adults with stroke. These studies were conducted in various countries and used different formats: some programmes were delivered in groups, others individually, and the length and content of the programmes varied. While some studies showed benefits for informal caregivers when they were included in self-management support, the outcomes were not always as positive for the older adults with stroke themselves. This contrast suggests that self-management programmes may need to be better adapted to the specific circumstances and abilities of older people.

This raises several important questions:

- Do older adults recover differently from stroke than younger people?
- Could cognitive challenges (memory or thinking difficulties) make it harder for older adults to benefit from self-management programmes?
- What social or practical barriers might prevent older adults from reconnecting with others or resume meaningful activities after stroke?

These questions are important for both clinical practice and future research, and they highlight the need to design more age-sensitive and personalised support for older adults recovering from stroke.

IDENTIFYING WHO NEEDS MORE SUPPORT: SCREENING FOR PSYCHOSOCIAL VULNERABILITY AFTER STROKE

Identifying older adults who may be struggling with psychosocial vulnerability after a stroke can help health professionals offer more tailored support, especially in relation to self-management and emotional wellbeing (Bragstad et al., 2020). The concept of sense of coherence, introduced by Antonovsky, describes a person's ability to manage stress and stay well, even in difficult situations. It reflects how well someone understands what is happening (comprehensibility), how capable they feel in managing it (manageability), and whether they see it as meaningful (meaningfulness) (Antonovsky, 1987). For older adults recovering from stroke, a strong sense of coherence can support motivation, coping, and emotional resilience. In contrast, those with a weaker sense of coherence may feel overwhelmed or powerless, which can make it harder to stay engaged in rehabilitation or manage everyday challenges. Recognising low sense of coherence early can help tailor support more effectively – such as adapting self-management approaches, involving informal caregivers, or providing additional psychological support. While it is important to recognise subgroups of people recovering from stroke, we believe that all older adults recovering from stroke can benefit from supportive self-management approaches. The main difference lies in the intensity and form of support needed to promote wellbeing, independence, and participation in daily life.

Recognising the Dyadic Unit

Low sense of coherence is not limited to older adults after stroke – it may also affect informal caregivers, who often face emotional stress, changes in roles, and health challenges of their own (Chumbler et al., 2004; Jaracz et al., 2024). In many cases, the informal caregiver is also an older adult and may struggle with physical limitations, cognitive strain, or social isolation. When a loved one has a stroke, the informal caregiver's everyday life is often profoundly affected. Routines are disrupted, and they must quickly adapt to new responsibilities while also providing emotional and practical support. This dual burden can make both members of the dyad – the older adult and the informal caregiver – psychosocially vulnerable, particularly in the early stages of recovery (Andersen et al., 2017). Recognising and addressing this shared vulnerability is essential to effective rehabilitation planning. This view is supported by recent rehabilitation guidelines, which emphasise the need to involve informal caregivers as an integral part of stroke recovery (Maribo, 2022; Stroke Foundation, 2022; Strokeguideline, 2023). Viewing older adults recovering from stroke and their informal caregiver as a dyadic unit – a connected pair rather than two separate individuals – has important implications for rehabilitation planning and delivered. Stroke rehabilitation should therefore be planned to support both individuals, taking into account their shared and individual needs. This includes providing support that enables each person to manage daily tasks, maintain emotional wellbeing, and stay socially connected through meaningful activities. Informal caregivers may be relatives, partners, friends, or neighbours who have a significant personal relationship with the older adult. They can be either primary or secondary carers, and may live with or separately from the person they support. While caregiving roles are often filled by spouses or close family members, any trusted individual designated by the older adult can take on this responsibility. If no such person is identified, rehabilitation services should help locate one – potentially through voluntary organisations or local networks.

In the next section, we provide practical guidance for delivering self-management support that reflects this interconnected reality – ensuring that both members of the dyad are supported throughout the rehabilitation process.

PRACTICAL GUIDANCE OF THE SELF-MANAGEMENT PROGRAMME FOR OLDER ADULTS AND THEIR INFORMAL CAREGIVERS

The implementation and delivery of the self-management programme are based on a set of guiding principles, why it matters and how to apply it (see Table 2.1).

The guiding principles of this self-management intervention reflect a humanistic approach, emphasising personalised and timely support to enhance its overall effectiveness. This approach values the lived experience, personal goals, and unique life context of both the older adult and their informal caregiver, aiming to sustain former lifestyles or support the development of new, meaningful perspectives. Furthermore, it recognises that recovery is not only about physical rehabilitation but also about emotional adjustment, rebuilding social connections, and regaining a sense of identity. By tailoring support to each person's priorities and readiness, the programme sought to create a safe and enabling environment in which both older adults and their informal caregivers could take an active role in the rehabilitation process.

RETHINKING ELIGIBILITY FOR SELF-MANAGEMENT SUPPORT

This chapter has focused on the role of self-management in stroke rehabilitation for adults aged 65 and older. While some studies show positive outcomes for informal caregivers, such as greater understanding and improved coping, the effects for older adults stroke recovering from stroke are less consistent. This discrepancy invites reflection on how older adults may differ from the general stroke population. Many studies include adults of all ages, yet older adults often live with additional challenges – such as multimorbidity, reduced cognitive or physical capacity, and limited social

TABLE 2.1
Back to Life: Six Guiding Principles

Guiding Principles	Why It Matters	How to Apply It
1: Apply a person-centred approach	It is essential to identify the older adult's pre-stroke identity. This understanding forms the basis for helping healthcare professionals preserve and support the individual's sense of self throughout rehabilitation and selecting appropriate actions. Gaining insight into the older adult's pre-stroke identity also supports a person-centred approach, guiding health professionals towards a rehabilitation strategy that emphasises the older adult's strengths and intrinsic motivations to regain lost abilities or develop new coping strategies.	• Use COPM (Canadian Occupational Performance Measure) to identify activity-related challenges. • Ask what matters most in the older adult's daily life. • Involve informal caregivers in discussions. • Use an interview or short form of open questions to guide the conversation. • Let the older adult choose which life areas to focus on (e.g., home, family, physical activity, friends, work, hobbies). • Keep the focus on the older adult's own priorities.

2. Building trusting relationships	Research indicates that a strong therapeutic relationship accounts for up to 80% of successful rehabilitation outcomes (Møller and Lerbech, 2010). While it is essential to focus stroke rehabilitation on the older adult's daily life and personal context, it is equally important to acknowledge the structural conditions and limitations of the healthcare system. Being systemic about these constraints fosters a relationship grounded in trust and authenticity, which in turn enhances engagement and promotes more effective rehabilitation.	• Start each session by asking about the older adult needs today.
		• Use open questions:
		  • *"What's been on your mind lately?"*
		  • *"What are you thinking about today?"*
		  • *"What's using up your energy right now?"*
		• Help the older adult set the focus for the day.
		• Encourage shared responsibility for the rehabilitation process.

3. Foster open dialogue	Successful communication is closely linked to the quality of therapeutic relationships and meaningful interactions. It is essential for health professionals to acknowledge and accept complex or distressing emotions expressed by the older adults. Older adults recovering from stroke often experience a range of difficult thoughts and feelings that can be challenging to process. Responding with empathy and an affective attuned approach helps validate the older adult's experience, building psychological safety and promoting a more trusting and supportive therapeutic environment.	• Show genuine interest and respect for the older adult's identity. • Be curious; help the older adult view topics from new angles. • Ask open, reflective questions (using words like *how*, *where*, *which*). • Respond to emotions with empathy. • Allow silence when needed – active listening can reveal important thoughts.

4: Engage informal caregivers	Most older adults recovering from stroke maintain close relationships with their family members and friends, making it essential to prioritise effective communication and collaboration with informal caregivers. Identifying key informal caregivers and understanding their preferred level of involvement can enhance the rehabilitation process. While many informal caregivers are willing to engage as partners in care, their interest and capacity to collaborate may vary. When appropriately involved, informal caregivers can help transfer of rehabilitation strategies into the older adult's daily life, supporting continuity and sustainability of care.	• Use network cards (simple visual tools for mapping a person's social connections) to make the older adult's supporting network visible.
		• Ask:
		  • *Who can support you, and in what way?"*
		  • *"How would you like your network to look in the future?"*
		• Recognise different support roles (emotional, practical, advisory).
		• Speak openly with informal caregivers about:
		  • Life after stroke
		  • New roles, expectations, and changes

(Continued)

TABLE 2.1 ***(Continued)***
Back to Life: Six Guiding Principles

Guiding Principles	Why It Matters	How to Apply It

5. Transfer learning to daily life	Transferring relearned or new activities and skills to the older adult's daily life and social context is a critical component of effective stroke rehabilitation. This process not only enhances the older adult's sense of security and confidence in their ability to re-engage with daily life and society, but also strengthens their capacity for self-management – the ability to navigate and take control of one's life independently. Ultimately, the successful integration of these skills into everyday routines serves as a key indicator of the stroke rehabilitation's long-term impact and indicates whether the therapeutic gains are sustained beyond the formal course of treatment.	• Encourage regular social contact to provide structure, meaning, and positive experiences.
		• Help the older adult stay connected despite the stroke's impact.
		• End each session with a reflection:
		  • *"What did you learn today?"*
		  • *"How can you use this in your daily life?"*
		• Use these reflections to strengthen learning and build motivation.

6. Practice active reflection (and homework)	Research demonstrates that rehabilitation is most effective when patients actively participate in developing solutions to the challenges they face (Maribo, 2022). This collaborative approach increases the likelihood that the strategies and techniques will be applied beyond the formal stroke rehabilitation setting. Consequently, therapists must adopt a flexible and responsive approach, showing respect for the older adult's ideas, preferences, and reflections. In addition, involving informal caregivers as partners in the stroke rehabilitation process can further support the successful transfer of training into the older adult's daily life, enhancing both continuity and engagement.	• Use open dialog to forester reflections
		• Encourage using a diary or calendar to track training, appointments, and goals.
		• Suggest keeping a logbook to increase self-awareness and track progress.
		• Include questions such as:
		  • *"What worked well today?"*
		  • *"What would you like to try differently?"*
		• Recommend trying new actions and noting their effects.

networks – that may influence their ability to benefit from conventional self-management interventions. Crucially, not all individuals with stroke are equally positioned to take on the role of a "self-manager." People with cognitive impairments – such as reduced insight, poor initiation, or unrealistic appraisals of their abilities – may face particular difficulties in navigating self-management independently. These realities challenge the assumption that all patients can or should take on responsibility for managing their own recovery without structured support.

In clinical practice, there is a risk that health professionals – often unintentionally – associate the "ideal" self-manager with characteristics such as high motivation, insight, and compliance. As a result, individuals who appear less organised, more dependent, or emotionally overwhelmed may be overlooked for self-management support. This risks excluding precisely those who might benefit the most, particularly if their challenges are misinterpreted as a lack of engagement rather than as signs of underlying cognitive or psychosocial vulnerability

From both our research and clinical experience, we propose a shift to dyadic thinking in stroke rehabilitation. This means moving away from viewing agency as something located solely within the individual, and instead understanding it as co-constructed – emerging in the relationship between the older adult with stroke, their informal caregiver, and the wider rehabilitation team. Importantly, we believe that informal caregivers should be included as part of the rehabilitation process, regardless of whether the older adult lives alone or not. The dyadic relationship is often central to how stroke is managed in everyday life, and its importance should be reflected in how rehabilitation services are designed and delivered. A special focus should also be given to the stressed dyad – where both the older adult with stroke and their informal caregiver are vulnerable, for example due to their own health problems, fatigue, or emotional strain. These are precisely the situations where well-designed self-management support can have the most impact, if it is delivered with sensitivity and tailored to fluctuating capacity. Finally, we recognise that self-management interventions may be more readily taken up by those who are already doing relatively well – for example, people who have prior experience with healthcare systems, higher health literacy, or stronger support networks. This raises the question of whether current eligibility criteria inadvertently reinforce inequalities, by primarily reaching those who are already more capable of managing on their own. In light of this, we call for a broader and more inclusive approach to self-management support – one that is flexible enough to accommodate varying levels of independence, evolving needs, and the shared efforts of dyads. Self-management should not be seen as something individuals either qualify for or not, but as something that can be scaled and shaped depending on the context, with both people in the dyad actively involved where possible. Ultimately, increasing the relevance and impact of self-management support requires more than individual motivation – it requires a system that acknowledges the complexity of stroke recovery, the role of close relationships, and the value of shared responsibility. These principles are echoed in current research, which supports co-design, co-production, and public involvement as vital strategies for developing meaningful and sustainable interventions.

REFERENCES

Amiri, F. S., Abolhassani, S., Alimohammadi, N. & Roghani, T. 2022. Investigating the effect of self-management program on stroke's patients' self-efficacy. *BMC Neurology*, 22, 1–10.

Andersen, C. W., Birtø, K. & Lawætz, M. 2017. *Fokus på pårørende i kommunal rehabilitering. Et oplæg til refleksion og handling*. København: Center for Kræft & Sundhed.

Antonovsky, A. 1987. *Unraveling the mystery of health: how people manage stress and stay well*. Jossey-Bass.

Bandura, A. 1977. Self-efficacy: toward a unifying theory of behavioral change. *Psychological Review*, 84, 191–215.

Bodenheimer, T., Macgregor, K. & Sharifi, C. 2005. *Helping patients manage their chronic conditions*. CA: California HealthCare Foundation.

Boger, E. J., Hankins, M., Demain, S. H. & Latter, S. M. 2015. Development and psychometric evaluation of a new patient -reported outcome measure for stroke self -management: The Southampton Stroke Self - Management Questionnaire (SSSMQ). *Health and Quality of Life Outcomes*, 13, 165–165.

Bragstad, L. K., Hjelle, E. G., Zucknick, M., Sveen, U., Thommessen, B., Bronken, B. A., Martinsen, R., Kitzmüller, G., Mangset, M., Kvigne, K. J., Hilari, K., Lightbody, C. E. & Kirkevold, M. 2020. The effects of a dialogue-based intervention to promote psychosocial well-being after stroke: a randomized controlled trial. *Clinical Rehabilitation*, 34, 1056–1071.

Chumbler, N. R., Rittman, M., Puymbroeck, M. V., Vogel, W. B. & Qnin, H. 2004. The sense of coherence, burden, and depressive symptoms in informal caregivers during the first month after stroke. *International Journal of Geriatric Psychiatry*, 19, 944–953.

Cramm, J. M., Strating, M. M. H., de Vreede, P. L., Steverink, N. & Nieboer, A. P. 2012. Validation of the Self-Management Ability Scale (SMAS) and development and validation of a shorter scale (SMAS-S) among older patients shortly after hospitalisation. *Health and Quality of Life Outcomes*, 10, 9–9.

Daneage Association (Ældre Sagen). 2025. *Arbejdsstyrke og beskæftigelse 2013–2023. Ældre i tal*. Ældre Sagen.

Danish Agency For Labour Market And Recruitment (STAR). 2025. *The state pension age now and in the future* [Online]. Available: https://star.dk/ydelser/pension-og-efterloen/folkepension-tidlig-pension-foertidspension-og-seniorpension/folkepension/folkepensionsalderen-nu-og-fremover?utm_source=chatgpt.com [Accessed].

Danish Health Authority. 2011. *Hjerneskaderehabilitering – En medicinsk teknologivurdering. Sammenfatning*. Sundhedsstyrelsen.

Danish Health Authority. 2024. *Fact sheet: stroke in Denmark*. Copenhagen: Danish Health Authority.

Danish Legal Information (Retsinformation). 2021. *Lov om social pension. Lov om højeste, mellemste, forhøjet almindelig og almindelig førtidspension m.v. Lov om delpension*. Schultz Information.

de Silva, D. 2011. Evidence: Helping people help themselves. *In:* Foundation, H. (ed.) *A review of the evidence considering whether it is worthwhile to support self-management*. The Health Foundation.

Feigin, V. L., Abdollahi, A., Abreu, L. G., et al. 2024. Global, regional, and national burden of stroke and its risk factors, 1990–2021: a systematic analysis for the Global Burden of Disease Study 2021. *Lancet Neurology*, 23, 973–1003.

Flachs, E. M. M. F. 2015. *Sygdomsbyrden i Danmark: Sygdomme*. Kbh., Sundhedsstyrelsen.

Fryer, C. E., Luker, J. A., Mcdonnell, M. N., Hillier, S. L. & Hillier, S. L. 2016. Self management programmes for quality of life in people with stroke. *Cochrane Database of Systematic Reviews*, 2019, CD010442.

Grøn, L. & Andersen, C. R. 2014. *Sårbarhed og handlekraft i alderdommen: et etnografisk feltarbejde blandt fagpersoner og ældre i Horsens og omegn*. Kora.

Hibbard, J. H., Stockard, J., Mahoney, E. R. & Tusler, M. 2004. Development of the Patient Activation Measure (PAM): conceptualizing and measuring activation in patients and consumers. *Health Services Research*, 39, 1005–1026.

Jaracz, K., Grabowska-Fudala, B., Jaracz, J., Moczko, J., Kleka, P., Pawlicka, A. & Górna, K. 2024. Caregiver burden after stroke: a 10-year follow-up study of Polish caregivers for stroke patients. *BMC Nursing*, 23, 589.

Jones, F., Partridge, C. & Reid, F. 2008. The Stroke Self-Efficacy Questionnaire: measuring individual confidence in functional performance after stroke. *Journal of Clinical Nursing*, 17, 244–252.

Knapp, P. 2000. Non-drug strategies to resolve psychosocial difficulties after stroke. *Age and Ageing*, 29, 23–30.

Lorig, K. R. & Holman, H. 2003. Self-management education: history, definition, outcomes, and mechanisms. *Annals of Behavioral Medicine*, 26, 1–7.

Macgillivray, S., Kroll, T., Oliver, T., Morris, J. & Bernhardt, J. A. 2012. The importance of psychological and social factors in influencing the uptake and maintenance of physical activity after stroke: a structured review of the empirical literature. *Stroke Research and Treatment*, 2012, 98–117.

Maribo, T. M. F. 2022. *White book on rehabilitation*. Rehabiliteringsforum Danmark.

Minshall, C., Castle, D. J., Thompson, D. R., Pascoe, M., Cameron, J., Mccabe, M., Apputhurai, P., Knowles, S. R., Jenkins, Z. & Ski, C. F. 2020. A psychosocial intervention for stroke survivors and carers: 12-month outcomes of a randomized controlled trial. *Topics in Stroke Rehabilitation*, 27, 563–576.

Møller, K. & Lerbech, L. 2010. Professionsdidaktiske reflektioner på baggrund af undersøgelse af kommunikation i indlæggelsessamtaler i klinisk praksis. *In:* Beedholm, I. K. & Greve, C. (eds.) *Professionsdidaktik: et særligt anliggende for professionshøjskolerne?* VIA Systime.

National Health Service England. 2021. *Measuring supported self-management: five steps to help teams choose approaches*. NHS England.

Pallesen, H., Pedersen, S. K. S., Srensen, S. L., Naess-Schmidt, E. T., Brunner, I., Nielsen, J. F. & Kjeldsen, S. S. 2025. "Stroke-65 plus. Continued active life." A randomized controlled trial of a self-management neurorehabilitation intervention for elderly people after stroke. *Disability and Rehabilitation*, 47, 104–113.

Pedersen, S. K. S., Sørensen, S. L., Stabel, H. H., Brunner, I. & Pallesen, H. 2020. Effect of self-management support for elderly people post-stroke: a systematic review. *Geriatrics (Basel)*, 5, 38.

Riazi, A., Aspden, T. & Jones, F. 2014. Stroke Self-efficacy Questionnaire: a Rasch-refined measure of confidence post stroke. *Journal of Rehabilitation Medicine*, 46, 406–412.

Ryan, P. & Sawin, K. J. 2009. The individual and family self-management theory: background and perspectives on context, process, and outcomes. *Nursing Outlook*, 57, 217–225.e6.

Sørensen, S. L., Pedersen, S. K. S. & Pallesen, H. 2019. Social psychological mechanisms and processes in a novel, health professional-led, self-management intervention for older stroke individuals: a synthesis and phenomenological study. *BMC Health Services Research*, 19, 320.

Stroke Foundation. 2022. *Clinical guidelines for stroke management. Chapter 7 of 8: discharge planning and transfer of care*. Stroke Foundation.

Strokeguideline. 2023. *National clinical guideline for stroke for United Kingdom and Ireland. Chapter 2: organisation of stroke services*. Royal College of Physicians.

Turner, B., Fleming, J., Cornwell, P., Worrall, L., Ownsworth, T., Haines, T., Kendall, M. & Chenoweth, L. 2007. A qualitative study of the transition from hospital to home for individuals with acquired brain injury and their family caregivers. *Brain Injury*, 21, 1119–1130.

Vluggen, T. P. M. M., Van Haastregt, J. C. M., Tan, F. E., Verbunt, J. A., Van Heugten, C. M. & Schols, J. M. G. A. 2021. Effectiveness of an integrated multidisciplinary geriatric rehabilitation programme for older persons with stroke: a multicentre randomised controlled trial. *BMC Geriatrics*, 21, 134.

World Health Organisation. 2002. *International classification of functioning, disability and health: ICF*. Danmarks Blindebibliotek.

World Health Organisation. 2014. *Global status report on noncommunicable diseases 2014*. World Health Organisation.

3 Fear of Movement and Avoidance Behaviour as Barriers for Effective Self-Management in Musculoskeletal Pain

Thomas Matheve and Liesbet De Baets

INTRODUCTION

Musculoskeletal disorders are the leading contributor to disability worldwide (Vos, 2017). Approximately 1.7 billion people suffer from musculoskeletal pain, with low back pain and osteoarthritis being the most prevalent and disabling conditions. Although acute musculoskeletal pain often resolves after a few weeks, a significant proportion of people will develop recurrent or chronic musculoskeletal pain. For example, after an episode of acute low back pain, up to 69% of persons experience low back pain recurrence within one year of recovery, and 15–25% of people will develop chronic low back pain (da Silva et al., 2019; Wallwork et al., 2024). The development and persistence of chronic musculoskeletal pain can be influenced by a myriad of factors, including biomechanical, psychological, social, and behavioural factors (Dunn et al., 2024; Vlaeyen et al., 2018). Due to this multidimensional nature, chronic musculoskeletal pain has been proven notoriously difficult to treat, with traditional rehabilitation programmes often resulting in limited long-term improvements in pain and disability (Jenkins et al., 2025; Lawford et al., 2024; Traweger et al., 2025). As such, there has been a paradigm shift from clinician-led treatment to self-management, where people predominantly manage their chronic musculoskeletal pain outside the healthcare system (Hutting, 2025; Kongsted et al., 2021).

Various definitions of self-management exist, but in essence, it refers to an individual's ability to actively participate and take responsibility in the management of the actual or potential impact of their condition (Barlow et al., 2002; Jonkman et al., 2016; Kongsted et al., 2021). The success of self-management depends on the individual's ability to engage in meaningful activities and manage symptoms in an independent and flexible manner (Kongsted et al., 2021). Although self-management is increasingly being recognized as an integral part of high-quality care for people with chronic musculoskeletal pain, current evidence for its effectiveness is limited, with systematic reviews reporting only small positive effects on pain and disability (Elbers et al., 2018; Oliveira et al., 2012; Rathnayake, Sparkes, & Sheeran, 2021; Wu et al., 2022). Moreover, self-management interventions do not seem to affect healthcare utilization in people with musculoskeletal pain (Grøn et al., 2025). However, current self-management programmes often have a narrow scope and fail to address all essential aspects of a comprehensive self-management approach, which may explain their limited effectiveness.

Recent work has provided guidance on self-management for people with chronic musculoskeletal pain (Diener, 2021; Hutting et al., 2019; Kongsted et al., 2021). One of the key elements is to identify and address the barriers to effective self-management. In this respect, fear of movement and avoidance behaviour have consistently been shown as such barriers in people with chronic

DOI: 10.1201/9781003599074-4

musculoskeletal pain (Darlow et al., 2025; Gilanyi et al., 2024; Grande et al., 2025; Kanavaki et al., 2017; Palazzo et al., 2016; Seven et al., 2024). This should come as no surprise as self-management in chronic musculoskeletal pain often includes an active behavioural component, such as performing home exercises, maintaining an active lifestyle, managing symptoms, continuing to engage in valued life activities despite the pain, or resuming these activities following a flare-up or relapse. Unfortunately, persons with chronic musculoskeletal pain often hold unhelpful beliefs about physical activity or lack the confidence to stay active while in pain, which can pose significant barriers to effective self-management (Caneiro, Bunzli, & O'Sullivan, 2021). Especially, when persons fear that physical activity might lead to negative outcomes—such as damage to the painful area or increased pain—they may choose to avoid it altogether.

In this chapter, we will discuss the following aspects: (1) a general introduction to fear of movement and avoidance behaviour in chronic musculoskeletal pain; (2) management of fear of movement and avoidance behaviour by exposure therapy *in vivo*; (3) fear of movement and avoidance behaviour as barriers to effective self-management; and (4) a clinical case study to provide guidance to support effective self-management in persons with chronic musculoskeletal pain by focusing on fear of movement and avoidance behaviours as barriers for self-management.

FEAR OF MOVEMENT AND AVOIDANCE BEHAVIOUR IN PERSONS WITH CHRONIC MUSCULOSKELETAL PAIN

In acute musculoskeletal pain, temporarily avoiding certain activities may be advisable to reduce the load on the affected tissues allowing them to heal (Hodges & Smeets, 2015). This is considered *helpful or adaptive behaviour*, as it promotes recovery. However, avoidance behaviour is also commonly seen in persons with chronic musculoskeletal pain. A hallmark characteristic of chronic musculoskeletal pain is the often poor association between findings on medical imaging and the presence of pain or the clinical presentation of the patient. This has been shown for many chronic musculoskeletal pain conditions, including low back pain (Brinjikji et al., 2015), neck pain (Farrell et al., 2019), shoulder pain (Tran et al., 2018), and knee (Culvenor et al., 2019) and hip osteoarthritis (Kim et al., 2015). Moreover, adequate levels of physical activity do not negatively impact medical imaging findings over time (e.g., progression of osteoarthritis (Jayabalan et al., 2019)). As such, when pain persists after tissues have healed, tissue (over)protection is no longer necessary and it is safe to move. In this context, avoidance behaviour becomes *unhelpful or maladaptive* and it can lead to the persistence of pain-related disability (Hodges & Smeets, 2015; Vlaeyen, Crombez, & Linton, 2016).

Fear and avoidance behaviour typically *generalize* to other tasks (Meulders, 2018; Sharpe et al., 2022; Vandael et al., 2023). For example, when a person experiences acute LBP after lifting an object with a bent back, it is adaptive that they initially avoid similar activities that may lead to re-injury or bodily damage, even when they have never been paired with pain (Meulders, 2018). This generalization is adaptive because it enables individuals to extrapolate predictions about the initial painful activity to other movements without the necessity to learn anew and experience pain again (Meulders, 2018). However, in people with chronic musculoskeletal pain, *overgeneralization* is often present (Vandael et al., 2023). This means that people will also fear and avoid a broad range of activities that are safe to perform, thereby increasing the disruption of daily life and the perceived disability.

To illustrate this, we present the case of Anne (Box 1).

Safety Behaviours

People with chronic musculoskeletal pain often do not completely avoid feared activities, but they use safety behaviours to complete a task (De Baets et al., 2023). Via safety behaviours, people

BOX 3.1 CASE STUDY

Two years ago, Anne experienced a sharp pain in her lower back while lifting her two-year-old child from the floor. Each time she attempted the same movement, she felt the same sharp pain. This led Anne to become fearful of lifting her child, as she believed the pain signalled a serious underlying problem in her back. She began to avoid this activity, primarily because she thought it would prevent worsening the perceived injury. Now, two years later, Anne continues to avoid lifting her child whenever possible. Moreover, she has also started avoiding a range of other activities, such as lifting groceries, gardening and manipulating loads in general—even without bending her back. As a result, Anne feels increasingly limited in her daily life activities and had to give up one of her hobbies (gardening).

aim to minimize the possibility that the feared outcome will occur (Sharpe et al., 2022). For example, when Anne lifts her child, she only does this with bent knees, a straight back and bracing of her back and abdominal muscles, as she believes this will prevent her spine from buckling (see Box 2 for more examples of safety behaviours). Especially, when overprotective behaviour generalizes to multiple contexts and activities—and becomes a stereotypical movement pattern—it will inappropriately load the musculoskeletal system (Falla et al., 2014). In turn, this can lead to peripheral tissue sensitization and persistent pain (Hoegh, 2022), which is likely to reinforce the unhelpful beliefs of the person and the persistence of avoidance behaviour (Bunzli et al., 2017; Darlow et al., 2025).

In Anne's case, the overprotective behaviour was consistently present during various daily life activities. For example, she consciously attempted to keep her back straight during sitting and bicycle rides, with overactivity of her lumbar extensor muscles. As such, even during low load activities, prolonged overactivity of the trunk muscle was present, leading to excessive compression on the spinal structures. The fact that even low load activities became painful over time convinced Anne that something had to be wrong with her lower back.

Safety behaviours should be interpreted in their context (Sharpe et al., 2022). In some cases, subtle safety behaviours may enable a person to remain engaged in valued life activities. For example, when a person has developed chronic ankle instability after multiple inversion traumas, it makes sense for this person to wear a brace during basketball games. Otherwise, there would be a high chance of a new inversion trauma with potentially serious consequences. In contrast, when a person only wants to walk outside the house with an ankle brace after recovering from an inversion trauma, such safety behaviour would be unhelpful.

BOX 3.2 EXAMPLES OF SAFETY BEHAVIOURS

A person with low back pain may only lift light weights with a straight back as they think this will prevent the disc from popping out.

A person with knee pain may only run with a knee brace as they are convinced this will prevent twisting the knee.

A person with shoulder pain may only travel by public transport when they are able to sit down, as standing up and holding on to a rail may cause severe pain in case of sudden or unexpected perturbations.

A patient may only be willing to perform exercises in the presence of a therapist, as they are convinced that without supervision, they will do something wrong and risk further harm to the painful area.

Safety Behaviour as Barriers to Effective Self-Management

The unjudicial and consistent use of safety behaviours may thus become a barrier to self-management for various reasons. First, a key aspect of self-management is about learning to cope in an independent and flexible manner (Hutting, 2025; Hutting et al., 2019; Kongsted et al., 2021). Safety behaviours can lock someone into rigid routines. For example, people may be convinced they can only engage in activities when they are able to control situations. A person may only be willing to go out for dinner when they are sure they can sit on a chair with a back rest. Second, safety behaviours maintain the individual's unhelpful beliefs by preventing them from being disconfirmed (Lovibond et al., 2009; Meulders, 2020). For example, when a person never goes out without an ankle brace, this will prevent them from experiencing and learning that it is safe to walk without the brace and that they will not sprain their ankle again. As a consequence, fear and avoidance behaviour will persist. Third, safety behaviours may reinforce fear as the behaviour itself can be a source of information, i.e., 'I avoid so it must be dangerous' (Gangemi, Mancini, & van den Hout, 2012). Finally, generalized safety behaviours can contribute to the persistence of pain by inappropriately loading the musculoskeletal system (Hodges & Smeets, 2015).

In sum, identifying safety behaviours during the patient interview and clinical examination, and addressing them during treatment is a first crucial step for effective self-management. The goal for effective long-term self-management is learning people with chronic musculoskeletal pain to recognize these safety behaviours during daily life activities and equipping people with the tools to adequately tackle them.

Motivational and Contextual Factors

Behaviour is strongly determined by a person's priorities and their motivation to achieve certain goals or to remain engaged in meaningful activities (Van Damme & Kindermans, 2015; Van Damme et al., 2012). A person may therefore persist in performing valued activities – despite experiencing pain – while avoiding other activities that are perceived as less important (De Baets et al., 2023). For example, Anne continues to lift her child regularly despite the pain, as caring for her child is a key priority in her life—one she considers more important than the discomfort it may cause in her lower back. In contrast, she has completely stopped weeding her garden. Although she dislikes the appearance of an untidy garden, this concern does not outweigh the pain she experiences during and after the activity. Therefore, it is essential to explore patients' priorities and motivational drivers to gain a clear understanding of their avoidance behaviour, as this will be essential to guide choices during self-management (De Baets et al., 2023).

The Acquisition of Fear of Movement

Fear of movement can be acquired via direct experience, instructional learning, observational learning or a combination of the previous (Meulders, 2018, 2020). We will consider the case of Anne to explain *direct experience*. Lifting her child was initially a neutral activity—one that she had performed numerous times before. At a certain moment, she experienced a sharp pain during this activity. When she later attempted to perform the same movement again, the pain reoccurred. As a result, Anne began to associate lifting her child with pain and started avoiding this activity, believing it to be harmful to her back. Whereas lifting was once a neutral activity, it had now become a conditioned stimulus, eliciting a conditioned response—namely, avoidance behaviour, which is a typical response to (anticipated) pain. Fear of movement can also be acquired via *instructional learning*, i.e., via written or verbal instructions, or information from various sources, such as (social) media, significant others or healthcare providers themselves. For example, when healthcare providers hold negative beliefs about chronic musculoskeletal pain, they may inadvertently transmit these beliefs to their patients. In *observational learning*, people learn pain-related behaviours—such as avoidance—by observing others engaging in these behaviours when confronted with pain.

It is important to recognize that many learning processes occur unconsciously, so people may be unaware of them. Therefore, discussing with the patient how fear can be acquired can provide them with greater insight into their problem, thereby facilitating the identification and management of certain barriers to effective self-management. For example, the patient's thoughts, emotions, and behaviours during a pain flare can be addressed, since increased pain (i.e., direct experience) may be a strong trigger for some individuals to relapse into prolonged avoidance behaviour. Increasing awareness may enable individuals to more readily recognize such a relapse into this unhelpful behaviour and manage it independently. Another example is to explore the cognitions and the role of a partner, as they may suggest that performing certain activities might not be advisable, thereby reinforcing fear of movement and avoidance behaviour instead of facilitating recovery.

Fear of Movement as a Mediator for Long-Term Treatment Success

Fear of movement is an important mediator to reduce pain-related disability after rehabilitation programmes for chronic musculoskeletal pain (Cashin et al., 2023; Lawford et al., 2023; Mansell et al., 2017; Murillo et al., 2022, 2023; Wood et al., 2023). This means that improvements in disability after rehabilitation programmes are partially caused by reductions in fear of movement. Although the mediating role of fear of movement in pain reduction after rehabilitation is less clear in the short term (Cashin et al., 2023; Holden et al., 2021; Lawford et al., 2023), it does seem to impact long-term treatment effects. In persons with chronic musculoskeletal pain who achieved clinically relevant reductions in pain intensity after a multidisciplinary rehabilitation programme, those with elevated levels of fear of movement at the end of the rehabilitation programme largely failed to maintain these treatment gains after one year follow-up (Moore et al., 2016). This shows that addressing fear of movement and avoidance behaviour—when present—is crucial for long-term treatment success.

MANAGING FEAR OF MOVEMENT AND AVOIDANCE BEHAVIOUR: EXPOSURE THERAPY IN VIVO

Exposure therapy in vivo is considered as the treatment of choice to tackle fear of movement and avoidance behaviour (den Hollander et al., 2022). The primary aim of EXP is to extinguish avoidance behaviour, so the patient is able to re-engage in their valued life activities. An important aspect for the patient to understand is that the focus is not on pain reduction, although this may eventually be achieved (e.g., by reducing stereotypical safety behaviours) (den Hollander et al., 2022).

During exposure therapy *in vivo*, patients are exposed to the feared activities, so they can experience and learn that the anticipated adverse consequences do not occur. For example, the intervertebral disc will not rupture when the spine is flexed. By repeatedly experiencing that their expectations are not fulfilled (i.e., *expectancy violation*) (Craske et al., 2014), patients can learn that the initially feared and avoided movements are safe to perform. It is important to note that the original associations (e.g., "bending is harmful") are not erased from memory. Instead, the aim is for the new associations (e.g., "bending is safe") to become stronger than the old ones, so that upon confrontation with the originally feared situation, the patient will engage in the new behaviour rather than the old avoidance pattern (Craske et al., 2014).

Patient Selection for Exposure Therapy in Vivo

Before initiating treatment, it is essential to determine whether the patient is a suitable candidate for exposure therapy *in vivo* (den Hollander et al., 2022). Important aspects to consider are: Fear of movement and avoidance behaviour should contribute to the person's pain-related disability; it should be physically safe for the patient to perform the feared movements; and patients must be

TABLE 3.1
Reasons Why People Fear and Avoid Physical Activities

Reasons	Explanation	Examples
Fear for pain	Fear that pain will increase during or after performing the task, which will lead to increased suffering.	Pain increase itself; emotions that may be triggered by pain increase
Fear for functional loss	Fear that a pain flare will negatively affect their ability to perform valuable tasks.	Not being able to go to work the day after; having to lie down afterwards; it will disrupt my whole week.
Fear for harm	Fear that activities may cause (further) damage to the painful body-part.	The intervertebral disc that might rupture; twisting the knee; rupturing a tendon after a tendon-repair

willing to participate in treatment, as confrontation with feared situations may be unpleasant and trigger (strong) emotional responses.

Understanding the patients' beliefs is crucial: which activities are avoided, what is the influence of contextual factors and what does the patient think will happen if they would perform the feared activity (De Baets et al., 2023)? People with chronic musculoskeletal pain fear and avoid physical activity (including exercises) for three main reasons: Fear for pain, fear for harm, fear for functional loss, or a combination of the previous (see Table 3.1) (Bunzli et al., 2015). Exposure therapy *in vivo* is typically used for patients who associate activities with harmful consequences because it should be possible to create an expectancy violation during exposure therapy *in vivo* (Craske et al., 2014). This may be more difficult to achieve in patients who fear pain itself (without fearing harm). Performing the feared movement without safety behaviours may be painful, and potentially more so than with safety behaviours. As a result, the patient's expectation—that the activity will be painful—will be confirmed rather than disproven, thereby preventing expectancy violation, and potentially strengthening the avoidance behaviour.

Contextual Factors Matter

Analogous to acquisition, the extinction of fear and avoidance behaviour is also context-specific (Vervliet, Craske, & Hermans, 2013). This specificity may be related to various aspects, such as movement characteristics of the activity itself (e.g., execution speed) or the environment (e.g., workplace vs. supervised treatment sessions) (Meulders, 2020). A (partial) generalization of the treatment effect can occur to activities that are similar to those to which the individual was exposed during exposure. As a rule, this generalization decreases as similarity decreases (Meulders, 2020). This implies that fear and avoidance behaviour may re-emerge when individuals are confronted with the initially feared activity in a new context (i.e., context renewal). For example, when a person has learned that lifting with a bent back is safe and they do not avoid it anymore, they may still be reluctant to perform the same activity with a bent and rotated back. This is essential for self-management, since it is impossible to expose patients to all relevant activities across all contexts. As such, we will need to provide home exercises to teach patients with chronic musculoskeletal pain the necessary skills to cope with these new situations independently.

Exposure *In Vivo* and Barriers to Self-Management

Exposing patients to feared activities holds various barriers to self-management. The focus is placed on improving functioning and disability rather than on reducing pain itself, which may not always align with the patient's expectations or preferences. In addition, exposure is not necessarily what patients anticipate from treatment, and it can be experienced as unpleasant or emotionally challenging, especially during initial treatment. Moreover, during behavioural experiments, exposure may temporarily increase pain, which can further complicate patients' engagement in the process. Discussing these aspects with patients and providing sufficient support to guide them through this process is fundamental, in particular when people are reluctant to this behaviour change.

FEAR OF MOVEMENT AND AVOIDANCE BEHAVIOUR AS BARRIERS TO EFFECTIVE SELF MANAGEMENT

In the previous section, we have already highlighted how fear of movement and avoidance behaviour can be barriers to effective self-management. A particular challenge for long-term self-management is that fear of movement and avoidance behaviour can re-occur, even after initial successful treatment (Gatzounis, den Hollander, & Meulders, 2021; Meulders, 2020). Besides context renewal, the regular pain relapses and pain-flares that are typical for chronic musculoskeletal pain deserve consideration. These new pain episodes may reinforce patient beliefs that something is wrong with their body or that they suffered a re-injury, which in turn may result in overprotective behaviour (Bunzli et al., 2015). This may happen when patients relate their new pain episode to the original painful and feared activity (re-acquisition), but also when such relationships are not present—for example, when patients cannot recall a specific reason for the new pain episode (reinstatement) (Meulders, 2018, 2020). Patients need to understand that these new pain episodes are common, are typically not a sign of re-injury in absence of a trauma, and will often resolve with the right approach.

Given the frequent pain flares and pain recurrences in chronic musculoskeletal pain (da Silva et al., 2019; Hsu et al., 2025; Kongsted et al., 2016; Suri et al., 2025; Thomas, Guillemin, & Neogi, 2022) and the continuous confrontation with new contexts, long-term self-management involves an ongoing process of learning and maintaining resilience despite setbacks and obstacles. Equipping patients to adequately deal with these setbacks and to overcome these obstacles is paramount for successful long-term self-management of chronic musculoskeletal pain.

Kongsted et al. (2021) provide a clinical framework to self-management for musculoskeletal pain. They identified three clinical processes of self-management (i.e., planning, delivery and evaluation), each consisting of multiple self-management components. For each of these components, we have mapped the main reasons why and how fear of movement and avoidance behaviour can be barriers to effective self-management (Table 3.2).

CLINICAL CASE STUDY

This case study illustrates how fear of movement can manifest in complex ways and how clinicians can assess and address it to support self-management. Key clinical actions related to treatment planning, delivery and evaluation are described to provide guidance to support effective self-management in persons with chronic musculoskeletal pain by focusing on fear of movement and avoidance behaviours as barriers for self-management.

CASE INTRODUCTION

Case History

Two years ago, Mr. B. (a 48-year-old office worker) presented with chronic pain in the left interscapular and shoulder region at the multidisciplinary pain centre. His first pain episode had occurred four years earlier. During this initial episode of shoulder pain, he visited a physiotherapist, who prescribed exercises to strengthen his shoulder and scapular muscles. Since these exercises aggravated the pain, he stopped doing them as he feared to damage his shoulder and he consulted a shoulder specialist. Mr. B. underwent medical imaging, but the scan revealed no findings that could explain his symptoms. Although the pain initially decreased when he became very protective and avoided using his arm to carry loads or move it overhead, he experienced several relapses following the first episode.

TABLE 3.2
Fear of Movement and Avoidance Behaviour as Barriers to Different Components of Self-Management

Clinical Process	Self-management Component	Fear of Movement and Avoidance Behaviour as Barriers
Planning	Management based on valued goals by patient	Pain reduction is often an important treatment goal of patients. However, pain reduction is not a primary treatment aim of exposure therapy *in vivo*, and pain may temporarily increase when people perform feared activities without safety behaviours.
	Shared decision-making about treatment plan	Exposure therapy *in vivo* is often not what people with chronic musculoskeletal pain expect to be offered during rehabilitation. People may also be unwilling to be exposed to feared and avoided activities, or they may be reluctant to re-engage in activities after a pain relapse or pain flare.
	Identify readiness to change	Avoidance behaviour may be rooted in strong personal convictions that may have been reinforced by other health care providers. Resistance to behaviour change can be strong, as people may be reluctant to perform feared activities.
Delivery	Making sense of problem	People may hold strong biomedical beliefs about chronic musculoskeletal pain, where they are convinced that their pain is a sign of damaged tissues that need protection.
	Skill teaching to solve daily life problems	Extinction of fear of movement and avoidance behaviour is context-specific. When people are confronted with the feared activity in a new context, fear and avoidance behaviour may reoccur (context-renewal). People need to be confident enough and be taught the skills to learn how to engage in feared activities in daily life contexts that have not been practiced during supervised treatment.
	Help patients experience success	People with chronic musculoskeletal pain often experience relapses or pain-flares, which are potent triggers for reoccurrence of fear of movement and avoidance behaviour. This may occur when pain recurs during the initially feared/painful task (re-acquisition) or when the pain re-emerges in the absence of a discernible trigger (reinstatement). Pain relapses and pain-flares may be experienced by patients as failure of the ability to self-manage their problem.
	Provide tools for symptom management (including emotions)	Engaging in feared activities may temporarily increase pain and may also provoke strong emotional responses.
Evaluation	Evaluate and discuss achievement and adjustment of treatment goals	When patients remain too focused on pain relief—which may not be able to achieve initially—it may seem that little improvement has been made. Patients may refuse progression even when objectively capable, fearing that "pushing it" will cause harm. Improvements made in the clinic may not generalize to daily life if fear prevents practicing in varied contexts, undermining the usefulness of goal adjustments.
	Evaluate patients' understanding of their problem	Even when patients have a correct understanding of their problem, their new views may be challenged over time by various factors (e.g., pain relapse or pain flares, information from significant others or other healthcare providers).
	Help patients in action planning	Reoccurrence of fear and avoidance behaviour can hamper the planning of people with chronic musculoskeletal pain to re-engage in valued life activities after a relapse or pain-flare, or to continue with these activities during such episodes.

This gradually evolved into rather continuous pain (rated 4/10) with frequent pain flares (6–7/10) over the following years. In the year before he visited the multidisciplinary pain centre, his pain had become continuous, rated 6–7/10 on a visual analogue scale for pain, and was described during the interview as both annoying and exhausting, leading to decreased function and reduced quality of life.

His primary therapeutic goal was to regain control over his life, which he defined as participating in activities with reduced pain and less exhaustion. He completed the multidisciplinary pain rehabilitation programme, which lasted six weeks (without any structured follow-up sessions or booster sessions) and included educational sessions, as well as modules on relaxation and mindfulness techniques. At the time, these modules were emphasized—rather than cognitive-behavioural approaches such as exposure *in vivo* therapy—because of his poor body awareness and maladaptive stress-coping strategies, which were considered key mechanisms underlying his chronic pain. At the end of the programme, Mr. B. reported that applying these techniques had been beneficial, leading to reduced pain interference in daily life, less exhaustion, and an enhanced quality of life. He also specifically emphasized that the techniques he had learned were life-changing and that he intended to continue practicing them in the future.

Current Situation

Currently—12 months after completing the multidisciplinary pain rehabilitation program—Mr. B. re-contacted the multidisciplinary pain centre. Over the past year, his pain had worsened, accompanied by avoidance of valued activities, not only due to severe pain-related fear but also due to a clear fear of damaging his shoulder (snapping his rotator cuff tendons), along with general exhaustion.

The interview and clinical examination revealed that he had continuously applied mindfulness techniques as part of his self-management strategy since the end of the multidisciplinary pain rehabilitation programme. However, from the interview and clinical examination, it emerged that Mr. B. had developed a rigid pattern of hyper-control over his body and environment, instead of cultivating present-moment awareness and acceptance. His "mindfulness" practice had become a mechanism for constant monitoring and avoidance of movements and activities. For example, although Mr. B. remained socially and professionally active, he relied on numerous safety behaviours.

These included bringing his own ergonomic chair to both work and social events, and continuously monitoring his posture—particularly the position of his left shoulder—to avoid potential harm if the arm were touched or moved by others. He also avoided shared transportation, where he could not control the driving, and modified his home environment to maintain postural and movement control. For instance, he had installed small steps throughout the house to avoid reaching beyond 60° of anteflexion when retrieving items from for example overhead kitchen cabinets. He described anteflexion until 60° as his 'safe arc of movement'. Mr. B. further reported avoiding crowded places to minimize the risk of unexpected movements. He would only attend the theatre if he knew the seating plan in advance and could sit with his wife on his left side to protect his arm. When traveling, he brought his own mattress and portable recliner, and cancelled trips if this was not possible. He also avoided spontaneous outings with colleagues due to their unpredictability, such as not knowing what type of chairs would be available at a bar.

Interestingly, Mr. B. mentioned he did not understand why his symptoms continued to get worse, as he was able to almost fully plan and control his environment. While Mr. B.'s narrative revealed a high degree of vigilance and control over his physical environment, he explicitly described this sense of control—particularly around planning and organizing his activities—as the key reason he believed he was successfully applying mindfulness in his daily life.

Case Interpretation

This misapplication of mindfulness—whose key aim is to cultivate present-moment awareness with an attitude of openness, curiosity, and acceptance—illustrates how self-management efforts, when not well planned, delivered, or evaluated, can inadvertently lead to maladaptive patterns, as seen in Mr. B.'s case, such as the need to control by applying rigid safety behaviours. These, in turn, may lead to sustained physical and mental arousal and increased psychological stress as well as inappropriate loading of the musculoskeletal system, triggering the sensitivity of the nociceptive system and contributing to the persistence of pain.

Mr. B.'s case exemplifies how fear of movement—as based on fear for pain and fear for harm—can result in strong avoidance behaviour, which in turn was reinforced by a perceived sense of safety by applying avoidance behaviours. His strategy of "mindful control" had become maladaptive, leading to increased disability and emotional distress. His hypervigilance and need for control were both cognitive and behavioural, maintained by internal (e.g., anxiety, attentional bias) and external (e.g., environmental unpredictability) factors. Although he continued to use relaxation techniques, these were insufficient to counteract the heightened arousal triggered by his need for control.

FEAR OF MOVEMENT AND AVOIDANCE BEHAVIOURS AS BARRIERS TO EFFECTIVE SELF-MANAGEMENT

In Mr. B.'s case, fear of movement and the resulting avoidance behaviours acted as central barriers to effective self-management following his participation in a multidisciplinary pain rehabilitation program. According to Kongsted et al. (2021), effective self-management requires attention to specific clinical processes during planning, delivery, and evaluation (see Table 3.2).

A critical omission occurred during the *planning phase* of Mr. B.'s programme. Although the multidisciplinary pain rehabilitation programme was tailored to his value-based goals through shared decision-making, his readiness to change was insufficiently addressed. In particular, his psychological flexibility—the ability to tolerate uncertainty, let go of excessive control, and adapt behaviour—was not explored. These factors are essential for behavioural change and for the integration of mindfulness and relaxation practices into daily life. As a result, Mr. B. developed a rigid, hyper-controlling approach toward his body and environment, reinforcing avoidance behaviours driven by fear of pain and harm. He misinterpreted this rigid control as successful mindfulness practice.

Furthermore, his beliefs about pain and movement while in pain were not investigated sufficiently during the *planning phase*, leaving maladaptive interpretations unchallenged. During the *delivery phase*, Mr. B. received appropriate structured education on pain mechanisms and participated in relaxation and mindfulness modules, designed to enhance his body awareness and improve his stress-coping strategies. He engaged actively and consistently applied the techniques throughout the six-week program. His initial improvements during the programme in pain interference, exhaustion, and quality of life confirmed the short-term relevance of the strategies provided.

However, in the *evaluation phase*, essential clinical processes were missing. Effective evaluation should include re-assessment of goals, the creation of a clear action plan for ongoing self-management, and exploration of the patient's evolving understanding of pain. None of these were sufficiently conducted. There was no structured re-evaluation of goals or behaviours, nor was a post-programme action plan established. Therefore, his interpretation of mindfulness as a tool for control, and his belief that pain could be avoided through rigid movement strategies (e.g., avoiding shoulder elevation above 60°), went unaddressed as these maladaptive patterns could not be detected and corrected. The absence of structured evaluation and ongoing support significantly contributed to the deterioration of his self-management. Regular check-ins would have enabled early identification of maladaptive patterns, reassessment of beliefs about pain and movement, and timely revision of goals and strategies. By missing these opportunities, the programme allowed rigid avoidance behaviours to persist and intensify, ultimately undermining the long-term effectiveness of the intervention.

NEW CARE PLAN FOR MR. B. TO ALLOW FOR EFFECTIVE SELF-MANAGEMENT

A new care plan was developed based on Mr. B.'s current understanding of pain and the beliefs underlying his behaviours. During the intake interview, the activities he avoided, the contextual factors influencing these behaviours, and his expectations of what might happen if he performed the feared activities were explored in depth. In this *planning phase*, his willingness to change his control strategies was also confirmed. Together with the therapist, several treatment priorities were agreed upon, all directed toward his overarching goal of re-engaging in valued activities with less exhaustion and pain. These priorities included pain education, exposure *in vivo* therapy, and the reframing of mindfulness practices. The aims of each part of the intervention were clearly explained to align with Mr. B.'s expectations.

PAIN EDUCATION

The pain education component focused on deepening his understanding of the relationship between his fear of pain, fear of harm, and the use of safety behaviours. It also addressed the short-term advantages and long-term disadvantages of such behaviours. Pain neuroscience education helped him to reframe his beliefs about preferred postures, movement avoidance, and the perceived vulnerability of his shoulder. A key message was that pain does not necessarily signal damage and that movement—even when uncomfortable—is safe. In addition, the disadvantages of hyper-control strategies for appropriate stress regulation were emphasized.

EXPOSURE THERAPY *IN VIVO*

Exposure *in vivo* therapy was integrated to extinguish Mr. B.'s avoidance behaviours, which included limiting shoulder elevation to 60° of anteflexion, keeping his left arm in a controlled position, bringing his own chair to control seating, avoiding being a passenger, and avoiding crowded places to minimize unexpected arm movements. Together with the therapist, a hierarchy of feared movements and situations was developed. Exposures to feared situations were conducted in random order to reduce predictability, and each exposure was paired with guided reflection in order to consolidate learning. During reflection, people are encouraged to consciously think and speak about what they did and what happened (or did not happen). Mr. B. learned that while performing the feared activities, the anticipated harm (e.g., tendon snapping) did not occur, thus violating his expectations. This provided strong opportunities to learn that the feared activities were safe to perform. At the same time, he experienced small temporary increases in pain, as explained during the education sessions, which reinforced the notion that discomfort did not mean damage.

To further support the exposure therapy, mindfulness practices were reframed. Mr. B. came to understand that mindfulness is not about control but about awareness and acceptance. It was emphasized to approach the observed painful sensations during exposure without judgment, allowing for discomfort to be present without reacting with avoidance or new control strategies. This shift from a control-based to an acceptance-based approach enhanced both the effectiveness of the exposure *in vivo* therapy and his adherence to it, including during home practice. At home, Mr. B. practised exposure independently with previously feared movements such as overhead reaching, sitting without controlling his arm position, and being a passenger while his wife drove. These exercises helped him to overcome fear of pain and movement and enabled him to re-engage in daily activities without reliance on safety behaviours.

To ensure proper *evaluation* and to strengthen self-management, Mr. B. kept a daily log and a "success journal" in which he recorded positive experiences, reinforcing competence and progress. His understanding of pain and movement with pain was re-evaluated regularly during exposure and mindfulness sessions. Following the eight-week programme, regular follow-up sessions were scheduled to review progress, provide space for dialogue and reflection, and adjust strategies if necessary. Relapse prevention strategies were also addressed by identifying personal triggers. In Mr. B.'s case, this involved an increased sense of responsibility for certain work tasks.

Therapy was concluded six months after the new care plan was initiated. Mr. B. was able to engage in previously avoided activities, which significantly improved his quality of life. Especially, the shift from the need for control to acceptance resulted in a reduction of exhaustion, as he did not feel the need any more to consistently focus on his arm, and he was able to relax and enjoy social activities again. He mentioned that the regular follow-up after the exposure programme was very helpful to support his self-management, as many barriers and triggers for relapse were present, such as pain flares or having to engage in activities that could not be practised under supervision (e.g., going to the theatre). Currently, pain-levels are mild (2/10) and pain-flares are far less common. Although long-term self-management was encouraged, Mr. B. was given the message that he could contact the pain centre in case of questions, uncertainties or clear changes in symptoms.

CONCLUSIONS

Persons with musculoskeletal pain often hold unhelpful beliefs about physical activity or lack the confidence to stay active while in pain, which can pose significant barriers to effective self-management. Especially, when persons fear that physical activity might lead to negative outcomes, they may choose to avoid it altogether. While fear of movement and avoidance behaviour have been identified as primary barriers to effective self-management in people with chronic musculoskeletal pain, it is also highly complex and strongly influenced by contextual factors. Understanding fear of movement and avoidance behaviour from an individual's perspective, and how it interferes with effective self-management, requires careful consideration of all potential contributing factors.

REFERENCES

Barlow, J., Wright, C., Sheasby, J., Turner, A., & Hainsworth, J. (2002). Self-management approaches for people with chronic conditions: A review. *Patient Educ Couns*, *48*(2), 177–187. https://doi.org/10.1016/s0738-3991(02)00032-0

Brinjikji, W., Luetmer, P. H., Comstock, B., Bresnahan, B. W., Chen, L. E., Deyo, R. A., Halabi, S., Turner, J. A., Avins, A. L., James, K., Wald, J. T., Kallmes, D. F., & Jarvik, J. G. (2015). Systematic literature review of imaging features of spinal degeneration in asymptomatic populations. *AJNR Am J Neuroradiol*, *36*(4), 811–816. https://doi.org/10.3174/ajnr.A4173

Bunzli, S., Smith, A., Schütze, R., Lin, I., & O'Sullivan, P. (2017). Making sense of low back pain and pain-related fear. *J Orthop Sports Phys Ther*, *47*(9), 628–636. https://doi.org/10.2519/jospt.2017.7434

Bunzli, S., Smith, A., Watkins, R., Schutze, R., & O'Sullivan, P. (2015). What do people who score highly on the Tampa Scale of Kinesiophobia really believe? *Pain*, *31*(7), 621–632. https://doi.org/10.1097/ajp.0000000000000143

Caneiro, J. P., Bunzli, S., & O'Sullivan, P. (2021). Beliefs about the body and pain: The critical role in musculoskeletal pain management. *Braz J Phys Ther*, *25*(1), 17–29. https://doi.org/10.1016/j.bjpt.2020.06.003

Cashin, A. G., Lee, H., Wand, B. M., Bagg, M. K., O'Hagan, E. T., Rizzo, R. R. N., Stanton, T. R., Moseley, G. L., & McAuley, J. H. (2023). Mechanisms of education and graded sensorimotor retraining in people with chronic low back pain: A mediation analysis. *Pain*, *164*(12), 2792–2800. https://doi.org/10.1097/j.pain.0000000000002978

Craske, M. G., Treanor, M., Conway, C. C., Zbozinek, T., & Vervliet, B. (2014). Maximizing exposure therapy: An inhibitory learning approach. *Behav Res Ther*, *58*, 10–23. https://doi.org/10.1016/j.brat.2014.04.006

Culvenor, A. G., Øiestad, B. E., Hart, H. F., Stefanik, J. J., Guermazi, A., & Crossley, K. M. (2019). Prevalence of knee osteoarthritis features on magnetic resonance imaging in asymptomatic uninjured adults: A systematic review and meta-analysis. *Br J Sports Med*, *53*(20), 1268–1278. https://doi.org/10.1136/bjsports-2018-099257

Darlow, B., Belton, J., Brown, M., Clark, J., Richards, D. P., Simick Behera, N., & Bunzli, S. (2025). Making sense of osteoarthritis: A narrative review. *Osteoarthr Cartil*, *33*(1), 17–26. https://doi.org/10.1016/j.joca.2024.09.012

da Silva, T., Mills, K., Brown, B. T., Pocovi, N., de Campos, T., Maher, C., & Hancock, M. J. (2019). Recurrence of low back pain is common: A prospective inception cohort study. *J Physiother*, *65*(3), 159–165. https://doi.org/10.1016/j.jphys.2019.04.010

De Baets, L., Meulders, A., Van Damme, S., Caneiro, J. P., & Matheve, T. (2023). Understanding discrepancies in a person's fear of movement and avoidance behaviour: A guide for musculoskeletal rehabilitation clinicians who support people with chronic musculoskeletal pain. *J Orthop Sports Phys Ther*, 1–29. https://doi.org/10.2519/jospt.2023.11420

den Hollander, M., Smeets, R., van Meulenbroek, T., van Laake-Geelen, C. C. M., Baadjou, V. A., & Timmers, I. (2022). Exposure in vivo as a treatment approach to target pain-related fear: Theory and new insights from research and clinical practice. *Phys Ther*, *102*(2). https://doi.org/10.1093/ptj/pzab270

Diener, I. (2021). Physiotherapy support for self-management of persisting musculoskeletal pain disorders. *S Afr J Physiother*, *77*(1), 1564. https://doi.org/10.4102/sajp.v77i1.1564

Dunn, M., Rushton, A. B., Mistry, J., Soundy, A., & Heneghan, N. R. (2024). The biopsychosocial factors associated with development of chronic musculoskeletal pain. An umbrella review and meta-analysis of observational systematic reviews. *PLoS One*, *19*(4), e0294830. https://doi.org/10.1371/journal.pone.0294830

Elbers, S., Wittink, H., Pool, J. J. M., & Smeets, R. (2018). The effectiveness of generic self-management interventions for patients with chronic musculoskeletal pain on physical function, self-efficacy, pain intensity and physical activity: A systematic review and meta-analysis. *Eur J Pain*, *22*(9), 1577–1596. https://doi.org/10.1002/ejp.1253

Falla, D., Gizzi, L., Tschapek, M., Erlenwein, J., & Petzke, F. (2014). Reduced task-induced variations in the distribution of activity across back muscle regions in individuals with low back pain. *Pain*, *155*(5), 944–953. https://doi.org/10.1016/j.pain.2014.01.027

Farrell, S. F., Smith, A. D., Hancock, M. J., Webb, A. L., & Sterling, M. (2019). Cervical spine findings on MRI in people with neck pain compared with pain-free controls: A systematic review and meta-analysis. *J Magn Reson Imaging*, *49*(6), 1638–1654. https://doi.org/10.1002/jmri.26567

Gangemi, A., Mancini, F., & van den Hout, M. (2012). Behavior as information: "If i avoid, then there must be a danger. *J Behav Ther Exp Psychiatry*, *43*(4), 1032–1038. https://doi.org/10.1016/j.jbtep.2012.04.005

Gatzounis, R., den Hollander, M., & Meulders, A. (2021). Optimizing long-term outcomes of exposure for chronic primary pain from the lens of learning theory. *J Pain*, *22*(11), 1315–1327. https://doi.org/10.1016/j.jpain.2021.04.012

Gilanyi, Y. L., Shah, B., Cashin, A. G., Gibbs, M. T., Bellamy, J., Day, R., McAuley, J. H., & Jones, M. D. (2024). Barriers and enablers to exercise adherence in people with nonspecific chronic low back pain: A systematic review of qualitative evidence. *Pain*, *165*(10), 2200–2214. https://doi.org/10.1097/j.pain.0000000000003234

Grande, G. H. D., Vidal, R. V. C., Salini, M. C. R., Christofaro, D. G. D., & Oliveira, C. B. (2025). Barriers and facilitators to physical activity and exercise among people with chronic low back pain: A qualitative evidence synthesis. *J Orthop Sports Phys Ther*, *55*(5), 312–330. https://doi.org/10.2519/jospt.2025.12905

Grøn, S., Johansson, M., Schiphof, D., Koes, B., & Kongsted, A. (2025). Do self-management supportive interventions reduce healthcare utilization for people with musculoskeletal pain conditions? – A systematic review. *Public Health*, *238*, 152–161. https://doi.org/10.1016/j.puhe.2024.10.021

Hodges, P. W., & Smeets, R. J. (2015). Interaction between pain, movement, and physical activity: Short-term benefits, long-term consequences, and targets for treatment. *Clin J Pain*, *31*(2), 97–107. https://doi.org/10.1097/AJP.0000000000000098

Hoegh, M. (2022). Pain science in practice (Part 3): Peripheral sensitization. *J Orthop Sports Phys Ther*, *52*(6), 303–306. https://doi.org/10.2519/jospt.2022.11202

Holden, S., Matthews, M., Rathleff, M. S., Kasza, J., & Vicenzino, B. (2021). How do hip exercises improve pain in individuals with patellofemoral pain? Secondary mediation analysis of strength and psychological factors as mechanisms. *J Orthop Sports Phys Ther*, *51*(12), 602–610. https://doi.org/10.2519/jospt.2021.10674

Hsu, T. C., Yimer, B. B., Whelan, P., Armitage, C. J., Druce, K., & McBeth, J. (2025). Associations between daily symptoms and pain flares in rheumatoid arthritis: Case-crossover mHealth study. *JMIR Mhealth Uhealth*, *13*, e64889. https://doi.org/10.2196/64889

Hutting, N. (2025). From passive care to self-management support: A new era in manual and musculoskeletal physiotherapy. *Musculoskelet Sci Pract*, *78*, 103370. https://doi.org/10.1016/j.msksp.2025.103370

Hutting, N., Johnston, V., Staal, J. B., & Heerkens, Y. F. (2019). Promoting the use of self-management strategies for people with persistent musculoskeletal disorders: The role of physical therapists. *J Orthop Sports Phys Ther, 49*(4), 212–215. https://doi.org/10.2519/jospt.2019.0605

Jayabalan, P., Kocherginsky, M., Chang, A. H., Rouleau, G. W., Koloms, K. L., Lee, J., Dunlop, D., Chang, R. W., & Sharma, L. (2019). Physical activity and worsening of radiographic findings in persons with or at higher risk of knee osteoarthritis. *Arthritis Care Res (Hoboken), 71*(2), 198–206. https://doi.org/10.1002/acr.23756

Jenkins, H. J., Corrêa, L., Brown, B. T., Ferreira, G. E., Nim, C., Aspinall, S. L., Wareham, D., Choi, J., Maher, C. G., & Hancock, M. J. (2025). Long-term effectiveness of non-surgical interventions for chronic low back pain: A systematic review and meta-analysis. *Lancet Rheumatol, 7*(9), e607–e617. https://doi.org/10.1016/s2665-9913(25)00064-5

Jonkman, N. H., Schuurmans, M. J., Jaarsma, T., Shortridge-Baggett, L. M., Hoes, A. W., & Trappenburg, J. C. (2016). Self-management interventions: Proposal and validation of a new operational definition. *J Clin Epidemiol, 80*, 34–42. https://doi.org/10.1016/j.jclinepi.2016.08.001

Kanavaki, A. M., Rushton, A., Efstathiou, N., Alrushud, A., Klocke, R., Abhishek, A., & Duda, J. L. (2017). Barriers and facilitators of physical activity in knee and hip osteoarthritis: A systematic review of qualitative evidence. *BMJ Open, 7*(12), e017042. https://doi.org/10.1136/bmjopen-2017-017042

Kim, C., Nevitt, M. C., Niu, J., Clancy, M. M., Lane, N. E., Link, T. M., Vlad, S., Tolstykh, I., Jungmann, P. M., Felson, D. T., & Guermazi, A. (2015). Association of hip pain with radiographic evidence of hip osteoarthritis: Diagnostic test study. *BMJ, 351*, h5983. https://doi.org/10.1136/bmj.h5983

Kongsted, A., Kent, P., Axen, I., Downie, A. S., & Dunn, K. M. (2016). What have we learned from ten years of trajectory research in low back pain? *BMC Musculoskelet Disord, 17*, 220. https://doi.org/10.1186/s12891-016-1071-2

Kongsted, A., Ris, I., Kjaer, P., & Hartvigsen, J. (2021). Self-management at the core of back pain care: 10 key points for clinicians. *Braz J Phys Ther, 25*(4), 396–406. https://doi.org/10.1016/j.bjpt.2021.05.002

Lawford, B. J., Hall, M., Hinman, R. S., Van der Esch, M., Harmer, A. R., Spiers, L., Kimp, A., Dell'Isola, A., & Bennell, K. L. (2024). Exercise for osteoarthritis of the knee. *Cochrane Database Syst Rev, 12*(12), Cd004376. https://doi.org/10.1002/14651858.CD004376.pub4

Lawford, B. J., Hinman, R. S., McManus, F., Lamb, K. E., Egerton, T., Keating, C., Brown, C., Oliver, K., & Bennell, K. L. (2023). How does exercise, with and without diet, improve pain and function in knee osteoarthritis? A secondary analysis of a randomized controlled trial exploring potential mediators of effects. *Arthritis Care Res (Hoboken), 75*(11), 2316–2327. https://doi.org/10.1002/acr.25140

Lovibond, P. F., Mitchell, C. J., Minard, E., Brady, A., & Menzies, R. G. (2009). Safety behaviours preserve threat beliefs: Protection from extinction of human fear conditioning by an avoidance response. *Behav Res Ther, 47*(8), 716–720. https://doi.org/10.1016/j.brat.2009.04.013

Mansell, G., Hill, J. C., Main, C. J., Von Korff, M., & van der Windt, D. (2017). Mediators of treatment effect in the back in action trial: Using latent growth modeling to take change over time into account. *Clin J Pain, 33*(9), 811–819. https://doi.org/10.1097/ajp.0000000000000463

Meulders, A. (2018). From fear of movement-related pain and avoidance to chronic pain disability: A state-of-the-art review. *Curr Opin Behav Sci, 26*, 130–136.

Meulders, A. (2020). Fear in the context of pain: Lessons learned from 100 years of fear conditioning research. *Behav Res Ther, 131*, 103635. https://doi.org/10.1016/j.brat.2020.103635

Moore, E., Thibault, P., Adams, H., & Sullivan, M. J. L. (2016). Catastrophizing and pain-related fear predict failure to maintain treatment gains following participation in a pain rehabilitation program. *Pain Rep, 1*(2), e567. https://doi.org/10.1097/pr9.0000000000000567

Murillo, C., Galán-Martín, M., Montero-Cuadrado, F., Lluch, E., Meeus, M., & Loh, W. W. (2023). Reductions in kinesiophobia and distress after pain neuroscience education and exercise lead to favourable outcomes: A secondary mediation analysis of a randomized controlled trial in primary care. *Pain, 164*(10), 2296–2305. https://doi.org/10.1097/j.pain.0000000000002929

Murillo, C., Vo, T. T., Vansteelandt, S., Harrison, L. E., Cagnie, B., Coppieters, I., Chys, M., Timmers, I., & Meeus, M. (2022). How do psychologically based interventions for chronic musculoskeletal pain work? A systematic review and meta-analysis of specific moderators and mediators of treatment. *Clin Psychol Rev, 94*, 102160. https://doi.org/10.1016/j.cpr.2022.102160

Oliveira, V. C., Ferreira, P. H., Maher, C. G., Pinto, R. Z., Refshauge, K. M., & Ferreira, M. L. (2012). Effectiveness of self-management of low back pain: Systematic review with meta-analysis. *Arthritis Care Res (Hoboken), 64*(11), 1739–1748. https://doi.org/10.1002/acr.21737

Palazzo, C., Klinger, E., Dorner, V., Kadri, A., Thierry, O., Boumenir, Y., Martin, W., Poiraudeau, S., & Ville, I. (2016). Barriers to home-based exercise program adherence with chronic low back pain:

Patient expectations regarding new technologies. *Ann Phys Rehabil Med*, *59*(2), 107–113. https://doi.org/10.1016/j.rehab.2016.01.009

Rathnayake, A. P. S., Sparkes, V., & Sheeran, L. (2021). What is the effect of low back pain self-management interventions with exercise components added? A systematic review with meta-analysis. *Musculoskelet Sci Pract*, *56*, 102469. https://doi.org/10.1016/j.msksp.2021.102469

Seven, B., Gökkurt, A., Koç, M., Küpeli, B., & Oskay, D. (2024). Investigation of the barriers to and functional outcomes of telerehabilitation in patients with hand injury. *J Hand Ther*, *37*(3), 378–387. https://doi.org/10.1016/j.jht.2023.10.003

Sharpe, L., Todd, J., Scott, A., Gatzounis, R., Menzies, R. E., & Meulders, A. (2022). Safety behaviours or safety precautions? The role of subtle avoidance in anxiety disorders in the context of chronic physical illness. *Clin Psychol Rev*, *92*, 102126. https://doi.org/10.1016/j.cpr.2022.102126

Suri, P., Korpak, A. M., Timmons, A. K., Tanus, A. D., Brubeck, H. F., Costa, N., Staab, C. A., Hodges, P. W., Daniels, C. J., Heagerty, P. J., & Jensen, M. P. (2025). Convergent validity of a person-dependent definition of a low back pain flare. *Pain*. https://doi.org/10.1097/j.pain.0000000000003703

Thomas, M. J., Guillemin, F., & Neogi, T. (2022). Osteoarthritis flares. *Clin Geriatr Med*, *38*(2), 239–257. https://doi.org/10.1016/j.cger.2021.11.001

Tran, G., Cowling, P., Smith, T., Bury, J., Lucas, A., Barr, A., Kingsbury, S. R., & Conaghan, P. G. (2018). What imaging-detected pathologies are associated with shoulder symptoms and their persistence? A systematic literature review. *Arthritis Care Res (Hoboken)*, *70*(8), 1169–1184. https://doi.org/10.1002/acr.23554

Traweger, A., Scott, A., Kjaer, M., Wezenbeek, E., Scattone Silva, R., Kennedy, J. G., Butler, J. J., Gomez-Florit, M., Gomes, M. E., Snedeker, J. G., Dakin, S. G., & Wildemann, B. (2025). Achilles tendinopathy. *Nat Rev Dis Primers*, *11*(1), 20. https://doi.org/10.1038/s41572-025-00602-9

Vandael, K., Vervliet, B., Peters, M., & Meulders, A. (2023). Excessive generalization of pain-related avoidance behavior: Mechanisms, targets for intervention, and future directions. *Pain*, *164*(11), 2405–2410. https://doi.org/10.1097/j.pain.0000000000002990

Van Damme, S., & Kindermans, H. (2015). A self-regulation perspective on avoidance and persistence behavior in chronic pain: New theories, new challenges. *Clin J Pain*, *31*(2), 115–122. https://doi.org/10.1097/AJP.0000000000000096

Van Damme, S., Van Ryckeghem, D. M. L., Wyffels, F., Van Hulle, L., & Crombez, G. (2012). No pain no gain? Pursuing a competing goal inhibits avoidance behavior. *Pain*, *153*(4), 800–804. https://doi.org/10.1016/j.pain.2011.12.015

Vervliet, B., Craske, M. G., & Hermans, D. (2013). Fear extinction and relapse: State of the art. *Annu Rev Clin Psychol*, *9*, 215–248. https://doi.org/10.1146/annurev-clinpsy-050212-185542

Vlaeyen, J. W., Crombez, G., & Linton, S. J. (2016). The fear-avoidance model of pain. *Pain*, *157*(8), 1588–1589. https://doi.org/10.1097/j.pain.0000000000000574

Vlaeyen, J. W. S., Maher, C. G., Wiech, K., Van Zundert, J., Meloto, C. B., Diatchenko, L., Battie, M. C., Goossens, M., Koes, B., & Linton, S. J. (2018). Low back pain. *Nat Rev Dis Primers*, *4*(1), 52. https://doi.org/10.1038/s41572-018-0052-1

Vos, T. (2017). Global, regional, and national incidence, prevalence, and years lived with disability for 328 diseases and injuries for 195 countries, 1990–2016: A systematic analysis for the Global Burden of Disease Study 2016. *Lancet*, *390*(10100), 1211–1259. https://doi.org/10.1016/s0140-6736(17)32154-2

Wallwork, S. B., Braithwaite, F. A., O'Keeffe, M., Travers, M. J., Summers, S. J., Lange, B., Hince, D. A., Costa, L. O. P., Menezes Costa, L. D. C., Chiera, B., & Moseley, G. L. (2024). The clinical course of acute, subacute and persistent low back pain: A systematic review and meta-analysis. *CMAJ*, *196*(2), E29–E46. https://doi.org/10.1503/cmaj.230542

Wood, L., Bejarano, G., Csiernik, B., Miyamoto, G. C., Mansell, G., Hayden, J. A., Lewis, M., & Cashin, A. G. (2023). Pain catastrophising and kinesiophobia mediate pain and physical function improvements with Pilates exercise in chronic low back pain: A mediation analysis of a randomised controlled trial. *J Physiother*, *69*(3), 168–174. https://doi.org/10.1016/j.jphys.2023.05.008

Wu, Z., Zhou, R., Zhu, Y., Zeng, Z., Ye, Z., Wang, Z., Liu, W., & Xu, X. (2022). Self-management for knee osteoarthritis: A systematic review and meta-analysis of randomized controlled trials. *Pain Res Manag*, *2022*, 2681240. https://doi.org/10.1155/2022/2681240

4 Capabilities for Community Living and Participation for Older Adults with Autism Spectrum Disorder

Elias Mpofu, Michał T. Tomczak, and Ganette Apeadu-Baah

INTRODUCTION

Older adults with autism are pushing for inclusive communities, which is, those communities where they are able to manage themselves based on their capabilities (Pellicano et al., 2022; Robeyns, 2016). Importantly, people with autism (hereafter autistics following identity first preference of the autism community (Cage et al., 2018; Scheeren et al., 2021)), advocate for and prefer a strengths rather than deficit model about their community living, of which they seek to be "accepted or appreciated as an autistic person, with Autism positively recognized and accepted by others and the self as an integral part of that individual" (Cage et al., 2018, p. 424). A strength-based approach aligns with the view that "what ... ability is valued or deemed important in ...autistic ...worlds" validating "autistic peoples' perspective" would contribute to their sense of unique community (Rosqvist, 2019; p. 170) to one's capabilities. Capabilities refer to the skills necessary for people to successfully engage in activities that result in the desired life outcomes (Nussbaum, 2011; Sen, 1985). Essentially, the capabilities that older autistic adults perceive to be within reach in their life situations influence their decisions, self-managing their community living and participation.

Self-managing community living requires initiatives and support for meeting present needs, and for optimizing their future selves. Autism is characterized by "persistent deficits in social communication and social interaction across multiple contexts" and "the presence of restricted, repetitive patterns of behavior, interests or activities" (American Psychiatric Association, 2013, p. 31), and manifest "in varying levels of severity, affecting development throughout the lifespan" (Chapman, 2020, p. 800). However, for older autistic adults, "the disabilities and dependencies that result from aging interact with those resulting from Autism" (Piven et al., 2011, p. 2151), impacting their self-managing everyday living to their best capabilities. The capabilities of older autistic adults for self-managing their life situations remain unexplored, in part due to the overemphasis on deficits portending what they cannot do and denying the older autistic adults their sense of agency. Conceivably, famous individuals across all fields of human endeavor would include countless adult autistics who have either chosen not to speak out about their autism or were unaware of their autism for contributing to autistic narratives of empowerment rather than deficiencies.

This chapter considers the intrinsic capabilities of older autistic adults for their community living and participation. It outlines the role of decisional capabilities of older autistic adults for self-managing life situations by older autistic adults, the interaction between intrinsic capabilities and life situations, with reference to a conceptual model. Moreover, the chapter discusses research and practice guidelines on how older autistic adults utilize their intrinsic capabilities for improved community living and participation with decisional authority. In the next section, we clarify autistic capabilities and community living and participation; to background the life situation demands and self-managing prospects, we consider the rest of this chapter.

 DOI: 10.1201/9781003599074-5

OLDER AUTISTIC ADULTS' COMMUNITY LIVING AND PARTICIPATION

As previously noted, older autistic adults report unmet community living and needs (Elichaoff, 2015). Yet, they would likely have under-utilized intrinsic capacities for self-managing their community participation. The World Health Organization (WHO) International Classification of Functioning, Disability and Health (WHO-ICF, 2001) defined participation as a person's "involvement in life situations" (p. 10) or the realities in people's lives. Participation refers to "being autonomous to some extent or being able to control one's own life, including to fulfill personal goals and societal roles" (Chang et al., 2013, p. 771), premised on intrinsic capacities (inherent personal capabilities: World Health Organization: WHO, 2020). Self-managing life situations depend on leveraging intrinsic capacities to change possibilities into actual actions in everyday living.

Autistic people are the most at risk for exclusion from their community living of all disability groups (Farley et al., 2018), denying them their life situation priorities and the actions for enriching their everyday living. These denials would exacerbate resulting from autism symptoms in the absence of evidence on how best to support them to achieve fulfilling lives (Uddin, 2022). Contrary to stereotypes, older autistic adults tend to be very community-engaged and also seek to help their communities rather than seeking help from community others (Lockwood et al., 2021). Nonetheless, what older autistic adults can do does not necessarily become what they do in their life situations. Yet, much depends on their capabilities for changing life situations to be who they can be with others in their lives.

Preliminary studies suggest that autistics prefer to self-manage their life worlds with decisional authority, their preference for close relationships with a small number of similar others on the spectrum (Chapman, 2019; Davis & Crompton, 2021), social robotics (Schweinberger et al., 2020), and virtual rather than physical community options only (Stendal & Balandin, 2015). Their decisional choices undergird how and what they engage self-managing their life situations for successful community living and participation.

Decisional Choices

A defining quality of autism is the uncertainty of otherwise self-evident intrinsic capacities (what the person can do), translating into performance (what the person does) (see also APA, 2013). This uncertainty in people with autism turning their intrinsic capacities into self-managing actions could diminish their community living and participation from underutilization of the intrinsic capacities (Asher et al., 2020). This is particularly significant, given the fact that older autistic adults report unmet community living needs (Elichaoff, 2015; Farley et al., 2018), which may be compounded by disabilities and dependencies that result from the aging process. Knowing how older autistic adults make decisions for self-managing is requisite for the resources and supports aimed at facilitating their community living and participation (Li & Chapman, 2013).

While older adults are more cautious in their decision making than younger adults (taking time to consider possible options) (Bruine de Bruin et al., 2012), they also have a strong track record in decision making drawing on their greater experience in managing life situations (Peters et al., 2007). For that reason, we would expect older autistic adults to make effective life situation decisions based on past experiences to provide appropriate guidance for their self-management. They also utilize their decision-making capabilities effectively about issues with which they had a higher emotional (affect) investment (Fujino et al., 2020). This suggests that emotion or affect acts as a prism for self-managing actions or choices, predisposing some pieces of information over competing others (Kahneman, 2011). There is evidence to suggest that, contrary to stereotyping autistics as having bland affect, affect regulation by older autistic adults was similar to that of neurotypical others (Bruggink et al., 2016; Peters et al., 2007), to suggest a need for caution in discounting their decisional choices premised on diagnosis only.

Like neurotypical others, older autistic adults require predictability in their life outcomes from their everyday decision outcomes, either independently or with the assistance of a partner or family, as opposed to a higher level of care (Maddox & Gaus, 2019; Perkins & Berkman, 2012). Yet, while decision making is a fundamental personal functioning or self-management capability, "hardly any studies have examined choice making by people with Autism considering best alternatives they perceive in their life situations" (Farmer et al., 2017, p. 1067). This, despite the importance of decision making in choice of a broad range of community living supports, "the extent to which... people with Autism experience difficulties with decision making, is unknown" (Luke et al., 2012, p. 614), while their risk for stigmatization by neurotypical others of their self-managing preferences remains high.

Stigmatization and Stereotyping Effects

The diagnostic characterization of autism as a difficulty with social interaction has often led to stereotypes of autistic people as asocial (Holt et al., 2022). Yet, "autism constitutes a different form of life, rather than being a deficit of mind" and "neurotypical individuals ... fail to read autistic states of mind, and rate them unfavourably" (Botha et al., 2022, p. 430). In other words, an understanding of "what social ability is valued or deemed important in different social contexts" in "autistic social worlds", validating "autistic peoples' perspective of sociality" contributes to valuing their unique "insights into alternative ways of conceptualizing sociality and community" (Rosqvist, 2019, p. 170). Self-managing their everyday lives, older autistic adults prefer a sociality difference orientation rather than a deficit regarding their community living and participation choices (Alkhaldi et al., 2019; Anderson-Chavarria, 2021). Older autistic adults would learn of alternative self-management resources and practices in use by similar others that might work for them, and for their relationship situations.

Regrettably, people with autism are stigmatized for their interactional discordance (Mitchell et al., 2021; Sasson et al., 2017), leaving them with feeling "not valued and unwanted, [and] perhaps ... a burden on society and that the world would be better off without them" (Mitchell et al., 2021, p. 2). While adult autistics valued interpersonal relationships as much as neurotypical others "autistic people describe belonging as a crucial aspect of their well-being, ...thwarted belonging is ...a far more common everyday experience for autistic people than it is for neurotypical people" (Mitchell et al., 2021, p. 2), from being denied their life situation capabilities self-mamaging their community living and participation.

However, not all autistic people want maximal involvement in normative or typical community living activities, even if they could (Mitchell et al., 2019). For instance, an adult autistic could be overly focused on a few areas of community living and participation, perhaps charitable work, physical exercise regimen, travel, and dieting. They may be thinking about something related to one of these core activity areas. While these fixations are accomplishments in themselves, they may be socially challenging. For instance, when an autistic adult wants to pursue their intense interests and is somewhat disinterested to engage in discussion about unrelated topics, others may still seek their opinion or participation. Evidently, autistics experience significantly less social engagement, family contact, and neighborhood inclusivity compared to neurotypical peers (Bishop-Fitzpatrick et al., 2016; Jones et al., 2019). Thus, aging with autism, community living alone does not translate to social inclusion (Bagatell, 2010; Bishop-Fitzpatrick et al., 2016; Turcotte et al., 2016), and older autistics would have learned along the life how to self-manage with camouflaging.

Camouflaging

"Camouflaging" involves hiding or masking aspects of oneself from others to "pass" in everyday social interactions (Bradley et al., 2021; Cage & Troxell-Whitman, 2019; Fombonne, 2020; Mitchell et al., 2019). Older autistic adults often have learned to manage by camouflaging their sociality to the social mores of neurotypical others for social acceptance (Cook et al., 2022). However, older autistic adults value social participation with family, friends, and society (Cage et al., 2018;

Chapman, 2019), and with less camouflaging who they are as autistics (Cage & Troxell-Whitman, 2019; Stendal & Balandin, 2015). Regrettably, some may "mask" certain social challenges with substance use, with unwanted risks to self-managing in their life situations (Miller et al., 2021). Evidence on "the role age may play in camouflaging" would "shed light on this potential effect" on their community living outcomes (Jorgenson et al., 2020, p. 4346). Moreover, in today's digital world, older autistic adults would have alternative self-representations for their self-managing in both real and virtual communities.

LIFE SITUATION CAPABILITIES

The concept of life situation is central to understanding the use of personal capabilities for managing typical or routine community life practices (Jurczyk et al., 2015). Capability theory (Nussbaum, 2011) considers life situations as opportunities for actions that would be beneficial, avoiding those that would be detrimental. In other words, people would act on capabilities aligned to their priority life choices with opportunity. Translated to community living and participation, the capabilities approach would suggest that older autistic adults would employ their intrinsic capacities (inherent abilities: WHO, 2020) to achieve life outcomes at a desired level, negotiating barriers to that end.

Intrinsic Capacities

As previously noted, judgment and decision-making processes are particularly significant intrinsic capacities for self-managing everyday life, and their importance increases at older ages. For older autistic adults, self-managing capabilities would be those that "best reflect issues that are of most relevance for the autistic community" (Scheeren et al., 2021, p. 11), and also how or whether capabilities "should be available differently" (Hiersteiner et al., 2017, p. 46). For instance, an older autistic adult may self-identify their productivity to be explained in part by their autism, as by their ability for prolonged focus on tasks resulting in successful long-term projects. Being able to focus on work tasks and projects for extended periods while with no distraction, tuning the rest of the world out, adult autistics have an intrinsic capability advantage for self-managing their productivity over the years. Conceivably, older autistic adults allocate their capabilities to priority life domains rather than evenly across life domains, presumably for attaining their optimal functioning within their reach, reducing the gap between their intrinsic capacities and achievements.

Older autistic adults' intrinsic capabilities would vary by severity and spread of symptoms, and health and function dependencies from the aging process. Autism is on a continuum of severity from low functioning to high functioning (APA, 2013). However, the emerging evidence on symptom presentation suggests that while older autistic adults were more likely to self-manage less well compared to younger autistics (Bishop-Fitzpatrick et al., 2015; Van Heijst & Geurts, 2015), they also report modest improvements in symptoms (Van Heijst & Geurts, 2015). This could be because the superimposition of age-related functional deterioration on autism symptoms could theoretically result in greater intrinsic capacities impairments than expected with age-related decline alone. Moreover, how well older autistic adults managed their community living outcomes would vary by life-situation histories, sociodemographic (see also Georgiades et al., 2013; Grzadzinski et al., 2013), also by their functional autism traits profiles.

Autism Traits Profiles

Well-documented autism intrinsic capacities include atypical social skills, communication (**Social**), attention switching, and attention to detail, imagination, and interest in numbers, dates, patterns, and categories of things (**Practical**). These fall on a continuum of severity, mediated by comorbid conditions, intellectual disability, and language ability (**Health and function**) (Mitchell et al., 2019; Rodogno et al., 2016).

"Age-related ill-health is the first step towards preventing health inequality for older adults on the autism spectrum" (Happé & Frith, 2020, p. 222). Autistic people are at high risk for co-morbid psychiatric disabilities interrupting their community living self-management (Hirvikoski et al., 2020; Marriage et al., 2009). While autism is not a psychiatric condition, about 28–89 percent of people aging with autism report diagnosable psychiatric conditions (Howlin & Magiati, 2017) at a rate of three to four times higher than neurotypical others (Cage, 2020). "At present, however, there is no formal way to designate the combined effect of these different aspects of autism on a person's life" (Waizbard-Bartov et al., 2023, p. 685). Nonetheless, these psychological conditions may be compounded by age-related declines in cognitive function.

Older autistic adults with comorbid psychiatric conditions had lower social wellbeing compared to those without a psychiatric condition (Rydzewska et al., 2018). They need dependable resources to manage their life situations, minimizing their vulnerabilities with the aging process. Thus, a "one-size-fits-all" self-managing capabilities approach would not explain the diversity in how older adults self-manage their life situations (Lombardo, 2021). Life situation capabilities would depend on the levels of support the older autistic adults perceived to require.

Support Level Needs

With appropriate support, older autistic adults would better translate their intrinsic capabilities into successful community living (Stendal & Balandin, 2015). Self-managing capabilities, people with autism are categorized based on the severity level and need for support: Level 3 (requiring very substantial support); Level 2 (requiring substantial support); and Level 3 (requiring support) (APA, 2013). On a continuum of symptom spread and severity, those presenting with more severe symptoms, with spread across life activities, would require more intensive community living supports for self-managing than their high-functioning peers (Farley et al., 2009). For instance, by their support level needs for self-managing, older autistic adults would vary in appraisal or material and belongingness support needs for converting their intrinsic capabilities of older autistic adults into actual community living and participation actions (see Figure 4.1).

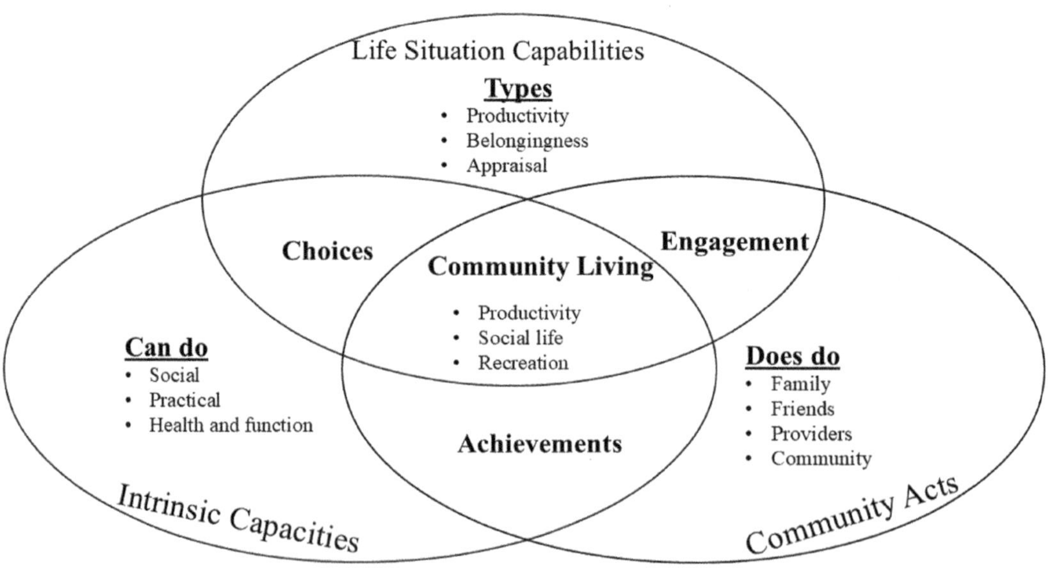

FIGURE 4.1 Intersection of capabilities, intrinsic capacities, and community actions

Appraisal Support refers to having the personal space to share private worries and fears. ***Belonging Support*** refers to opportunities to get invited to do things with others, while ***Tangible Support*** refers to the availability of help for physical and material wellness (Hedley et al., 2017). For older autistic adults, their wellbeing is premised on the predictability of support for self-managing in the community by themselves, and/or with the help of either a partner or with family, as opposed to a higher level of care (Maddox & Gaus, 2019; Moss et al., 2019; Perkins & Berkman, 2012). However, autistics have difficulty in describing their emotion (Alexithymia: Hogeveen & Grafman, 2021), which can be challenging in a marriage, from being unable to convey emotions to a partner and to identify with a partner's emotions, seeming to be uncaring. They also may lose what limited relationship supports they have with the death or incapacity of their parents or siblings. In addition, because surviving older parents may also need care, older autistic adults may lose the customary relationship systems developed over a lifetime (Dudley et al., 2019), in the absence of compensatory support resources for satisfying living outcomes.

Satisfaction with Life

Satisfaction with life is premised on self-managing by the ability to "read" the social subtext of neurotypical others, who often are "widely inaccurate" in their understanding regarding the social motives of the person with Autism (Milton, 2012, p. 884). Undeniably, the support capability actions of older autistic adults would make for improved relationships with family, friends, neighbors, strangers, and service providers, premised on the opportunities older autistic adults perceive. Moreover, older autistic adults self-managing for satisfying life outcomes are presaged by their ability to leverage personal capabilities to access, transact, or exchange information for desired life goals (Lozier et al., 2014). Conceivably, there would be more life situation capabilities for successful community living, providing room for self-exploration of options in present life situation as well as by the influences of social disparities by sociodemographic, autism symptoms, and health and function, for example.

SOCIODEMOGRAPHIC AND LIVING ARRANGEMENT EFFECTS

Sociodemographics of age, gender, race/ethnicity, and their inter-sectionalities would moderate the relationship between the intrinsic capabilities of older autistic adults for self-managing their community living outcomes. Likewise, where and with whom the older autistic adults lived would influence their opportunities for translating intrinsic capabilities into the community living outcomes they desire.

Sociodemographics

Race/ethnicity and gender health disparities in the general population were prevalent in older autistic adults (Benevides et al., 2021; Schott et al., 2022), which would impair self-managing their community living outcomes. For instance, females with autism had more severe autism symptoms than males (Cage & Troxell-Whitman, 2019). However, females are more successful at passing as neurotypical (Cage & Troxell-Whitman, 2019). In the United States, Hispanic, Black, Asian/Pacific, American Indian/Native Americans, and women tend not to have access to Autism diagnostic services or to be misdiagnosed with other conditions (i.e., intellectual disabilities, conduct disorders) (Bargiela et al., 2016; Mandell et al., 2007). Risk for multiple functional disabilities is higher among older adult racial/ethnic minorities in the United States (Moore et al., 2020), suggesting diminished self-managing capabilities in the absence of targeted supports. Moreover, the intersection between multiple comorbidities and socio-demographic inequities would hamper the translation of what may be apparent capabilities into successful community living outcomes.

Across these inter-sectionalities, older autistic adults self-manage through their unique life experiences and comfort, and fit into their daily routines, and community living arrangements. "Many will show evidence of some kind of deficit in mentalizing over the lifespan, while others may not show any difficulty or may simply mask the difficulty via compensatory mechanisms" (Lombardo et al., 2016, p. 2).

Community Living Arrangements

Community living is defined by "engagement in all aspects of an activity as judged against contemporary …community standards and resulting in maximal involvement of the person in the activity" (Thompson et al., 2015, p. 13). Increasingly, people inhabit physical living arrangements and digital or virtual communities, often a combination of these two.

Living Arrangements

Of U.S. older autistic adults, for instance, about eight percent lived in their own homes, which is a lower rate compared to those with other developmental disabilities (Hewitt et al., 2017). About 25–50 percent lived in residential placement (Crompton et al., 2020; Gray et al., 2014). Older autistic adults lived with family (Gray et al., 2014; Hewitt et al., 2017). Over 70 percent of older autistic adults were under a guardianship arrangement (Hewitt et al., 2017). The rest of older autistic adults were likely to live in group homes or other institutional settings (Hewitt et al., 2017). These living arrangements portend differences in opportunities for older autistic adults, translating their intrinsic capabilities into actions for the end goals they desire.

Family living settings may be helpful for the social engagement of older autistic adults (Orsmond et al., 2009), while they also carry the risk of overprotectiveness by family, which may deny the use of capabilities for inclusive community living options by older adults with ASD (Krauss et al., 2005). However, while the severity and number of traits associated with Autism may influence relationship satisfaction (Bishop-Fitzpatrick et al., 2016), this was not the case with older autistic adults who were satisfied with their marital relationships despite their partner's symptomatic profile.

Some studies suggest that older adults living independently prefer social relationships with friends rather than family (Mpofu et al., 2024), while those in long-term care facilities reported lower satisfaction with relationship needs overall compared to those living independently or with family (Gray et al., 2014). Older autistics may also experience difficulties making casual friendships such as with strangers or people new to them. For instance, initiating small talk with a stranger may seem overly demanding, perceiving that they may never encounter the person again. They may struggle with small talk about something they have no interest in and present as blunt affect when they do not mean to be rude.

Guardianship (assisted) capability decision settings appear to take away from independent living choices, aging with autism, potentially widening the gap with the opportunity to perform the actions premised on the decisions in which one is invested (Hiersteiner et al., 2017). Nonetheless, long-term care facility living and guardianship arrangements that provided participatory decision making would empower older autistic adults to recognize and utilize their capabilities for improved community living (Bari et al., 2018).

It is a reasonable presupposition that living arrangements influence the later life course trajectory in intrinsic capacities of older autistic adults for their community living actions. They may experience improvement, plateauing, or a decline in their use of intrinsic capacities for improved community living and participation. Moreover, it would be a reasonable presumption that older autistic adults' community living outcomes would depend in part on present living arrangements or as they transition into new living arrangements, as may be necessitated by their changing life situations (Crompton et al., 2020), including partaking of digital or virtual communities.

Digital Living

Increasingly, digital technologies are ubiquitous for community living and participation of older adults (Ballantyne et al., 2010), and older autistic adults are no exception (Martinez-Martin et al., 2020). Autistics used digital technologies more than other disability groups, other than those with attention deficit hyperactive disorder: ADHD (Johansson et al., 2021). In the present digital age, older autistic adults would leverage technology for self-managing their community living and participation more than was the case in previous times. Thus, digital tools are central to everyday relationship participation, and older autistic adults would use them for self-management of everyday living needs.

Among older autistic adults, age cohort effects would influence decisional choices for use of digital technologies for community living, so that younger-older adults (55–64 years) would likely use digital technologies more than the middle-older adults (65 to 80 years) or older-old adults (81 years and above) (Zheng et al., 2022). The lag in digital technology literacy by the middle-older to older-old adults would influence their choices for digital tools supported everyday living, as would the interaction between age cohort effects, any chronic health conditions they may, autism symptom severity spread (low; high), living arrangement (independent, family, assisted), and decisional authority (autonomous versus guardianship) (Colombo-Dougovito et al., 2021). Moreover, access-use of digital devices by older autistic adults would change over time from emerging needs for self-management of their relationships in priority life domains.

Moreover, while older autistic adults used digital tools to assist their home keeping and self-care, their sustainable community living and participation decisional choices would vary by the digital tools their life situations (Mpofu et al., 2022). For instance, an autistic may be hypersensitive to bright lighting which may be a feature digital tool they are using, bringing about sensory overload. Similarly, they may be overly sensitive to digital tools' sounds. Both these types of sensory overload would be disruptive to their overall mental health while seeming ordinary to others in their life situations. Others may wonder why the autistic adult seemed somewhat agitated, being unaware of the role of digital tool functional qualities on their self-management in everyday situations. The unintentional disconnect from use of some digital tools with risk of sensory overload may be compounded by the fact that autistics rarely make eye contact with others, as frequent eye contact is sensory overload for people with autism, unless an activity they are keenly interested in. Regrettably, fewer studies have reported on digital tools use appropriateness and effectiveness self-managing everyday life by older autistic adults (Hrabal et al., 2023).

IMPLICATIONS FOR RESEARCH AND PRACTICE

As previously noted, self-managing community living ultimately rests on decision choices and competencies for desired outcomes. In this sense, capabilities-oriented self-management of older autistic adults would be likely, with a focus on the "more immediate and direct impact on the daily lives of autistic people and their families, especially related to services and supports" (Pellicano et al., 2018, p. 82). This is not to deny the importance of improving the community and policy environment barriers to the unmet community living and participation of older autistic adults compared to the general population (Chapman, 2020; Milton, 2012). It is, however, increasingly clear that capitalizing on the older autistic adults' intrinsic capabilities is an essential component of their community living self-management. This capabilities orientation calls for studies on older autistic intrinsic capabilities, the development of a practice framework to guide interventions aimed at improving their community living and participation based on their information framing and reference points, behavioral norm incentivizing, and direct guidance of targeted behaviors.

Information Framing and Reference Points

Presumably, the primary influence on intrinsic capabilities utilization by older autistic adults is the information available to them, and especially how it is framed or contextualized. For instance, older autistic adults would have priorities for everyday living and reference points. Such community living information framing and reference points would include possible choices, knowledge about own intrinsic capacities, and available support. This would be so, given the fact that consequential real-world decisions about community living options are based on "a subjective measure like utility is used to assign the relative desirability of each choice" (Gold & Shadlen, 2007, p. 560). That being the case, older autistic adults' self-management would be influenced by their perceptions of their own life situation demands, and behavioral incentives for the choices they would consider in their prevailing life situation demands to meet their aspirations.

Behavioral Norm Incentivizing

The incentives older autistic adults perceive for use of their intrinsic capabilities for meeting their everyday living would depend on the cost-benefits based on current and prospective use of specific capabilities. For instance, older autistic adults, perhaps like neurotypical others, may decide on capabilities they perceive as dependability, and fit with meeting daily community living routines and with unobtrusiveness. They may also consider the relative advantage to capabilities important to attaining life satisfaction and aspirations in both the neurotypical and autistic communities. Regarding the significance to the autistic community of the behavioral incentivizing norm, older autistic adults would likely prioritize the use of capabilities they perceived to be aligned with those of social referent group others in a similar choice situation. They would do so believing the social others to be a credible source of accurate information about the appropriate behavior for the context.

"Autism acceptance from others could be important for autistics" (Cage et al., 2017, p. 474) and would allow autistic adults to reclaim a sense of "autistic agency and community" (Parsloe, 2015, p. 336). Older autistic adults would benefit from exploring other possible selves, self-managing their lives. Importantly, older autistic adults have a lived culture over many years, transacting both the mainstream culture and their autism community culture, which is often unrecognized by neurotypical people, compounding their sense of social exclusion (Chapman, 2020; Milton, 2012). There is emerging evidence to suggest that autism acceptance is beneficial to the well-being of both the people with autism (Cage, 2020; Cage et al., 2018), their families, and service providers (Da Paz et al., 2018). This could be by the fact that improved acceptance likely comes with recognition and validation of autistic capabilities (Chapman, 2020). Even then, older autistic adults would likely utilize a holistic decisional framework for their capabilities to deliver to their community living and participation needs self-managing their choices.

Direct Guidance of Target Behaviors

Decisions by older autistic adults to use intrinsic capabilities for successful community living and participation would be from a sense of control they perceive of the capability utilization, usage cues, and desirability in their environment, current or default usage experiences, and recommendations by family, friends, as well as service providers. For instance, there is evidence to suggest that older autistic adults would utilize a resource if they perceived a sense of control, and less demand to implement based on previous experience, and with support from caregivers or service providers (Brewer et al., 2017). Of self-initiated autistic behaviors is repetitive behavior, which is an asset to completing time-consuming long-term projects with the discipline to religiously self-schedule to routinized days on end to achieve wanted work outcomes. Additionally, the predisposition to repetitious behavior helps health wellbeing self-management, adhering to physical fitness exercise, for example, that requires sticking to a predetermined schedule. However, behavior does not always match the intention (Milkman, 2021), and there are apparent downsides related to repetitive behaviors, as when the autistic adults may experience significant distress when their predetermined schedule is inadvertently disrupted. Family and friends may never fully understand the degree of distress that interrupting a few hours of a routinized personal schedule would seriously deplete the adult autistics sense of wellbeing. Nonetheless, capability to use decisions based on cues and prompts in the environment, personal experience, and support by significant others would be important to the community living and participation outcomes of older autistic adults. Moreover, older autistic adults would be predisposed to use community living and participation choices that minimize cost to capability resources depletion, and for fulfillment of their aspired life participation. For instance, in self-managing their repetition of behavior avoiding potential conflicts that can arise as a result, adult autistics may diarize their social commitments on the calendar to minimize risk for what may come as unforeseen or unanticipated disruption of work-related endeavors they find to provoke anxiety.

Importantly, "autism cannot avoid being related to the cultural norms of a social, empathic, and engaged individual" and what is problematic is the bias by professional services to "demarcate, locate, and treat particular discontents and impairments that have appeared" (Verhoeff, 2015, p. 21). These approaches inherently marginalize the intrinsic capacities of older autistic adults with inestimable cost to their community living outcomes. Moreover, the ongoing lack of clarity between what self-management behaviors are at different ages and for different genders and cultures would influence initiatives to improve on the life outcomes of older autistic adults (de Leeuw et al., 2020). Direct guidance of targeted self-management behaviors of older autistic adults should build on their capabilities employing participatory approaches for their sustained commitment.

CONCLUSION

Older autistic adults experience limited community living and participation from avoidable gaps between their intrinsic capacities and actual community living actions. The variability in community life trajectories for autistic individuals is huge, by the interaction between their intrinsic capabilities and the levels of support they may require for self-managing their community living and participation. This is part because social interaction difficulties in autism are not an absolute or inherent characteristic of the individual, and there is more of a difference in how they may express their capabilities for self-managing their successful community living and participation. Moreover, simply having a capability (or capabilities) does not guarantee use by older autistic adults for their community living and participation. However, many older autistic adults would utilize their intrinsic capacities for the community living and participation they desire with ongoing support from family (spouses, children, grandchildren, and friends) and service providers.

Increasingly, community living and participation include digital or virtual communities and older autistic adults utilize digital tools for translating their personal capabilities into community living and participation outcomes. Older autistic adults would use information sources and priorities and would likely engage in actions they perceive for managing their priority community living and participation outcomes. There is an urgent need to explore and discover older autistic adults' intrinsic capabilities to self-manage their community living, and the benefits they perceive from the use of specific capabilities to present needs in their lives. Conceivably, adopting a capabilities approach, more autistics will achieve a thriving adulthood less encumbered by disablement stereotypes. The intrinsic capabilities approach to community living and participation we proposed in this chapter would benefit older autistic adults to self-manage their social worlds with less need to camouflage their true interests and with the ability to seek the company they enjoy for satisfying community lives.

REFERENCES

Alkhaldi, R. S., Sheppard, E., & Mitchell, P. (2019). Is there a link between autistic people being perceived unfavorably and having a mind that is difficult to read? *Journal of Autism and Developmental Disorders, 49*(10), 3973–3982. https://doi.org/10.1007/s10803-019-04101-1

American Psychiatric Association. (2013). *Diagnostic and Statistical Manual of Mental Disorders: DSM-5.* (5th ed.). American Psychiatric Publishing. https://doi.org/10.1176/appi.books.9780890425596

Anderson-Chavarria, M. (2021). The autism predicament: Models of autism and their impact on autistic identity. *Disability & Society, 37*(8), 1321–1341. https://doi.org/10.1080/09687599.2021.1877117

Asher, M., Kauffmann, A., & Aderka, I. M. (2020). Out of sync: Nonverbal synchrony in social anxiety disorder. *Clinical Psychological Science, 8*(2), 280–294. https://doi.org/10.1177/2167702619894566

Bagatell, N. (2010). From cure to community: Transforming notions of autism. *Ethos, 38*(1), 33–55. https://doi.org/10.1111/j.1548-1352.2009.01080.x

Ballantyne, A., Trenwith, L., Zubrinich, S., & Corlis, M. (2010). 'I feel less lonely': What older people say about participating in a social networking website. *Quality in Ageing and Older Adults, 11*(3), 25–35. https://doi.org/10.5042/qiaoa.2010.0526

Bargiela, S., Steward, R., & Mandy, W. (2016). The experiences of late-diagnosed women with autism spectrum conditions: An investigation of the female autism phenotype. *Journal of Autism and Developmental Disorders, 46*(10), 3281–3294. https://doi.org/10.1007/s10803-016-2872-8

Bari, S., Tisci, R., Burlando, R., & Keller, R. (2018). Caring for autistic adults: A qualitative analysis under the lens of capability approach. *Italian Sociological Review, 8*(2), 243–264. https://doi.org/10.13136/isr.v8i2.189

Benevides, T. W., Carretta, H. J., Rust, G., & Shea, L. (2021). Racial and ethnic disparities in benefits eligibility and spending among adults on the autism spectrum: A cohort study using the Medicare Medicaid Linked Enrollees Analytic Data Source. *PloS One, 16*(5), e0251353.

Bishop-Fitzpatrick, L., Hong, J., Smith, L. E., Makuch, R. A., Greenberg, J. S., & Mailick, M. R. (2016). Characterizing objective quality of life and normative outcomes in adults with autism spectrum disorder: An exploratory latent class analysis. *Journal of Autism and Developmental Disorders, 46*, 2707–2719. https://doi.org/10.1007/s10803-016-2816-3

Bishop-Fitzpatrick, L., Mazefsky, C. A., Minshew, N. J., & Eack, S. M. (2015). The relationship between stress and social functioning in adults with autism spectrum disorder and without intellectual disability. *Autism Research, 8*(2), 164–173. https://doi.org/10.1002/aur.1433

Botha, M., Dibb, B., & Frost, D. M. (2022). Autism is me": An investigation of how autistic individuals make sense of autism and stigma. *Disability & Society, 37*(3), 427–453.

Bradley, L., Shaw, R., Baron-Cohen, S., & Cassidy, S. (2021). Autistic adults' experiences of camouflaging and its perceived impact on mental health. *Autism in Adulthood, 3*(4), 320–329. https://doi.org/full/10.1089/aut.2020.0071

Brewer, N., Young, R. L., & Barnett, E. (2017). Measuring theory of mind in adults with autism spectrum disorder. *Journal of Autism and Developmental Disorders, 47*(7), 1927–1941. https://doi.org/10.1007/s10803-017-3150-0

Bruggink, A., Huisman, S., Vuijk, R., Kraaij, V., & Garnefski, N. (2016). Cognitive emotion regulation, anxiety and depression in adults with autism spectrum disorder. *Research in Autism Spectrum Disorders, 22*, 34–44. https://www.sciencedirect.com/science/article/pii/S1750946715300027

Bruine de Bruin, W., Parker, A. M., & Fischhoff, B. (2012). Explaining adult age differences in decision-making competence. *Journal of Behavioral Decision Making, 25*(4), 352–360. https://doi.org/10.1002/bdm.712

Cage, E. (2020) Autism acceptance and mental health. In: F. Volkmar (Ed.), *Encyclopedia of Autism Spectrum Disorders.* Springer. https://doi.org/10.1007/s10803-017-3342-7

Cage, E., Di Monaco, J., & Newell, V. (2018). Experiences of autism acceptance and mental health in autistic adults. *Journal of Autism and Developmental Disorders, 48*(2), 473–484. https://doi.org/10.1007/s10803-017-3342-7

Cage, E., & Troxell-Whitman, Z. (2019). Understanding the reasons, contexts and costs of camouflaging for autistic adults. *Journal of Autism and Developmental Disorders, 49*(5), 1899–1911. https://doi.org/10.1007/s10803-018-03878-x

Chang, F. H., Coster, W. J., & Helfrich, C. A. (2013). Community participation measures for people with disabilities: A systematic review of content from an international classification of functioning, disability and health perspective. *Archives of Physical Medicine and Rehabilitation, 94*(4), 771–781. https://doi.org/10.1016/j.apmr.2012.10.031

Chapman, R. (2019). Autism as a form of life: Wittgenstein and the psychological coherence of autism. *Metaphilosophy*, *50*(4), 421–440. https://doi.org/10.1111/meta.

Chapman, R. (2020). The reality of autism: On the metaphysics of disorder and diversity. *Philosophical Psychology*, *33*(6), 799–819. https://doi.org/10.1080/09515089.2020.1751103

Colombo-Dougovito, A. M., Blagrave, A. J., & Healy, S. (2021). A grounded theory of adoption and maintenance of physical activity among autistic adults. *Autism*, *25*(3), 627–641. https://doi.org/abs/10.1177/1362361320932444

Cook, J., Crane, L., Hull, L., Bourne, L., & Mandy, W. (2022). Self-reported camouflaging behaviours used by autistic adults during everyday social interactions. *Autism*, *26*(2), 406–421. https://doi.org/10.1177/13623613211026754

Crompton, C. J., Michael, C., Dawson, M., & Fletcher-Watson, S. (2020). Residential care for older autistic adults: Insights from three multi-expert summits. *Autism in Adulthood*, *2*(2), 121–127. https://doi.org/10.1089/aut.2019.0080

Da Paz, N. S., Siegel, B., Coccia, M. A., & Epel, E. S. (2018). Acceptance or despair? Maternal adjustment to having a child diagnosed with autism. *Journal of Autism and Developmental Disorders*, *48*(6), 1971–1981. https://doi.org/10.1007/s10803-017-3450-4

Davis, R., & Crompton, C. J. (2021). What do new findings about social interaction in autistic adults mean for neurodevelopmental research? *Perspectives on Psychological Science*, *16*(3), 649–653. https://doi.org/10.1177/1745691620958010

de Leeuw, A., Happé, F., & Hoekstra, R. A. (2020). A conceptual framework for understanding the cultural and contextual factors on autism across the globe. *Autism Research*, *13*(7), 1029–1050. https://doi.org/10.1002/aur.2276

Dudley, K. M., Klinger, M. R., Meyer, A., Powell, P., & Klinger, L. G. (2019). Understanding service usage and needs for adults with ASD: The importance of living situation. *Journal of Autism and Developmental Disorders*, *49*(2), 556–568. https://doi.org/10.1007/s10803-018-3729-0

Elichaoff, F. (2015). What's it like being you? Growing old(er) with autism spectrum conditions – A scoping study. *The European Journal of Social and Behavioural Sciences*, *13*(2), 231–246. https://doi.org/10.15405/ejsbs.166

Farley, M., Cottle, K. J., Bilder, D., Viskochil, J., Coon, H., & McMahon, W. (2018). Mid-life social outcomes for a population-based sample of adults with ASD. *Autism Research*, *11*(1), 142–152. https://doi.org/10.1002/aur.1897

Farley, M. A., McMahon, W. M., Fombonne, E., Jenson, W. R., Miller, J., Gardner, M., ... & Coon, H. (2009). Twenty-year outcome for individuals with autism and average or near-average cognitive abilities. *Autism Research*, *2*(2), 109–118. https://doi.org/full/10.1002/aur.69

Farmer, G. D., Baron-Cohen, S., & Skylark, W. J. (2017). People with autism spectrum conditions make more consistent decisions. *Psychological Science*, *28*(8), 1067–1076. https://doi.org/10.1177/0956797617694867

Fombonne, E. (2020). Camouflage and autism. *Journal of Child Psychology and Psychiatry*, *61*(7), 735–738. https://doi.org/full/10.1111/jcpp.13296

Fujino, J., Tei, S., Itahashi, T., Aoki, Y. Y., Ohta, H., Kubota, M., & Takahashi, H. (2020). Impact of past experiences on decision-making in autism spectrum disorder. *European Archives of Psychiatry and Clinical Neuroscience*, *270*, 1063–1071. https://doi.org/10.1007/s00406-019-01071-4

Georgiades, S., Szatmari, P., & Boyle, M. (2013). Importance of studying heterogeneity in autism. *Neuropsychiatry*, *3*(2), 123. https://doi.org/10.2217/NPY.13.8

Gold, J. I., & Shadlen, M. N. (2007). The neural basis of decision making. *Annual. Review of. Neuroscience*, *30*(1), 535–574. https://doi.org/10.1146/annurev.neuro.29.051605.113038

Gray, K. M., Keating, C. M., Taffe, J. R., Brereton, A. V., Einfeld, S. L., Reardon, T. C., & Tonge, B. J. (2014). Adult outcomes in autism: Community inclusion and living skills. *Journal of Autism and Developmental Disorders*, *44*(12), 3006–3015. 10.1007/s10803-014-2159-x

Grzadzinski, R., Huerta, M., & Lord, C. (2013). DSM-5 and autism spectrum disorders (ASDs): An opportunity for identifying ASD subtypes. *Molecular Autism*, *4*(1), 1–6. 10.1186/2040-2392-4-12

Happé, F., & Frith, U. (2020). Annual research review: Looking back to look forward–changes in the concept of autism and implications for future research. *Journal of Child Psychology and Psychiatry*, *61*(3), 218–232. https://doi.org/10.1111/jcpp.13176

Hedley, D., Uljarević, M., Wilmot, M., Richdale, A., & Dissanayake, C. (2017). Brief report: Social support, depression and suicidal ideation in adults with autism spectrum disorder. *Journal of Autism and Developmental Disorders*, *47*(11), 3669–3677. 10.1007/s10803-017-3274-2

Hewitt, A. S., Stancliffe, R. J., Hall-Lande, J., Nord, D., Pettingell, S. L., Hamre, K., & Hallas-Muchow, L. (2017). Characteristics of adults with autism spectrum disorder who use residential services and supports through adult developmental disability services in the United States. *Research in Autism Spectrum Disorders*, *34*, 1–9. https://doi.org/10.1016/j.rasd.2016.11.007

Hiersteiner, D., Bradley, V., Ne'eman, A., Bershadsky, J., & Bonardi, A. (2017). Putting the research in context: The life experience and outcomes of adults on the autism spectrum receiving services in 29 States. *Inclusion*, *5*(1), 45–59. https://www.tandfonline.com/journals/tinc20

Hirvikoski, T., Boman, M., Chen, Q., D'Onofrio, B. M., Mittendorfer-Rutz, E., Lichtenstein, P., Bölte, S., & Larsson, H. (2020). Individual risk and familial liability for suicide attempts and suicide in autism: A population-based study. *Psychological Medicine*, *50*(9), 1463–1474. https://doi.org/10.1017/S0033291719001405

Hogeveen, J., & Grafman, J. (2021). Alexithymia. In: *Handbook of Clinical Neurology* 183,47–62). Elsevier. https://doi.org/10.1016/B978-0-12-822290-4.00004-9

Holt, A., Bounekhla, K., Welch, C., & Polatajko, H. (2022). "Unheard minds, again and again": Autistic insider perspectives and theory of mind. *Disability and Rehabilitation*, *44*(20), 5887–5897. https://doi.org/10.1080/09638288.2021.1949052

Howlin, P., & Magiati, I. (2017). Autism spectrum disorder: Outcomes in adulthood. *Current Opinion in Psychiatry*, *30*(2), 69–76. https://doi.org/10.1097/YCO.0000000000000308

Hrabal, J. M., Davis, T. N., & Wicker, M. R. (2023). The use of technology to teach daily living skills for adults with autism: A systematic review. *Advances in Neurodevelopmental Disorders*, *7*(3), 443–458. 10.1007/s41252-022-00255-9

Johansson, S., Gulliksen, J., & Gustavsson, C. (2021). Disability digital divide: The use of The internet, smartphones, computers and tablets among people with disabilities in Sweden. *Universal Access in the Information Society*, *20*(1), 105–120. 10.1007/s10209-020-00714-x

Jones, E. A., Fiani, T., Stewart, J. L., Sheikh, R., Neil, N., & Fienup, D. M. (2019). When one sibling has autism: Adjustment and sibling relationship. *Journal of Child and Family Studies*, *28*(5), 1272–1282. 10.1007/s10826-019-01374-z

Jorgenson, C., Lewis, T., Rose, C., & Kanne, S. (2020). Social camouflaging in autistic and neurotypical adolescents: A pilot study of differences by sex and diagnosis. *Journal of Autism and Developmental Disorders*, *50*(12), 4344–4355. 10.1007/s10803-020-04491-7

Jurczyk, K., Voß, G. G., & Weihrich, M. (2015). Conduct of everyday life in subject-oriented sociology: Concept and empirical research. In: *Psychology and the Conduct of Everyday Life* (pp. 34–64). Routledge. https://doi.org/10.4324/9781315746890-3

Kahneman, D. (2011). *Thinking, Fast and Slow*. Macmillan.

Krauss, M. W., Seltzer, M. M., & Jacobson, H. T. (2005). Adults with autism living at home or in non-family settings: Positive and negative aspects of residential status. *Journal of Intellectual Disability Research*, *49*(Pt 2), 111–124. https://doi.org/10.1111/j.1365-2788.2004.00599.x

Li, M., & Chapman, G. B. (2013). Nudge to health: Harnessing decision research to promote health behavior. *Social and Personality Psychology Compass*, *7*(3), 187–198. https://doi.org/10.1111/spc3.12019

Lockwood, P. L., Abdurahman, A., Gabay, A. S., Drew, D., Tamm, M., Husain, M., & Apps, M. (2021). Aging increases prosocial motivation for effort. *Psychological Science*, *32*(5), 668–681. https://doi.org/10.1177/0956797620975781.

Lombardo, M. V. (2021). Prototyping as subtyping strategy for studying heterogeneity in autism. *Autism Research*, *14*(10), 2224. https://doi.org/10.1002/aur.2535

Lombardo, M. V., Lai, M. C., Auyeung, B., Holt, R. J., Allison, C., Smith, P., & Baron-Cohen, S. (2016). Unsupervised data-driven stratification of mentalizing heterogeneity in autism. *Scientific Reports*, *6*(1), 35333. https://www.nature.com/articles/srep35333

Lozier, L. M., Vanmeter, J. W., & Marsh, A. A. (2014). Impairments in facial affect recognition associated with autism spectrum disorders: A meta-analysis. *Development Psychopathology*, *26*(4Pt1), 933–945. https://doi.org/10.1017/S0954579414000479

Luke, L., Clare, I. C., Ring, H., Redley, M., & Watson, P. (2012). Decision-making difficulties experienced by adults with autism spectrum conditions. *Autism*, *16*(6), 612–621. https://doi.org/10.1177/1362361311415876

Maddox, B. B., & Gaus, V. L. (2019). Community mental health services for autistic adults: Good news and bad news. *Autism in Adulthood*, *1*(1), 15–19. https://doi.org/10.1089/aut.2018.0006

Mandell, D. S., Ittenbach, R. F., Levy, S. E., & Pinto-Martin, J. A. (2007). Disparities in diagnoses received prior to a diagnosis of autism spectrum disorder. *Journal of Autism and Developmental Disorders*, *37*(9), 1795–1802. 10.1007/s10803-006-0314-8

Marriage, S., Wolverton, A., & Marriage, K. (2009). Autism spectrum disorder grown up: A chart review of adult functioning. *Journal of the Canadian Academy of Child and Adolescent Psychiatry*, *18*(4), 322–328. https://pmc.ncbi.nlm.nih.gov/articles/PMC2765385/

Martinez-Martin, E., Escalona, F., & Cazorla, M. (2020). Socially assistive robots for older adults and people with autism: An overview. *Electronics*, *9*(2), 367. https://doi.org/10.3390/electronics9020367.

Milkman, K. (2021). *How to Change: The Science of Getting from Where You Are to Where You Want to Be.* Penguin.

Miller, D., Rees, J., & Pearson, A. (2021). "Masking is life": Experiences of masking in autistic and nonautistic adults. *Autism in Adulthood, 3*(4), 330–338. https://doi.org/abs/10.1089/aut.2020.0083

Milton, D. (2012). On the ontological status of autism: The "double empathy problem". *Disability & Society, 27*(6), 883–887. https://doi.org/full/10.1080/09687599.2012.710008

Mitchell, P., Cassidy, S., & Sheppard, E. (2019). The double empathy problem, camouflage, and the value of expertise from experience. *Behavioral and Brain Sciences, 42*, e100. https://doi.org/10.1017/S0140525X18002212

Mitchell, P., Sheppard, E., & Cassidy, S. (2021). Autism and the double empathy problem: Implications for development and mental health. *British Journal of Developmental Psychology, 39*(1), 1–18. https://doi.org/10.1111/bjdp.12350

Moore, A. R., Bohm-Jordan, M., Amey, F., & Mpofu, E. (2020). Correlates of single versus multiple functional disabilities among aging Americans: Race/ethnicity and region of birth. *Gerontology and Geriatric Medicine, 6*, 2333721420914785.

Moss, P., Eirinaki, V., Savage, S., & Howlin, P. (2019). Growing older with autism–The experiences of adult siblings of individuals with autism. *Research in Autism Spectrum Disorders, 63*, 42–51. https://doi.org/10.1016/j.rasd.2018.10.005

Mpofu, E., Tomczak, M. T., Hutson, N., Gafford, L., & Zhan, R. (2022). Context of digitalized employment for older adults with autism spectrum disorder in the new normal. In: *Managing Human Resources: The New Normal* (pp. 269–289). Springer International Publishing. 10.1007/978-3-031-09803-1_15

Mpofu, E., Zhan, R. F., Yin, C., & Brock, K. (2024). Qualities of older adults' family and friendship relationships and their association with life satisfaction. *Geriatrics, 9*(2), 49. https://doi.org/10.3390/geriatrics9020049

Nussbaum, M. C. (2011). *Creating Capabilities: The Human Development Approach.* Harvard University Press.

Orsmond, G. I., Kuo, H.-Y., & Seltzer, M. M. (2009). Siblings of individuals with an autism spectrum disorder: Sibling relationships and wellbeing in adolescence and adulthood. *Autism, 13*(1), 59–80. https://doi.org/10.1177/1362361308097119

Parsloe, S. M. (2015). Discourses of disability, narratives of community: Reclaiming an autistic identity online. *Journal of Applied Communication Research, 43*(3), 336–356. doi/full/10.1080/00909882.2015.1052829

Pellicano, E., Fatima, U., Hall, G., Heyworth, M., Lawson, W., Lilley, R., & Stears, M. (2022). A capabilities approach to understanding and supporting autistic adulthood. *Nature Reviews Psychology, 1*(11), 624–639. https://www.nature.com/articles/s44159-022-00099-z

Pellicano, L., Mandy, W., Bölte, S., Stahmer, A., Lounds Taylor, J., & Mandell, D. S. (2018). A new era for autism research, and for our journal. *Autism*, 22(2), 82–83. https://doi.org/full/10.1177/1362361317748556

Perkins, E. A., & Berkman, K. A. (2012). Into the unknown: Aging with autism spectrum disorders. *American Journal on Intellectual and Developmental Disabilities, 117*(6), 478–496. https://doi.org/10.1352/1944-7558-117.6.478.

Peters, E., Hess, T. M., Västfjäll, D., & Auman, C. (2007). Adult age differences in dual information processes: Implications for the role of affective and deliberative processes in older adults' decision making. *Perspectives on Psychological Science, 2*(1), 1–23.

Piven, J., & Rabins, P., & Autism-in-Older Adults Working Group. (2011). Autism spectrum disorders in older adults: Toward defining a research agenda. *Journal of the American Geriatrics Society, 59*(11), 2151–2155. https://doi.org/10.1111/j.1532-5415.2011.03632.x

Robeyns, I. (2016). Conceptualising well-being for autistic persons. *Journal of Medical Ethics, 42*(6), 383–390.

Rodogno, R., Krause-Jensen, K., & Ashcroft, R. E. (2016). 'Autism and the good life': A new approach to the study of well-being. *Journal of Medical Ethics, 42*(6), 401–408. https://jme.bmj.com/content/42/6/401.short

Rosqvist, H. B. (2019). Doing things together: Exploring meanings of different forms of sociality among autistic people in an autistic workspace. *Alter, 13*(3), 168–178. https://doi.org/10.1016/j.alter.2019.03.003

Rydzewska, E., Hughes-McCormack, L. A., Gillberg, C., Henderson, A., MacIntyre, C., Rintoul, J., & Cooper, S. A. (2018). Prevalence of long-term health conditions in adults with autism: Observational study of a whole country population. *BMJ Open, 8*(8), e023945. https://doi.org/10.1136/bmjopen-2018-023945

Sasson, N. J., Faso, D. J., Nugent, J., Lovell, S., Kennedy, D. P., & Grossman, R. B. (2017). Neurotypical peers are less willing to interact with those with autism based on thin slice judgments. *Scientific Reports, 7*(1), 1–10. https://www.nature.com/articles/srep40700

Scheeren, A. M., Buil, J. M., Howlin, P., Bartels, M., & Begeer, S. (2021). Objective and subjective psychosocial outcomes in adults with autism spectrum disorder: A 6-year longitudinal study. *Autism*, 26(1), 243–255.

Schott, W., Tao, S., & Shea, L. (2022). Co-occurring conditions and racial-ethnic disparities: Medicaid enrolled adults on the autism spectrum. *Autism Research*, *15*(1), 70–85. https://doi.org/10.1002/aur.2644

Schweinberger, S. R., Pohl, M., & Winkler, P. (2020). Autistic traits, personality, and evaluations of humanoid robots by young and older adults. *Computers in Human Behavior*, *106*, 106256. https://doi.org/10.1016/j.chb.2020.106256

Sen, A. (1985). *Commodities and Capabilities*. North-Holland.

Stendal, K., & Balandin, S. (2015). Virtual worlds for people with autism spectrum disorder: A case study in second life. *Disability and Rehabilitation*, *37*(17), 1591–1598. https://doi.org/10.3109/09638288.2015.1052577

Thompson, J. R., Bryant, B. R., Schalock, R. L., Shogren, K. A., Tassé, M. J., Wehmeyer, M. L., Campbell, E. M., Craig, E. M., Hughes, C., & Rotholz, D. A. (2015). *Supports Intensity Scale — Adult Version: User's Manual*. American Association on Intellectual and Developmental Disabilities.

Turcotte, P., Mathew, M., Shea, L. L., Brusilovskiy, E., & Nonnemacher, S. L. (2016). Service needs across the lifespan for individuals with autism. *Journal of Autism and Developmental Disorders*, *46*(7), 2480–2489. https://doi.org/10.1007/s10803-016-2787-4

Uddin, L. Q. (2022). Exceptional abilities in autism: Theories and open questions. *Current Directions in Psychological Science*, *31*(6), 509–517. 10.1177/09637214221113760

Van Heijst, B. F., & Geurts, H. M. (2015). Quality of life in autism across the lifespan: A meta-analysis. *Autism*, *19*(2), 158–167. https://doi.org/abs/10.1177/1362361313517053

Verhoeff, B. (2015). Fundamental challenges for autism research: The science–practice gap, demarcating autism and the unsuccessful search for the neurobiological basis of autism. *Medicine, Health Care and Philosophy*, *18*(3), 443–447. 10.1007/s11019-015-9636-7

Waizbard-Bartov, E., Fein, D., Lord, C., & Amaral, D. G. (2023). Autism severity and its relationship to disability. *Autism Research*, *16*(4), 685–696. https://doi.org/10.1002/aur.2898

World Health Organization. (2001). *International Classification of Functioning, Disability and Health* (WHO-ICF, 2001). https://www.who.int/standards/classifications/international-classification-of-functioning-disability-and-health

World Health Organization. (2020). *Healthy Aging and Functional Ability*. https://www.who.int/news-room/questions-and-answers/item/healthy-ageing-and-functional-ability

Zheng, L., Foley, K. R., Grove, R., Elley, K., Brown, S. A., Leong, D. J., & Hwang, Y. I. (2022). The use of everyday and assistive technology in the lives of older autistic adults. *Autism*, *26*(6), 1550–1562. https://doi.org/abs/10.1177/13623613211058519

5 Self-Management for People with Chronic Inflammatory Arthritis

Christina Merete Tvede Madsen, Kirsten Lykke Knak, Astrid Jensen Damgaard, and Jette Primdahl

INTRODUCTION

The prevalence of chronic inflammatory arthritis diseases varies in published studies and with geographically variance. Rheumatoid arthritis is the most frequent disease affecting approximately 0.2–0.41% in Europe and 0.6% in the US (Finckh et al., 2022), while psoriatic arthritis affects about 0.13% of the population (Scotti et al., 2018) and estimates for the prevalence of axial spondyloarthritis ranges widely from 0.3 to1.4% (Sieper and Poddubnyy, 2017). Together these diagnoses are referred to as chronic inflammatory arthritis.

Despite the primary focus of treatment on mitigating inflammation in people with inflammatory arthritis, a substantial proportion continue to endure significant disease-related impairments (Ishida et al., 2018a; Smolen, 2016; Smolen et al., 2014). Furthermore, even those patients who attain remission or a state of low disease activity frequently confront considerable physical, psychological, and social challenges (Smolen et al., 2018). These challenges encompass pain, fatigue, sleep disturbances, physical disability, anxiety, depression, and restrictions in social participation, including occupational engagement (Gwinnutt et al., 2020; Hider et al., 2019; Ishida et al., 2018b; Primdahl et al., 2019). Consequently, effective management of these multifaceted challenges necessitates comprehensive support to empower people with inflammatory arthritis to manage the challenges and to know when and where to seek professional support (self-management support). Self-management support should be coordinated in the team of health professionals in rheumatology to ensure coherence of the interventions (Damgaard et al., 2023a). This is in line with the World Health Organization's recommendation of coherence in rehabilitation across healthcare sectors (World Health Organization, 2017). Huge differences exist across i.e. European countries in whether patients with inflammatory arthritis have access to support from other health professionals than a rheumatologist. Notably, existing evidence regarding well-defined outpatient self-management support involving interdisciplinary teams remains limited, underscoring the imperative for evidence from innovative strategies to enhance the effectiveness of patient care for those with inflammatory arthritis (Damgaard et al., 2023a).

The European Alliance of Associations for Rheumatology recommends implementation of self-management strategies in the treatment of people with inflammatory arthritis to enhance the empowerment of their own care (Nikiphorou et al., 2021). The recommendations on self-management strategies include promoting patient engagement, offering comprehensive education, integrating problem-solving and goal setting into routine care, advocating for physical activity and a healthy lifestyle, regularly assessing mental health, cognitive behavioural therapy, facilitating discussions about work, recognizing the potential of digital healthcare tools, and signposting patients to relevant resources of self-management (Nikiphorou et al., 2021).

Self-efficacy is closely connected to self-management and encompasses an individual's belief in their abilities to address specific challenges and achieve desired outcomes (Bandura, 1977b).

DOI: 10.1201/9781003599074-6

It influences goal selection, effort, and persistence, and is shaped by personal experiences, observing others, verbal encouragement, and emotional feedback, factors that vary depending on the context and task (Bandura, 1977b). Strengthening self-efficacy supports behaviour change and encourages active involvement in care (Bandura, 1977b), particularly when individuals perceive strategies as personally relevant and attainable (Bandura, 2004). This underscores the importance of designing rehabilitation interventions that not only support behavioural change, but also align with the individual's values and preferences. Therefore, such interventions should be based on a person-centred approach and shared decision-making which is a collaborative process between healthcare providers and patients to make informed choices (Elwyn et al., 2016). A person-centred approach is defined by tailoring interventions to the patient's values (Mccormack et al., 2015). Furthermore, rehabilitation is grounded in a biopsychosocial approach, and aims to optimize functioning and promote a meaningful life (World Health Organization, 2017). The World Health Organization defines it as a set of interventions that reduce disability and enhance functioning in interaction with the individual's environment (World Health Organization, 2017). This holistic perspective highlights the importance of strategies that are both clinically effective and personally relevant.

In the following, four rehabilitation interventions based on a self-management approach are described. The self-management approach in the interventions is based on Barlow et al.'s definition of self-management as the capacity to navigate the multifaceted challenges of chronic conditions, including symptom management and lifestyle adaptations (Barlow et al., 2002b). In addition, a person's ability to know when and how to access professional support if needed (Barlow et al., 2002b). Furthermore, all four interventions build upon a cognitive behavioural approach. The approach utilized is Acceptance and Commitment Therapy or Focused Acceptance and Commitment Therapy (Aisbett and Harris, 2010; Strosahl et al., 2012). Focused Acceptance and Commitment Therapy is a promising condensed version of the evidence-based approach Acceptance and Commitment Therapy, designed for clinical settings with time constraints (Strosahl et al., 2012). Both approaches emphasize support to lead a meaningful life despite variable symptoms like pain and fatigue. Acceptance and Commitment Therapy comprises six core processes:

1. Acceptance (acceptance of unchangeable life situations to conserve energy for pursuing what truly matters, rather than resisting what cannot be changed).
2. Cognitive defusion (to promote a flexible mindset by recognizing that thoughts are not facts and should not dictate behaviour).
3. Present-moment awareness (a neutral non-judging exploration of sensations and thoughts).
4. Self-as-context (a transcendent, observing perspective from which individuals can notice their thoughts, emotions, and experiences without feeling defined or limited by them)
5. Values identification (awareness of one's own life values and the extent to which one is living in alignment with them
6. Committed action (how to initiate a behaviour consciously aligned with one's life values

This approach aims to enhance psychological flexibility and collectively guide individuals in aligning their behaviours with their values despite adverse experiences (Aisbett and Harris, 2010; Strosahl et al., 2012).

The four interventions have been co-created based on the British Medical Research Council framework for developing and evaluating complex interventions (Skivington et al., 2024). The interventions synthesize insights gathered from the literature, theories, relevant stakeholders - including patient research partners - and a research team (Skivington et al., 2024).

THE FOUR INTERVENTIONS

INSELMA

In response to the need for an interdisciplinary coordinated approach to support self-management in people with inflammatory arthritis, we developed the Interdisciplinary Nurse-coordinated SELf-MAnagement (INSELMA) intervention (Primdahl et al., 2024) within the TASEMA – TArgeted SElf-MAnagement in People with Inflammatory Arthritis - programme. INSELMA is an outpatient rehabilitation offer focusing on self-management targeting people with inflammatory arthritis who experience substantial disease impact, despite the pharmacological treatment.

The INSELMA intervention aims to enhance peoples' self-management capabilities, self-efficacy, and quality of life while reducing the psychosocial and physical impacts of inflammatory arthritis. The research team comprised two rheumatologists, a physiotherapist, three nurses, and two patient research partners representing two hospitals and research units (Primdahl et al., 2024). The stakeholders involved in the co-creation encompassed rheumatologists, rheumatology nurses, physiotherapists, occupational therapists, a social worker, health professionals from various municipalities, researches, patient research partners and other patient representatives.

Apart from self-management, guiding theories to support the intervention are self-efficacy (Bandura, 1977b), Acceptance and Commitment Therapy (Aisbett and Harris, 2010) and health literacy (Bröder et al., 2018). Health literacy encompasses the personal competencies and situational resources necessary for individuals to access, comprehend, evaluate, and utilize health information and services (Bröder et al., 2018). Challenges with health literacy bear importance for specific aspects of self-management, i.e. adherence, communication and navigating the healthcare system (van der Gaag et al. 2022). Recently, challenges in health literacy have been found to be associated to poorer physical and mental health, poorer work outcomes, decreased chance of being on immune-modulating treatment and greater comorbidity burden in people with inflammatory arthritis (Dey et al., 2025).

The INSELMA Intervention

INSELMA is a Danish multicentre study. The intervention is structured as a six-month outpatient intervention. Each participant is paired with a coordinating rheumatology nurse who facilitates an initial consultation including a biopsychosocial assessment (Blum et al., 2025; Primdahl et al., 2024). Participants identify up to five significant daily activities that presents challenges for them in their everyday life, using the Patient Specific Functional Scale (Horn et al., 2012). The coordinating rheumatology nurse collaborates with the participant to establish short- and long-term goals, coordinate support from various professionals, including physiotherapists, occupational therapists and a social worker, to enhance self-management skills through communication strategies derived from Acceptance and Commitment Therapy and principles of health literacy. The intervention is depicted in Figure 5.1 (Blum et al., 2025).

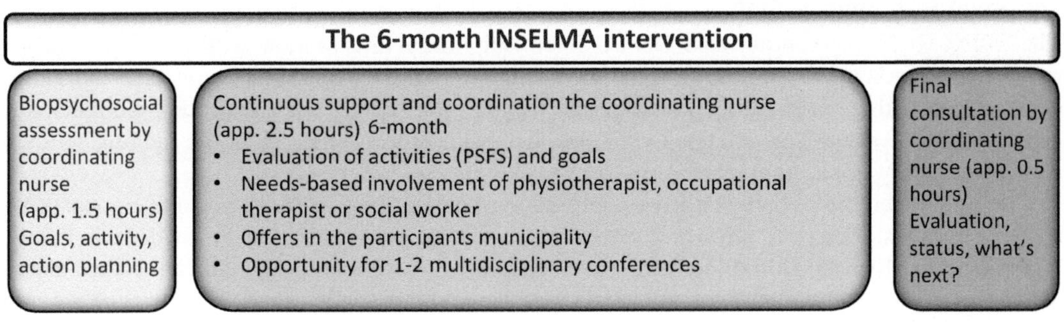

FIGURE 5.1 The six-month INSELMA intervention.

Each participant received approximately eight hours support during six months from the health professionals. We saw a tendency towards an increase in the participants' quality of life, mental well-being and self-efficacy, and a decrease in symptoms of anxiety, depression, fatigue, and pain (Blum et al., 2025). Individual interviews with participants revealed that they experienced the INSELMA intervention as a great opportunity to reduce long-held challenges, they had fought alone until now (Blum et al., 2024). They felt the intervention was adapted to their specific needs and considered the empathic and goal-oriented support from the same coordinating rheumatology nurse and from physiotherapists and occupational therapists, to be essential. This gave them renewed hope for the future. It was important for the participants with time in between consultations to work towards goals. Overall, the participants experienced decreased impact of their disease and an improved self-management ability (Blum et al., 2024). Interviews with the health professionals showed that they experienced the new roles and tasks as challenging in the beginning, but considered the INSELMA intervention to be meaningful and an opportunity to increase coherence in the patients' pathways (Madsen et al., 2025a). Based on these very positive results, we consider the intervention as feasible, meaningful and promising. At present, we aim to confirm these proof-of-concept findings in a larger randomized trial including a socioeconomic evaluation.

SPINCODE

Individuals with axial spondyloarthritis still face a substantial disease burden despite achievement of low disease activity (Liu et al., 2021) and people with non-radiographic axial spondyloarthritis present similar disease burden as people with radiographic axial spondyloarthritis (Mogard et al., 2020). This underscores the need for comprehensive rehabilitation programs with effective self-management strategies for people with chronic low back pain with suspected axial spondyloarthritis.

SPINCODE is an outpatient physiotherapist-coordinated rehabilitation intervention focusing on self-management in people with suspected axial spondyloarthritis. The overall aim of the SPINCODE intervention is to enhance health-related quality of life and improve daily activities considered troublesome by the patients, by providing goal-based tailored counselling and by enhancing physical activity and self-management.

The involved stakeholders in SPINCODE encompass the interdisciplinary team from the Danish Hospital for Rheumatic Diseases (two physiotherapists, one social worker, one occupational therapist, one nursing assistant, and two nurses, all with experience in rheumatology rehabilitation), physiotherapists from primary care, and patient research partners. The theories and approaches to support the intervention encompassed: (i) Self-management (Barlow et al., 2002a; Grady and Gough, 2014) and self-efficacy (Bandura, 1977a), (ii) Shared decision-making (Elwyn et al., 2017), a person-centred approach (Mccormack et al., 2015), and (iii) focused acceptance and commitment therapy (Strosahl et al., 2012).

The SPINCODE Intervention

The SPINCODE intervention is a Danish interdisciplinary intervention with a duration of six months conducted at the Danish Hospital for Rheumatic Diseases. It consists of three individual consultations with a coordinating physiotherapist, two group-based patient education seminars, and needs-based individual consultations with various health professionals from the interdisciplinary team (Figure 5.2) (Knak et al., 2024).

The aim of the three visits with the coordinating physiotherapist are to perform a biopsychosocial assessment, objective physical assessments, agree on goal setting, and provide individually tailored counselling guided by the theories. Additionally, the aim is to facilitate coherence across health professionals at the hospital and across healthcare sectors. The aims of the two group seminars are to promote peer learning and enhance the participants' self-management ability through patient education on axial spondyloarthritis, pharmacological treatment, exercise/physical activity,

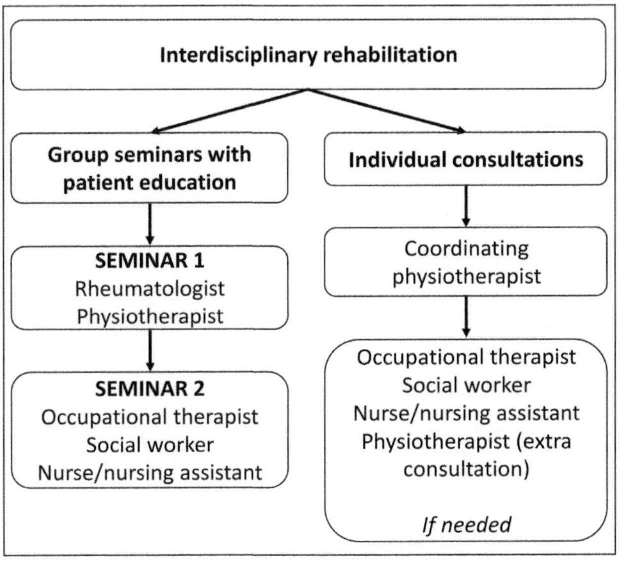

FIGURE 5.2 The SPINCODE intervention. (Knak et al., 2024)

and disease management in everyday life with a focus on work, daily activities, and energy management delivered by a physiotherapist, a rheumatologist, an occupational therapist, a nurse/nursing assistant, and a social worker. If needed, additional visits with the interdisciplinary team are possible with the aim of providing self-management support on physical activity and exercise (physiotherapist), work and daily activities (occupational therapist), pain, fatigue, sleep, and understanding of chronic disease (nurse/nursing assistant), and how to get additional support within the social, educational, and labour market areas (social worker) (in total, a maximum of six hours).

COMFI

Despite advances in pharmacological treatment, more than two thirds of people with inflammatory arthritis continue to experience a substantial and persistent burden of fatigue (Beckers et al., 2023). People with inflammatory arthritis frequently describe fatigue as overwhelming, unpredictable, difficult to manage and as deeply disruptive to everyday life including work, and participation in daily activities (Beckers et al., 2023). The need for support in managing fatigue and its far-reaching effects is requested by people with inflammatory arthritis (Dures et al., 2020). Beyond the personal toll, inflammatory arthritis-related fatigue contributes to limitations in physical activity and high levels of absenteeism and work disability, resulting in considerable economic and societal costs (Dures et al., 2020; Gwinnutt et al., 2020). This underlines the urgent need for effective, person-centred interventions to reduce the severity and impact of fatigue. Based on the 2023 recommendations from the European Alliance of Associations for Rheumatology for the management of fatigue, the management should include tailored physical activity and psycho-educational interventions (Dures et al., 2023). However, the effect of a group-based intervention combining a cognitive behavioural approach and physical activity has not been explored in people with inflammatory arthritis.

The COMbined Fatigue Intervention (COMFI) study is a multi-centre study conducted in Denmark and Sweden. The group-based outpatient COMFI combines physical activity and focused acceptance and commitment therapy. The overall aim of COMFI is to enhance self-management of fatigue and thus reduce fatigue severity and impact for people with inflammatory arthritis. The development of COMFI involved a wide range of stakeholders including patient research partners, patient representatives, relatives, health professionals, and researchers. Notably, five patient research partners were active members of the project group, ensuring that the patient perspective was incorporated throughout all phases of the project. COMFI was developed based on focused acceptance and commitment therapy, self-management principles, self-efficacy (Bandura, 1977a; Barlow et al., 2002a; Grady and Gough, 2014; Strosahl et al., 2012), and considerations related to group-based delivery.

The COMFI Intervention

The duration of COMFI is 24 weeks, and it consists of (Damgaard et al., 2025):

1. **Six group sessions over a period of 12 weeks** focusing on understanding and management of fatigue and related factors, management of physical activity, trying out physical activity recommended to reduce fatigue impact, mindfulness, energy management, and fostering peer support.
2. **A seventh booster session** in week 24 to reinforce learning and the process towards a value-based life.
3. **An optional individual session** is offered for tailored support.
4. **A support telephone line/online consultation** is available during weeks 13–23 to address ongoing challenges.
5. **Optional participation of relatives:** participants' relatives are invited to participate in group session one and six to enhance their understanding of fatigue, support the patient, and take care of themselves as a relative to a person experiencing fatigue. The relatives have the opportunity to attend both a session together with the patient participants and a secluded session with relatives only.

The intervention is visual presented in Figure 5.3.

Work-On

Up to 40% of people diagnosed with inflammatory arthritis lose their employment within the first few years following diagnosis (Sokka et al., 2010; Verstappen et al., 2010). The risk of unemployment is influenced by multiple factors, including prolonged sick leave, disease activity, type of job, individual characteristics, and socioeconomic status (Escorpizo et al., 2020). Once unemployed, people with inflammatory arthritis face reduced chances of re-entering the workforce (Boonen et al., 2022). Consequently, early identification of reduced work ability and implementation of targeted vocational rehabilitation close to the patient's everyday life is essential to help people with inflammatory arthritis maintain paid employment (Boonen et al., 2022; Kirkeskov and Bray, 2023).

Therefore, we developed and feasibility tested a six-month outpatient vocational rehabilitation intervention, WORK-ON, for people with inflammatory arthritis who consider themselves to be

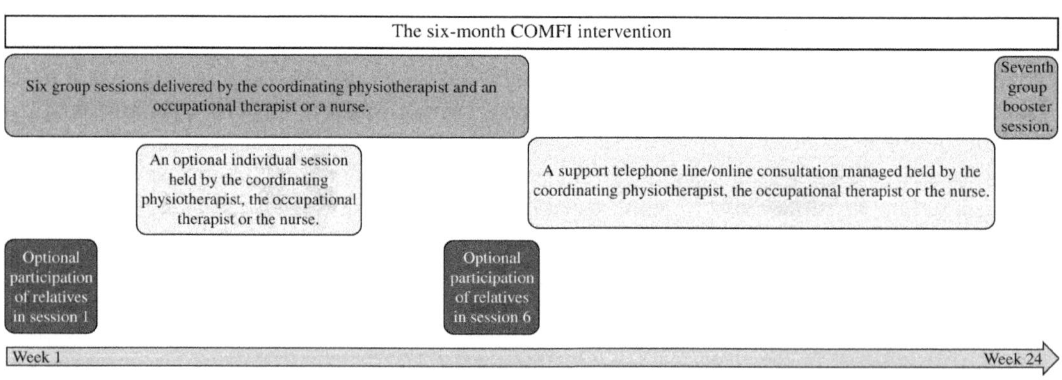

FIGURE 5.3 The COMFI intervention.

at risk of losing their job within the following two years (Madsen et al., 2023, 2024a). The aim of WORK-ON is to increase work ability, reduce sick leave, and prevent job loss.

The development of WORK-ON included a broad range of stakeholders such as patient research partners, occupational therapists, physiotherapists, a social worker, and nurses all holding extensive experience with rheumatology rehabilitation, researchers, and health professionals from municipality job centres. WORK-ON is based on self-management (Barlow et al., 2002a; Grady and Gough, 2014), shared decision-making (Elwyn et al., 2016), occupational balance (Eklund et al., 2017), and focused acceptance and commitment therapy (Aisbett and Harris, 2010; Strosahl et al., 2012). The WORK-ON intervention has been feasibility tested in 19 participants at the Danish Hospital for Rheumatic Diseases. WORK-ON was feasible to deliver and the participants were satisfied with the intervention. A process evaluation showed that the participants especially valued the continuity of health professionals throughout the six months of the intervention and the opportunity for peer support (Madsen et al., 2025b). The health professionals valued the opportunity for interdisciplinary cooperation through an extended time period. The self-management approach added an important aspect in the vocational rehabilitation to people with inflammatory arthritis in managing everyday life including work.

Before the present testing of the efficacy of the WORK-ON intervention in a randomized trial, the intervention was adapted by including a fourth group session and increased focus on fatigue management and employer involvement (Madsen et al., 2024b).

The Adjusted WORK-ON Intervention

The adjusted six-month WORK-ON intervention is tested in a single-centre randomized trial study in Denmark. The intervention consists of three parts: (1) an initial assessment and goal setting with a coordinating occupational therapist and, additional sessions with the coordinating occupational therapist for self-management support throughout the intervention for follow-up. (2) Four group sessions for peer support held by a social worker, a physiotherapist, an occupational therapist, and a nurse. (3) Need-based individual consultations with a physiotherapist, a nurse, and a social worker (Figure 5.4).

The coordinating occupational therapist assesses and guides the participants regarding potential need for hand exercises, small aids and bandages, and guidance on ergonomic positions in relation to work, pain and sleep. The participants are encouraged to involve their employer.

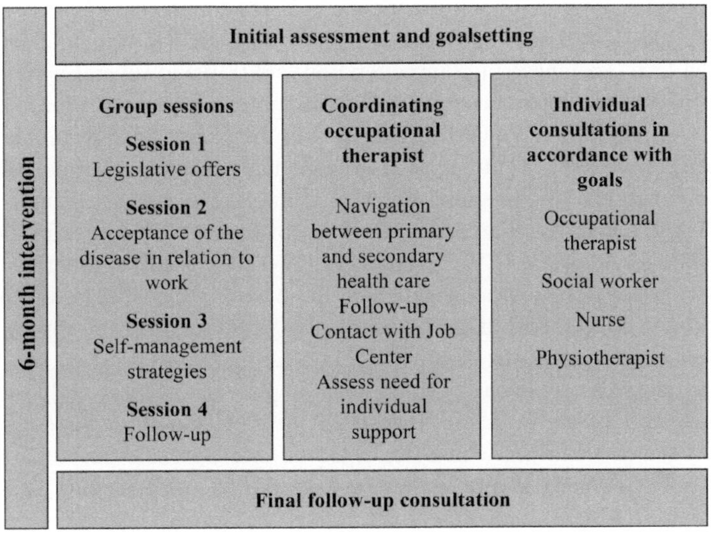

FIGURE 5.4 Content of WORK-ON. (Madsen et al., 2023)

A final follow-up consultation with the participant and relevant partners (e.g. social workers, consultants from the municipal jobcentre, employers, and relatives) are planned to evaluate and to discuss future needs for rehabilitation or self-management support. Six months after the final consultation, the coordinating occupational therapist and the participant have a follow-up consultation by phone.

DISCUSSION

The need for effective rehabilitation interventions that emphasize self-management for individuals with inflammatory arthritis is critical to support their biopsychosocial functioning, and facilitating participation in daily activities including work. This chapter aims to explore self-management within the context of novel rehabilitation interventions. Currently, the SPINCODE and COMFI interventions are undergoing feasibility testing. The INSELMA and WORK-ON interventions have completed the feasibility testing and demonstrated promising results. These interventions are now being evaluated for efficacy in larger randomized trials compared to a control group. While previous feasibility studies have yielded encouraging results, further investigation is essential to establish the efficacy of these interventions in larger randomized studies.

The four interventions described herein were developed in accordance with the British Medical Research Council's framework, which ensures systematic development, testing, adaption, and implementation of interventions in clinical practice (Skivington et al., 2024). Their development involved co-creation with relevant stakeholders, grounded in specific theoretical and conceptual approaches, and tested through in feasibility studies (INSELMA, WORK-ON, SPINCODE, and COMFI) prior to their inclusion in larger efficacy studies (INSELMA and WORK-ON). Although co-creation may seem to consume significant time and resources, this approach is expected to lead to effective interventions through co-creation, testing, and adaptation informed by relevant stakeholders, including patient research partners. Feasibility testing provides a vital opportunity to adapt interventions before testing in larger studies or broader implementation. Other approaches for co-creation, such as citizen science, participatory design, and action research, can also be considered (Citizen Science Association, 2016; Clark et al., 2020; Rothmann et al., 2016). The involvement of patient research partners adheres to the European Alliance of Associations for Rheumatology recommendations (de Wit et al., 2024) and the collaboration can be documented using the tool GRIPP 2 (Staniszewska et al., 2017).

As part of the implementation of self-management interventions, competence development and training of health professionals are important to ensure fidelity in delivering the intervention. Health professionals often face challenges in comprehending and utilising several new theories and tools while also providing self-management support. Furthermore, opportunities for feedback and supervision should be facilitated to enhance learning during the testing of novel interventions. Precise description and documentation of interventions is essential to ensure transparency, facilitate replication and broader application. The rehabilitation interventions presented have employed a self-management approach and have utilized the Template for Intervention Description and Replication (Hoffmann et al., 2014), and/or the PRECIS 2 tool (Loudon et al., 2015) to describe the interventions.

A person-centred approach, characterized by collaboration, shared decision-making and a biopsychosocial approach, is essential in the four described interventions to support the participants' self-management abilities and skills. Thus, the coordinating health professionals aim to agree on goals and plan the interventions in close collaboration with each participant based on the persons' values, preferences and needs in accordance with the Focused Acceptance and Commitment Therapy approach and goal setting which was Specific, Measureable, Achievable, Relevant, and Time-based (SMART) (Wade, 2009). However, negative attitudes among health professionals may impede participants' self-management efforts and adversely impact their self-efficacy, fostering feelings of blame or imposing unrealistic expectations regarding intervention outcomes (Bandura, 1977b).

To facilitate optimal shared decision-making and effective outcomes of self-management interventions, health literacy is highly relevant. Health literacy encompasses patients' ability to seek, understand, critically assess, and act upon health information (Kickbusch et al., 2013). A scoping review has underscored the importance of health literacy in self-management, specifically concerning medical management, patient-provider communication, and knowledge acquisition in patients with chronic diseases (van der Gaag et al., 2022). A focus on how to support the patients' health literacy will be necessary for further implementation in interventions based on a self-management approach. In the INSELMA intervention, the coordinating rheumatology nurse can utilize the Conversation of Health Literacy Tool (Jensen et al., 2021)to explore challenges in health literacy, guide participants toward resources, and facilitate their understanding and use of health-related information, thereby potentially addressing social inequities (Dey and Nikiphorou, 2025). Nonetheless, health professionals often encounter difficulties in identifying diverse patient profiles that present varying challenges in health literacy (Bakker et al., 2021, 2022).

Unfortunately, in many self-management studies, the self-management concept is not clearly defined (Damgaard et al., 2023b). As there is no agreement on a single definition of self-management, it is important to state what it includes as both an approach and outcome as it will affect the content and opportunity for replication. When this being said, there is a large variety in the use of outcome measures in studies on self-management and there is an urgent need to develop a core outcome set to measure self-management in rheumatology (Hansen et al., 2022). It may be difficult to measure self-management, therefore proxies for self-management are used such as the Pain Self-Efficacy Questionnaire (Errebo et al., 2024) or Self-Efficacy for Managing Chronic Disease 6-itemScale (Christiansen et al., 2023). It is important to consider self-efficacy not merely as an endpoint but as a mechanism that enables behavioural change; thus, self-management intervention outcomes frequently incorporate additional factors, including pain, fatigue, and overall quality of life (Hansen et al., 2022).

Apart from self-efficacy, self-management relates to other concepts such as self-care, self-monitoring, and symptom management (Richard and Shea, 2011). Self-care can be understood as a broad overall concept encompassing the other concepts and may be defined as activities to achieve, maintain, or promote maximum health (Richard and Shea, 2011). Self-monitoring is considered part of self-management and symptom management is considered part of self-management and self-monitoring if performed by the patient (Richard and Shea, 2011). In addition to Barlow's definition of self-management (Barlow et al., 2002a, 2002b), Wilkinson and Whitehead define self-management as "the ability of the individual, in conjunction with family, community, and health professionals, to manage symptoms, treatments, lifestyle changes, and psychosocial, cultural, and spiritual consequences of chronic diseases" (Wilkinson and Whitehead, 2009). This definition emphasizes the collaboration with health professionals, emphasizing that individuals should not bear the sole responsibility for managing their symptoms and challenges.

PERSPECTIVES

Looking ahead, the field of self-management in rehabilitation for inflammatory arthritis is increasingly shaped by the use of digital health technologies and individually tailored interventions (Barnett et al., 2023; Moe and Vliet Vlieland, 2024; Mollard and Michaud, 2021).

Self-management support in rehabilitation interventions signifies the integration of multi-dimensional data streams, including wearable sensor outputs, patient-reported outcomes, and psychosocial profiles (including health literacy), to deliver adaptive, personalized self-management interventions. Artificial intelligence-driven algorithms may assist in tailoring goal setting, monitoring adherence, and prompting early interventions when the disease burden increases. Online and physical environments hold potential for self-management support that addresses both physical and psychological dimensions of living with inflammatory arthritis (Vlad et al., 2025). Digital self-management interventions, such as mobile applications, web-based platforms, and wearable biosensors, are emerging as scalable solutions with proven utility in inflammatory arthritis (Mollard and Michaud, 2021). Mobile health applications in RA have been associated with reductions in disease activity and improvements in patient-reported outcomes, including pain and physical function (Mollard and Michaud, 2021). Future efforts should emphasize the application of self-management support, behavioural and motivational theories as part of application design, coupled with theoretically grounded co-design with patients to enhance usability and relevance (Barnett et al., 2023). Successful adoption of these innovations to facilitate self-management depends on their integration into coordinated, interdisciplinary care frameworks. The European Alliance of Associations for Rheumatology recognizes the possibility of digital health applications to empower self-management in individuals with inflammatory arthritis and has recommendations for the development, evaluation and implementation of digital health applications to foster self-management in this patient population (Najm et al., 2019). The European Alliance of Associations for Rheumatology has recommended the following points to consider (Najm et al., 2019):

- Applications need an overarching conceptual framework and adherence to data protection.
- Self-management applications must provide information that is current, scientifically valid, user-friendly, and evidence-based when relevant.
- Applications should be tailored to the individual's needs; relevant stakeholders including patients and health professionals, need to be involved in the development of applications.
- Applications need to be transparent, should not cause harm, and may support communication with health professionals.
- Applications should be generalizable to the general patient population, considerations if social network is embedded in the application, and cost-benefit considerations.

Self-management support as part of rehabilitation in rheumatology needs to evolve beyond isolated interventions towards collaboration across sectors and health professionals such as rheumatologists, physiotherapists, occupational therapists, social workers, and psychologists supported by digital records and shared outcome monitoring dashboards (Vlad et al., 2025).

Future research in self-management needs to focus on innovative designs and implementation strategies, with an emphasis on long-term effectiveness, equity, and scalability (Moe and Vliet Vlieland, 2024). Alternative trial designs (e.g. interrupted time series, hybrid effectiveness-implementation trials), mixed-methods, or process evaluations can elucidate how self-management interventions work, for whom, and under which contextual factors. Particular attention should be paid to health literacy, digital equity and access, especially among older adults or underserved populations, and to train health professionals' competencies in how to support patients with digital and organizational health literacy challenges and how to support behavioural change (Moe and Vliet Vlieland, 2024).

Together, all this points toward a future where self-management support for inflammatory arthritis is data-informed, participant-driven, and systemically embedded, enhancing long-term quality of life and functional autonomy for individuals with chronic inflammatory arthritis.

REFERENCES

Aisbett, B. & Harris, R. 2010. *Lykkefælden [The happiness trap].* Dansk Psykologisk Forlag.

Bakker, M. M., Putrik, P., Dikovec, C., Rademakers, J., Vonkeman, H. E., Kok, M. R., Voorneveld-Nieuwenhuis, H., Ramiro, S., De Wit, M., Buchbinder, R., Batterham, R., Osborne, R. H. & Boonen, A. 2022. Exploring discordance between health literacy questionnaire scores of people with RMDs and assessment by treating health professionals. *Rheumatology (Oxford)*, 62, 52–64.

Bakker, M. M., Putrik, P., Rademakers, J., Laar, M., Vonkeman, H., Kok, M. R., Voorneveld-Nieuwenhuis, H., Ramiro, S., Wit, M., Buchbinder, R., Batterham, R., Osborne, R. H. & Boonen, A. 2021. Addressing health literacy needs in rheumatology: Which patient health literacy profiles need the attention of health professionals? *Arthritis Care and Research (Hoboken)*, 73, 100–109.

Bandura, A. 1977a. Self-efficacy: toward a unifying theory of behavioral change. *Psychological Review*, 84, 191–215.

Bandura, A. 1977b. Self-efficacy: toward a unifying theory of behavioral change. *Psychological Review*, 84, 24.

Bandura, A. 2004. Health promotion by social cognitive means. *Health Education & Behavior*, 31, 143–164.

Barlow, J., Wright, C., Sheasby, J., Turner, A. & Hainsworth, J. 2002a. Self-management approaches for people with chronic conditions: a review. *Patient Education and Counseling*, 48, 177–187.

Barlow, J. H., Cullen, L. A. & Rowe, I. F. 2002b. Educational preferences, psychological well-being and self-efficacy among people with rheumatoid arthritis. *Patient Education and Counseling*, 46, 11–19.

Barnett, R., Clarke, C., Sengupta, R. & Rouse, P. C. 2023. Protocol for a systematic literature review of smartphone apps to support the self-management of rheumatic and musculoskeletal diseases: development strategies, theoretical underpinnings and barriers to engagement. *Systematic Reviews*, 12, 129.

Beckers, E., Hermans, K., Van Tubergen, A. & Boonen, A. 2023. Fatigue in patients with rheumatic and musculoskeletal diseases: a scoping review on definitions, measurement instruments, determinants, consequences and interventions. *RMD Open*, 9, e003056.

Blum, N. S., Esbensen, B. A., Bremander, A., Hendricks, O., Østergaard, M., Latocha, K. M., Andersen, L., Jensen, K. V. & Primdahl, J. 2025. Feasibility of INSELMA: an interdisciplinary nurse-coordinated self-management intervention for people with inflammatory arthritis and substantial disease impact. *EULAR Rheumatology Open*, 1, 137–146.

Blum, N. S., Esbensen, B. A., Østergaard, M., Bremander, A., Hendricks, O., Lindgren, L. H., Andersen, L., Jensen, K. V. & Primdahl, J. 2024. Patients' experience of a novel interdisciplinary nurse-led self-management intervention (INSELMA)—a qualitative evaluation. *BMC Rheumatology*, 8, 10–12.

Boonen, A., Webers, C., Butink, M., Barten, B., Betteridge, N., Black, D. C., Bremander, A., Boteva, B., Brzezińska, O., Chauhan, L., Copsey, S., Guimarães, V., Gignac, M., Glaysher, J., Green, F., Hoving, J. L., Marques, M. L., Smucrova, H., Stamm, T. A. & Verstappen, S. M. M. 2022. 2021 EULAR points to consider to support people with rheumatic and musculoskeletal diseases to participate in healthy and sustainable paid work. *Annals of the Rheumatic Diseases*, 82, 57–64.

Bröder, J., Chang, P., Kickbusch, I., Dlevin-Zanin, D., Mcelhinney, E., Nutbeam, D., Okar, O., Osborne, R., Pelikan, J., Rotman, I., Rowlands, G., Nunes-Saoga, L., Simmons, R., Sørensen, K., van der Brouck, S., Velardo, S. & Wills, J. 2018. IUHPE position statement on health literacy: a practical vision for a health literate world. *Global Health Promotion*, 25, 9.

Christiansen, M. G., Lund-Jacobsen, T., Jarden, M., Pappot, H. & Piil, K. 2023. Danish translation and linguistic validation of a self-efficacy questionnaire. *Danish Medical Journal*, 70, A09220682.

Citizen Science Association, I. B. 2016. *Citizen science: theory and practice*. Ubiquity Press.

Clark, J. S., Porath, S., Thiele, J. & Jobe, M. 2020. *Action research*. New Prairie Press.

Damgaard, A., Dures, E., Bremander, A., Lindqvist, E., Mogard, E., Knak, K., Krarup, H., Graversgaard, J. & Primdahl, J. 2025. OP0112-HPR THE DEVELOPMENT OF A COMBINED FATIGUE INTERVENTION (COMFI) FOR PEOPLE WITH INFLAMMATORY ARTHRITIS. *Annals of the Rheumatic Diseases*, 84, 100.

Damgaard, A. J., Primdahl, J., Esbensen, B. A., Latocha, K. M. & Bremander, A. 2023a. Self-management support needs of patients with inflammatory arthritis and the content of self-management interventions: a scoping review. *Seminars in Arthritis and Rheumatism*, 60, 152203.

Damgaard, A. J., Primdahl, J., Esbensen, B. A., Latocha, K. M. & Bremander, A. 2023b. Self-management support needs of patients with inflammatory arthritis and the content of self-management interventions: a scoping review. *Seminars in Arthritis and Rheumatism*, 60, 152203–152203.

de Wit, M., Aouad, K., Elhai, M., Benavent, D., Bertheussen, H., Blackburn, S., Böhm, P., Duarte, C., Falahee, M., Karlfeldt, S., Kiltz, U., Mateus, E. F., Richards, D. P., Rodríguez-Carrio, J., Sagen, J., Shumnalieva, R., Stones, S. R., Tas, S. W., Tillett, W., Vieira, A., Wilhelmer, T.-C., Zabalan, C., Primdahl, J., Studenic, P. & Gossec, L. 2024. EULAR recommendations for the involvement of patient research partners in rheumatology research: 2023 update. *Annals of the Rheumatic Diseases*, 83(11), 1443–1453.

Dey, M. & Nikiphorou, E. 2025. Health equity and causes of disparities in rheumatological management. *Joint Bone Spine*, 92, 105902.

Dey, M., Norton, S., Cope, A., Buch, M., Osborne, R., Galloway, J. & Nikiphorou, E. 2025. Health literacy associates with clinical, treatment and work status in people with inflammatory arthritis: results from a national cohort. *Annals of the Rheumatic Diseases*, 84(Suppl. 1), 23–24. EULAR. doi: 10.1016/j.ard.2025.08.018

Dures, E., Cramp, F., Hackett, K. & Primdahl, J. 2020. Fatigue in inflammatory arthritis. *Best Practice and Research Clinical Rheumatology*, 34, 101526.

Dures, E., Farisoğullari, B., Santos, E. J. F., Molto, A., Feldthusen, C., Harris, C., Elling-Audersch, C., Connolly, D., Elefante, E., Estévez-López, F., Bini, I., Primdahl, J., Hoeper, K., Urban, M., Van De Laar, M. A. F. J., Redondo, M., Böhm, P., Amarnani, R., Hayward, R. & Machado, P. M.. 2023. 2023 EULAR recommendations for the management of fatigue in people with inflammatory rheumatic and musculoskeletal diseases. *Annals of the Rheumatic Diseases*, 83(10), 1260–1267.

Eklund, M., Orban, K., Argentzell, E., Bejerholm, U., Tjörnstrand, C., Erlandsson, L.-K. & Håkansson, C. 2017. The linkage between patterns of daily occupations and occupational balance: applications within occupational science and occupational therapy practice. *Scandinavian Journal of Occupational Therapy*, 24*(1)*, 41–56.

Elwyn, G., Durand, M. A., Song, J., Aarts, J., Barr, P. J., Berger, Z., Cochran, N., Frosch, D., Galasiński, D., Gulbrandsen, P., Han, P. K. J., Härter, M., Kinnersley, P., Lloyd, A., Mishra, M., Perestelo-Perez, L., Scholl, I., Tomori, K., Trevena, L. & Van Der Weijden, T. 2017. A three-talk model for shared decision making: multistage consultation process. *BMJ: British Medical Journal*, 359, j4891.

Elwyn, G., Frosch, D. L. & Kobrin, S. 2016. Implementing shared decision-making: consider all the consequences. *Implementation Science*, 11, 114.

Errebo, M., Oxfeldt, M., Tegner, H. & Christensen, J. 2024. Psychometric evaluation of the Danish version of the Pain Self-Efficacy Questionnaire in patients with subacute and chronic low back pain. *Scandinavian Journal of Pain*, 24(1), 20240032.

Escorpizo, R., Burghardt, E. & Richards, C. 2020. Type of job, personal factors, and disease status are important contextual factors when measuring worker productivity in people with arthritis: a Delphi study. *Disability and Rehabilitation*, 42, 3496–3503.

Finckh, A., Gilbert, B., Hodkinson, B., Bae, S.-C., Thomas, R., Deane, K. D., Alpizar-Rodriguez, D. & Lauper, K. 2022. Global epidemiology of rheumatoid arthritis. *Nature Reviews Rheumatology*, 18, 591–602.

Grady, P. A. & Gough, L. L. 2014. Self-management: a comprehensive approach to management of chronic conditions. *American Journal of Public Health (1971)*, 104, e25–e31.

Gwinnutt, J. M., Leggett, S., Lunt, M., Barton, A., Hyrich, K. L., Walker-Bone, K., Verstappen, S. M., Rams & Co-Investigators, B. 2020. Predictors of presenteeism, absenteeism and job loss in patients commencing methotrexate or biologic therapy for rheumatoid arthritis. *Rheumatology*, 59, 2908–2919.

Hansen, C. W., Esbensen, B. A., De Thurah, A., Christensen, R., De Wit, M. & Cromhout, P. F. 2022. Outcome measures in rheumatology applied in self-management interventions targeting people with inflammatory arthritis: a systematic review of outcome domains and measurement instruments. *Seminars in Arthritis and Rheumatism*, 54, 151995.

Hider, S. L., Muller, S., Helliwell, T., Prior, J. A., Scott, I., Lawton, S. A., Zwierska, I., van Schaardenburg, D., van der Helm-Van Mil, A., Raza, K. & Mallen, C. D. 2019. Symptoms associated with inflammatory arthritis are common in the primary care population: results from the joint symptoms survey. *Rheumatology (Oxford)*, 58, 2009–2014.

Hoffmann, T. C., Glasziou, P. P., Boutron, I., Milne, R., Perera, R., Moher, D., Altman, D. G., Barbour, V., Macdonald, H., Johnston, M., Lamb, S. E., Dixon-Woods, M., Mcculloch, P., Wyatt, J. C., Chan, A.-W. & Michie, S. 2014. Better reporting of interventions: Template for intervention description and replication (TIDieR) checklist and guide. *BMJ: British Medical Journal*, 348, g1687–g1687.

Horn, K. K., Jennings, S., Richardson, G., Vliet, D. V., Hefford, C. & Abbott, J. H. 2012. The patient-specific functional scale: Psychometrics, clinimetrics, and application as a clinical outcome measure. *Journal of Orthopaedic and Sports Physical Therapy*, 42, 30–42.

Ishida, M., Kuroiwa, Y., Yoshida, E., Sato, M., Krupa, D., Henry, N., Ikeda, K. & Kaneko, Y. 2018a. Residual symptoms and disease burden among patients with rheumatoid arthritis in remission or low disease activity: a systematic literature review. *Modern Rheumatology*, 28, 789–799.

Ishida, M., Kuroiwa, Y., Yoshida, E., Sato, M., Krupa, D., Henry, N., Ikeda, K. & Kaneko, Y. 2018b. Residual symptoms and disease burden among patients with rheumatoid arthritis in remission or low disease activity: a systematic literature review. *Modern Rheumatology*, 28, 789–799.

Jensen, N. H., Aaby, A., Ryom, K. & Maindal, H. T. 2021. A CHAT about health literacy – a qualitative feasibility study of the Conversational Health Literacy Assessment Tool (CHAT) in a Danish municipal healthcare centre. *Scandinavian Journal of Caring Sciences*, 35, 1250–1258.

Kickbusch, I., Pelikan, J. M., Tsouros, F. A. & Agis, D. 2013. *Health literacy: the solid facts*. World Health Organization Regional Office for Europe.

Kirkeskov, L. & Bray, K. 2023. Employment of patients with rheumatoid arthritis – a systematic review and meta-analysis. *BMC Rheumatology*, 7, 41–41.

Knak, K. L., Primdahl, J., Kröber, G., Fongen, C., Graversgaard, J. & Bremander, A. 2024. Development of a physiotherapist-coordinated interdisciplinary rehabilitation intervention for people with suspected axial spondyloarthritis: The SPINCODE rehabilitation intervention. *Journal of Clinical Medicine*, 13, 1234.

Liu, V., Fong, W., Kwan, Y. H. & Leung, Y. Y. 2021. Residual disease burden in patients with axial spondyloarthritis and psoriatic arthritis despite low disease activity States in a multiethnic Asian population. *The Journal of Rheumatology*, 48, 677–684.

Loudon, K., Treweek, S., Sullivan, F., Donnan, P., Thorpe, K. E. & Zwarenstein, M. 2015. The PRECIS-2 tool: designing trials that are fit for purpose. *BMJ: British Medical Journal*, 350, h2147.

Madsen, C. M. T., Christensen, J. R., Bremander, A., Eggen, L. & Primdahl, J. 2024a. Feasibility test of WORK-ON: a vocational rehabilitation intervention for people with chronic inflammatory arthritis. *BMC Musculoskeletal Disorders*, 25, 755.

Madsen, C. M. T., Esbensen, B. A., Blum, N. S., Rønne, P. F., Bremander, A., Hendricks, O., Østergaard, M., Andersen, L. & Primdahl, J. 2025a. Health professionals' experiences delivering an interdisciplinary nurse-coordinated self-management intervention for patients with inflammatory arthritis. *Disability and Rehabilitation*, 47(22), 5905–5913.

Madsen, C. M. T., Knak, K. L., Bremander, A. & Primdahl, J. 2025b. Patients' experiences on participating in WORK-ON – a vocational rehabilitation intervention. *Annals of the Rheumatic Diseases*, 84, 1468.

Madsen, C. M. T., Primdahl, J., Bremander, A., Eggen, L. & Christensen, J. R. 2023. Developing a complex vocational rehabilitation intervention for patients with inflammatory arthritis: the WORK-ON study. *BMC Health Services Research*, 23(1), 739. doi: 10.1186/s12913-023-09780-2.PMID: 37422649

Madsen, C. M. T., Primdahl, J. & Christensen, J. R. 2024b. Testing the efficacy of WORK-ON: vocational rehabilitation for people with chronic inflammatory arthritis in Denmark—protocol for a randomised controlled trial. *BMJ Open*, 14, e089050.

Mccormack, B., Borg, M., Cardiff, S., Dewing, J., Jacobs, G., Janes, N., Karlsson, B., Mccance, T., Mekki, T. E. & Porock, D. 2015. Person-centredness-the 'state'of the art. *International Practice Development Journal*, 5, 1.

Moe, R. H. & Vliet Vlieland, T. P. M. 2024. Current and future challenges for rehabilitation for inflammatory arthritis. *Journal of Clinical Medicine*, 13, 1808.

Mogard, E., Olofsson, T., Bergman, S., Bremander, A., Kristensen, L. E., Kvistgaard Olsen, J., Wallman, J. K. & Lindqvist, E. 2020. Chronic pain and assessment of pain sensitivity in patients with axial spondyloarthritis: Results from the SPARTAKUS cohort. *The Journal of Rheumatology*, 47(10), 1521–1528.

Mollard, E. & Michaud, K. 2021. Self-management of rheumatoid arthritis: mobile applications. *Current Rheumatology Reports*, 23, 2.

Najm, A., Nikiphorou, E., Kostine, M., Richez, C., Pauling, J. D., Finckh, A., Ritschl, V., Prior, Y., Balážová, P., Stones, S., Szekanecz, Z., Iagnocco, A., Ramiro, S., Sivera, F., Dougados, M., Carmona, L., Burmester, G., Wiek, D., Gossec, L. & Berenbaum, F. 2019. EULAR points to consider for the development, evaluation and implementation of mobile health applications aiding self-management in people living with rheumatic and musculoskeletal diseases. *RMD Open*, 5, e001014.

Nikiphorou, E., Santos, E. J. F., Marques, A., Böhm, P., Bijlsma, J. W., Daien, C. I., Esbensen, B. A., Ferreira, R. J. O., Fragoulis, G. E., Holmes, P., Mcbain, H., Metsios, G. S., Moe, R. H., Stamm, T. A., De Thurah, A., Zabalan, C., Carmona, L. & Bosworth, A. 2021. 2021 EULAR recommendations for the implementation of self-management strategies in patients with inflammatory arthritis. *Annals of the Rheumatic Diseases*, 80, 1278–1285.

Primdahl, J., Bremander, A., Hendricks, O., Østergaard, M., Latocha, K. M., Andersen, L., Jensen, K. V. & Esbensen, B. A. 2024. Development of a complex interdisciplinary nurse-coordinated SELf-MAnagement (INSELMA) intervention for patients with inflammatory arthritis. *BMC Health Services Research*, 24, 87.

Primdahl, J., Hegelund, A., Lorenzen, A. G., Loeppenthin, K., Dures, E. & Appel Esbensen, B. 2019. The experience of people with rheumatoid arthritis living with fatigue: a qualitative metasynthesis. *BMJ Open*, 9, e024338.

Richard, A. A. & Shea, K. 2011. Delineation of self-care and associated concepts. *Journal of Nursing Scholarship*, 43, 255–264.

Rothmann, M. J., Danbjørg, D. B., Myhre Jensen & Clemensen, J. 2016. Participatory design in health care – participation, power and knowledge. *Proceedings of the 14th Participatory Design Conference*, 2, 127–128. doi: 10.1145/2948076.294810

Scotti, L., Franchi, M., Marchesoni, A. & Corrao, G. 2018. Prevalence and incidence of psoriatic arthritis: a systematic review and meta-analysis. *Seminars in Arthritis and Rheumatism*, 48, 28–34.

Sieper, J. & Poddubnyy, D. 2017. Axial spondyloarthritis. *Lancet*, 390, 73–84.

Skivington, K., Craig, N., Craig, P., Rycroft-Malone, J., Matthews, L., Simpson, S. A. & Moore, L. 2024. Introducing the revised framework for developing and evaluating complex interventions: a challenge and a resource for nursing research. *International Journal of Nursing Studies*, 154, 104748.

Smolen, J. S. 2016. Treat-to-target as an approach in inflammatory arthritis. *Current Opinion in Rheumatology*, 28, 297–302.

Smolen, J. S., Aletaha, D., Barton, A., Burmester, G. R., Emery, P., Firestein, G. S., Kavanaugh, A., Mcinnes, I. B., Solomon, D. H., Strand, V. & Yamamoto, K. 2018. Rheumatoid arthritis. *Nature Reviews Disease Primers*, 4, 18001.

Smolen, J. S., Braun, J., Dougados, M., Emery, P., Fitzgerald, O., Helliwell, P., Kavanaugh, A., Kvien, T. K., Landewe, R., Luger, T., Mease, P., Olivieri, I., Reveille, J., Ritchlin, C., Rudwaleit, M., Schoels, M., Sieper, J., Wit, M., Baraliakos, X. & van der Heijde, D. 2014. Treating spondyloarthritis, including ankylosing spondylitis and psoriatic arthritis, to target: recommendations of an international task force. *Annals of the Rheumatic Diseases*, 73, 6–16.

Sokka, T., Kautiainen, H., Pincus, T., Verstappen, S. M. M., Aggarwal, A., Alten, R., Andersone, D., Badsha, H., Baecklund, E., Belmonte, M., Craig-Müller, J., Da Mota, L. M. H., Dimic, A., Fathi, N. A., Ferraccioli, G., Fukuda, W., Géher, P., Gogus, F. & Hajjaj-Hassouni, N. 2010. Work disability remains a major problem in rheumatoid arthritis in the 2000s: data from 32 countries in the QUEST-RA study. *Arthritis Research and Therapy*, 12, R42.

Staniszewska, S., Brett, J., Simera, I., Seers, K., Mockford, C., Goodlad, S., Altman, D. G., Moher, D., Barber, R., Denegri, S., Entwistle, A., Littlejohns, P., Morris, C., Suleman, R., Thomas, V. & TYSALL, C. 2017. GRIPP2 reporting checklists: tools to improve reporting of patient and public involvement in research. *BMJ (Online)*, 358, j3453.

Strosahl, K. D., Robinson, P. J. & Gustavsson, T. 2012. *Brief interventions for radical change: principles and practice of focused acceptance and commitment therapy*. New Harbinger Publications.

van der Gaag, M., Heijmans, M., Spoiala, C. & Rademakers, J. 2022. The importance of health literacy for self-management: a scoping review of reviews. *Chronic Illness*, 18, 234–254.

Verstappen, S. M. M., Watson, K. D., Lunt, M., Mcgrother, K., Symmons, D. P. M., Hyrich, K. L., Register, B. S. R. B. & On Behalf Of The, B. S. R. B. R. 2010. Working status in patients with rheumatoid arthritis, ankylosing spondylitis and psoriatic arthritis: results from the British Society for Rheumatology Biologics Register. *Rheumatology*, 49, 1570–1577. doi: 10.1136/ard-2022-222678

Vlad, A. L., Popazu, C., Lescai, A.-M., Voinescu, D. C. & Baltă, A. A. Ș. 2025. Where do we stand in the management of rheumatoid arthritis ahead of EULAR/ACR 2025? *Clinical Practice*, 15(6), 103.

Wade, D. T. 2009. Goal setting in rehabilitation: an overview of what, why and how. *Clinical Rehabilitation*, 23, 291–295.

Wilkinson, A. & Whitehead, L. 2009. Evolution of the concept of self-care and implications for nurses: a literature review. *International Journal of Nursing Studies*, 46(8), 1143–1147.

World Health Organization. 2017. *Rehabilitation in health systems*. World Health Organization.

6 Supportive Self-Management and Stroke

Frances Horgan, Olive Lennon, Mary O'Neill,
Sarah-Jane Byrne, Patricia Hall, Geraldine O'Callaghan,
Molly Manning, Anne Hickey, and Clíodhna Ní Bhroin

INTRODUCTION

STROKE

A stroke is the commonest cause of adult-acquired long-term disability internationally and can affect someone physically, emotionally, cognitively, and socially (INAS 2020/SAFE 2020). It can rob people of the power of speech, sight, and swallow; can cause paralysis, incontinence, and life-long dependency on others to carry out the smallest, most personal tasks. Even mild or moderate stroke can result in complex physical, communication, cognitive, and psychological difficulties with life changing impact. The societal costs of stroke are significant with disability-related healthcare costs after stroke in Europe estimated at €15.9 billion (35% of the total stroke costs) and additional productivity losses estimated at €4 billion (Wafa et al., 2020). Numbers of people living with the consequences of stroke are ever growing and the need for effective management strategies is critical. By 2035, a 34% increase in total stroke events in the European Union (EU) is expected, and by 2047, a 27% rise in prevalent cases in the community is projected (Steven et al., 2017).

The European Stroke Organisation (ESO) Action Plan for Stroke 2018–2030 outlines a range of supports adults need after stroke that build on existing national strategies and guidelines for stroke management (National Clinical Guidelines for Stroke for UK and Ireland, 2023). These span emergency care and acute management of stroke (including thrombolysis), access to multi-disciplinary team (MDT) management, and early rehabilitation in organised stroke units to longer-term care. Follow-on care encompasses a documented plan for community rehabilitation, self-management support for all stroke patients with residual difficulties and their carers on discharge from hospital and follow-up reviews of rehabilitation and other needs at three to six months and annually thereafter (European Stroke Organisation https://actionplan.eso-stroke.org/domains/stroke-rehabilitation). High-quality evidence suggests self-management, in the context of rehabilitation delivered soon after the stroke event, results in short-term (< 1 year) improvements in basic and extended activities of daily living, and a reduction in poor outcomes (dependence/death), with further evidence that problem-solving interventions can facilitate reintegration into the community (Parke et al., 2015).

Importantly, self-management is highlighted as a research and development priority for longer-term rehabilitation after stroke (Norrving et al., 2018). This is a period where stroke survivors and their families are known to use trial and error in everyday activities to co-construct a new life after stroke, a strategy that tests their self-management capabilities and skills (Satink et al., 2016).

Many un-met needs are evidenced at this time (McKevitt et al., 2011) most notably associated with social and emotional matters (Moura et al., 2023). Stroke survivors frequently report feeling "abandoned" after leaving hospital and "falling off a cliff edge" with few formal community-based supports available despite wide-ranging, complex, ongoing or changing needs (Abrahamson and Wilson, 2019). During this time, family members often become carers by default, providing unseen and unacknowledged support during recovery (Woodford et al., 2018), often without knowledge, training or support that causes extensive stress on relationships, employment, and finances

DOI: 10.1201/9781003599074-7

(Moura et al., 2023). Fragmentation of rehabilitation services or lack of access when combined with limited understanding of the needs and wishes of stroke survivors and those of their caregivers can curb their rehabilitation and self-management potential (Hartford et al., 2019). Good communication and collaboration systems between hospital and community stakeholders helps to build bridges between services that enhances the continuum of care and work towards ongoing community solutions (Yang et al., 2022).

STROKE AND SELF-MANAGEMENT

While the goal of self-management can be broadly defined as: "The actions individuals and caregivers take for themselves, their children, their families and others to maintain good physical and mental health; meet social and psychological needs; prevent illness or accidents; care for minor ailments and long-term conditions; and maintain health and wellbeing after an acute illness or discharge from hospital" (UK Department of Health, 2005), stroke is a sudden occurrence with significant consequences and requires considerable adjustment after the event. In this way it can differ from other long-term conditions and their self-management and is required to dovetail with active rehabilitation. In its simplest form, supporting self-management in stroke rehabilitation involves educating people about their condition, how to manage the effects of their stroke and motivating them to be able to look after themselves to the best of their ability (Hancock et al., 2023) and helping people to understand the risk of stroke recurrence and to make healthy lifestyle choices (Lennon et al., 2021). However, this is challenging to enact. It requires an enabling healthcare system with flexibility to meet needs that emerge over time for stroke survivors (Jones et al., 2017), that supports decision-making, and integrates self-management into a broader, personalised care model using person-centred approaches, education and training on stroke management, access to health data, and connections to support networks including family and peer support and health coaching to build knowledge, skills, and confidence (Smets et al., 2024; Satink et al., 2016) during the rehabilitation journey and in everyday life after stroke. Thus, self-management in stroke should be understood within a framework of supported self-management (SSM) where rehabilitation does not end and self-management begins but rather it evolves as a dynamic partnership that values the person's agency while providing tailored supports to optimise their independence.

Supported self-management (SSM) in stroke is commonly underpinned by social cognitive theory. This foregrounds the concept of self-efficacy, a concept described as a person's belief in their ability to succeed (Bandura, 1991), as broadly applicable to both rehabilitation and condition management contexts. In rehabilitation, this includes developing problem-solving skills, setting and working toward meaningful goals, managing setbacks, and sustaining motivation throughout what is often an unpredictable recovery trajectory (Jones et al., 2017; Jones and Brimicombe, 2014). The Bridges self-management programme in stroke is one such example that incorporates supported self-management into rehabilitation and supports shared decision making. It uses a whole system approach requiring three core elements: (1) the uniqueness of each person with stroke is considered; (2) staff are trained with specialist skills; and (3) the organisation supports the self-management ethos (Jones and Brimicombe, 2014). The latter is important as integrating individual models of supported self-management in everyday care requires organisational leadership and change (Hancock et al., 2023).

Stroke survivors are typically introduced to the concept of supported self-management when they are medically stable and rehabilitation begins, ideally in a specialist, stroke-specific rehabilitation unit and/or an early supported discharge (ESD) team to maximise recovery potential through multidisciplinary care. In preparing for discharge, patients and their family support network need to have already built foundational self-management skills to be well-prepared for assuming greater levels of responsibility in overseeing all aspects of the condition. This requires enhanced communication and support during the transition from hospital to home, including onward referrals to help individuals "live well after stroke" by continuing to address ongoing needs, promote recovery and independence and improve their outcomes (National Stroke Strategy 2022–2027, Health Service Executive (HSE) of Ireland).

PROBLEMATISING SELF-MANAGEMENT AS A CONCEPT IN STROKE

The language of self-management is important. The term itself "self-management" can suggest a solitary process where a person is left to manage alone, without recognising the need for ongoing support and partnership. Using terms like "teaching people to self-manage" speaks to directive paternalistic practices rather than personalised models of care with shared emphasis on improving the knowledge, skills, and confidence of people to live well and manage their condition. Suggesting outcomes from self-management such as "people looking after themselves better" has judgemental connotations, implying the person with stroke is not managing well and "could do better".

Issues of equity are also critical to the successful design and implementation of supported self-management and to achieving positive health outcomes after stroke. Therefore, supported self-management intervention design must consider the influence of social determinants such as health literacy, socio-economic status, language, and culture, all of which shape an individual's capacity and resources to engage with SSM and navigate stroke support systems with autonomy (Hale et al., 2022; van der Gaag et al., 2005).

The concept of treatment burden, defined as the workload of healthcare for patients and its impact on well-being, is particularly relevant in stroke care (Gallacher et al., 2013). Stroke survivors often face significant demands in managing their condition, including understanding symptoms, setting goals, managing emotions, interacting with professionals and social networks, attending appointments, adhering to medications, adjusting psychologically, managing finances, and coordinating home care (Gallacher et al., 2013, 2018). This burden is exacerbated by fragmented care, poor communication, lack of psychosocial support, inaccessible information, inadequate signposting, paternalistic practices, and poor continuity of care (Gallacher et al., 2013, 2018). Broader life demands and environmental factors also influence the experience of treatment burden and these can shift dynamically over time (Gallacher et al., 2018).

Treatment burden and self-management capacity are strongly shaped by how services are provided and must be accounted for in self-management interventions (Gallacher et al., 2018). Working within constrained stroke rehabilitation services can limit clinicians' ability to deliver effective and personalised SSM, and organisational cultural shifts are needed to create the conditions that support both patients and healthcare providers (Kidd et al., 2024). Real-world implementation must therefore be considered not only at the level of patient-practitioner interactions but also in terms of broader systemic factors. Certain groups including ethnic minorities and people with post-stroke aphasia (language problems after stroke) or cognitive difficulties experience inequities in care delivery and/or poorer outcomes post-stroke (Emmett et al., 2025; Fluck et al., 2023; Hilari, 2011; Thompson et al., 2022).

ETHNICITY

Ethnic minority status is frequently associated with poorer outcomes post-stroke, and the dominant Western biomedical model of stroke rehabilitation often fails to accommodate diverse cultural perspectives (Emmett et al., 2025; Hale et al., 2022; Thompson et al., 2022). The concept of "self"-management may additionally conflict with the values of collectivist cultures, where health decisions are made within the context of family or community (Hale et al., 2022).

APHASIA

People with aphasia are commonly excluded from stroke related research, including SSM interventions, negatively impacting the external validity of the evidence generated (Brady et al., 2013; Shiggins et al., 2024; Vaughan and Manning, 2023; Wray et al., 2018). Given the complex and pervasive psychosocial ramifications of aphasia, SSM interventions may require additional attention to communication strategies, psychological wellbeing, social identity, and relationships. A number of SSM programmes are under development and evaluation. For example, The Living with Aphasia programme, has been co-produced with people with lived experience and clinicians, and is underpinned by behaviour change theory communication (Wray et al., 2021, 2025). It incorporates clinician training and an implementation toolkit; information for friends and family members including communication and coping strategies and signposting to additional support services; and an accessible guide for people with aphasia including stories from other people with aphasia, and strategies for managing low mood, fatigue and communication (Wray et al., 2021, 2025). The intervention additionally emphasises active goal setting, reflection and planning by the person with aphasia (Wray et al., 2025).

Cognitive Impairment

Post-stroke cognitive impairment (PSCI) is common (Mellon et al., 2015; Sexton et al., 2021), and approximately 10% of stroke survivors go on to develop new dementia in the first year after stroke (El Husseini et al., 2023; Kuźma et al., 2018; Pendlebury and Rothwell, 2009). PSCI typically affects several domains with resulting attention and concentration difficulties, memory impairment, executive dysfunction, fatigue, and mood disturbance. These can compromise someone's capacity to take on responsibility for day-to-day management of care, including medication adherence, monitoring symptoms, managing comorbidity, engagement with healthcare appointments, and engagement with rehabilitation. These self-management activities involve memory, problem-solving, interacting with healthcare providers and decision-making (Schmaderer et al., 2021). Data suggest that stroke survivors with PSCI receive considerable support from family members and caregivers with self-management tasks (e.g., taking medications) (Rohde et al., 2017), with higher levels of reported carer burden (Atteih et al., 2015; Dankner et al., 2016; Rohde et al., 2019). There is a dearth of research on promoting and supporting self-management in stroke survivors with PSCI, with many excluded from studies of self-management supports (Klockar et al., 2023; Sun et al., 2022). Strategies recommended to support stroke survivors with PSCI engage in self-management activities are largely drawn from those developed for people with dementia (Rees et al., 2021) and include management of fatigue and emotional well-being, tailored goal-setting, specific strategies for improving memory, attention, and executive function (Dobe et al., 2023; Moran et al., 2025), simplifying routines, integrating the use of memory aids and assistive technologies in day-to-day self-management activities, and building in support from others (e.g., family members) where needed.

CLÍODHNA'S STORY

Clíodhna is a co-author of this chapter and a Patient and Public Involvement (PPI) representative across several research projects addressing stroke care and ongoing support pathways to enable survivors to live a meaningful life after stroke. Clíodhna's story of lived experience of supported self-management in stroke rehabilitation shares insights into its role in her recovery over time. The voice of people with lived experience and their families can help enrich our understanding of what supported self-management feels like and how it can help to reimagine and rebuild a life after stroke. Clíodhna was 32 years old when she had her stroke on the 4th of May 2017 as a result of an arterial dissection. Following admission to hospital, she had a thrombectomy and two ten-centimetre clots were removed. Clíodhna was in acute care for two and a half weeks. She was discharged to rehabilitation for six weeks and then discharged home. She prefers to be referred to as "a person with stroke" and finds terms like "stroke survivor" or "stroke victim" unsettling.

What did supported self-management look like to me? In the beginning (Week 3, when I moved to a rehabilitation hospital) it looked like choosing what to wear, dressing myself and making my bed. The steps started small and had to be things I could realistically manage. When I wasn't eating or attending therapies I was sleeping for three hours a day and nine hours at night. Fatigue was and remains my constant companion. My stroke took a lot from me and I had a lot to relearn, I couldn't look any further than self-care tasks. At that stage I was only beginning to recover my words and realise that I had lost my inner monologue.

The stroke plunged me and my family into a medical world that we knew very little about. My family had to 'upskill' in interfacing with medical professionals while protecting and reassuring me, taking on various therapy tasks that were recommended to encourage my recovery. My family was an essential part of my early recovery, along with my neurologist setting the tone that there was no end date to my possible recovery. I was told there was no time limit to what I could achieve. Neuroplasticity would allow my brain to rewire itself and 8 years on this is still happening...over 7.5 years after I left the rehabilitation hospital.

At a gradual pace I learned to manage my self-care, medication and my 'extra treats' like painting my nails. Things that were achievable with the help of my OT led me to feeling more like myself and I even got a name for painting the nails of any interested patient on my ward. These little human touches let me (and us!) feel more like who we were before the strokes changed our lives. I like to think it helped us make peace with how our lives have changed but that we still had lots to reconnect us to "the before times". The autonomy I enjoyed by making my own bed was empowering and led me to strive for more. I can't emphasise how monumental the stroke was, I had to discover that I was essentially the same person with a few added extras. Like fatigue, overstimulation, aphasia, executive dysfunction and, really, invisible disabilities that would accompany me for the rest of my life. This all happened while I was managing to walk to my therapy appointments instead of being collected, I had learned how to navigate around the hospital and as my confidence grew so did my ambition. I saw that I could live a good life, albeit a little differently.

I've learned to problem solve better than my non-brain injured family and friends, I can break problems down, plan and test solutions better than I ever could before. I am less anxious and less afraid of doing the wrong thing. The confidence and bravery I had to build within myself before I could take on a new challenge in my self-management was monumental. I had to fight against my fear of failure and become a recovering perfectionist which was personally challenging. However, the personal growth made all my efforts worthwhile to date. I've incorporated rehabilitation and recovery into my daily life.

The stroke took my life as I knew it but recovering has allowed me to form my post-stroke life into something meaningful.

SELF-MANAGEMENT ACROSS TRANSITIONS IN STROKE REHABILITATION

Transitions in stroke care are defining moments in the rehabilitation journey. Whether moving from the hospital to home, into early supported discharge, or across phases of community-based care, each transition brings both challenges and opportunities. These transitions can be informed by Bridges Transition Model to understand and manage the personal aspects of change well (Miller, 2017). Embedding self-management support at these critical junctures can empower individuals to take greater control of their recovery, enhance functional outcomes, and navigate the long-term realities of life after stroke.

Key elements of effective self-management support across transitions include:

Person-centred Education – the Right Information at the Right Time

Personalised education is a key foundation for supporting people to manage life after stroke (Hancock et al., 2023). At each transition point, individuals and their families need more than just information about the condition or recovery timelines. They need practical, tailored guidance on how to live well after stroke. To be effective, information should be given at the right time, repeated as needed, and adapted to suit each person's needs, readiness, and cognitive ability. It also needs to be clear and accessible, using written plans, visual tools, or coaching approaches like teach-back

(Lindblom et al., 2023). When linked to personal goals, this kind of education helps build confidence and supports meaningful change (Finch et al., 2021).

Collaborative Goal Setting

Establishing shared, realistic goals helps individuals focus on "what matters most" to them, whether that's improving physical ability, managing fatigue, or returning to work (Heredia-Callejón et al., 2023; Sarre et al., 2014). When goals are co-developed and broken down into achievable steps, they can foster a sense of progress and autonomy. This can make goals feel more relevant, increases motivation and ownership (Chen et al., 2020), and when healthcare professionals act as partners and facilitators, rather than experts, goal setting can become a more dynamic, empowering process. When stroke survivors experience poststroke fatigue, practical advice and strategies to manage this may be helpful along with support from family, peers, and the wider stroke network (Delbridge et al., 2023). In busy healthcare environments, challenges for healthcare professionals include limited time and a lack of confidence or training in collaborative goal setting. Training and reflective practice have been identified as ways to build these skills among staff and support better outcomes for people with stroke (Hancock et al., 2023).

Building Self-Efficacy

Rehabilitation teams play a key role in helping people with stroke to strengthen self-efficacy. Supporting individuals with stroke to build everyday skills, such as pacing, problem solving, and navigating the healthcare system, is a vital part of stroke recovery. When people feel confident, they're more likely to stay motivated and manage setbacks. That confidence grows through coaching, encouragement, and seeing themselves or others succeed (Satink et al., 2016). In contrast, when expectations are unclear or healthcare professionals become overly directive, it can undermine progress and reduce an individual's sense of empowerment (Hartford et al., 2019). Thus, trusting relationships and a supported self-management approach are key to fostering readiness, confidence, and active engagement in recovery following stroke (Heredia-Callejón et al., 2023).

Emotional and Peer Support

Transitions after stroke often bring uncertainty that can result in a loss of confidence and emotional distress (Chen et al., 2021). Recognising this and embedding psychological support into care is essential. Peer support can facilitate social learning and meaning-making by exchanging information and knowledge with other stroke survivors. This form of social learning and comparison is likely to improve resilience and psychosocial outcomes after stroke (Sadler et al., 2017). Peer support, whether through structured groups, one-to-one connections, or informal networks, offers safe spaces to share advice, reduce isolation, and feel seen. It is further noted to help with problem-solving and normalising the challenges of recovery (O'Callaghan et al., 2024a). However, access to peer support is often limited by practical barriers like transport, timing, or availability. Services that weave emotional support into routine care tend to see better engagement and outcomes (O'Callaghan et al., 2024a). Emotional support should be viewed not as optional, but as a core part of recovery and supported self-management.

Integrated, Ongoing Support

Supported self-management is not a one-off intervention. It requires reinforcement across settings using a coordinated approach. Early supported discharge teams, community rehabilitation services, and primary care providers all have a role in revisiting goals, monitoring progress, and re-engaging individuals when needs change (O'Callaghan et al., 2024b). Integration and collaboration across health and social services is critical for smooth transitions and instilling confidence and trust, as is

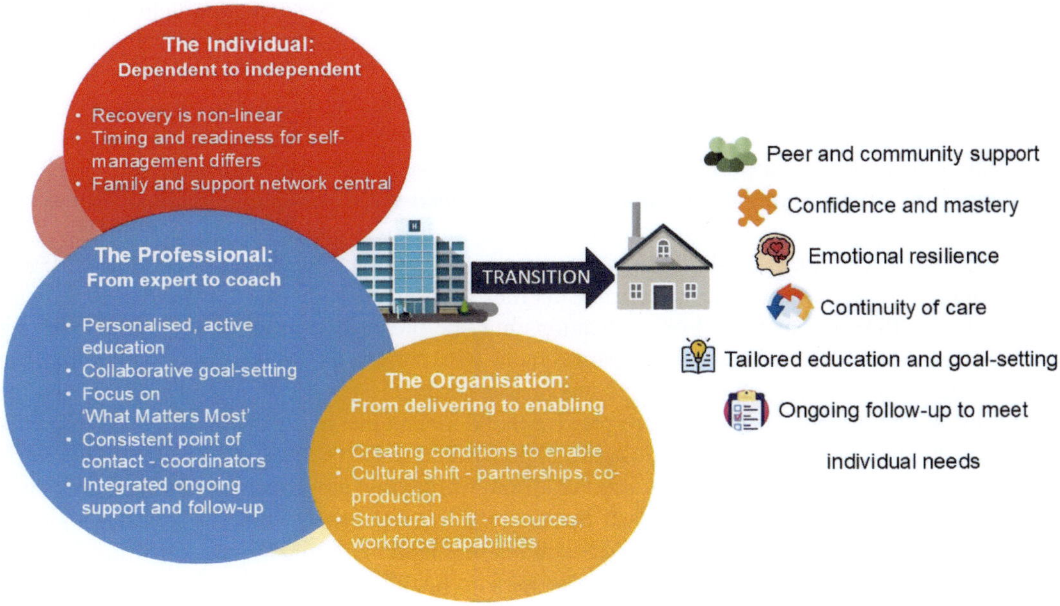
The Individual:
Dependent to independent
• Recovery is non-linear
• Timing and readiness for self-management differs
• Family and support network central
The Professional:
From expert to coach
• Personalised, active education
• Collaborative goal-setting
• Focus on 'What Matters Most'
• Consistent point of contact - coordinators
• Integrated ongoing support and follow-up
The Organisation:
From delivering to enabling
• Creating conditions to enable
• Cultural shift - partnerships, co-production
• Structural shift - resources, workforce capabilities
TRANSITION
Peer and community support
Confidence and mastery
Emotional resilience
Continuity of care
Tailored education and goal-setting
Ongoing follow-up to meet individual needs

FIGURE 6.1 Transition infographic with the individual, professional, and organisational enablers to transition home and link with community support services.

continuity of key professionals (O'Callaghan et al., 2024a). Stroke coordinators or link workers can act as consistent points of contact, while technology, like remote check-ins or virtual rehabilitation, can also play a key role in providing ongoing support (O'Callaghan et al., 2024a). Successful self-management in rehabilitation is about more than independence, it's about enabling people to live well with their condition. When services align (hospital, community/primary care, rehabilitation, advocacy groups, social and peer support networks) around supporting autonomy and "what matters most", and when transitions are treated as key intervention points rather than handovers, we lay the groundwork for sustainable, person-led recovery (Figure 6.1).

MANAGING HEALTH AND LIFESTYLE AFTER A STROKE

Evaluating one's lifestyle after stroke and addressing behaviours that are not helpful is an important aspect of supported self-management to optimise recovery and future health and wellness, as reflected in the Stroke Action Plan for Europe to 2030 (Norrving et al., 2018). Data suggest that people with stroke often have less healthy lifestyle habits than the general population (Bailey et al., 2019; Lennon et al., 2021; Redfern et al., 2000; Von Sarnowski et al., 2013) and up to a third of people after stroke either discontinue or do not correctly take one or more of their prescribed medications (Al AlShaikh et al., 2016; Bushnell et al., 2010; Khan et al., 2010; Klein et al., 2021). Lifestyle-related behaviours (e.g., smoking, vaping, not being physically active enough, eating an unhealthy diet, ineffective stress management) or health beliefs (e.g., "I don't need to take blood pressure medication because I feel fine" or "exercise is not for me") are often long-standing, entrenched and difficult to change for the better after stroke.

Making changes to one's lifestyle or health behaviours so that those changes become part of the everyday life is challenging and is influenced by complex social, environmental and cultural factors (Michie and Abraham, 2004). Effective change requires an understanding of risk-related behaviours and how to best go about changing them. Important mediators that can act as barriers or facilitators to effective behaviour change include intentions and goals, self-efficacy, motivation, outcome expectancies, perceived susceptibility/severity, and social influences (Conner and Norman, 2017). Supported self-management of risk behaviours after stroke is required, but it must be underpinned by behaviour change theory and contextualised to the capacities and personal priorities of individuals with stroke (Lawrence et al., 2019) to make meaningful change, cognisant of other challenges that arise in the context of stroke including cognition, vision and physical challenges, polypharmacy use (a number of medications at the same time), and financial issues (Fleming et al., 2023; Gadkari and McHorney, 2012).

Medications from several classes are typically prescribed to aid recovery and reduce future cardiovascular risk after stroke. The type and dose of medication is often adjusted to get the best result in each situation (Fleming et al., 2023) As examples, antiplatelet agents, antihypertensives, and statins may be prescribed, where appropriate, as they can substantially reduce the risk of a recurrent stroke (Rothwell et al., 2011) or medications may be prescribed to address muscle spasticity to allow easier movement. Medication management (Chapman and Bogle, 2014) requires stroke survivors (and their wider support systems where appropriate) to obtain their medications from the pharmacy, organise medications correctly, read and understand the medication label, and remember to take the medications at the correct dosage and prescribed times (Neville et al., 2020). Therefore, self-management of medications goes beyond simply following prescriptions and bringing them to the pharmacy to be filled. Effective self-management requires stroke survivors to monitor their condition, understand the medications, associated side effects, and understand when medications may need to be altered, discuss issues or concerns with healthcare professionals, build and maintain routines, and seek assistance by the appropriate service should an issue arise. Studies have shown that supported self-management of medications during in-patient rehabilitation using active information provision that increases stroke survivors' medication knowledge and joint planning of daily medication routines and planning for discharge results in significantly better medication management capacity in everyday life after stroke (Neville et al., 2020). Following discharge to primary care, behavioural interventions (that address medication adherence as a health behaviour and that reduce medication concerns) and structured self-management interventions have shown in meta-analyses to improve adherence with prescribed medications after stroke (Al AlShaikh et al., 2016; Hall et al., 2024a; Kronish et al., 2013; Lawrence et al., 2015; Redfern et al., 2006; Sakakibara et al., 2017). Figure 6.2 provides helpful questions for stroke survivors to ask; helpful information

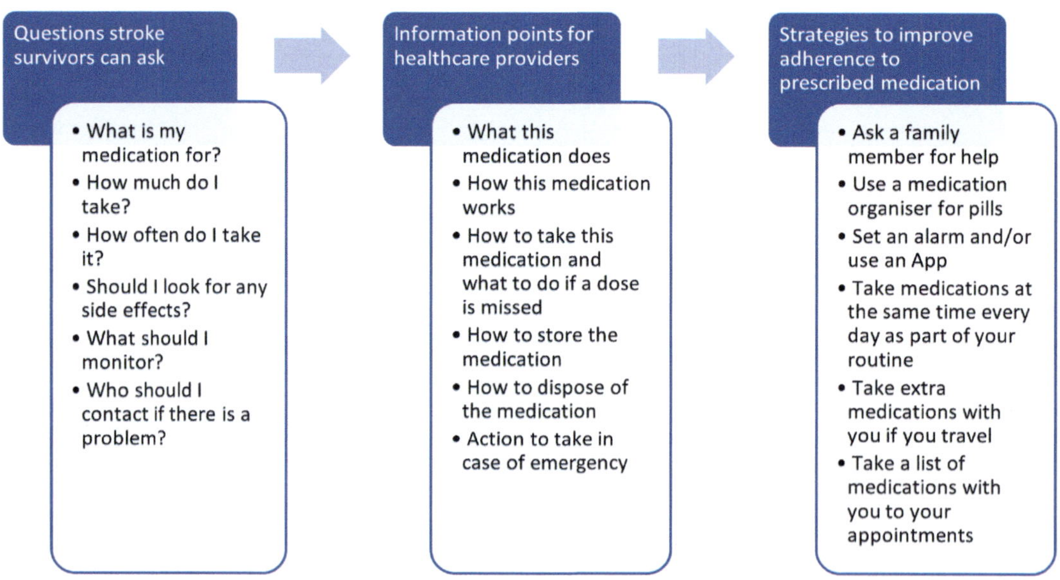

FIGURE 6.2 Supporting medication adherence.

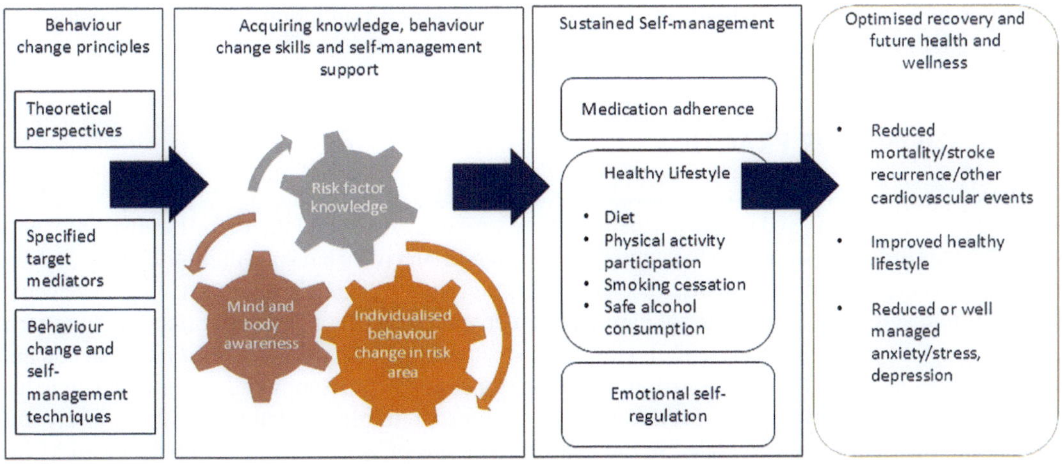

FIGURE 6.3 Supported self-management model for risk reducing behaviours after stroke.

points for healthcare providers to support self-management and strategies to help improve adherence to prescribed medications. Supporting and improving other healthy lifestyle habits after stroke is beneficial for long-term health and well-being in everyday life and in reducing the risk of another stroke as shown in Figure 6.3.

Modifiable risk factors for stroke, such as an unhealthy diet, low levels of physical activity, and substance misuse (e.g. unsafe alcohol consumption), often go unmanaged after someone experiences a stroke. Simple supported self-management strategies have been shown to improve medication adherence and reduce psychological distress after stroke (Sakakibara et al., 2017; Wan et al., 2021), but changes in longstanding health behaviours require both the person with stroke and their healthcare practitioners to understand behaviour-change processes and to address mediators that affect behaviour change (Redfern et al., 2006). Stroke survivors have identified this as something that they figure out over time and in the context of their lives but is helped by being equipped by knowledge and good social supports and using reminders and reinforcements to keep good behaviours going (Hall et al., 2025). Health beliefs, self-identity, and perceived ability to change behaviour were further noted by people after stroke to assert both positive and negative influences on health behaviours, alongside aspects for supported self-management that include the need for family support, goal setting, skills development, resources, and positive messaging (Hall et al., 2025; Lawrence et al., 2010, 2016).

Complex (multimodal lifestyle-based) health interventions for stroke secondary prevention often include targeted health education, behavioural counselling, and/or behaviour change skills acquisition, with evidence that supports their role in increasing physical activity participation and improving healthy eating post-stroke (Hall et al., 2024b). Specific theory-informed behaviour change constructs with an established evidence base for reducing lifestyle-related risks after stroke include Knowledge (the awareness of the existence of something), Beliefs about Consequences (the acceptance of the truth, reality, or validity about outcomes of a behaviour in a given situation) and Emotions (the complex reaction pattern, involving experiential, behavioural, and physiological elements, by which the individual attempts to deal with a personally significant matter or event) (Cane et al., 2012; Hall et al., 2024b). Successful interventions targeting stroke knowledge are noted to provide interactive and tailored information on risk reducing behaviours; offer self-management information and support in goal setting to improve lifestyle habits; and provide information on self-monitoring in relation to maintaining behaviour change (Hall et al., 2024b). Interventions targeting people's health beliefs about the consequences of risk-related behaviours are successful in influencing adherence to preventive medications by correcting misperceptions. Successful interventions addressing and supporting people's emotions after stroke help acquisition of emotional self-regulation skills after stroke which can have many additional benefits for managing other health risk behaviours.

IMPLICATIONS FOR PRACTICE

Stroke is sudden in onset and its associated sequelae are many, negatively impacting aspects of physical, cognitive, emotional, and social wellbeing. Many stroke survivors and their families live with these consequences of stroke, some of which emerge over time as survivors navigate daily life following discharge from hospital and rehabilitative services. This highlights the importance of having an effective stroke system across the continuum of care from emergency admission, rehabilitation and long-term care and support (Martins et al., 2023). How to best support people after stroke to have agency and self-fulfilment in life after stroke is still not clear (Legg et al., 2023). Supported self-management has a clear role to play however clinicians need sufficient time and training to deliver SSM effectively, and collaborative care must be embedded in the culture and ethos of stroke rehabilitation (Duncan Millar et al., 2023; Kidd et al., 2024). The design and implementation of SSM interventions must critically consider wider contexts, such as a lack of representation in the existing stroke evidence base and inequities in healthcare access and resources, to avoid exacerbating health disparities. There is a pressing need for inclusive and culturally responsive approaches that acknowledge these limitations and work in partnership with diverse communities to co-design effective SSM interventions (MacFarlane et al., 2024; Wray et al., 2021). A realist understanding of how SSM interventions function in specific service contexts and with specific individuals and/or communities is also essential, as is ensuring that knowledge translation efforts reflect these nuances (Kidd et al., 2024).

REFERENCES

Abrahamson, V., and Wilson, P. (2019) Positioning the six-month review in the recovery process post-stroke: The ideology of personal responsibility. *Health Soc Care Community*, 27, 249–259. doi:10.1111/hsc.12677.

Al AlShaikh, S., Quinn, T., Dunn, W., Walters, M., and Dawson, J. (2016) Predictive factors of non-adherence to secondary preventative medication after stroke or transient ischaemic attack: A systematic review and meta-analyses. *Eur Stroke J*, 1(2), 65–75. doi:10.1177/2396987316647187.

Atteih, S., Mellon, L., Hall, P., Brewer, L., Horgan, F., Williams, D., and Hickey, A. (2015) ASPIRE-S study group. Implications of stroke for caregiver outcomes: Findings from the ASPIRE-S study. *Int J Stroke*, 10(6), 918–23. doi:10.1111/ijs.12535.

Bailey, R. R., Phad, A., McGrath, R., and Haire-Joshu, D. (2019) Prevalence of five lifestyle risk factors among US adults with and without stroke. *Disabil Health*, 12(2), 323–7. doi:10.1016/j.dhjo.2018.11.003.

Bandura, A. (1991) Social cognitive theory of self-regulation. *Organiz Behav Human Decis Process*, 50, 248–287. doi:10.1016/0749-5978(91)90022-L.

Brady, M. C., Fredrick, A., and Williams, B. (2013) People with aphasia: Capacity to consent, research participation and intervention inequalities. *International Journal of Stroke*, 8(3), 193–196. doi:10.1111/j.1747-4949.2012.00900.x.

Bushnell, C. D., Zimmer, L. O., Pan, W., Olson, D. M., Zhao, X., Meteleva, T., Schwamm, L., Ovbiagele, B., Williams, L., Labresh, K. A., and Peterson, E. D. (2010) Persistence with stroke prevention medications 3 months after hospitalization. *Arch Neurol*, 67, 1456–1463.

Butler, E. N., and Evenson, K. R. (2014) Prevalence of physical activity and sedentary behavior among stroke survivors in the United States. *Top. Stroke Rehabil*, 21, 246–255. doi:10.1310/tsr2103-246.

Cane, J., O'Connor, D., and Michie, S. (2012) Validation of the theoretical domains framework for use in behaviour change and implementation research. *Implement Sci*, 24(7), 37. doi:10.1186/1748-5908-7-37.

Chapman, B., and Bogle, V. (2014) Adherence to medication and self-management in stroke patients. *Br J Nurs*, 23, 158–166. doi:10.12968/bjon.2014.23.3.158.

Chen, L., Xiao, L. D., and Chamberlain, D. (2020) An integrative review: Challenges and opportunities for stroke survivors and caregivers in hospital to home transition care. *J Adv Nurs*, 76, 2253–2265. doi:10.1111/jan.14446.

Chen, L., Xiao, L. D., Chamberlain, D., and Newman, P. (2021) Enablers and barriers in hospital-to-home transitional care for stroke survivors and caregivers: A systematic review. *J Clin Nurs*, 30, 2786–2807. doi:10.1111/jocn.15807.

Conner, M., and Norman, P. (2017) Health behaviour: Current issues and challenges. *Psychol Health*, 32(8), 895–906. doi:10.1080/08870446.2017.1336240.

Dankner, R., Bachner, Y. G., Ginsberg, G., Ziv, A., Ben, D. H., Litmanovitch-Goldstein, D., Chodick, G., Balicer, R., Tanne, D., and Greenberg, D. (2016) Correlates of well-being among caregivers of long-term community-dwelling stroke survivors. *Int J Rehabil Res*, 39(4), 326–330. doi:10.1097/MRR.0000000000000192.

Delbridge, A., Davey, J., Galloway, M., Drummond, A., Lanyon, L., Olley, N., Mason, G., English, C., and Simpson, D. B. (2023) Exploring post-stroke fatigue from the perspective of stroke survivors: What strategies help? A qualitative study. *Disabil Rehabil*. 1–7. doi:10.1080/09638288.2023.2266363.

Department of Health. (2005) *UK Promoting Self-Management in Stroke Rehabilitation*. https://www.myotspot.com/self-management-stroke-rehab/

Dobe, J., Gustafsson, L., Walder, K., Bower, K., and Lachman, R. (2023) Co-creation of self-management support during inpatient stroke rehabilitation. *PEC Innov*, 10(3), 100191. doi:10.1016/j.pecinn.2023.100191.

Duncan Millar, J., Mason, H., and Kidd, L. (2023) What is important in supporting self-management in community stroke rehabilitation? A Q methodology study. *Disabil Rehabil*, 45(14), 2307–2315. doi:10.1080/09638288.2022.2087766.

El Husseini, N., Katzan, I. L., Rost, N. S., Blake, M. L., Byun, E., Pendlebury, S. T., Aparicio, H. J., Marquine, M. J., Gottesman, R. F., and Smith, E. E. (2023) Cognitive impairment after ischemic and hemorrhagic stroke: A scientific statement from the American Heart Association/American Stroke Association. *Stroke*, 54(6), e272–e291. doi:10.1161/STR.0000000000000430.

Emmett, E. S., O'Connell, M. D. L., Pei, R., Douiri, A., Wyatt, D., Bhalla, A., Wolfe, C. D. A., and Marshall, I. J. (2025) Trends in ethnic disparities in stroke care and long-term outcomes. *JAMA Netw Open*, 8(1), e2453252. doi:10.1001/jamanetworkopen.2024.53252.

European Stroke Organisation (ESO) Action Plan for Stroke 2018–2030. European Stroke Organisation. doi:10.1177/2396987318808719 https://actionplan.eso-stroke.org/domains/stroke-rehabilitation

European Stroke Organisation (ESO) and Stroke Alliance for Europe (SAFE). (2018) *The Stroke Action Plan for Europe (SAP-E) 2018–2030*. European Stroke Organisation. https://eso-stroke.org/projects/stroke-action-plan/

Finch, E., Foster, M., and Fleming, J. (2021) Disrupted biographies: Making sense of minor stroke after hospital discharge. *Disabil Rehabil*, 43(18), 2632–2639. doi:10.1080/09638288.2019.1708980.

Fleming, T. K., Schwartz, J. K., Belagaje, S. R., Katz, L. W., and Strow, J. T. (2023) Medication management after stroke. *Arch Phys Med Rehabil*, 104(10), 1739–1744.

Fluck, D., Fry, C. H., Gulli, G., Affley, B., Robin, J., Kakar, P., Sharma, P., and Han, T. S. (2023) Adverse stroke outcomes amongst UK ethnic minorities: A multi-centre registry-based cohort study of acute stroke. *Neurol Sci*, 44(6), 2071–2080. doi:10.1007/s10072-023-06640-z.

Gadkari, A. S., and McHorney, C. A. (2012) Unintentional non-adherence to chronic prescription medications: How unintentional is it really? *BMC Health Serv Res*, 12, 98. doi:10.1186/1472-6963-12-98.

Gallacher, K., Morrison, D., Jani, B., Macdonald, S., May, C. R., Montori, V. M., Erwin, P. J., Batty, G. D., Eton, D. T., Langhorne, P., and Mair, F. S. (2013) Uncovering treatment burden as a key concept for stroke care: A systematic review of qualitative research. *PLoS Med*, 10(6), e1001473. doi:10.1371/journal.pmed.1001473.

Gallacher, K. I., May, C. R., Langhorne, P., and Mair, F. S. (2018) A conceptual model of treatment burden and patient capacity in stroke. *BMC Fam Pract*, 19(1), 9. doi:10.1186/s12875-017-0691-4.

Hale, L., Oosman, S., and Stewart, A. V. (2022) Editorial: Challenging the concept of self-management support in unique and diverse populations. *Front Rehabil Sci*, 3, 999528. doi:10.3389/fresc.2022.999528.

Hall, P., da Cruz Peniche, P., Hickey, J., and Lennon, O. (2025) Identifying mediators of healthy lifestyle adoption after stroke: A focus group study using a theoretical domains framework guided analysis. *BMC Neurol*, 25, 135. doi:10.1186/s12883-025-04144-1.

Hall, P., Lawrence, M., Blake, C., and Lennon, O. (2024a) Interventions for behaviour change and self-management of risk in stroke secondary prevention: An overview of reviews. *Cerebrovasc Dis*, 53(1), 1–13. doi:10.1159/000531138.

Hall, P., Lawrence, M., Kroll, T., Blake, C., Matthews, J., and Lennon, O. (2024b) Reducing risk behaviours after stroke: An overview of reviews interrogating primary study data using the theoretical domains framework. *PLOS ONE*, 19(4), e0302364. https://doi.org/10.1371/journal.pone.0302364

Hancock, N. J., Houghton, J., and Jones, F. (2023) Integrating an approach to personalised self-management support in stroke and neurorehabilitation service contexts: People1st – A quality improvement initiative. *Disability and Rehabilitation*, 45(19), 3034–3045. doi:10.1080/09638288.2022.2127930.

Hartford, W., Lear, S., and Nimmon, L. (2019) Stroke survivors' experiences of team support along their recovery continuum. *BMC Health Serv Res*, 19(1), 723. doi:10.1186/s12913-019-4533-z.

Heredia-Callejón, A., García-Pérez, P., Armenta-Peinado, J. A., Infantes-Rosales, M., and Rodríguez-Martínez, M. C. (2023) Influence of the therapeutic alliance on the rehabilitation of stroke: A systematic *review of qualitative studies. J Clin Med*, 12, 4266. doi:10.3390/jcm12134266.

Hilari, K. (2011) The impact of stroke: Are people with aphasia different to those without? *Disabil Rehabil*, 33(3), 211–218. doi:10.3109/09638288.2010.508829.

Jones, and Brimicombe (2014) Every interaction counts: The 'Bridges' approach to stroke self-management. *Int J Ther Rehabil*, 21(4), 158–159. www.bridgesselfmanagement.org.uk

Jones, F., McKevitt, C., Riazi, A., and Liston, M. (2017) How is rehabilitation with and without an integrated self-management approach perceived by UK community dwelling stroke survivors? A qualitative process evaluation to explore implementation and contextual variations. *BMJ Open*, 7, e014109. doi:10.1136/bmjopen-2016014109.

Jones, F., Postges, H., and Brimicombe, L. (2016) Building bridges between healthcare professionals, patients and families: A coproduced and integrated approach to self-management support in stroke. *NeuroRehabilitation*, 39471–480. doi:10.3233/NRE-161379.

Khan, N. A., Yun, L., Humphries, K., and Kapral, M. (2010) Antihypertensive drug use and adherence after stroke: Are there sex differences. *Stroke*, 41, 1445–1449. doi:10.1161/strokeaha.110.579375.

Kidd, L., Brown, J., Mason, H., Quinn, T., Gallacher, K. I., Jones, F., Fisher, R., Lebedis, T., Barber, M., Brennan, K., Gilmour, B., Fraser, C., Mooney, P., and Taggart, A. (2024). A realist evaluation of mechanisms and contexts for facilitating the implementation of supported self-management in community stroke care (The IMPETUS study). *Health Soc Care Community*, 2024(1), 9198768. doi:10.1155/2024/9198768.

Klein, A. P., Yarbrough, K., and Cole, J. W. (2021) Stroke, smoking and vaping: The no-good, the bad and the ugly. *Ann Public Health Res*, 8(1), 1–21.

Klockar, E., Kylén, M., Gustavsson, C., Finch, T., Jones, F., and Elf, M. (2023) Self-management from the perspective of people with stroke – An interview study. *Patient Educ Couns*, 112, 107740. doi:10.1016/j.pec.2023.107740.

Kronish, I. M., Diefenbach, M. A., Edmondson, D. E., Phillips, L. A., Fei, K., and Horowitz, C. R. (2013) Key barriers to medication adherence in survivors of strokes and transient ischemic attacks. *J Gen Intern Med*, 28, 675–682. doi:10.1007/s11606-012-2308-x.

Kuźma, E., Lourida, I., Moore, S. F., Levine, D. A., Ukoumunne, O. C., and Llewellyn, D. J. (2018) Stroke and dementia risk: A systematic review and meta-analysis. *Alzheimers Dement*, 14(11), 1416–1426. doi:10.1016/j.jalz.2018.06.3061.

Lawrence, M., Asaba, E., Duncan, E., Elf, M., Eriksson, G., Faulkner, J., Guidetti, S., Johansson, B., Kruuse, C., Lambrick, D., and Longman, C. (2019) Stroke secondary prevention, a non-surgical and non-pharmacological consensus definition: Results of a Delphi study. *BMC Res Notes*, 12, 1–6. doi:10.1186/s13104-019-4857-0.

Lawrence, M., Kerr, S., Watson, H., Paton, G., and Ellis, G. (2010) An exploration of lifestyle beliefs and lifestyle behaviour following stroke: Findings from a focus group study of patients and family members. *BMC Fam Pract*, 11(1), 97. doi:10.1186/1471-2296-11-97.

Lawrence, M., Pringle, J., Kerr, S., Booth, J., Govan, L., and Roberts, N. J. (2015) Multimodal secondary prevention behavioral interventions for TIA and stroke: A systematic review and meta-analysis. *PLoS ONE*, 10, e0120902.

Lawrence, M., Pringle, J., Kerr, S., and Booth, J. (2016) Stroke survivors' and family members' perspectives of multimodal lifestyle interventions for secondary prevention of stroke and transient ischemic attack: A qualitative review and meta-aggregation. *Disabil Rehabil*, 38(1), 11–21. doi:10.3109/09638288.2015.1031831.

Legg, L., Stevens, E., McKevitt, C., and Wolfe, C. (2023) *The Unmet Needs of Stroke Survivors in Europe: a Scoping Review of the Literature on Life after Stroke: A Life Saved Is a Life Worth Living.* Stroke Alliance for Europe. https://www.safestroke.eu/wp-content/uploads/2023/03/A-life-saved-is-a-live-worth-living-unmet-needs-of-stroke-survivors-in-Europe_lay-version_final.pdf

Lennon, O., Hall, P., and Blake, C. (2021) Predictors of adherence to lifestyle recommendations in stroke secondary prevention. *Int J Environ Res Public Health*, 18(9), 4666. doi:10.3390/ijerph18094666.

Lindblom, S., Ytterberg, C., Flink, M., Carlsson, A. C., Stenberg, U., Tistad, M., von Koch, L., and Laska, A. C. (2023) The use of teach back at Hospital discharge to support self-management of prescribed medication for secondary prevention after stroke—Findings from a feasibility study. *Healthcare*, 11(3), 391. doi:10.3390/healthcare11030391.

MacFarlane, A., Huschke, S., Marques, M. J., Gama, A., Kinaan, W., Hassan, A., Papyan, A., Phelan, H., Severoni, S., Kumar, B., and Dias, S. (2024) Normalising participatory health research approaches in the WHO European region for refugee and migrant health: A paradigm shift. *Lancet Reg Health Eur*, 41. doi:10.1016/j.lanepe.2024.100837.

Martins, S. C. O., Secchi, T. L., Molina, C., and Nogueira, R. (2023) Editorial: 'Development of stroke systems of care across the globe'. *Front Neurol*, 14, 1292036. doi:10.3389/fneur.2023.1292036.

McKevitt, C., Fudge, N., Redfern, J., Sheldenkar, A., Crichton, S., Rudd, A. R., Forster, A., Young, J., Nazareth, I., Silver, L. E., Rothwell, P. M., and Wolfe, C. D. (2011) Self-reported long-term needs after stroke. *Stroke*, 42(5), 1398–403. doi:10.1161/strokeaha.110.598839.

Mellon, L., Brewer, L., Hall, P., Horgan, F., Williams, D., Hickey, A., and ASPIRE-S study group. (2015) Cognitive impairment six months after ischaemic stroke: A profile from the ASPIRE-s study. *BMC Neurol*, 15, 31. doi:10.1186/s12883-015-0288-2.

Michie, S., and Abraham, C. (2004) Identifying techniques that promote health behaviour change: Evidence based or evidence inspired. *Psychol Health*, 19, 29–49.

Miller, J. L. (2017) *Managing Transitions: Using William Bridges' Transition Model and A Change Style Assessment Instrument to Inform Strategies and Measure Progress in Organizational Change Management* (Scholarship and Professional Work, 74). https://digitalcommons.butler.edu/librarian_papers/74

Moran, C. N., Pender, N., Williams, D. J., Bennett, K., Merriman, N. A., Horgan, F., Kelly, P. J., Pendlebury, S. T., Johnson, M., Faky, M., Oglesby, M., McGlinchey, J., Murray, M., and Hickey, A. (2025) stroke-Cog-r: Protocol for a pilot randomised controlled trial evaluating the feasibility and acceptability of a novel cognitive rehabilitation intervention for post-stroke cognitive impairment. *HRB Open Res*, 8, 59. doi:10.12688/hrbopenres.14144.1.

Moura, A., Magalhães, P., Castanheira Pais, S., and Alves, E. (2023) Adaptation processes of survivors and informal caregivers after stroke: A scoping review through the Lens of educational sciences. *Am J Health Educ*, 54(4), 305–316. doi:10.1080/19325037.2023.2209614.

National Clinical Guideline for Stroke for the UK and Ireland. (2023) London: Intercollegiate Stroke Working Party, 2023 May 4. www.strokeguideline.org.

National Office of Clinical Audit. (2020) *Irish National Audit of Stroke (INAS) National Report 2020 (NOCA)*. National Office of Clinical Audit.

Neville, H., Sehgal, C., MacMillan, K., Kooka, C., Haire, M., Harding, C., MacFarlane-Conrad, M., MacKay, S., Mountain, A., Nodwell, L., Short, C., and Kelly White, J. (2020) Improving patient medication management capacity through a self-medication program in a rehabilitation inpatient setting. *Arch Phys Med Rehabil*, 101(11), e54–e54. doi:10.1016/j.apmr.2020.09.162.

Norrving, B., Barrick, J., Davalos, A., Dichgans, M., Cordonnier, C., and Guekht, A. (2018) Action plan for stroke in Europe 2018–2030. *Eur Stroke J*, 3(4), 309–336. doi:10.1177/2396987318808719.

O'Callaghan, G., Fahy, M., O'Meara, S., Lindblom, S., von Koch, L., Langhorne, P., Galvin, R., and Horgan, F. (2024a) DOI: Experiences and preferences of people with stroke and caregivers, around supports provided at the transition from hospital to home: A qualitative descriptive study. *BMC Neurology*, 24, 251. doi:10.1186/s12883-024-03767-0.

O'Callaghan, G., Fahy, M., O'Meara, S., Chawke, M., Waldron, E., Corry, M., Gallagher, S., Coyne, C., Lynch, J., Kennedy, E., Walsh, T., Cronin, H., Hannon, N., Fallon, C., Williams, D. J., Langhorne, P., Galvin, R., and Horgan, F. (2024b) Transitioning to home and beyond following stroke: A prospective cohort study of outcomes and needs. *BMC Health Serv Res*, 24(1), 449. doi:1186/s12913-024-10820-8.

Parke, H. L., Epiphaniou, E., Pearce, G., Taylor, S. J. C., Sheikh, A., Griffiths, C. J., Greenhalgh, T., and Pinnock, H. (2015) Self-management support interventions for stroke survivors: A systematic meta-review. *PLoS ONE*, 10(7), e0131448. doi:10.1371/journal.pone.0131448.

Pendlebury, S. T., and Rothwell, P. M. (2009) Prevalence, incidence, and factors associated with pre-stroke and post-stroke dementia: A systematic review and meta-analysis. *Lancet Neurol*, 8(11), 1006–1118. doi:10.1016/S1474-4422(09)70236-4.

Redfern, J., McKevitt, C., Dundas, R., Rudd, A. G., and Wolfe, C. D. (2000) Behavioral risk factor prevalence and lifestyle change after stroke: A prospective study. *Stroke*, 31, 1877–1881. doi:10.1161/01.str.31.8.1877.

Redfern, J., McKevitt, C., and Wolfe, C. D. A. (2006) Development of complex interventions in stroke care: A systematic review. *Stroke*, 37(9), 2410–9. doi:10.1161/01.STR.0000237097.00342.a9.

Rees, J., Tuijt, R., Burton, A., Walters, K., and Cooper, C. (2021) Supporting self-care of long-term conditions in people with dementia: A systematic review. *Int J Nurs Stud*, 16, 103432. doi:10.1016/j.ijnurstu.2019.103432.

Rohde, D., Gaynor, E., Large, M., Conway, O., Bennett, K., Williams, D. J., Callaly, E., Dolan, E., and Hickey, A. (2019) Stroke survivor cognitive decline and psychological wellbeing of family caregivers five years post-stroke: A cross-sectional analysis. *Top Stroke Rehabil*, 26(3), 180–186. doi:10.1080/10749357.2019.1590972.

Rohde, D., Merriman, N. A., Doyle, F., Bennett, K., Williams, D., and Hickey, A. (2017) Does cognitive impairment impact adherence? A systematic review and meta-analysis of the association between cognitive impairment and medication non-adherence in stroke. *PLoS One*, 12(12), e0189339. doi:10.1371/journal.pone.0189339.

Rothwell, P. M., Algra, A., and Amarenco, P. (2011) Medical treatment in acute and long-term secondary prevention after transient ischaemic attack and ischaemic stroke. *Lancet*, 377, 1681–1692. doi:10.1016/s0140-6736(11)60516-3.

Sadler, E., Sarre, S., Tinker, A., Bhalla, A., and McKevitt, C. (2017) Developing a novel peer support intervention to promote resilience after stroke. *Health Soc Care Communit*, 25(5), 1590–1600. doi:10.1111/hsc.12336.

Sakakibara, B. M., Kim, A. J., and Eng, J. J. (2017) A systematic review and meta-analysis on self-management for improving risk factor control in stroke patients. *Int. J. Behav. Med*, 24, 42–53. doi:10.1007/s12529-016-9582-7.

Sarre, S., Redlich, C., Tinker, A., Sadler, E., Bhalla, A., and McKevitt, C. (2014) A systematic review of qualitative studies on adjusting after stroke: Lessons for the study of resilience. *Disabil Rehabil*, 36(9), 716–726. doi:10.3109/09638288.2013.814724.

Satink, T., Josephsson, S., Zajec, J., Cup, E. H. C., de Swart, B. J. M., and Nijhuis-van der Sanden, M. W. G. (2016) Negotiating role management through everyday activities: Narratives in action of two stroke survivors and their spouses. *Disabil Rehabil*, 38(24), 2354–2364. doi:10.3109/09638288.2015.1129442.

Schmaderer, M., Struwe, L., Linton, N., and Zimmerman, L. (2021) Self-management strategies differ by level of cognition in multimorbid patients. *Appl Nurs Res*, 58, 151407. doi:10.1016/j.apnr.2021.151407.

Scottish Intercollegiate Guidelines Network (SIGN) and the National Clinical Programme for Stroke, Ireland. (2023) *National Clinical Guideline for Stroke for the United Kingdom and Ireland. The British and Irish Association of Stroke Physicians.* BIASP. https://www.strokeguideline.org/

Sexton, E., Donnelly, N. A., Merriman, N. A., Hickey, A., Wren, M. A., O'Flaherty, M., Bandosz, P., Guzman-Castillo, M., Williams, D. J., Horgan, F., Pender, N., Feeney, J., de Looze, C., Kenny, R. A., Kelly, P., and Bennett, K. (2021) strokeCog markov model: Projected prevalent and incident cases of stroke and poststroke cognitive impairment to 2035 in Ireland. *Stroke*, 52(12), 3961–3969. doi:10.1161/STROKEAHA.121.034005.

Shiggins, C., Ryan, B., Dewan, F., Bernhardt, J., O'Halloran, R., Power, E., Lindley, R. I., McGurk, G., and Rose, M. L. (2024) Inclusion of people with aphasia in stroke trials: A systematic search and review. *Arch Phys Med Rehabil*, 105(3), 580–592. doi:10.1016/j.apmr.2023.06.010.

Smets, E. M. A., Menichetti, J., Lie, H. C., and Gerwing, J. (2024) What do we mean by "tailoring" of medical information during clinical interactions? *Patient Educ Couns*, 119, 108092. doi:10.1016/j.pec.2023.108092.

Stevens, E., Emmett, E., Wang, Y., McKevitt, C., and Wolfe, C. (2017) *The Burden of Stroke in Europe Report. King's college London for the Stroke Alliance for Europe (SAFE).* Stroke Alliance for Europe. www.strokeeurope.eu/downloads/TheBurdenOfStrokeInEuropeReport.pdf

Sun, Y., Liu, C., Zhang, N., Yang, D., Ma, J., Ma, C., and Zhang, X. (2022) Effect of self-management of stroke patients on rehabilitation based on patient-reported outcome. *Front Neurosci*, 16, 929646. doi:10.3389/fnins.2022.929646.

The Stroke Alliance for Europe. (2020) *SAFE Annual Report 2019.* The Stroke Alliance for Europe. https://www.safestroke.eu/wp-content/uploads/2020/01/SAFEAnnual-Report-2019-03012020FINAL.pdf

Thompson, S. G., Barber, P. A., Gommans, J. H., Cadilhac, D. A., Davis, A., Fink, J. N., Harwood, M., Levack, W., McNaughton, H., Feigin, V. L., Abernethy, V., Girvan, J., Denison, H., Corbin, M., Wilson, A., Douwes, J., and Ranta, A. (2022) The impact of ethnicity on stroke care access and patient outcomes: A new zealand nationwide observational study. *Lancet Reg Health West Pac*, 20, 100358. doi:10.1016/j.lanwpc.2021.100358.

van der Gaag, A., Smith, L., Davis, S., Moss, B., Cornelius, V., and Mowles, C. (2005) Therapy and support services for people with long-term stroke and aphasia and their relatives: A six-month follow-up study. *Clin Rehabil*, 19(4), 372–380. doi:10.1191/0269215505cr785oa.

Vaughan, E., and Manning, M. X. (2023) Are people with aphasia included in stroke trials? A systematic review and narrative synthesis. *Clin Rehabil*, 37(10), 1375–1385. doi:10.1177/02692155231172009.

Von Sarnowski, B., Putaala, J., Grittner, U., Gaertner, B., Schminke, U., Curtze, S., Huber, R., Tanislav, C., Lichy, C., Demarin, V., Basic-Kes, V., Ringelstein, E. B., Neumann-Haefelin, T., Enzinger, C., Fazekas, F., Rothwell, P. M., Dichgans, M., Jungehulsing, G. J., Heuschmann, P. U., Kaps, M., Norrving, B., Rolfs, A., Kessler, C., and Tatlisumak, T. (2013) Lifestyle risk factors for ischemic stroke and transient ischemic attack in young adults in the Stroke in Young Fabry Patients Study. *Stroke*, 44, 19–125. doi:10.1161/strokeaha.112.665190.

Wafa, H. A., Wolfe, C. D., Emmett, E., Roth, G. A., Johnson, C. O., and Wang, Y. (2020) Burden of stroke in Europe: Thirty-year projections of incidence, prevalence, deaths, and disability-adjusted life years. *Stroke*, 51(8), 2418–2427. doi:10.1161/strokeaha.120.029606.

Wan, X., Chau, J. P. C., Mou, H., and Liu, X. (2021) Effects of peer support interventions on physical and psychosocial outcomes among stroke survivors: A systematic review and meta-analysis. *Int J Nurs Stud*, 121, 104001. doi:10.1016/j.ijnurstu.2021.104001.

Woodford, J., Farrand, P., Watkins, E. R., and Llewellyn, D. J. (2018) "I don't believe in leading a life of my own, I lead his life": A qualitative investigation of difficulties experienced by informal caregivers of stroke survivors experiencing depressive and anxious symptoms. *Clin Gerontol*, 41(4), 293–307. doi:10.1080/07317115.2017.1363104.

Wray, F., Clarke, D., Cruice, M., and Forster, A. (2021) Development of a self-management intervention for stroke survivors with aphasia using co-production and behaviour change theory: An outline of methods and processes. *PloS One*, 16(11), e0259103. doi:10.1371/journal.pone.0259103.

Wray, F., Clarke, D., and Forster, A. (2018) Post-stroke self-management interventions: A systematic review of effectiveness and investigation of the inclusion of stroke survivors with aphasia. *Disabil Rehabil*, 40(11), 1237–1251. doi:10.1080/09638288.2017.1294206.

Wray, F., Cruice, M., Kellar, I., and Forster, A. (2025) Protocol for a feasibility study evaluating a supported self-management intervention for stroke survivors with aphasia (StarStep study). *Pilot Feasibility Stud*, 11(1), 11. doi:10.1186/s40814-024-01589-y.

Yang, C. L., Labbe, D., Sakakibara, B. M., Vissers, J., and Bird, M. L. (2022) World café-A community conversation: A Canadian perspective on stroke survivors needs for community integration. *Top Stroke Rehabil*, 29(5), 392–400. doi:10.1080/10749357.2021.1928839.

7 Integrating Self-Management Strategies Supported by Digital Technologies in Post-Stroke Rehabilitation

Ann Marie Hestetun-Mandrup, Anne Lund, Anne Catrine Trægde Martinsen, and Minna Pikkarainen

INTRODUCTION

Self-management has become a cornerstone in post-stroke rehabilitation, particularly in the later phases after hospital discharge. However, its definition and conceptualization vary widely across disciplines and contexts (Fletcher et al., 2019). As a component of person-centered philosophy, self-management empowers individuals with stroke to take an active and operational role in managing their rehabilitation, making decisions, and developing skills and knowledge needed for recovery. This integration has established self-management as a hallmark of quality care at both political and practical levels (Linnet Olesen and Jørgensen, 2023).

A recent scoping review demonstrates that stroke survivors' use of self-management strategies is multifaceted, complicated, and involve different approaches; however, more research is needed to fully understand their use of self-management strategies in stroke rehabilitation (Rahman et al., 2023). Previous research in rehabilitation spans from addressing specific and holistic properties of an individual to recognizing the person as an expert in their own care, emphasizing active participation, or even framing it as a legal and human right (Leplege et al., 2007). This chapter explores self-management as an extension of person-centered rehabilitation, with a particular focus on the role of digital technologies. By drawing on qualitative interviews with stroke survivors (Hestetun-Mandrup et al., 2026a) and multidisciplinary healthcare professionals (Hestetun-Mandrup et al., 2026b) as case examples, it explores how individuals navigate post-stroke changes and leverage digital technologies to enhance their recovery. The interviews were conducted in Norway between June 2022 and January 2023. The chapter highlights and discuss key self-management strategies, such as problem-solving, decision-making, and goal-setting, alongside the role of self-efficacy in strengthening these practices (Dobe et al., 2023; Lorig and Holman, 2003; Wang et al., 2025). We argue that while self-management offers opportunities for individuals with stroke, it is also a complex and challenging process. While digital technologies offer opportunities to support self-management, the chapter also considers the challenges of balancing autonomy for stroke survivors with professional healthcare support in healthcare settings.

REHABILITATION AND SELF-MANAGEMENT CONCERNING CHANGING BEHAVIOR

The essence of rehabilitation involves achieving behavioral change, and self-management strategies play a key role in facilitating these changes, aligning closely with this concept (Wade, 2005). Self-management encompasses the actions individuals take to manage their health and life after a stroke, spanning mainly the three elements of medical, behavioral, and emotional dimensions

DOI: 10.1201/9781003599074-8

(Dobe et al., 2023; Lorig and Holman, 2003). Rooted in person-centered approaches, it emphasizes tailoring care to the individual's unique needs, values, and preferences (Jesus et al., 2016; Leplege et al., 2007). At its core, it encourages active participation in the recovery journey, fostering autonomy, resilience, and long-term adaptation to physical, psychological, emotional, and social challenges.

Corbin and Strauss' seminal work on chronic illness (Corbin and Strauss, 1988) highlights that self-management spans across medical, behavioral role, and emotional *doings* (Lorig and Holman, 2003). Importantly, even a stroke survivors' decision not to actively engage in rehabilitation reflects a management style, reinforcing the idea that self-management is an unavoidable part of life after a stroke (Lorig and Holman, 2003). The important remaining question that will be addressed in this chapter is how self-management strategies are used in general and assisted by digital technologies. Originating from rehabilitation practices for chronically ill children, modern self-management has since evolved into a framework for managing chronic illnesses, including stroke (Henry et al., 2022; Lorig and Holman, 2003). While managing chronic conditions like stroke often involves alternating foregrounds of the illness and the health like Paterson (Paterson, 2001) explained, self-management ultimately aims to keep wellness and health at the forefront of an individual's life (Lorig and Holman, 2003).

CAN DIGITAL TECHNOLOGIES ENHANCE THE USE OF SELF-MANAGEMENT STRATEGIES?

Digital technologies provide innovative opportunities to operationalize self-management in rehabilitation. They offer tools for self-training, enabling individuals to regulate the intensity, duration, and mode of their rehabilitation activities, thereby maximizing engagement and outcomes (Ding et al., 2025; Gåsvær et al., 2023). Furthermore, technologies such as virtual reality (VR) (Adams et al., 2023; Hernandez et al., 2022), robotics (Aprile et al., 2022), gaming (Allegue et al., 2022; Cramer et al., 2019; Gauthier et al., 2022) in combination with telerehabilitation for stroke survivors, not only support task-specific training for the user but also reflect a broader shift in the therapeutic relationship, where individuals take on more responsibility for their care, supported by healthcare professionals in a more contractual and informational role (Leplege et al., 2007).

Despite their potential, digital technologies are often ambiguously referenced in stroke guidelines. While resource utilization as part of a self-management strategy is frequently mentioned, descriptions of how digital technologies should be employed to support self-management are lacking (Henry et al., 2022). Self-management strategies – such as problem-solving, decision-making, using resources, taking action, and building partnership with healthcare professionals (Dobe et al., 2023; Lorig and Holman, 2003; Parke et al., 2015) – can be enhanced by digital technologies (Hestetun-Mandrup et al., 2026a), however their practical application requires further exploration. Additionally, recent studies have expanded self-management frameworks to include behavior change techniques like goal-setting, knowledge-sharing, and reintegration into the community, although their unique components overlap (Henry et al., 2022).

Self-efficacy is frequently discussed in connection with self-management. Scholars widely recognize self-efficacy as a mediator that enhances the potential of self-management programs (Dobe et al., 2023; Lorig and Holman, 2003; Wang et al., 2025), while some argue that it serves as the foundational concept of self-management (Henry et al., 2022). Despite its recognized importance, self-efficacy is rarely emphasized in stroke guidelines, with only one making explicit recommendations (Henry et al., 2022). For stroke survivors, self-efficacy can strengthen self-management by improving self-control and reducing impulsive behaviors (Wang et al., 2025). Developing a short-term action plan that aligns with the individual's confidence to achieve it is a key strategy for fostering self-efficacy (Lorig and Holman, 2003).

In this chapter, we discuss the challenges and tensions inherent in self-management. Despite its potential to empower individuals, self-management is often criticized for prioritizing autonomy and individual responsibility while overlooking the relational and collaborative aspects of care

(Fletcher et al., 2019; Mol, 2008). Scholars argue for a more practice-based, relational approach that integrates support from healthcare professionals and acknowledges the fluctuating nature of self-management in real-life contexts. This is particularly relevant in stroke rehabilitation, where self-management of the stroke survivors often requires a dynamic interplay between independent actions and support from healthcare professionals. Self-management can be argued within stroke guidelines as both something that should be practiced outside formal therapy (Henry et al., 2022) and as a process where social support, an important influencing factor, is integrated into formal therapeutic practices (Jiang et al., 2025).

In the following sections, the chapter examines the complexities of self-management in the digital context from stroke survivors' and health care personnels' perspectives. Grounded in the practical applicability of cases from our stroke studies, it seeks to unravel the nuances of self-management as a concept and practice, offering insights into how it can be effectively integrated into person-centered and technology-supported rehabilitation.

SELF-MANAGEMENT FROM THE USER'S PERSPECTIVE

Stroke Survivors

Our recent study highlighted that digital technologies can act as valuable motivators for self-management, especially when access to post-stroke rehabilitation is limited (Hestetun-Mandrup et al., 2026a). Participants in the study used various technologies, such as video-consultations, wearables, and virtual reality, to support knowledge acquisition, self-management, and communication. These technologies were seen as beneficial for exercising and gaining information. The participants also emphasized the importance of personal contact and shared responsibility in digital rehabilitation setups. These findings demonstrate that using self-managed digital technologies in rehabilitation can empower stroke survivors and make rehabilitation more interactive and personalized. However, it is important to consider the challenges stroke survivors may face, such as changing energy and capacity levels after a stroke, which affect their ability to use digital technologies.

"I'll Manage": Adapting to a New Sense of Self through Post-Stroke Rehabilitation

A recurring theme in our study, which was not included in the original publication, is how stroke survivors adapt to a new sense of self through rehabilitation, both in a general sense without linking it specifically to digital technology and in contexts where digital technologies are applied. This theme sheds light on the lived experiences of managing a changed identity while navigating post-stroke challenges and highlights the long-term journey toward personal growth and self-acceptance.

In the theme, experiences of managing a new self after stroke were present but noticeable on various levels. For many participants, self-management was tied to a process of acknowledging and adapting to a transformed sense of self. One participant, "John", expressed how this journey toward acceptance, despite transforming him, unfolded over several years:

> The task of rehabilitation is to accept that you have damages. It took me three years before I accepted it. You know what, I'll remain "John". But I will not be the same as I was. I become a new "John".

This cognitive process in changing behavior and accepting a new self was often described as a significant challenge but also a source of resilience and personal growth. Both self-management strategies of problem-solving and acting were rhetorically articulated through phrases such as *"a different life"*, *"not the one I used to be"*, *"to come out of"*, or *"a fight"*, emphasizing the emotional and behavioral dimensions of adapting to their new circumstances. The face value of managing on your own and facets of self-discipline is often referred to as "specialist bodies of knowledge" (Fletcher et al., 2019).

Self-management was also seen as an integral concept of rehabilitation, which at its core revolves around changing behavior. "Fred" reflected on how rehabilitation provided a self-managed purpose and motivation:

> The aim and the motive for appreciating returning to [rehabilitation] is because I still would like to be, should I say, awaken, by needing some movement, we need activities, we need something to sustain a certain standard of living.
>
> **("Fred")**

This comment suggests that self-management spans multiple levels, from bodily functions and meaningful activities to broader life recognition and expectations. The term "awakened" captures both the physical and cognitive dimensions of rehabilitation, reflecting a deeper level of awareness and engagement.

The Balance between Support and Independence

Participants frequently described how healthcare professionals and their social networks influenced their self-management journey. For some, interactions with healthcare professionals served as pivotal moments that fostered independence. "Jack" recounted how direct advice from a therapist reshaped his approach:

> "If you want to get somewhere you better start working", or, "Mister, if you want to be a part of this society, you better speed up".

These provocations, though direct, motivate participants to take greater responsibility for their rehabilitation. This sense of ownership often extended to discovering new treatment options or utilizing digital technologies for self-management. Examples like using Fitbit watches to track their walking distance as a rehabilitation goal, increased their motivation to continue to self-manage, particularly during the COVID-19 pandemic when formal rehabilitation services were limited (Hestetun-Mandrup et al., 2026a).

Interestingly, self-management as a behavioral practice often first became apparent after experiencing a stroke. "Jen" contextualized this behavioral change in managing daily activities, where she created new meaningful life roles:

> Because that sense of self-mastery, I probably took it for granted before. Back then, you did everything, and everything was just a given. But now, you feel incredibly happy when you realize, "Oh, I managed it! I didn't need to ask for help."

> I've gone from having home help twice a week to getting assistance from my sister and brother-in-law to create a weekly plan on the fridge. Now, I do a little bit every day, so by the weekend, I have a clean and tidy flat, and I've done it all myself. And that feeling, I promise you, is immense. So, being as independent as possible and managing things on my own, that's my goal.

In our study, many participants were familiar with using digital technologies in everyday life and during rehabilitation, which made continued use easier. As a part of this, they embraced full responsibility for their post-stroke rehabilitation, with statements like "*Because it is what I make of it*" ("Eric") (Hestetun-Mandrup et al., 2026a). While a few felt abandoned after intensive rehabilitation, most preferred taking ownership of their recovery, describing it as '*being their own captain*' ("Al") or '*triggering their own well-being.*' Stubbornness frequently emerged as a self-reflective trait, with some participants using metaphors like "Pippi Longstocking" to symbolize resilience and a willingness to face new challenges, echoing her mantra, "*I haven't done this before, but I'll manage*" ("John").

In contrast, self-management was not always a straightforward process of empowerment and health in the foreground. For most, it involved navigating feelings of uncertainty, resignation, or loss. "Emma" described the social challenge of presenting a "manageable" self to others while grappling with internal struggles and being in the middle of the process of overcoming this self-reconstruction. Adapting to the new circumstances post-stroke was important for the participants because experiencing a stroke was considered an emotional journey toward self-management and self-acceptance.

> It is a little challenging when people ask, 'How are you doing?' and 'are you doing well?' I'm just; Eh! How I'm doing?? At that time, I feel like replying 'What do you think??

This highlights the emotional complexity of self-management, where individuals must balance their personal realities with societal expectations.

The Dynamic Partnership between Stroke Survivors and Healthcare Professionals

Although many participants recognized that they bore the main responsibility for their rehabilitation process and self-management, they also acknowledged the importance of continued collaboration with healthcare professionals. The healthcare professional role was understood as to assist and facilitate the process. Consequently, using digital technologies became more pronounced during their rehabilitation period by video-conferences or webinars with healthcare professionals or others with stroke (Hestetun-Mandrup et al., 2026a). Especially, this partnership was seen as essential for navigating transitions from hospital to home and for maintaining progress in rehabilitation. "Anne" reflected on the challenges of this transition:

> It has gone well, but there have been some transitions. At least I have felt a bit left to manage on my own. Finding a physiotherapist myself. Knowing who is good. Many of the initiatives I have received have been my own suggestions.

Still, before the participants activated their need for independence, they called for a collaborative process with therapist, sometimes to gain medical knowledge and management, like "Luke" expressed in understanding the actual processes:

> Because you do get a bit skeptical when you've had a stroke in what is going on in your brain. So, I'm very interested in knowing this, and respond to it (.) The matter of which part of the brain is damaged – I have no qualifications to assess this.

Participants often described wanting accessible and ongoing support, such as a direct line of communication with healthcare professionals, rather than going through intermediaries like general practitioners. "John" referred to this concept as having the rehabilitation center "*in your pocket*", suggesting a need for seamless and responsive support systems. Such a collaboration with healthcare professionals was especially important in the many cases where stroke participants wished to use self-managed digital programs, but lacked available tools for self-managing (Hestetun-Mandrup et al., 2026a).

HEALTHCARE PROFESSIONALS' PERSPECTIVES ON SELF-MANAGEMENT

In a separate study involving healthcare professionals, self-management was often linked to encouraging motivation through collaboration (Hestetun-Mandrup et al., 2026b). Goal-setting was highlighted as a critical tool for fostering self-management strategies, with some therapists wanting to use digital resources to encourage proactive behavior. One occupational therapist explained:

> I wish we could have a bit more follow-up along the way, mostly for the patient's sake, because it is quite easy to put that binder in a drawer when you get home, and then you have, in a sense, "free time" until they come back. When we say that goal-setting is so important, I wish we could have a bit more communication along the way. (.) if they almost got a push notification through an app.

This comment highlights the importance of integrating continuous support into the self-management process, ensuring that rehabilitation does not stop when formal therapy ends. Digital technologies, such as apps with push notifications, were seen as promising solutions for maintaining patient engagement and motivation in the home setting. The principle of involving patients in rehabilitation focused on addressing their existential needs, which healthcare professionals recognized as central to the essence of rehabilitation.

Self-management in the eyes of healthcare professionals was often linked to motivation. One nurse implied that digital pre-conversations with their patients helped engage motivation to manage.

> There were quite a few patients who didn't fully understand what they were coming to, and some maybe had no self-motivation, some who really didn't want to come, and many types of things. I see that these pre-conversations are important.

As therapists also bear responsibility of establishing a personal relationship without trying to hide behind a façade (Leplege et al., 2007), respecting the person behind the disease is an important part of creating self-management. A speech therapist described the importance of interacting outside the clinical nature of a hospital setting, such as in a digital context, to create a natural and relaxed environment for interaction, while demonstrating empathy and using humor as part of a supportive strategy for self-management.

> Just giving them the time and space to express themselves, joking a lot. I use a lot of humor with the patients and try to show some understanding of their situation. But I find that if you can mention relevant life experiences, I think it's a good way to build relationships, to dare to open up a bit, so we're not just sitting there as rigid authority figures, making it a one-sided conversation.

This relational approach underscores the need for healthcare professionals to move beyond traditional, top-down models of care and instead adopt a collaborative and empathetic stance that respects the individual's experiences and autonomy.

SELF-MANAGEMENT AS A COMPLEX AND EVOLVING PROCESS

Despite its potential to empower individuals, self-management is not without challenges. Participants and healthcare professionals alike acknowledged the tensions between fostering independence and providing necessary support. While some stroke survivors embrace self-management strategies as a pathway to autonomy, others describe it as a burdensome responsibility, particularly when formal support systems were perceived as insufficient.

This tension is further complicated by societal expectations and healthcare structures, where people with strokes avoid being a nuisance to the healthcare system. As one participant, "Hank", explained:

> For they sit at different distribution offices and say that Mrs. Olsen is managing fine, Hansen is managing fine, but that one, she needs a little bit of help. And then Olsen and Hansen are left to manage on their own. It shouldn't be like that. Because we humans say we're fine, but that's not always the case.

Such perspectives highlight the limitations of self-management when it is framed solely as an individual responsibility, without adequate structural and professional support. This is particularly evident in the transition from hospital to home, where many participants reported feeling abandoned or left to navigate their rehabilitation independently. In the future, digital technologies, such as videoconferencing software or apps, might help prepare for the transition from hospital to the home as shown in stroke studies (English et al., 2023; Lumprom et al., 2025; Spalding et al., 2026; Willems et al., 2022).

THE ROLE OF SOCIAL NETWORKS IN SELF-MANAGEMENT

The process of self-management often extends beyond the individual to include their social networks. In our studies, family members and close companions were described as integral to the self-management journey, with participants referring to their cohabitants as "partners" and equally involved in the process. These relationships were central to managing the practical and emotional challenges of stroke recovery, with expressions such as "getting lives to fit" reflecting the collaborative nature of adapting to a new situation, where digital technologies could invite to these social networks.

However, these dynamics also revealed complexities. Some participants described how their networks narrowed post-stroke, leading to feelings of isolation, while others emphasized the importance of shared resilience within their core support systems. This interplay between individual self-management and social support underscores the need for rehabilitation approaches that consider the broader social context of recovery.

DISCUSSION

This chapter shows the multifaceted nature of self-management. Drawing on the different cases, the analysis revealed how stroke survivors navigate through identity reconstruction, emotional adaptation, and behavior changes. Themes emerged around the evolving sense of self, the dynamic interplay between independence and support, and the integration of digital technologies as facilitators of self-management.

As we have seen in this chapter, there are several tensions between individual self-management, technology, and its' unclear collaborative involvement with healthcare professionals. First of all, living with a chronic condition like stroke provokes many emotional situations where empowerment and health, as these cases show, are not in constant prominent foreground. Moreover, the emotional impact of living with a chronic condition is important due to that it can change how individuals perceive their future, where experiences of anger, fear, frustration, and depression make emotional regulation an essential part of managing the condition effectively (Lorig and Holman, 2003). Understanding selfhood is essential to recognizing that, despite emotional and cognitive changes, a person retains their personal identity or self. While aspects of the socially constructed self may diminish due to how others interact with the individual, their core personhood, autonomy, and dignity must always be respected (Laghezza, 2024). Second, as stroke survivors are prone to adverse psychological states because of cognitive impairment, physical disability and lack of social support (Jiang et al., 2023), it clashes with the opportunistic inherent foundations based on positive psychology. As a solution, resilience, also when using technology, has been proven to alleviate the negative emotions for individuals with chronic diseases (Jiang et al., 2023). A study of individuals with other neurological conditions than stroke, demonstrated that VR-training at home for people with traumatic brain injury was easy to use, motivating, engaging and they created new routines in everyday life (Johansen et al., 2025). Thus, these participants also addressed the importance of therapeutic involvement for individual tailoring of the intervention.

Although it is challenging for the scientific community to disentangle how self-management encompasses both a process of self-efficacy and a partnership with healthcare professionals (Nott et al., 2021), here illustrated in "*what I make of it*" and having the rehabilitation centers "*in your pocket*", this partnership remains crucial. In relation to self-managed digital technologies, the participants in our study called for solutions, like app-based exercise programs to manage on their own (Hestetun-Mandrup et al., 2026a). Other stroke survivors used so-called everyday technologies, like smartphones, smartwatches, and gaming consoles, which are now rapidly being integrated into healthcare systems whereby remotely synchronized data enhance holistic treatment (Hayre et al., 2019). However, the most used digital solutions in hospital to home transitions are videoconferencing software and hospital-owned apps, where the support from healthcare professionals might be maintained, but where the technologies ironically do not belong to the stroke user. This collaboration is particularly important both initially and continuously to develop effective self-management strategies, balancing personal autonomy with professional support. However, as Lorig and Holman notes, a prerequisite for the stroke survivor is the ability to accurately report the trends and tempo of the disease, make informed choices about rehabilitation and discuss with healthcare professionals (Lorig and Holman, 2003). This is difficult in cases where stroke survivors, as we have revealed in this chapter, appear "just fine". In other situations, the incitement to self-manage can be present, but the resources and opportunities to do so with digital technologies can be scarce. For instance, using ICT is not necessarily inherent within all healthcare organizations. Everyday technologies, as readily available and consumer-owned solutions, offer potential for how this technology can be used in rehabilitation (Hayre et al., 2019). The increasing digitalization and consumerization of healthcare further complicate the landscape of self-management. As technology becomes increasingly accessible and affordable, it is likely to play a pivotal role to users in improving the health outcomes that self-management entails (Hayre et al., 2019). While digital technologies offer new opportunities for engagement, they also introduce a logic of choice, often overwhelming patients with information and options without necessarily providing the support and scaffolding needed for meaningful decisions, highlighting the need for greater focus on care (Mol, 2008). Participants in this study appreciated the flexibility and accessibility of digital technologies but also expressed a desire for relational continuity and human connection.

There are many complex sides of self-management both related to using digital technologies or in general, which are tied up with power and control after a stroke, eventually either in cases where self-management empowers people or control and restricts individuals. A study by Fletcher et al. (2019) found that stroke self-management was evident as rhetorical, personal, hierarchical and mutual power. In this chapter, self-management was mainly related to becoming self-efficient, where rhetorical, personal and the importance of mutual forms of self-management by collaboration with healthcare professionals were exhibited. The importance of rhetorical self-management shapes how patients and practitioners perceive their roles, potentially offering avenues for patients to acquire lay expertise. Stroke survivors are in positions to possess knowledge about their condition, which can empower ownership over their recovery process, but while professional expertise remains essential, a collaborative relationship with survivors can promote decision-making and a balanced dynamic (Fletcher et al., 2019).

Although self-management span over several types of management, the main focus of the participants in these empirical studies was less on medical management, such as adherence to diet and exercise, but more about role and emotional management. This aligns with the foundations of person-centeredness, where it is related to health as a wholeness rather than reducing it to biological and physical dominance (Killingback and Naylor, 2024). For instance, the shift in role management was highlighted by one participant who described focusing on maintaining a clean apartment after her stroke, in contrast to her previous role as a truck driver, where the self-management strategies only became necessary following the stroke. Such narratives underscore that self-management after stroke is deeply embedded in the reconfiguration of everyday life and personal roles. Still, these findings also point to the limitations of self-management as a universal solution. Indeed, the aim of self-management is less in focus especially for stroke individuals with severe cognitive impairments, as self-management rely on cognitive problem-solving processes (Fletcher et al., 2019). Ironically, this population is typically excluded from stroke research due to ethical difficulties in gaining informed consent, which blurs the realistic picture of practice. These tensions highlight the need for a more nuanced understanding of self-management that accounts for fluctuating capacities, relational dependencies, and the socio-emotional context of recovery.

Finally, the social and practical implications of integrating self-management strategies with digital technologies for post-stroke practice outline a comprehensive focus; not just on medical management but maybe even more relevant – role and emotional management. The findings emphasize the importance of contextual, relational, and motivational factors, highlighting both the empowering and challenging aspects of self-managed rehabilitation and the need for better digital support. As opposed to the impersonal, automated, mechanical procedures which can result from a technology focus, a transformational change with humanizing healthcare in working with patients and relevant stakeholders is highlighted by the International Experience Exchange for Patient Organizations (Killingback and Naylor, 2024). Healthcare professionals can encourage patient activation, enhance resilience, and foster a positive environment of social support to improve self-management among stroke survivors. Often, current stroke rehabilitation practices are grounded in the ICF model and early versions of person-centered care, emphasizing specific and holistic properties. Although being focused on abilities, level of functioning, social support, and the individuals' lives and identities (Leplege et al., 2007), it is no wonder why most stroke rehabilitation practices fail to embrace the full-scale self-management strategies by implying both problem-solving, decision-making, using resources, taking action, and building partnership with healthcare professionals (Lorig and Holman, 2003). An ethical aspect of self-management in relation to technology emphasizes that solely framing humans through medical science and technology is limiting (Killingback and Naylor, 2024; Laghezza, 2024). Instead, it highlights the importance of approaching patient interactions through embodied perspectives and human dialogue (Killingback and Naylor, 2024). The intersection of technology and person-centered practices, involving self-management, can enhance person-centered technology-based rehabilitation (Killingback and Naylor, 2024).

CONCLUSION

Self-management in post-stroke rehabilitation is a multifaceted and evolving concept that encompasses behavioral changes, collaboration with family members and healthcare professionals, and the integration of digital technologies. By drawing on the lived experiences of stroke survivors and the perspectives of healthcare professionals, this chapter highlights both the opportunities and challenges inherent in promoting self-management. While digital technologies provide innovative avenues for supporting autonomy and motivation, they must be paired with empathetic, collaborative approaches that address the emotional and relational aspects of recovery. Although using technologies for self-managing seems acceptable among stroke survivors, there are still lessons to be learned regarding the digital interface and its practical applicability to maximize its potential for self-management.

In this chapter, we underscore the importance of balancing independence with the need for professional and social support, particularly during critical transitions in the rehabilitation process. As self-management continues to gain prominence as a cornerstone of person-centered care, it is essential to ensure that it is not reduced to an individual responsibility but is instead framed as a shared endeavor between stroke survivors, their networks, and healthcare professionals. Helping stroke survivors to develop self-management strategies can enhance their resilience and resourcefulness, supporting them in rebuilding their lives over the long term.

REFERENCES

Adams, R. J., Ellington, A. L., Kuccera, K. A., Leaman, H., Smithson, C. & Patrie, J. T. 2023. Telehealth-guided virtual reality for recovery of upper extremity function following stroke. *OTJR: Occupation, Participation and Health*. https://doi.org/10.1177/15394492231158375

Allegue, D. R., Higgins, J., Sweet, S. N., Archambault, P. S., Michaud, F., Miller, W., Tousignant, M. & Kairy, D. 2022. Rehabilitation of upper extremity by telerehabilitation combined with exergames in survivors of chronic stroke: Preliminary findings from a feasibility clinical trial. *JMIR Rehabilitation and Assistive Technologies*, 9(2), e34105.

Aprile, I., Gallotti, M., Schirru, M., Insalaco, S., Germanotta, M., Di Luzio, F. S., Vollero, L. & Zollo, L. 2022. Robotic telerehabilitation: a feasibility study in patients with stroke. *Gait and Posture*, 97(Supplement 2), 25–26.

Corbin, J. M. & Strauss, A. 1988. *Unending work and care: managing chronic illness at home*. Jossey-Bass.

Cramer, S., Lucy, D., Le, V., Jill, S., Renee, A., Alison, M., Robert, Z., Nina, C., Walt, S., Megan, S., Barrett, A., Chae, J., Edwards, D., Agrawal, K., Ngo, K., Roth, E., Tirschwell, D., Woodbury, M., Zafonte, R. & Wolf, S. 2019. Telerehabilitation in the home versus therapy in-clinic for patients with stroke. *European Stroke Journal*, 3, 590–591.

Ding, K., Ma, Y., Zhang, L., Gu, Y., Pan, H., Gu, Z.-E. & Zhang, H. 2025. Patient-centered insights into virtual reality rehabilitation for stroke: a systematic review and qualitative meta-synthesis. *Journal of Neuroengineering and Rehabilitation*, 22, 124.

Dobe, J., Gustafsson, L., Walder, K., Bower, K. & Lachman, R. 2023. Co-creation of self-management support during inpatient stroke rehabilitation. *PEC Innovation*, 3, 100191.

English, C., Ramage, E. R., Attia, J., Bernhardt, J., Bonevski, B., Burke, M., Galloway, M., Hankey, G. J., Janssen, H., Lindley, R., Lynch, E., Oldmeadow, C., Said, C. M., Spratt, N. J., Zacharia, K., Macdonald-Wicks, L. & Patterson, A. 2023. Secondary prevention of stroke. A telehealth-delivered physical activity and diet pilot randomized trial (ENAbLE-pilot). *International Journal of Stroke*, 19, 199–208.

Fletcher, S., Kulnik, S. T., Demain, S. & Jones, F. 2019. The problem with self-management: problematising self-management and power using a Foucauldian lens in the context of stroke care and rehabilitation. *PloS One*, 14, e0218517.

Gåsvær, J. I., Jepsen, R., Heldal, I. & Sudmann, T. 2023. Supporting collaboration in rehabilitation trajectories with information and communication technologies: scoping review. *JMIR Rehabilitation and Assistive Technologies*, 10, e46408.

Gauthier, L. V., Nichols-Larsen, D. S., Uswatte, G., Strahl, N., Simeo, M., Proffitt, R., Kelly, K., Crawfis, R., Taub, E., Morris, D., Lowes, L. P., Mark, V. & Borstad, A. 2022. Video game rehabilitation for outpatient stroke (VIGoROUS): a multi-site randomized controlled trial of in-home, self-managed, upper-extremity therapy. *eClinicalMedicine*, 43, 101237.

Hayre, C. M., Muller, D. & Scherer, M. 2019. *Everyday technologies in healthcare*. CRC Press.

Henry, L., Leahy, S., Mccurtin, A. & Boland, P. 2022. Evaluation of the evidence for self-management post-stroke within clinical practice guidelines for people with stroke: a systematic review. *British Journal of Occupational Therapy*, 85, 923–946.

Hernandez, A., Bubyr, L., Archambault, P. S., Higgins, J., Levin, M. F. & Kairy, D. 2022. Virtual reality-based rehabilitation as a feasible and engaging tool for the management of chronic poststroke upper-extremity function recovery: randomized controlled trial. *JMIR Serious Games*, 10, e37506.

Hestetun-Mandrup, A. M., Hamre, C., Lund, A., Martinsen, A. C. T., He, H.-G. & Pikkarainen, M. 2026a. Exploring people with stroke's perceptions of digital technologies in post-stroke rehabilitation – a qualitative study. *Disability and Rehabilitation*, 48(2), 359–368. https://doi.org/10.1080/09638288.2025.2504615

Hestetun-Mandrup, A. M., Hamre, C., Lund, A., Martinsen, A. C. T., He, H.-G. & Pikkarainen, M. 2026b. Exploring the influence of digitalisation on multidisciplinary post-stroke rehabilitation practice: a qualitative study. *JMIR Rehabilitation and Assistive Technologies*, 13, e77753. https://doi.org/10.2196/77753

Jesus, T. S., Bright, F., Kayes, N. & Cott, C. A. 2016. Person-centred rehabilitation: what exactly does it mean? Protocol for a scoping review with thematic analysis towards framing the concept and practice of person-centred rehabilitation. *BMJ Open*, 6, e011959.

Jiang, N., Feng, L., Song, N., Ye, Y., Wei, B., Tian, T., Chen, N., Li, Y. & Jiang, X. 2025. Stroke survivors' patient activation and self-management: the serial mediating role of social support and resilience. *Geriatric Nursing*, 63, 16–25.

Jiang, N., Xv, Y., Sun, X., Feng, L., Wang, Y. B. & Jiang, X. L. 2023. Study on self-management of real-time and individualized support in stroke patients based on resilience: a protocol for a randomized controlled trial. *Trials, [Electronic Resource]*, 24, 493.

Johansen, T., Matre, M., Tornås, S., Løvstad, M., Ponsford, J. L., Olsen, A. & Lund, A. 2025. i thought it would be difficult, but this is actually something i can do–experiences with virtual reality-based cognitive training in persons with TBI. *Annals of Medicine*, 57, 2490218.

Killingback, C. & Naylor, J. 2024. Emerging technologies in healthcare: Interpersonal and client-based perspectives. In C. M. Hayre, D. Muller, M. Scherer, P. M. W. Hackett, & A. Gordley-Smith (Eds.), *Emerging technologies in healthcare interpersonal and client based perspectives*. CRC Press. https://doi.org/10.1201/9781003272786-1

Laghezza, A. 2024. Technology in the home: an ethical discussion about aging adults with cognitive changes. *In: Emerging technologies in healthcare*. CRC Press.

Leplege, A., Gzil, F., Cammelli, M., Lefeve, C., Pachoud, B. & Ville, I. 2007. Person-centredness: conceptual and historical perspectives. *Disability and Rehabilitation*, 29, 1555–1565.

Linnet Olesen, M. & Jørgensen, R. 2023. Impact of the person-centred intervention guided self-determination across healthcare settings—an integrated review. *Scandinavian Journal of Caring Sciences*, 37, 37–59.

Lorig, K. R. & Holman, H. R. 2003. Self-management education: history, definition, outcomes, and mechanisms. *Annals of Behavioral Medicine*, 26, 1–7.

Lumprom, O., Kritpracha, C., Kocakabak, C. & Latour, J. M. 2025. eHealth technologies in transitional care interventions for stroke survivors and caregivers: a scoping review. *Florence Nightingale Journal of Nursing*, 33, 1–23.

Mol, A. 2008. *The logic of care: Health and the problem of patient choice*. Routledge.

Nott, M., Wiseman, L., Seymour, T., Pike, S., Cuming, T. & Wall, G. 2021. Stroke self-management and the role of self-efficacy. *Disability and Rehabilitation*, 43, 1410–1419.

Parke, H. L., Epiphaniou, E., Pearce, G., Taylor, S. J., Sheikh, A., Griffiths, C. J., Greenhalgh, T. & Pinnock, H. 2015. Self-management support interventions for stroke survivors: a systematic meta-review. *PloS One*, 10, e0131448.

Paterson, B. L. 2001. The shifting perspectives model of chronic illness. *Journal of Nursing Scholarship*, 33, 21–26.

Rahman, M. S., Peng, W., Adams, J. & Sibbritt, D. 2023. The use of self-management strategies for stroke rehabilitation: a scoping review. *Topics in Stroke Rehabilitation*, 30, 552–567.

Spalding, K., Gustafsson, L., Hodson, T., Shirota, C., & Brough, R. (2026). Home is "a different planet" when transitioning from hospital after acquired brain injury: can digital technology help bridge the two worlds? *Disability and Rehabilitation*, 48(2), 395–402. https://doi.org/10.1080/09638288.2025.2508406

Wade, D. T. 2005. *Describing rehabilitation interventions*. SAGE Publications.

Wang, X., Jiang, H., Zhao, Z., Lin, B., Wang, T., Ruan, Z., Ping, Z., Chen, S. & Zhang, Z. 2025. The relationship between self-efficacy and self-management: A moderated mediation model of self-control and emotion regulation among stroke survivors. *Disability and Rehabilitation*, 1–12.

Willems, E. M., Vermeulen, J., Van Haastregt, J. C. & Zijlstra, G. R. 2022. Technologies to improve the participation of stroke patients in their home environment. *Disability and Rehabilitation*, 44, 7116–7126.

8 Rehab in Your Pocket
Reimagining Low Back Pain Rehabilitation and Self-Management via Smartphone Apps

Claudia Didyk, Belinda Lange and Lucy Kate Lewis

INTRODUCTION: OVERVIEW OF LOW BACK PAIN AND ITS IMPACT

Low back pain (LBP) is an indiscriminate (Maher and Ferreira, 2022) complex biopsychosocial symptom involving the interaction between biological, psychological and social factors that can lead to, and result from, injury (Chang et al., 2024; Knezevic et al., 2021). Low back pain is experienced between the lower border of the 12th ribs and the buttock creases (Dionne et al., 2008). It may include pain or neurological leg symptoms either bilaterally or unilaterally and can range from acute (<6 weeks) to chronic (>12 weeks). However, in 85% of cases it does not have a specific disease (such as cancer) or structural cause (fracture or organ referral) (Finucane et al., 2020; Hartvigsen et al., 2018; Maher et al., 2017; Mesner et al., 2016). Recurrence is likely and currently not consistently or reliably predictable (Da Silva et al., 2017). Low back pain often presents in conjunction with other comorbidities (Hartvigsen et al., 2018); however, modifiable risk factors have been identified, including high body mass index (BMI), ergonomic factors related to the workplace and smoking (Ferreira et al., 2023).

Low back pain is the leading cause of disability globally, based on prevalence (Vos et al., 2020). In 2020, the estimated number of people experiencing LBP was 619 million (Ferreira et al., 2023). Low back pain increases with age and is most prevalent in women (Li et al., 2024) potentially resulting from oestrogen deficiency in peri/menopause (Pang et al., 2023; Wang, 2017). Oestrogen deficiency can cause disk degeneration and osteoporosis, with resultant spinal fractures resulting in LBP (Pang et al., 2023; Wang, 2017). Low-middle-income countries showed the highest years lived with disability (YLD) related to LBP (Kahere and Ginindza, 2020). Years lived with disability ranked highest in people aged 45 to 54 years due to the impact on quality of life and working life (Chen et al., 2022). Disability related to LBP can vary between geographical areas and is affected by social and health systems (Hartvigsen et al., 2018), as such country-specific LBP management is required (Buchbinder et al., 2018; Hartvigsen et al., 2018). Increased longevity, resulting in an aging population globally, adds to the growing number of people experiencing LBP and the socioeconomic burden (Chang et al., 2024).

The global costs of LBP are significant with the United States of America (USA) ranking the highest at approximately USD 70 billion in direct costs (cost associated with diagnosis and treatment), and USD 395 billion in indirect costs (reduced quality of life, loss of productivity and early retirement) annually (Chang et al., 2024). The loss of work productivity not only increases the economic burden of LBP for individuals, contributing to the cycle of poverty and social inequality (Buchbinder et al., 2020), but also for society (Lancet Rheumatology, 2023). Low back pain is also one of the costliest chronic conditions per capita (Chang et al., 2024). Although guidelines recommend LBP be managed and rehabilitated in primary care (Cieza et al., 2020; Oliveira et al., 2018), and evidence recommends a positive health approach utilising self-management (Huber et al., 2016), LBP often results in costly hospitalisation (Edwards et al., 2017; Melman et al., 2023) which increases the burden on the public

DOI: 10.1201/9781003599074-9

health system and is often low value care (Buchbinder et al., 2018). Recent research into LBP management in the emergency department has been undertaken in the United Kingdom (Downie et al., 2019) and Australia (Flanagan et al., 2024). Although findings suggest that triaging of people with LBP directly to physiotherapists can reduce hospital length of stay (Downie et al., 2019; Flanagan et al., 2024) and likelihood of opioid prescription (Flanagan et al., 2024), LBP is best managed and rehabilitated in primary care (Oliveira et al., 2018). Unfortunately, private health costs have risen globally, whilst private health insurance memberships have fallen, adding to the personal financial burden on those with LBP accessing care privately in primary care (Willis Tower Watson [WTW], 2022). The focus globally continues to be on developing interventions for common causes of death rather than those that result in disability, such as LBP (Vos et al., 2020). As a result, novel, low cost and effective interventions are required to manage the burden of LBP (Vos et al., 2020).

REHABILITATION – A GLOBAL HEALTH REQUIREMENT

Rehabilitation is increasingly being recognised as a universal need across the lifespan, rather than only a requirement for those with a disability (Cieza et al., 2020). Rehabilitation is described as the care required when a person is limited in daily function by ageing, injuries, trauma and chronic diseases or disorders (Cieza, 2019) such as LBP. Although rehabilitation is an essential component of health systems, aimed at reducing disability and improving function, it is underutilised (Cieza et al., 2020). The Rehabilitation 2030 Initiative, launched by the World Health Organisation in 2017, aimed to address the rehabilitation needs of those living with chronic conditions (WHO, 2017) such as LBP (Cieza et al., 2020). Musculoskeletal disorders account for two thirds of the rehabilitation needs, with LBP the leading health condition in 134 countries (Cieza et al., 2020), for which the largest number of people could benefit from rehabilitation (WHO, 2023). One of the aims of the Initiative was to improve and increase equitable rehabilitation access, particularly in primary care, for the one in three people globally that may require rehabilitation (Cieza et al., 2020). Low-cost digital rehabilitation options that require minimal resources, can be effective in improving health outcomes, particularly in low and middle-income countries (Cieza et al., 2020). Smartphone apps could fill this need, improve pain, function (Lara-Palomo et al., 2022) and self-management based rehabilitation potential (Didyk et al., 2022a, 2022b).

Understanding Low Back Pain and the Need for Self-Management-Based Rehabilitation

Low back pain disability varies between countries and is influenced by social norms and local health care (Hartvigsen et al., 2018). Low back pain is one of the most common reasons for primary care visits (Britt et al., 2016; Fatoye et al., 2023; Paridaens et al., 2024; Vader et al., 2022). Although telehealth adoption surged during the global COVID-19 pandemic (Koonin et al., 2020; Shaver, 2022; Wong et al., 2023) and continues to be a viable option (Lara-Palomo et al., 2022), face-to-face management of LBP remains the standard (Madsen et al., 2023; Tabacof et al., 2022) due to limited digital infrastructure, particularly in low and middle-income countries (Chhabra et al., 2023). However, regular face-to-face consults with health professionals can be costly (Fatoye et al., 2023; Paridaens et al., 2024), particularly in the current economic climate, and inaccessible or impractical for those in rural and remote locations. Low back pain guidelines recommend non-invasive treatment options that encourage self-management, address individual psychosocial factors and aim to improve function as best practice (Australian Commission on Safety and Quality in Health Care [ACSQHC], 2022a; National Institute for Health and Care Excellence [NICE], 2016). Although guideline recommendations are based on the systematic analysis of the most up to date research and summarised for useability, there are barriers to their use (Foster et al., 2018). Barriers include time constraints, lack of clinician knowledge and ineffective payment models for psychological or physical treatment options which can impact the care received (Foster et al., 2018). Guideline recommended treatment options include: a biopsychosocial approach that is patient specific and encourages a graduated return to normal activity, non-pharmacological management options, limited use of imaging and surgery, psychological-based treatment options for those with chronic symptoms and education (Foster et al., 2018).

Low back pain education to dispel unhealthy beliefs around LBP and educate at the population level was the focus of a 1997 media campaign in Australia (Buchbinder et al., 2001). Unfortunately, lack of clinician knowledge of guideline recommendations continues, maintaining the gap between evidence and practice (ACSQHC, 2022a; Madsen et al., 2023). This gap needs addressing (Foster et al., 2018) to reduce potentially detrimental LBP related fear and beliefs (Edwards et al., 2017). Low back pain is one of the most feared conditions (ACSQHC, 2022a), which may explain why it is one of the most common reasons for hospital emergency department presentations globally (Edwards et al., 2017). Fear avoidance beliefs are high in the early stages of LBP (Coudeyre et al., 2007) and can predict chronicity (Yihunie et al., 2023). Health professionals equipped with the knowledge and skills to reduce LBP related fear-avoidance beliefs are essential, particularly in the acute stages, to reduce disability, pain and fear avoidance behaviour (Bunzli et al., 2017). Globally, countries such as Australia, Canada and the United Kingdom (UK) have launched LBP national clinical care standards and guidelines to assist health professionals in the management of LBP (ACSQHC, 2022a; Alves et al., 2024). Clinical practice guidelines provide evidence-based management recommendations whilst clinical care standards focus on clinical implementation and evaluation of the recommendations in clinical settings (Alves et al., 2024). Clinical practice guidelines and clinical care standards aim to reduce the provision of conflicting management advice provided to people with LBP, with the intention to reduce progression to chronicity (ACSQHC, 2022a; Alves et al., 2024). The guidelines discourage management options that can hinder recovery such as imaging, rest and medication and encourage rehabilitation options including pain education, active rehabilitation and self-management (ACSQHC, 2022a; Alves et al., 2024).

Self-management requires a person to actively participate in the management of the medical, behavioural and emotional requirements of their condition (Lorig and Holman, 2003) by monitoring symptoms, managing their wellbeing, undertaking health-promoting activities and following treatment plans (Dwarswaard and Van De Bovenkamp, 2015). Self-management aims to improve quality of life (Lorig and Holman, 2003) by developing a person's capacity to manage day-to-day. Consumer self-management differs between individuals, as self-management plans require discussions and shared decision making between health professionals and consumers to ensure validation and incorporation of preferences and needs (ACSQHC, 2022a). Shared decision making allows consumers the confidence to return to usual activities, control pain, modify contributing lifestyle factors and navigate barriers (ACSQHC, 2022b). Self-management is recommended by current LBP guidelines (Meroni et al., 2021) as it encourages participation in usual activity and work, to improve quality of life by better daily management of LBP (Lorig and Holman, 2003). Interventions that are targeted, personalised and address biopsychosocial factors, such as kinesiophobia (fear of movement), physical activity catastrophising, disability and depression, have been shown to reduce LBP disability and pain intensity (Du et al., 2017) with small to medium effects (Banerjee et al., 2022). However, adherence to self-management programs can be impacted by resources and access to the health system as well as health status and environmental and personal characteristics (Battersby et al., 2010; Schulman-Green et al., 2016).

Individual differences, preferences and circumstances require consideration in self-management behaviour change interventions (Stieger et al., 2020). Self-management, health behaviour and a person's openness to change can be impacted by ethnic differences (Hartvigsen et al., 2018) and personality traits (Baum et al., 2004; Chapman et al., 2014; Stieger et al., 2020). Those who are more emotionally resilient and able to manage stress well (emotional stability), thoughtful and able to control impulses (conscientiousness), cooperative (agreeableness), open to new experiences (openness) and assertive and sociable (extroversion), are more likely to self-manage better and undertake self-management health promoting activities (Dietmaier et al., 2022; Hampson et al., 2016; Mendoza-Catalán et al., 2022; Power and Pluess, 2015; Sirois and Hirsch, 2015; Zhang et al., 2019). Some personality traits in the general population have been shown to be associated with increased use of physical activity apps (Petersen et al., 2020), where increased adherence is required for improved outcomes (Schaller et al., 2017). However, the personality traits directly outlined in Petersen et al. (2020) do not align with those mentioned previously. Self-management programs specific to LBP have been shown to achieve moderate reductions in disability and pain intensity (Du et al., 2017; Oliveira et al., 2012; Van Tulder et al., 2000). Although challenging (Schaller et al., 2017), adherence is an important component of behaviour change (Prochaska et al., 1992) and successful self-management (Schaller et al., 2017). Smartphone apps have the capacity to improve disability (Shebib et al., 2019) and pain outcomes (Bailey et al., 2020; Cavanagh et al., 2019; Thurnheer et al., 2018). They are used extensively in the developed world (Statista, 2020), reducing barriers to rehabilitation care for those with LBP and offering a portable, cost-effective and scalable option for self-management-based rehabilitation (Merolli et al., 2022; Murray et al., 2016).

THE ROLE OF SMARTPHONE APPS IN LOW BACK PAIN SELF-MANAGEMENT-BASED REHABILITATION AND EVIDENCE OF EFFECTIVENESS

Smartphones are ubiquitous and smartphone users are predicted to surpass eight billion by 2029 (Figure 8.1) (Exploding Topics, 2025). Mobile app downloads are projected to surpass 180 billion annually by 2026 (Statista, 2025) (Figure 8.1). The revenue for mobile health apps (mHealth) is expected to exceed 82 billion USD in 2025 up from 67.4 billion USD in 2024 (Figure 8.1), a compound annual growth rate of over 23 percent (Business Research Company [BRC], 2025). Medical apps make up the largest share of this revenue (Fact.MR, 2022).

Digital technologies in health care are crucial to deliver health interventions and address public health concerns (Cucciniello et al., 2021; El Benny et al., 2021; Stark et al., 2022). This was highlighted during the COVID-19 pandemic (Petracca et al., 2020; Stark et al., 2022) where remote care options, such as telehealth, were indispensable when face-to-face care was limited (Accenture, 2020; Merolli et al., 2022). Digital health interventions are web-based computer programs and apps that can be accessed via computers or handheld devices, such as mobile phones (Nicholl et al., 2017). Smartphone apps can provide guidance on self-management (Nicholl et al., 2017) and digital health intervention research has shown efficacy for their use (Hewitt et al., 2020; Marcolino et al., 2018). Smartphone apps for LBP self-management have been shown to be effective for pain and disability outcomes (Bailey et al., 2020; Cavanagh et al., 2019; Du et al., 2020; Rintala et al., 2022; Shebib et al., 2019; Thurnheer et al., 2018). Recent systematic reviews have shown that smartphone apps are an effective adjunct for self-management of LBP with comparable results to

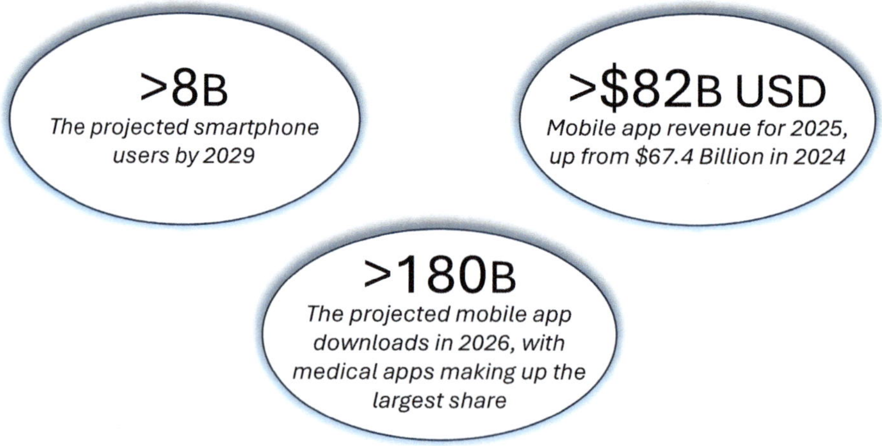

FIGURE 8.1 Smartphone app users, downloads and revenue.

usual care, with or without health professional input (Didyk et al., 2022b; Tayshete et al., 2025). Additionally, apps have potential to reduce barriers to care by offering a scalable cost-effective and portable option for people with LBP (Merolli et al., 2022; Murray et al., 2016).

CLINICAL IMPLICATIONS FOR REHABILITATION PRACTICE

Current management of LBP is high cost, low value care that is a waste of resources, unaffordable and unsustainable as an ongoing management option for LBP self-management, particularly in lower-income countries (Foster et al., 2018). Cost has been found to be a barrier to access of high value care (Dickson et al., 2024). High value care is considered care that delivers the best value and where the benefits outweigh the costs (Gleadhill et al., 2023). The LBP series Working Group for the Lancet have highlighted the urgent need for scalable, cost-effective LBP management options (Foster et al., 2018). The SPINE20 advocacy group was established in 2019 to raise global awareness about spine disorders and develop evidence-based policy recommendations for G20 governments regarding access to care, economy and rehabilitation (Chhabra et al., 2023). The SPINE20 advocacy group made recommendations to G20 countries to implement cost-effective, evidence-based practice for digital transformation in spine care for self-management, prevention as well as measurements of practice and outcomes (Chhabra et al., 2023). Smartphone apps have the potential to fill this global need as they are a readily available (Statista, 2023) option that can address resource constraints (Bennell et al., 2017). Apps are easy to access, affordable, scalable and have shown effectiveness in reducing LBP disability and pain (Bailey et al., 2020; Cavanagh et al., 2019; Du et al., 2020; Rintala et al., 2022; Shebib et al., 2019; Thurnheer et al., 2018).

Smartphone apps can improve access to evidence-based guidance and provide cost-effective guideline-based recommendations for self-management and rehabilitation (Iyengar et al., 2020; Murray et al., 2016; Stark et al., 2022; Stec et al., 2019; Whitelaw et al., 2020). Unfortunately, apps used in research are often not freely available for consumer use, reducing their benefit (Didyk et al., 2022a). It is difficult to reach conclusions on consumer-level app effectiveness due to limited and heterogeneous research and lack of studies into consumer-level apps (Didyk et al., 2022a, 2022b). However, research has shown that commercially available LBP self-management apps are of average to good quality, although few were designed to address and support self-management and behaviour change, which may impact their effectiveness and requires stricter regulation (Didyk et al., 2022a). With the accelerated integration of digital health use (Accenture, 2020; Merolli et al., 2022; Windisch et al., 2020), consumers have adapted and shown a desire for digital health management options (Accenture, 2020; Merolli et al., 2022), guided by trusted health professionals (Accenture, 2020; Byambasuren et al., 2020). However, despite consumer desire for digital health options, the uptake of smartphone apps for LBP self-management and rehabilitation is limited (Gordon et al., 2020) and may be due to barriers experienced by health professionals within the clinic (Gordon et al., 2020; Sarradon-Eck et al., 2021).

Digital health interventions offer convenience that consumers find appealing (Byambasuren et al., 2020; Deloitte, 2018). However, concerns have been raised by consumers regarding the potential for lower quality care resulting in less personalisation and professionalism, which requires addressing (Deloitte, 2018). The useability of apps by older consumers has been outlined as a barrier to app use, and as consumers look to health professionals for guidance on app recommendations (Accenture, 2020; Byambasuren et al., 2020), health professionals must also have the knowledge and tools to offer the support (Byambasuren et al., 2020). Only a small percentage of health professionals (11 percent) recommend digital health management tools despite over half of consumers reporting an interest in receiving digital health care from their usual providers (Accenture, 2020). A number of perceived barriers to the recommendation of LBP self-management apps have been outlined in the literature (ACSQHC, 2022a; Didyk et al., 2025b; Foster et al., 2018; Gleadhill et al., 2023; Sarradon-Eck et al., 2021).

Lack of knowledge of commercially available apps and app effectiveness has been outlined by health professionals as a perceived barrier to LBP self-management app recommendation for rehabilitation and requires addressing to reduce their underutilisation (Didyk et al., 2025b). Time constraints are an ongoing health system challenge that can impact high value care, particularly with the current fee for service structure that encourages short duration appointments (ACSQHC, 2022a; Foster et al., 2018; Gleadhill et al., 2023; Sarradon-Eck et al., 2021), and be a barrier to the adoption of novel health management options. Additionally, medical liability and data protection concerns can impact uptake of digital health options such as smartphone apps (Sarradon-Eck et al., 2021). However, research is lacking in this area and is required to reduce the barriers to smartphone app uptake in the self-management and rehabilitation of LBP.

Recent research aimed at understanding health professional app choice and use, found that health professionals used apps that were not condition specific for LBP self-management (Didyk et al., 2025b) and differed from those assessed in previous research to provide clinical guideline based recommendations (Didyk et al., 2022a, 2022b). This preference may have offered consumers an app with broader reach for personalisation to specific needs such as education and exercise (Didyk et al., 2025b). However, health professionals valued behaviour change options such as advice, goal setting, monitoring and social supports (Didyk et al., 2025b). Recommendation of self-management options for LBP by health professionals is crucial for outcome improvement (Foster et al., 2018). Recent research reported a lack of knowledge of LBP clinical guideline self-management recommendations by health professionals (Didyk et al., 2025b) and presents a challenge when managing people with LBP. This is of particular importance when facilitating return to work, as LBP is a leading cause of early retirement and can negatively impact wealth levels at retirement (Schofield et al., 2012). Improving self-management in clinical practice has been the subject of numerous research (Adam et al., 2020; Banerjee et al., 2022; Chala et al., 2022; Kongsted et al., 2021). A recent survey of Australian health professionals found that Physiotherapists with less than ten years of experience were more likely to recommend apps for health promotion and education and self-management (Didyk et al., 2025b). Those newer to the workforce may have increased technology literacy that can allow for easier integration of digital health options into clinical care (Didyk et al., 2025b; Keep et al., 2021; Konttila et al., 2019).

Apps can offer a self-management option in LBP rehabilitation that can increase access to health guidance and reduce health inequities as well as the economic and personal burden associated with LBP. However, current limited comparable research makes it difficult to determine what apps work best and with whom. Research delving into the personality traits and associated self-efficacy and self-management may help identify those that may benefit most from LBP self-management apps. Findings suggest that those with higher personality trait scores also reported higher self-efficacy, self-managed well (Burgess et al., 2010) and may not require additional self-management options. However, for those with lower personality trait scores and associated lower self-efficacy (Ambiel and Noronha, 2016; Brown and Cinamon, 2016; Delgado-Rodríguez et al., 2018; Hayat et al., 2020), smartphone apps may offer an alternative personalisable option to assist with improving self-management to assist with LBP rehabilitation.

CO-DESIGNING EFFECTIVE LOW BACK PAIN SELF-MANAGEMENT TECHNOLOGIES

Self-management interventions should be targeted and personalised (Banerjee et al., 2022). The World Health Organisation (2022) launched guidelines for self-care interventions and encouraged self-management toolkits. Population-based toolkits can address self-management education on a large scale. Although toolkits currently exist for the purpose of health professional education, they are not designed for consumers, and although they recommend patient education, the education provided is at the discretion of each health professional (NSW Agency for Clinical Innovation [NSWACI], 2016; Royal Australian College of General Practitioners [RACGP], 2013). It is unrealistic to expect health professionals to dedicate the time required to wade through all available evidence and choose appropriate education options to guide consumers, and this could result in inconsistent and inappropriate consumer education. Many separate toolkits used for research exist for app quality assessment and assessment of behaviour change and self-management potential (Azad-Khaneghah et al., 2021; Devan et al., 2019; Lewis, 2013; McKay et al., 2019; McMillan et al., 2016). None of these tools assess all three components, which reduces their applicability for use by time poor health professionals.

Consumer specific primary care toolkits for LBP self-management could provide consumers with evidence-based self-management advice and guidance on activity maintenance, LBP self-management apps, pain education, the nature of LBP and when to seek medical assistance. The use of co-design would allow for the integration of key stakeholder views in the development of interventions. The recent co-design and development of an app assessment tool, the LBP-SMART (Table 8.1), provides consumers and health professionals an efficient and effective method for choosing appropriate LBP self-management apps for LBP rehabilitation (Didyk et al., 2025a). The tool is divided into seven categories that were identified by participants as requirements for an LBP app assessment tool.

- *Safety*
- *Download process*
- *Look, function and feel*
- *Customisation*
- *Goals and Self-monitoring*
- *Enabling Sharing*
- *Additional Features*

Each category addressed a range of features related to quality and self-management and behaviour change potential (Figure 8.2). The breakdown of which features relate to quality, self-management or behaviour change are provided at the end of the LBP-SMART (Table 8.1).

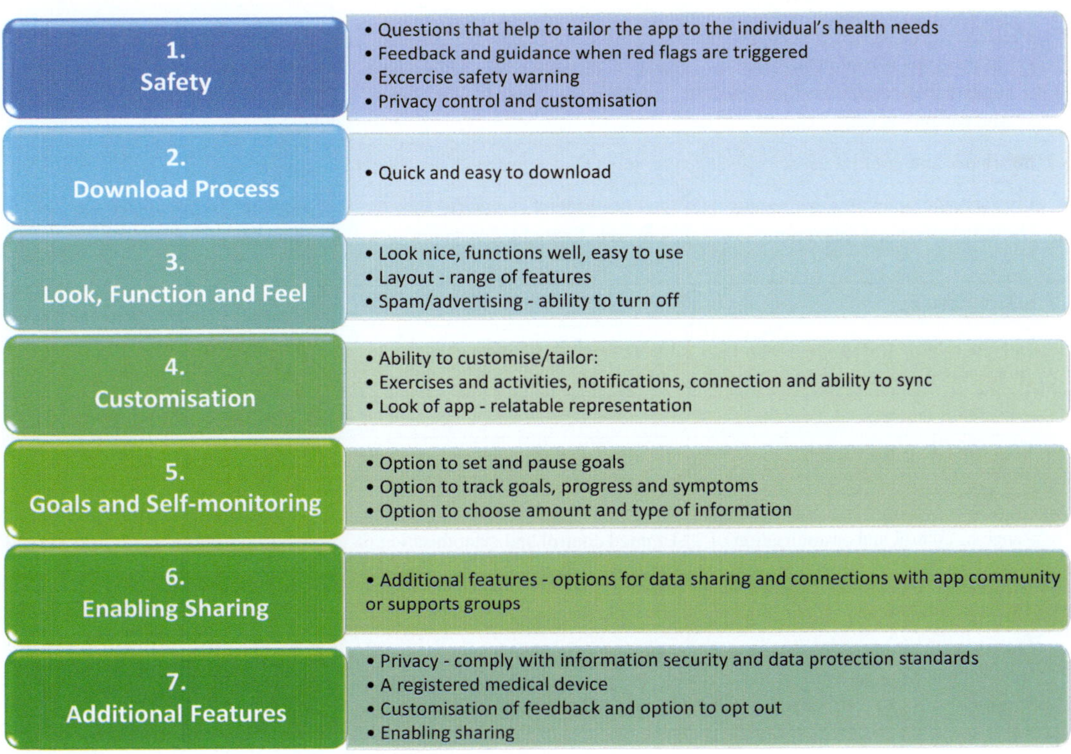

FIGURE 8.2 App assessment categories LBP-SMART. (Adapted from Didyk et al., 2025.)

TABLE 8.1
Preliminary LBP Self-Management App Review Tool (LBP-SMART)

Low Back Pain Self-Management App Review Tool (LBP-SMART)

It is recommended that, prior to using an app, you seek advice and oversight from a trusted health professional on:

- If the app suits your needs
- Managing possible risks to your health, e.g. Situations to avoid/aggravating factors
- Guidance and planning for changes to your symptoms
- Benefits and cautions of using the app
- Recommendations and suggestions to achieve your goals

Particularly if you have other conditions that may affect your ability to exercise or use the app.

Circle the most appropriate category for each row in the table

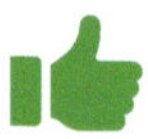	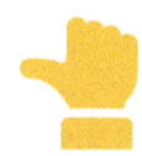	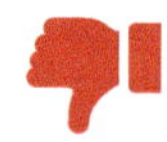
Safety		
1. Questions that help to tailor the app to the individual's health needs		
1.1 Thorough, relevant personalised health analysis questions	Somewhat personalised – some standard non-specific health questions	Not personalised at all – limited, general or irrelevant health questions
1.2 Information collected is used to customise effective and safe exercise prescription	Exercises somewhat customised	Exercises not customised
1.3 Information is continually used to update the exercises according to the person's needs	General progressions – some data used but not tailored to the person	General exercises without tailoring the person
2. Feedback and guidance when specific symptoms that require medical follow-up are triggered		
Lists specific symptoms that require health professional follow-up	Outlines general symptoms and provides limited guidance for follow-up	No specific symptoms or guidance provided
3. Safety warning		
Specific safety warning and checklist to clear that you are safe to exercise	General safety warning before exercising	No safety warning
4. Additional features		
A registered medical device		Not a registered medical device
5. Privacy		
Range of control and customisation of your own data	Limited control and customisation of your own data	No customisation
6. Additional features		
Comply with information security and data protection standards • Privacy policy		Comply with information security and data protection standards • No privacy policy

(Continued)

TABLE 8.1 *(Continued)*
Preliminary LBP Self-Management App Review Tool (LBP-SMART)

Low Back Pain Self-Management App Review Tool (LBP-SMART)		
Download process		
7. Download process		
Quick and easy to download without issues	Slow to download and/or with minor issues	Slow to download and/or major issues
Look, function and feel		
8. Looks nice		
Appealing modern, colourful and professional. App logo is related, colourful and easy to identify	Somewhat appealing – somewhat modern, somewhat professional looking, app logo is related to content	Not appealing – not modern, professional or colourful, logo is hard to identify
9. Functions well, easy to use		
Guidance on app gestures for use when required, know where you need to go next	Limited guidance	No guidance
10. Layout		
Range of layout features, e.g. Essential content on initial screen, easy to navigate menus, not overcrowded, fit the layout of screen	A few features but not all	Not many features
11. Spam, advertising		
Ability to be turned off	Limited ability to be turned off	No ability to be turned off
Customisation		
12. Exercises and activities		
12.1 Range of appropriate exercises and ability to pick and choose	Limited range of exercise and/or options to adapt	Fixed set of exercises and/or limited options to adapt
12.2 Range of activities and ability to pick and choose, e.g. emotional wellness, mindfulness, relaxation, breathing	Limited range of activities and/or limited options to adapt	No activities and/or limited options to adapt
12.3 Ability to modify the activities/exercises according to the individual's needs, e.g. type, amount and frequency	Limited ability to modify the activities/exercises	No ability to modify the activities/exercises
12.4 Range of formats available – video, written, verbal, pictorial	limited range of formats available	Only one format available
13. Tailoring of notifications and emails		
Ability to customise the type and amount of information provided	Able to have notifications but can't customise	No option to turn off notifications or customise
14. Look of app – representation of people in the app		
Range of options to customise avatar and or images, e.g. age, gender, level of fitness, body shape, clothing, culture, language	Limited options to customise the look	No options to customise the look

(Continued)

TABLE 8.1 *(Continued)*
Preliminary LBP Self-Management App Review Tool (LBP-SMART)

Low Back Pain Self-Management App Review Tool (LBP-SMART)		
15. Additional features		
Option for feedback		No option for feedback
16. Additional features		
Option for feedback • Option to opt out		Option for feedback • No option to opt out
Additional features		
17. Connection and ability to sync to other devices or programs		
Range of options for connections and syncing	Limited options	No options
Goals and self-monitoring		
18. Option to set goals		
Set goals with guidance	Set goals but no guidance	No option to set goals
19. Option to pause goals		
Without resetting to baseline	Option to pause goals but resets to baseline	No option to pause goals
20. Option to track progress and symptoms		
20.1 Progress reports – with simple visual representation of progress, e.g. graph, interactive, targets, rewards or gamification	Progress reports – no or complex and difficult to understand visual representation	No progress reports
20.2 Tracking of different measures, e.g. Pain, exercise tolerance, wellbeing, function, sleep, stress, readiness for change	One or more outcomes measured but not tracked over time	Not measured
20.3 Tracking with scale and text description	Tracking with scale only	No scale
21. Options for amount and type of information topics • Pain education – mild pain and exercise Activity pacing • Medication use • Problem solving – dealing with changes to your symptoms • Thought and behavioural management • Wellbeing • Distraction techniques **Types** • blog, video, written **Levels** • basics • evidence summary • links to research		
Self-tailoring of relevant, general information supported by research with different topics, types and levels	Limited generic information supported by research – not specific or tailored	No information or information not supported by research

(Continued)

TABLE 8.1 *(Continued)*
Preliminary LBP Self-Management App Review Tool (LBP-SMART)

Low Back Pain Self-Management App Review Tool (LBP-SMART)		
Enabling sharing		
22. Additional features		
Option for in app data sharing • Option to switch off		Option for in app data sharing No option to switch off
23. Additional features		
Option for progress sharing with app community Option to switch off		Option for progress sharing with app community • No option to switch off
24. Additional features		
Option to connect to social support group (blog) • Option to switch off personal data sharing		Option to connect to social support group (blog) • No option to switch off personal data sharing
Features		
Self-management – Items 2,3,18, 20.2, 20.3, 21, 24 Behaviour change – Items 1.1, 1.2, 1.3, 12–15, 17, 19, 20, 23 Quality – Items 5, 7–11 Additional features – Items 4, 6, 16, 22		

Source: Adapted from (Didyk et al., 2025).

Although the LBP-SMART requires pilot testing and further development of a measurable scale rather than the current simple rating system, it assesses not only app quality but also behaviour change and self-management potential and could be included in an LBP self-management and rehabilitation toolkit. The LBP-SMART was designed for LBP self-management app assessment; however, the behaviour change and quality categories are not specific to LBP and may be generalisable to other conditions. Further research would be required to explore this. The LBP toolkit could be delivered on a large scale to educate consumers at a population level, allowing for effortless integration into clinical practice to assist health professionals with implementation and adoption of LBP self-management apps. However, future research would be required to co-design and test an appropriate toolkit as such a toolkit, does not currently exist.

FUTURE DIRECTIONS IN LOW BACK PAIN SELF-MANAGEMENT AND SMARTPHONE APPS

A clear need for rigorous research, such as randomised controlled trials (RCTs), exploring commercially available LBP self-management app effectiveness has been identified. However, considering the rate at which apps are developed, updated and removed from apps stores (IQVIA Institute for Human Data [IQVIA], 2021; Larsen et al., 2016; Patrick et al., 2016), costly and slow RCTs may reduce the timely translation of app use into clinical practice (Murray et al., 2016; Patrick et al., 2016) and may not be appropriate for assessing the quality, behaviour change and self-management potential of commercially available apps. Additionally, perhaps RCT level of evidence may not be required for specific apps, and the inclusion of self-management and behaviour change features may appropriately support their use to potentially improve outcomes. Health professionals may gain confidence in low-risk app use recommendation, if the promotion of healthy lifestyle behaviours, such as activity maintenance for LBP, provides evidence of effectiveness and the benefits of app use outweigh the risks. Alternative assessment methods may be more appropriate (Didyk et al., 2025a) such as guiding app development to include self-management and behaviour change features and follow guideline based recommendations.

Various countries including Europe, the USA and Australia, have attempted to regulate health apps by implementing processes to ensure app quality at the development phase (ADHA, 2022; NICE, 2022; WHO, 2018). Despite this, health and wellness apps continue to be poorly regulated globally. Australia has developed an mHealth framework to assist developers in the app design process, and educate consumer choice on credible mHealth apps to encourage the uptake of app use in clinical practice (ADHA, 2022). However, the framework is aimed at developers and not consumers and requires the voluntary and paid participation of app developers to undergo a four-stage assessment process, the results of which are then listed in an app library with endorsement and a star rating for that particular application (ADHA, 2022). Although a positive step in improving confidence in app quality, the process is time consuming and does not allow for quick integration into clinical practice to improve app use, and apps remain underutilised for LBP self-management and rehabilitation (Gordon et al., 2020).

Consumers and health professionals would benefit from an easy to use, relevant checklist of necessary app features, based on stakeholder views (Ioannidis, 2016), to guide LBP self-management app assessment. This would allow for increased consumer confidence and reduced liability for health professionals as the recommendation of a specific app would not be required (Sarradon-Eck et al., 2021). Such a tool could result in increased uptake of app use for LBP self-management and rehabilitation and potentially reduce the economic and personal burden globally. Additionally, consumer and health professional education is required to increase knowledge of apps for LBP self-management to improve outcomes and app use (ACSQHC, 2022a; Foster et al., 2018). Consumer education could reduce incorrect beliefs, conflicting advice and fear associated with LBP that can perpetuate fear avoidance behaviour and progression to chronicity (Bunzli et al., 2017).

Consumers rely on health professional guidance (Accenture, 2020), and as such, education of health professionals on LBP self-management options, such as apps, is imperative (ACSQHC, 2022a) to allow them to appropriately guide consumers on evidence based options. Additionally, knowledge of, and use of, evidence based LBP self-management options and guidelines will allow health professionals to adhere to their required codes of conduct and fulfil insurance requirements (Australian Health Practitioner Regulation Agency [AHPRA], 2023). However, limited implementation of guideline-based care is widespread across health care generally (Foster et al., 2018; Qumseya et al., 2021). This may be a result of health professionals not being adequately exposed to guidelines in their undergraduate training or ongoing professional development (Derghazarian and Simmonds, 2011; Qumseya et al., 2021; Synnott et al., 2015) and requires addressing. Training and continuing education courses should be required to address and include guideline-based evidence as part of meeting accreditation. Additionally, although clinical guidelines are considered best practice (Foster et al., 2018), health professionals have reported that they find them to be restrictive of professional autonomy and not patient specific (Slade et al., 2016). Likewise, education regarding apps should also be provided in undergraduate and postgraduate education to encourage use and easier integration into clinical care.

CONCLUSION

Rehabilitation is centred on restoring function and improving quality of life for those affected by age-related decline, chronic illness or injury such as LBP. Digital health options, like smartphone apps, offer an adjunct rehabilitation intervention option to improve rehabilitation outcomes.

Smartphone apps are personalisable, offer feedback in real-time, track progress, provide education and can support self-management. Apps can make rehabilitation more accessible and engaging for people with LBP and extend the reach of clinic-based rehabilitation services. Innovative tools such as the LBP-SMART support people with LBP to choose quality, appropriate behaviour change and self-management apps to enhance rehabilitation. Smartphone apps offer an inclusive, efficient, scalable and sustainable, forward-thinking option for LBP rehabilitation. Smartphone apps are an option that embraces technology and innovation, remains grounded in evidence-based practice and meets the needs of diverse populations.

REFERENCES

Accenture. 2020. *Accenture 2020 consumer research on digital health* [Online]. Available: https://www.accenture.com/content/dam/accenture/final/a-com-migration/pdf/pdf-130/accenture-2020-digital-health-consumer-survey-us.pdf#zoom=40 [Accessed].

ACSQHC (Australian Commission on Safety and Quality in Health Care). 2022a. *Low back pain clinical care standards* [Online]. Available: https://www.safetyandquality.gov.au/sites/default/files/2022-08/low_back_pain_clinical_care_standard.pdf [Accessed].

ACSQHC (Australian Commission on Safety and Quality in Health Care). 2022b. *A novel approach to break the cycle of low back pain* [Online]. Available: https://www.safetyandquality.gov.au/about-us/latest-news/media-releases/novel-approach-break-cycle-low-back-pain#_edn2 [Accessed].

Adam, W. A. G., Lisa, R., Jonathan, H., Nadine, E. F., Lucy, Y., Elaine, H., Beth, S., David, T., Gareth, G., Frances, W., Lorraine, D., Alannah, M., Stephanie, H., Sarah, B., Stephanie, B.-W., Simon, W., Gemma, M., Linda, L. & Paul, L. 2020. Supporting self-management of low back pain with an internet intervention in primary care: a protocol for a randomised controlled trial of clinical and cost-effectiveness (SupportBack 2). *BMJ Open*, 10, e040543.

ADHA (Australian Digital Health Agency). 2022. *Assessment framework for mHealth apps* [Online]. Available: https://www.digitalhealth.gov.au/sites/default/files/documents/adha-mhealth-assessment-framework-dec.pdf [Accessed].

AHPRA (Australian Health Practitioner Regulation Agency). 2023. *Shared code of conduct principles* [Online]. Available: https://www.ahpra.gov.au/Resources/Code-of-conduct/Resources-to-help-health-practitioners/Shared-Code-of-conduct-principles.aspx [Accessed].

Alves, G. S., Vera, G. E. Z., Maher, C. G., Ferreira, G. E., Machado, G. C., Buchbinder, R., Pinto, R. Z. & Oliveira, C. B. 2024. Clinical care standards for the management of low back pain: a scoping review. *Rheumatology International*, 44, 1197–1207.

Ambiel, R. A. M. & Noronha, A. P. P. 2016. Professional choice self-efficacy: predicting traits and personality profiles in high school students. *Psicologia, Reflexão e Crítica*, 29, 1–8.

Azad-Khaneghah, P., Neubauer, N., Miguel Cruz, A. & Liu, L. 2021. Mobile health app usability and quality rating scales: a systematic review. *Disability and Rehabilitation: Assistive Technology*, 16, 712–721.

Bailey, J. F., Agarwal, V., Zheng, P., Smuck, M., Fredericson, M., Kennedy, D. J. & Krauss, J. 2020. Digital care for chronic musculoskeletal pain: 10,000 participant longitudinal cohort study. *Journal of Medical Internet Research*, 22, e18250–e18250.

Banerjee, A., Hendrick, P. & Blake, H. 2022. Predictors of self-management in patients with chronic low back pain: a longitudinal study. *BMC Musculoskeletal Disorders*, 23, 1071.

Battersby, M., Von Korff, M., Schaefer, J., Davis, C., Ludman, E., Greene, S. M., Parkerton, M. & Wagner, E. H. 2010. Twelve evidence-based principles for implementing self-management support in primary care. *The Joint Commission Journal on Quality and Patient Safety*, 36, 561–570.

Baum, A., Johnston, M. & Sutton, S. 2004. *The SAGE handbook of health psychology*. SAGE.

Bennell, K. L., Nelligan, R., Dobson, F., Rini, C., Keefe, F., Kasza, J., French, S., Bryant, C., Dalwood, A., Abbott, J. H. & Hinman, R. S. 2017. Effectiveness of an internet-delivered exercise and pain-coping skills training intervention for persons with chronic knee pain: a randomized trial. *Annals of Internal Medicine*, 166, 453–462.

BRC (Business Research Company). 2025. *mHealth apps global market report 2025 – by app type (disease and treatment management, wellness management, other app types), by connected medical devices (heart rate meters, wearable fitness sensor device, blood pressure monitors, pulse oximeters, other connected medical devices), by application (monitoring services, fitness solutions, diagnostic services, treatment services, other applications), by end-user (physicians, patients, insurance companies, research centers, pharmacy, biopharmaceutical companies, government, tech companies, other end-users) – market size, trends, and global forecast 2025–2034* [Online]. Available: https://www.thebusinessresearchcompany.com/report/mhealth-apps-global-market-report [Accessed].

Britt, H., Miller, G. C., Bayram, C., Henderson, J., Valenti, L., Harrison, C., Pan, Y., Charles, J., Pollack, A. J., Chambers, T., Gordon, J. & Wong, C. 2016. *A decade of Australian general practice activity 2006–07 to 2015–16*. Sydney University Press.

Brown, D. & Cinamon, R. G. 2016. Personality traits' effects on self-efficacy and outcome expectations for high school major choice. *International Journal for Educational and Vocational Guidance*, 16, 343–361.

Buchbinder, R., Jolley, D. & Wyatt, M. 2001. Population based intervention to change back pain beliefs and disability: three part evaluation. *BMJ*, 322, 1516–1520.

Buchbinder, R., Underwood, M., Hartvigsen, J. & Maher, C. G. 2020. The lancet series call to action to reduce low value care for low back pain: an update. *PAIN*, 161(Suppl 1), S1–S3.

Buchbinder, R., Van Tulder, M., Öberg, B., Costa, L. M., Woolf, A., Schoene, M., Croft, P., Buchbinder, R., Hartvigsen, J., Cherkin, D., Foster, N. E., Maher, C. G., Underwood, M., Van, Tulder, M., Anema, J. R., Chou, R., Cohen, S. P., Menezes Costa, L., Croft, P., Ferreira, M., Ferreira, P. H., Fritz, J. M., Genevay, S., Gross, D. P., Hancock, M. J., Hoy, D., Karppinen, J., Koes, B. W., Kongsted, A., Louw, Q., Öberg, B., Peul, W. C., Pransky, G., Schoene, M., Sieper, J., Smeets, R. J., Turner, J. A. & Woolf, A. 2018. Low back pain: a call for action. *The Lancet*, 391, 2384–2388.

Bunzli, S., Smith, A., Schütze, R., Lin, I. & O'sullivan, P. 2017. Making sense of low back pain and pain-related fear. *The Journal of Orthopaedic and Sports Physical Therapy*, 47, 628–636.

Burgess, L., Irvine, F. & Wallymahmed, A. 2010. Personality, stress and coping in intensive care nurses: a descriptive exploratory study. *Nursing in Critical Care*, 15, 129–140.

Byambasuren, O., Beller, E., Hoffmann, T. & Glasziou, P. 2020. Barriers to and facilitators of the prescription of mHealth apps in Australian general practice: qualitative study. *JMIR Mhealth Uhealth*, 8, e17447.

Cavanagh, R., Bhargava, A., Gleason, A., Micheel, L., Ciulla, R. & Hoyt, T. 2019. Use of health technologies for low back pain in the military health system. *Journal of Technology in Behavioral Science*, 4, 360–371.

Chala, M. B., Miller, J., Ghahari, S., Wondie, Y., Abebe, A. & Donnelly, C. 2022. Health care providers' understanding of self-management support for people with chronic low back pain in Ethiopia: an interpretive description. *BMC Health Services Research*, 22, 194.

Chang, D., Lui, A., Matsoyan, A., Safaee, M. M., Aryan, H. & Ames, C. 2024. Comparative review of the socioeconomic burden of lower back pain in the United States and globally. *Neurospine*, 21, 487–501.

Chapman, B. P., Hampson, S. & Clarkin, J. 2014. Personality-informed interventions for healthy aging: conclusions from a national institute on aging work group: conscientiousness and healthy aging. *Developmental Psychology*, 50, 1426–1441.

Chen, S., Chen, M., Wu, X., Lin, S., Tao, C., Cao, H., Shao, Z. & Xiao, G. 2022. global, regional and national burden of low back pain 1990–2019: a systematic analysis of the Global Burden of Disease Study 2019. *Journal of Orthopaedic Translation*, 32, 49–58.

Chhabra, H. S., Tamai, K., Alsebayel, H., Aleissa, S., Alqahtani, Y., Arand, M., Basu, S., Blattert, T. R., Bussières, A., Campello, M., Costanzo, G., Côté, P., Darwano, B., Franke, J., Garg, B., Hasan, R., Ito, M., Kamra, K., Kandziora, F., Kassim, N., Kato, S., Lahey, D., Mehta, K., Menezes, C. M., Muehlbauer, E. J., Mullerpatan, R., Pereira, P., Roberts, L., Ruosi, C., Sullivan, W., Shetty, A. P., Tucci, C., Wadhwa, S., Alturkistany, A., Busari, J. O., Wang, J. C., Teli, M. G. A., Rajasekaran, S., Mulukutla, R. D., Piccirillo, M., Hsieh, P. C., Dohring, E. J., Srivastava, S. K., Larouche, J., Vlok, A. & Nordin, M. 2023. SPINE20 recommendations 2023: one earth, one family, one future WITHOUT spine DISABILITY. *Brain and Spine,*, 3, 102688.

Cieza, A. 2019. Rehabilitation the health strategy of the 21st century, really? *Archives of Physical Medicine and Rehabilitation*, 100, 2212–2214.

Cieza, A., Causey, K., Kamenov, K., Hanson, S. W., Chatterji, S. & Vos, T. 2020. Global estimates of the need for rehabilitation based on the Global Burden of Disease Study 2019: a systematic analysis for the Global Burden of Disease Study 2019. *The Lancet (British Edition)*, 396, 2006–2017.

Coudeyre, E., Tubach, F., Rannou, F., Baron, G., Coriat, F., Brin, S., Revel, M. & Poiraudeau, S. 2007. Fear-avoidance beliefs about back pain in patients with acute LBP. *The Clinical Journal of Pain*, 23, 720–725.

Cucciniello, M., Petracca, F., Ciani, O. & Tarricone, R. 2021. Development features and study characteristics of mobile health apps in the management of chronic conditions: a systematic review of randomised trials. *NPJ Digital Medicine*, 4, 144–144.

Da Silva, T., Mills, K., Brown, B. T., Herbert, R. D., Maher, C. G. & Hancock, M. J. 2017. Risk of recurrence of low back pain: a systematic review. *Journal of Orthopaedic and Sports Physical Therapy*, 47, 305–313.

Delgado-Rodríguez, N., Hernández-Fernaud, E., Rosales, C., Díaz-Vilela, L., Isla-Díaz, R. & Díaz-Cabrera, D. 2018. Contextual performance in academic settings: the role of personality, self-efficacy, and impression management. *Revista de Psicología del Trabajo y de las Organizaciones*, 34, 1–6.

DELOITTE. 2018. *Consumers are on board with virtual health options: can the health care system deliver?* [Online]. Available: https://www2.deloitte.com/content/dam/insights/us/articles/4631_Virtual-consumer-survey/DI_Virtual-consumer-survey.pdf [Accessed].

Derghazarian, T. & Simmonds, M. J. 2011. Management of low back pain by physical therapists in Quebec: how are we doing? *Physiotherapy Canada*, 63, 464–473.

Devan, H., Farmery, D., Peebles, L. & Grainger, R. 2019. Evaluation of self-management support functions in apps for people with persistent pain: systematic review. *JMIR mHealth and uHealth*, 7, e13080-e13080.

Dickson, C., De Zoete, R. M. J., Berryman, C., Weinstein, P., Chen, K. K. & Rothmore, P. 2024. Patient-related barriers and enablers to the implementation of high-value physiotherapy for chronic pain: a systematic review. *Pain Med*, 25, 104–115.

Didyk, C., Kate, L. L. & And Lange, B. 2025a. Development of the low back pain self-management app review tool (LBP-SMART) for consumers to assess the quality, behaviour change and self-management potential of LBP smartphone apps. *Disability and Rehabilitation*, 47, 5319–5327.

Didyk, C., Lewis, L. K. & Lange, B. 2022a. Availability, content and quality of commercially available smartphone applications for the self-management of low back pain: a systematic assessment. *Disability and Rehabilitation*, 44, 7600–7609.

Didyk, C., Lewis, L. K. & Lange, B. 2022b. Effectiveness of smartphone apps for the self-management of low back pain in adults: a systematic review. *Disability and Rehabilitation*, 44, 7781–7790.

Didyk, C., Lewis, L. K. & Lange, B. 2025b. Health professionals' use of smartphone apps for clients with low back pain: an observational study. *Prim Health Care Research and Development*, 26, e14.

Dietmaier, J.-M., Von Dem Knesebeck, O., Heesen, C. & Kofahl, C. 2022. Personality and its association with self-management in multiple sclerosis. *Multiple Sclerosis and Related Disorders*, 61, 103752–103752.

Dionne, C. E., Dunn, K. M., Croft, P. R., Nachemson, A. L., Buchbinder, R., Walker, B. F., Wyatt, M., Cassidy, J. D., Rossignol, M., Leboeuf-Yde, C., Hartvigsen, J., Leino-Arjas, P., Latza, U., Reis, S., Del Real, M. T. G., Kovacs, F. M., Oberg, B., Ceaschi, C., Bouter, L. M., Koes, B., Picavet, H. S. J., Van Tulder, M. W., Burton, K., Foster, N. E., Macfarlane, G. J., Thomas, E., Underwood, M., Waddell, G., Shekelle, P., Volinn, E. & Korff, M. H. 2008. A consensus approach toward the standardization of back pain definitions for use in prevalence studies. *Spine (Philadelphia, Pa. 1976)*, 33, 95–103.

Downie, F., McRitchie, C., Monteith, W. & Turner, H. 2019. Physiotherapist as an alternative to a GP for musculoskeletal conditions: a 2-year service evaluation of UK primary care data. *British Journal of General Practice*, 69, e314–e320.

Du, S., Liu, W., Cai, S., Hu, Y. & Dong, J. 2020. The efficacy of e-health in the self-management of chronic low back pain: a meta analysis. *International Journal of Nursing Studies*, 106, 103507–103507.

Du, S. R. N. M. I. N., Hu, L. B. I. C. M., Dong, J. M. I. P., Xu, G. R. N. P. D., Chen, X. R. N. P. D., Jin, S. R. N. P. D., Zhang, H. R. N. P. D. & Yin, H. R. N. M. I. N. 2017. Self-management program for chronic low back pain: a systematic review and meta-analysis. *Patient Education and Counseling*, 100, 37–49.

Dwarswaard, J. & Van De Bovenkamp, H. 2015. Self-management support: a qualitative study of ethical dilemmas experienced by nurses. *Patient Education and Counseling*, 98, 1131–1136.

Edwards, J., Hayden, J., Asbridge, M., Gregoire, B. & Magee, K. 2017. Prevalence of low back pain in emergency settings: a systematic review and meta-analysis. *BMC Musculoskeletal Disorders*, 18, 143.

El Benny, M., Kabakian-Khasholian, T., El-Jardali, F. & Bardus, M. 2021. Application of the eHealth literacy model in digital health interventions: scoping review. *Journal of Medical Internet Research*, 23, e23473.

FACT.MR. 2022. *mHealth apps market analysis by product type (medical apps, fitness app), and by region – global market insights 2022 to 2032* [Online]. Available: https://www.factmr.com/report/mhealth-apps-market [Accessed].

Fatoye, F., Gebrye, T., Ryan, C. G., Useh, U. & Mbada, C. 2023. Global and regional estimates of clinical and economic burden of low back pain in high-income countries: a systematic review and meta-analysis. *Front Public Health*, 11, 1098100.

Ferreira, M. L., Luca, K. D., Haile, L. M., Gbd, L. B. P. C., Steinmetz, J. D., Culbreth, G. T., Cross, M., Kopec, J. A., Ferreira, P. H., Blyth, F. M., Buchbinder, R., Hartvigsen, J., Wu, A.-M., Safiri, S., Woolf, A. D., Collins, G. S., Ong, K. L., Vollset, S. E., Smith, A. E., Cruz, J. A., Fukutaki, K. G., Abate, S. M., Abbasifard, M., Abbasi-Kangevari, M., Abbasi-Kangevari, Z., Abdelalim, A., Abedi, A., Abidi, H., Estiningtyas Sakilah Adnani, Q., Ahmadi, A., Olusola Akinyemi, R., Tadesse Alamer, A., Zeleke Alem, A., Alimohamadi, Y., Alshehri, M. A., Alzahrani, H., Amini, S., Amiri, S., Amu, H., Liliana Andrei,

C., Andrei, T., Antony, B., Arabloo, J., Arulappan, J., Arumugam, A., Ashraf, T., Athari, S. S., Awoke, N., Azadnajafabad, S. & Winfried Bärnighausen, T. 2023. Global, regional, and national burden of low back pain, 1990–2020, its attributable risk factors, and projections to 2050: a systematic analysis of the Global Burden of Disease Study 2021. *The Lancet Rheumatology*, 5, e316–e329.

Finucane, L. M., Downie, A., Mercer, C., Greenhalgh, S. M., Boissonnault, W. G., Pool-Goudzwaard, A. L., Beneciuk, J. M., Leech, R. L. & Selfe, J. 2020. International framework for red flags for potential serious spinal pathologies. *The Journal of Orthopaedic and Sports Physical Therapy*, 50, 350–372.

Flanagan, P., Waller, R., Lin, I., Richards, K., Truter, P., Machado, G. C. & Cavalheri, V. 2024. Interventions to improve the quality of low back pain care in emergency departments: a systematic review and meta-analysis. *Internal and Emergency Medicine*, 19, 2057–2076.

Foster, N. E., Anema, J. R., Cherkin, D., Chou, R., Cohen, S. P., Gross, D. P., Ferreira, P. H., Fritz, J. M., Koes, B. W., Peul, W., Turner, J. A., Maher, C. G., Buchbinder, R., Hartvigsen, J., Cherkin, D., Foster, N. E., Maher, C. G., Underwood, M., Van Tulder, M., Anema, J. R., Chou, R., Cohen, S. P., Menezes Costa, L., Croft, P., Ferreira, M., Ferreira, P. H., Fritz, J. M., Genevay, S., Gross, D. P., Hancock, M. J., Hoy, D., Karppinen, J., Koes, B. W., Kongsted, A., Louw, Q., Öberg, B., Peul, W. C., Pransky, G., Schoene, M., Sieper, J., Smeets, R. J., Turner, J. A. & Woolf, A. 2018. Prevention and treatment of low back pain: evidence, challenges, and promising directions. *The Lancet (British Edition)*, 391, 2368–2383.

Gleadhill, C., Dooley, K., Kamper, S. J., Manvell, N., Corrigan, M., Cashin, A., Birchill, N., Donald, B., Leyland, M., Delbridge, A., Barnett, C., Renfrew, D., Lamond, S., Boettcher, C. E., Chambers, L., Maude, T., Davis, J., Hodgson, S., Makaroff, A., Wallace, J. B., Kotrick, K., Mullen, N., Gallagher, R., Zelinski, S., Watson, T., Davidson, S., Viana Da Silva, P., Mahon, B., Delore, C., Manvell, J., Gibbs, B., Hook, C., Stoddard, C., Meers, E., Byrne, M., Schneider, T., Bolsewicz, K. & Williams, C. M. 2023. What does high value care for musculoskeletal conditions mean and how do you apply it in practice? A consensus statement from a research network of physiotherapists in New South Wales, Australia. *BMJ Open*, 13, e071489.

Gordon, W. J., Landman, A., Zhang, H. & Bates, D. W. 2020. Beyond validation: getting health apps into clinical practice. *NPJ Digital Medicine*, 3, 14–14.

Hampson, S. E., Edmonds, G. W., Barckley, M., Goldberg, L. R., Dubanoski, J. P. & Hillier, T. A. 2016. A Big Five approach to self-regulation: personality traits and health trajectories in the Hawaii longitudinal study of personality and health. *Psychology, Health & Medicine*, 21, 152–162.

Hartvigsen, J., Hancock, M. J., Kongsted, A., Louw, Q., Ferreira, M. L., Genevay, S., Hoy, D., Karppinen, J., Pransky, G., Sieper, J., Smeets, R. J., Underwood, M., Buchbinder, R., Hartvigsen, J., Cherkin, D., Foster, N. E., Maher, C. G., Underwood, M., Van Tulder, M., Anema, J. R., Chou, R., Cohen, S. P., Menezes Costa, L., Croft, P., Ferreira, M., Ferreira, P. H., Fritz, J. M., Genevay, S., Gross, D. P., Hancock, M. J., Hoy, D., Karppinen, J., Koes, B. W., Kongsted, A., Louw, Q., Öberg, B., Peul, W. C., Pransky, G., Schoene, M., Sieper, J., Smeets, R. J., Turner, J. A. & Woolf, A. 2018. What low back pain is and why we need to pay attention. *The Lancet (British Edition)*, 391, 2356–2367.

Hayat, A. A., Kohoulat, N., Amini, M. & Faghihi, S. A. A. 2020. The predictive role of personality traits on academic performance of medical students: the mediating role of self-efficacy. *Medical Journal of the Islamic Republic of Iran*, 34, 77.

Hewitt, S., Sephton, R. & Yeowell, G. 2020. The effectiveness of digital health interventions in the management of musculoskeletal conditions: systematic literature review. *Journal of Medical Internet Research*, 22, e15617.

Huber, M., Van Vliet, M., Giezenberg, M., Winkens, B., Heerkens, Y., Dagnelie, P. C. & Knottnerus, J. A. 2016. Towards a 'patient-centred' operationalisation of the new dynamic concept of health: a mixed methods study. *BMJ Open*, 6, e010091.

Ioannidis, J. P. A. 2016. Why most clinical research is not useful. *PLoS Medicine*, 13, e1002049.

IQVIA. 2021. *Digital health trends 2021* [Online]. Available: https://www.iqvia.com/insights/the-iqvia-institute/reports/digital-health-trends-2021 [Accessed].

Iyengar, K., Upadhyaya, G. K., Vaishya, R. & Jain, V. 2020. COVID-19 and applications of smartphone technology in the current pandemic. *Diabetes & Metabolic Syndrome Clinical Research & Reviews*, 14, 733–737.

Kahere, M. & Ginindza, T. 2020. Mapping evidence on the prevalence, incidence, risk factors and cost associated with chronic low back pain among adults in Sub-Saharan Africa: a systematic scoping review protocol. *Systematic Reviews*, 9, 57–57.

Keep, M., Janssen, A., McGregor, D., Brunner, M., Baysari, M. T., Quinn, D. & Shaw, T. 2021. Mapping eHealth education: review of eHealth content in health and medical degrees at a metropolitan tertiary institute in Australia. *JMIR Med Educ*, 7, e16440.

Knezevic, N. N., Candido, K. D., Vlaeyen, J. W. S., Van Zundert, J. & Cohen, S. P. 2021. Low back pain. *The Lancet*, 398, 78–92.

Kongsted, A., Ris, I., Kjaer, P. & Hartvigsen, J. 2021. Self-management at the core of back pain care: 10 key points for clinicians. *Revista brasileira de fisioterapia (São Carlos (São Paulo, Brazil))*, 25, 396–406.

Konttila, J., Siira, H., Kyngäs, H., Lahtinen, M., Elo, S., Kääriäinen, M., Kaakinen, P., Oikarinen, A., Yamakawa, M., Fukui, S., Utsumi, M., Higami, Y., Higuchi, A. & Mikkonen, K. 2019. Healthcare professionals' competence in digitalisation: a systematic review. *Journal of Clinical Nursing*, 28, 745–761.

Koonin, L. M., Hoots, B., Tsang, C. A., Leroy, Z., Farris, K., Jolly, B., Antall, P., McCabe, B., Zelis, C. B. R., Tong, I. & Harris, A. M. 2020. Trends in the use of telehealth during the emergence of the COVID-19 pandemic — United States, January–March 2020. *MMWR. Morbidity and Mortality Weekly Report*, 69, 1595–1599.

Lara-Palomo, I. C., Gil-Martínez, E., Ramírez-García, J. D., Capel-Alcaraz, A. M., García-López, H., Castro-Sánchez, A. M. & Antequera-Soler, E. 2022. Efficacy of e-health interventions in patients with chronic low-back pain: a systematic review with meta-analysis. *Telemedicine Journal and e-Health*, 28, 1734–1752.

Larsen, M. E., Nicholas, J. & Christensen, H. 2016. Quantifying app store dynamics: longitudinal tracking of mental health apps. *JMIR Mhealth Uhealth*, 4, e96.

Lewis, T. L. 2013. A systematic self-certification model for mobile medical apps. *Journal of Medical Internet Research*, 15, e89.

Li, Y., Zou, C., Guo, W., Han, F., Fan, T., Zang, L. & Huang, G. 2024. Global burden of low back pain and its attributable risk factors from 1990 to 2021: a comprehensive analysis from the global burden of disease study 2021. *Frontiers in Public Health*, 12, 1480779.

Lorig, K. R. & Holman, H. 2003. Self-management education: history, definition, outcomes, and mechanisms. *Annals of Behavioral Medicine*, 26, 1–7.

Madsen, S. D., Morsø, L., Vach, W., Andersen, M. K., Lykkegaard, J., Schiøttz-Christensen, B. & Stochkendahl, M. J. 2023. Exploring usual care for patients with low back pain in primary care: a cross-sectional study of general practitioners, physiotherapists and chiropractors. *BMJ Open*, 13, e071602.

Maher, C. & Ferreira, G. 2022. Time to reconsider what Global Burden of Disease studies really tell us about low back pain. *Annals of the Rheumatic Diseases*, 81, 306–308.

Maher, C. P., Underwood, M. P. & Buchbinder, R. P. 2017. Non-specific low back pain. *The Lancet (British Edition)*, 389, 736–747.

Marcolino, M. S., Oliveira, J. A. Q., D'agostino, M., Ribeiro, A. L., Alkmim, M. B. M. & Novillo-Ortiz, D. 2018. The impact of mHealth interventions: systematic review of systematic reviews. *JMIR mHealth and uHealth*, 6, e23.

McKay, F. H., Slykerman, S. & Dunn, M. 2019. The app behavior change scale: creation of a scale to assess the potential of apps to promote behavior change. *JMIR mHealth and uHealth*, 7, e11130.

McMillan, B., Hickey, E., Patel, M. G. & Mitchell, C. 2016. Quality assessment of a sample of mobile app-based health behavior change interventions using a tool based on the National Institute of Health and Care Excellence behavior change guidance. *Patient Education and Counseling*, 99, 429–435.

Melman, A., Lord, H., Coombs, D., Zadro, J., Maher, C. & Machado, G. 2023. Global prevalence of hospital admissions for low back pain: a systematic review with meta-analysis. *BMJ Open*, 13, e069517.

Mendoza-Catalán, G., Rodríguez-Santamaría, Y., Domínguez-Chávez, C. J., Juárez-Medina, L. L., Villa-Rueda, A. A., González-Ramírez, J. & Gutiérrez-Valverde, J. M. 2022. Personality traits and self-care behaviors in adults with type 2 diabetes mellitus. *Diabetes, Metabolic Syndrome and Obesity*, 15, 1–6.

Merolli, M., Gray, K., Choo, D., Lawford, B. J. & Hinman, R. S. 2022. Use, and acceptability, of digital health technologies in musculoskeletal physical therapy: a survey of physical therapists and patients. *Musculoskeletal Care*, 20, 641–659.

Meroni, R., Piscitelli, D., Ravasio, C., Vanti, C., Bertozzi, L., De Vito, G., Perin, C., Guccione, A. A., Cerri, C. G. & Pillastrini, P. 2021. Evidence for managing chronic low back pain in primary care: a review of recommendations from high-quality clinical practice guidelines. *Disability and Rehabilitation*, 43, 1029–1043.

Mesner, S. A., Foster, N. E. & French, S. D. 2016. Implementation interventions to improve the management of non-specific low back pain: a systematic review. *BMC Musculoskeletal Disorders*, 17, 258.

Murray, E., Hekler, E. B., Andersson, G., Collins, L. M., Doherty, A., Hollis, C., Rivera, D. E., West, R. & Wyatt, J. C. 2016. Evaluating digital health interventions: key questions and approaches. *American Journal of Preventive Medicine*, 51, 843–851.

NICE (National Institute of Health and Care Excellence). 2016. Low back pain and sciatica in over 16s: assessment and management [Online]. National Institute for Health and Care Excellence (NICE). Available: https://www.nice.org.uk/guidance/ng59/chapter/Recommendations [Accessed].

NICE (National Institute of Health and Care Excellence). 2022. *Evidence standards for health and care excellence* [Online]. Available: https://www.nice.org.uk/about/what-we-do/our-programmes/evidence-standards-framework-for-digital-health-technologies [Accessed].

Nicholl, B. I., Sandal, L. F., Stochkendahl, M. J., McCallum, M., Suresh, N., Vasseljen, O., Hartvigsen, J., Mork, P. J., Kjaer, P., Søgaard, K. & Mair, F. S. 2017. Digital support interventions for the self-management of low back pain: a systematic review. *Journal of Medical Internet Research*, 19, e179.

NSWACI (NSW Agency for Clinical Innovation). 2016. *Management of people with acute low back pain: model of care.* [Online]. Available: https://aci.health.nsw.gov.au/__data/assets/pdf_file/0007/336688/acute-low-back-pain-moc.pdf [Accessed].

Oliveira, C. B., Maher, C. G., Pinto, R. Z., Traeger, A. C., Lin, C. C., Chenot, J. F., Van Tulder, M. & Koes, B. W. 2018. Clinical practice guidelines for the management of non-specific low back pain in primary care: an updated overview. *European Spine Journal*, 27, 2791–2803.

Oliveira, V. C., Ferreira, P. H., Maher, C. G., Pinto, R. Z., Refshauge, K. M. & Ferreira, M. L. 2012. Effectiveness of self-management of low back pain: systematic review with meta-analysis. *Arthritis Care & Research*, 64, 1739–1748.

Pang, H., Chen, S., Klyne, D. M., Harrich, D., Ding, W., Yang, S. & Han, F. Y. 2023. Low back pain and osteoarthritis pain: a perspective of estrogen. *Bone Research*, 11, 42–42.

Paridaens, R., Vaes, B., Van Den Bulck, S. & Soetaert, J. 2024. Benchmarks for low back pain in general practice in Flanders: electronic audit of INTEGO. *BMC Primary Care*, 25, 431.

Patrick, K., Hekler, E. B., Estrin, D., Mohr, D. C., Riper, H., Crane, D., Godino, J. & Riley, W. T. 2016. The pace of technologic change: Implications for digital health behavior intervention research. *American Journal of Preventive Medicine*, 51, 816–824.

Petersen, J. M., Kemps, E., Lewis, L. K. & Prichard, I. 2020. Psychological mechanisms underlying the relationship between commercial physical activity app use and physical activity engagement. *Psychology of Sport and Exercise*, 51, 101719.

Petracca, F., Ciani, O., Cucciniello, M. & Tarricone, R. 2020. Harnessing digital health technologies during and after the COVID-19 pandemic: context matters. *Journal of Medical Internet Research*, 22, e21815.

Power, R. A. & Pluess, M. 2015. Heritability estimates of the Big Five personality traits based on common genetic variants. *Translational Psychiatry*, 5, e604.

Prochaska, J. O., Diclemente, C. C. & Norcross, J. C. 1992. In search of how people change: applications to addictive behaviors. *The American Psychologist*, 47, 1102–1114.

Qumseya, B., Goddard, A., Qumseya, A., Estores, D., Draganov, P. V. & Forsmark, C. 2021. Barriers to clinical practice guideline implementation among physicians: a physician survey. *Int J Gen Med*, 14, 7591–7598.

RACGP (Royal Australian College of General Practitioners). 2013. *Handbook of Non-Drug Interventions (HANDI)* [Online]. Available: https://www.racgp.org.au/clinical-resources/clinical-guidelines/handi [Accessed].

Rheumatology, T. L. 2023. *The global epidemic of low back pain* [Online]. Elsevier. Available: https://doi.org/10.1016/S2665-9913(23)00133-9 [Accessed].

Rintala, A., Rantalainen, R., Kaksonen, A., Luomajoki, H. & Kauranen, K. 2022. mHealth apps for low back pain self-management: scoping review. *JMIR mHealth and uHealth*, 10, e39682.

Sarradon-Eck, A., Bouchez, T., Auroy, L., Schuers, M. & Darmon, D. 2021. Attitudes of general practitioners toward prescription of mobile health apps: qualitative study. *JMIR mHealth and uHealth*, 9, e21795.

Schaller, A., Petrowski, K., Pfoertner, T.-K. & Froboese, I. 2017. Effectiveness of A theory-based multicomponent intervention (movement coaching) on the promotion of total and domain-specific physical activity: a randomised controlled trial in low back pain patients. *BMC Musculoskeletal Disorders*, 18, 431.

Schofield, D. J., Callander, E. J., Shrestha, R. N., Percival, R., Kelly, S. J., Passey, M. E. & Med, B. 2012. Labor force participation and the influence of having back problems on income poverty in Australia. *Spine (Philadelphia, Pa. 1976)*, 37, 1156–1163.

Schulman-Green, D., Jaser, S. S., Park, C. & Whittemore, R. 2016. A metasynthesis of factors affecting self-management of chronic illness. *Journal of Advanced Nursing*, 72, 1469–1489.

Shaver, J. 2022. The state of telehealth before and after the COVID-19 pandemic. *Primary Care*, 49, 517–530.

Shebib, R., Bailey, J. F., Smittenaar, P., Perez, D. A., Mecklenburg, G. & Hunter, S. 2019. Randomized controlled trial of a 12-week digital care program in improving low back pain. *NPJ Digital Medicine*, 2, 1–1.

Sirois, F. M. & Hirsch, J. K. 2015. Big Five traits, affect balance and health behaviors: a self-regulation resource perspective. *Personality and Individual Differences*, 87, 59–64.

Slade, S. C., Kent, P., Patel, S., Bucknall, T. & Buchbinder, R. 2016. Barriers to primary care clinician adherence to clinical guidelines for the management of low back pain: a systematic review and metasynthesis of qualitative studies. *The Clinical Journal of Pain*, 32, 800–816.

Stark, C., Cunningham, J., Turner, P., Johnson, M. A. & Bäcker, H. C. 2022. App-based rehabilitation in back pain, a systematic review. *Journal of Personalized Medicine*, 12, 1558.

STATISTA. 2020. *Number of smartphone users worldwide from 2016 to 2021 (in billions)* [Online]. Available: https://www.statista.com/statistics/330695/number-of-smartphone-users-worldwide/ [Accessed].

STATISTA. 2023. *Number of smartphone subscriptions worldwide from 2016 to 2021, with forecasts from 2022 to 2027* [Online]. Available: https://www.statista.com/statistics/330695/number-of-smartphone-users-worldwide/ [Accessed].

STATISTA. 2025. *Mobile app downloads worldwide from 2021 to 2026, by store (in billions)* [Online]. Available: https://www.statista.com/statistics/1010716/apple-app-store-google-play-app-downloads-forecast/ [Accessed].

Stec, M. A., Arbour, M. W. & Hines, H. F. 2019. Client-centered mobile health care applications: using the mobile application rating scale instrument for evidence-based evaluation. *Journal of Midwifery & Women's Health*, 64, 324–329.

Stieger, M., Robinson, S. A., Bisson, A. N. & Lachman, M. E. 2020. The relationship of personality and behavior change in a physical activity intervention: the role of conscientiousness and healthy neuroticism. *Personality and Individual Differences*, 166, 110224.

Synnott, A., O'keeffe, M., Bunzli, S., Dankaerts, W., O'sullivan, P. & O'sullivan, K. 2015. Physiotherapists may stigmatise or feel unprepared to treat people with low back pain and psychosocial factors that influence recovery: a systematic review. *Journal of Physiotherapy*, 61, 68–76.

Tabacof, L., Baker, T. S., Durbin, J. R., Desai, V., Zeng, Q., Sahasrabudhe, A., Herrera, J. E. & Putrino, D. 2022. Telehealth treatment for nonspecific low back pain: a review of the current state in mobile health. *PM & R*, 14, 1086–1098.

Tayshete, I., McCarthy, C., Ademoyegun, A., Gebrye, T., Fatoye, F. & Mbada, C. 2025. Effectiveness of smartphone-based applications in low-back pain rehabilitation: a systematic review and meta-analysis. *Bulletin of Faculty of Physical Therapy*, 30, 29.

Thurnheer, S. E., Gravestock, I., Pichierri, G., Steurer, J. & Burgstaller, J. M. 2018. Benefits of mobile apps in pain management: systematic review. *JMIR mHealth and uHealth*, 6, e11231.

Topics, E. 2025. *How many people own smartphones? (2025–2029)* [Online]. Available: https://explodingtopics.com/blog/smartphone-stats [Accessed].

Vader, K., Donnelly, C., French, S. D., Grady, C., Hill, J. C., Tripp, D. A., Williams, A. & Miller, J. 2022. Implementing a new physiotherapist-led primary care model for low back pain: a qualitative study of patient and primary care team perspectives. *BMC Primary Care*, 23, 201.

Van Tulder, M. W., Ostelo, R., Vlaeyen, J. W. S., Linton, S. J., Morley÷, S. J. & Assendelft, W. J. J. 2000. Behavioral treatment for chronic low back pain: a systematic review within the framework of the Cochrane Back Review Group. *Spine*, 25, 2688–2699.

Vos, T., Lim, S. S., Abbafati, C., et al. 2020. Global Burden of 369 Diseases and injuries in 204 countries and territories, 1990–2019: a systematic analysis for the Global Burden of Disease Study 2019. *The Lancet*, 396, 1204–1222.

Wang, Y. X. J. 2017. Menopause as a potential cause for higher prevalence of low back pain in women than in age-matched men. *Journal of Orthopaedic Translation*, 8, 1–4.

Whitelaw, S., Mamas, M. A., Topol, E. & Van Spall, H. G. C. 2020. Applications of digital technology in COVID-19 pandemic planning and response. *The Lancet (British Edition)*, 2, e435–e440.

WHO (World Health Organization). 2017. *The need to scale up rehabilitation* [Online]. Available: https://iris.who.int/handle/10665/331210 [Accessed].

WHO (World Health Organization). 2018. *Classification of digital health interventions v1.0: a shared language to describe the uses of digital technology for health* [Online]. Available: https://apps.who.int/iris/handle/10665/260480 [Accessed].

WHO (World Health Organization). 2022. *WHO guideline on self-care interventions for health and well-being, 2022 revision* [Online]. Available: https://www.who.int/publications/i/item/9789240052192 [Accessed].

WHO (World Health Organization). 2023. *Low back pain* [Online]. Available: https://www.who.int/news-room/fact-sheets/detail/low-back-pain [Accessed].
Windisch, O., Zamberg, I., Zanella, M.-C., Gayet-Ageron, A., Blondon, K., Schiffer, E. & Agoritsas, T. 2020. Using mHealth to increase the reach of local guidance to health professionals as part of an institutional response plan to the COVID-19 outbreak: usage analysis study. *JMIR mHealth and uHealth*, 8, e20025.
Wong, H., Razvi, Y., Hamid, M. A., Mistry, N. & Filler, G. 2023. Age and sex-related comparison of referral-based telemedicine service utilization during the COVID-19 pandemic in Ontario: a retrospective analysis. *BMC Health Serv Res*, 23, 1374.
WTW (Willis Towers Watson) 2022. *Global medical trends survey report* [Online]. Available: https://www.wtwco.com/en-AU/Insights/2021/11/2022-global-medical-trends-survey-report [Accessed].
Yihunie, M., Abich, Y., Demissie, S. F., Kassa, T., Ranganathan, P. & Janakiraman, B. 2023. Fear-avoidance beliefs for physical activity among chronic low back pain: a multicenter cross-sectional study. *Journal of Pain Research*, 16, 233–243.
Zhang, G., Chen, X., Xiao, L., Li, Y., Li, B., Yan, Z., Guo, L. & Rost, D. H. 2019. The relationship between big five and self-control in boxers: a mediating model. *Frontiers in Psychology*, 10, 1690.

9 The 'Connected We St@nd' Online Programme for Haemodialysis Self-Management

Translating Evidence into Practice

Helena Sousa, Oscar Ribeiro, and Daniela Figueiredo

KIDNEY FAILURE AND HAEMODIALYSIS: CLINICAL PRESENTATION

Chronic kidney disease (CKD) is a growing global public health challenge, affecting about 700 to 850 million people worldwide, with an estimated prevalence of 8–14% (Kovesdy, 2022). Due to its high prevalence and incidence, CKD is predicted to become the fifth leading cause of death by 2040 (GBD Chronic Kidney Disease Collaboration, 2020).

Kidney failure, also known as end-stage renal disease (ESRD), is the final stage of CKD and is diagnosed when the estimated glomerular filtration rate (eGFR) falls below 15 mL/min per 1.73 m^2, accompanied by evidence of progressive and irreversible kidney damage over the preceding three months (The Kidney Disease: Improving Global Outcomes [KDIGO], 2013). At this stage, the kidneys can no longer perform their vital functions and, therefore, people living with this serious health condition cannot survive without undergoing life-sustaining kidney replacement therapy, namely dialysis (haemodialysis or peritoneal dialysis) or kidney transplantation (KDIGO, 2013).

Worldwide, in-centre haemodialysis is the primary treatment for adults with kidney failure (Himmelfarb et al., 2020). This kidney therapy requires patients to travel to specialized dialysis centres three times a week, with each session lasting about four hours (Torreggiani et al., 2023). During haemodialysis, the patient's blood circulates through an extracorporeal purification circuit that uses a dialysis machine, dialysis fluid, and a haemodialyser – a device that replicates the filtering function of the kidneys (KDIGO, 2013). Access to the bloodstream is gained through a surgically implanted vascular access (arteriovenous fistula or central venous catheter) placed before starting regular treatments (Lok et al., 2020).

Due to its rigid schedule of attendance to treatment sessions and other adherence requirements (e.g., strict diet and fluid restrictions), haemodialysis is considered one of the most burdensome medical treatments, negatively impacting personal, family, and social activities and requiring a significant degree of self- and family-management efforts (Buemi et al., 2020).

SELF-MANAGEMENT CHALLENGES IN HAEMODIALYSIS

Self-management refers to the ability of the individual, together with his/her family, community, and healthcare professionals, to handle the symptoms, treatments, physical and psychosocial consequences, and lifestyle changes inherent in living with a medical condition (Barlow et al., 2002; Lorig and Holman, 2003).

DOI: 10.1201/9781003599074-10

Self-management in haemodialysis poses unique challenges, given the chronic, invasive, and life-sustaining nature of this kidney therapy (Li et al., 2021). Overall, this treatment requires a solid understanding of dialysis, the adoption of complex health-related behaviours, and the management of frequent and distressing physical symptoms (Sousa et al., 2024a). Ongoing coping efforts are also necessary, not only to improve adherence and long-term survival but also to support the psychosocial adjustment of patients and their caregivers (Buemi et al., 2020).

Considering the specificities of haemodialysis, the Corbin and Strauss Self-Management Framework (1988) offers a comprehensive and practically relevant perspective for understanding the demands of this treatment. According to the model, successful self-management involves three main tasks: (i) medical management (covering practical aspects of the disease and its treatments), (ii) behavioural management (referring to adopting and maintaining health behaviours that promote well-being and enhance the effectiveness of medical treatments), and (iii) emotional management (encompassing the psychosocial aspects of living with chronic illness) (Corbin and Strauss, 1988; Sousa et al., 2024a; Sousa, 2025b).

Figure 9.1 presents the self-management tasks proposed by Corbin and Strauss (1988) applied to the haemodialysis context.

Given the vital role of family support in managing kidney failure, it is important to consider the experiences of individuals on haemodialysis through a broader developmental lens – one that includes those providing informal care. Family caregivers, i.e., close relatives or friends who ensure unpaid support and assistance to a significant other, often play a key role in helping to manage the demands of kidney therapy (Stall et al., 2019). Their responsibilities may include communicating with the healthcare team, preparing meals, managing fluid intake and complex medication regimens, ensuring transportation to and from dialysis units, coordinating medical appointments, encouraging treatment adherence, and providing emotional support (Hoang et al., 2018; Sousa et al., 2022a).

In this context, Jablonski's (2004) adaptation of Rolland's (1987) Family Systems Illness Model provides a valuable framework for understanding the medical, behavioural, and emotional challenges faced by people with kidney failure and their families over time. According to this model,

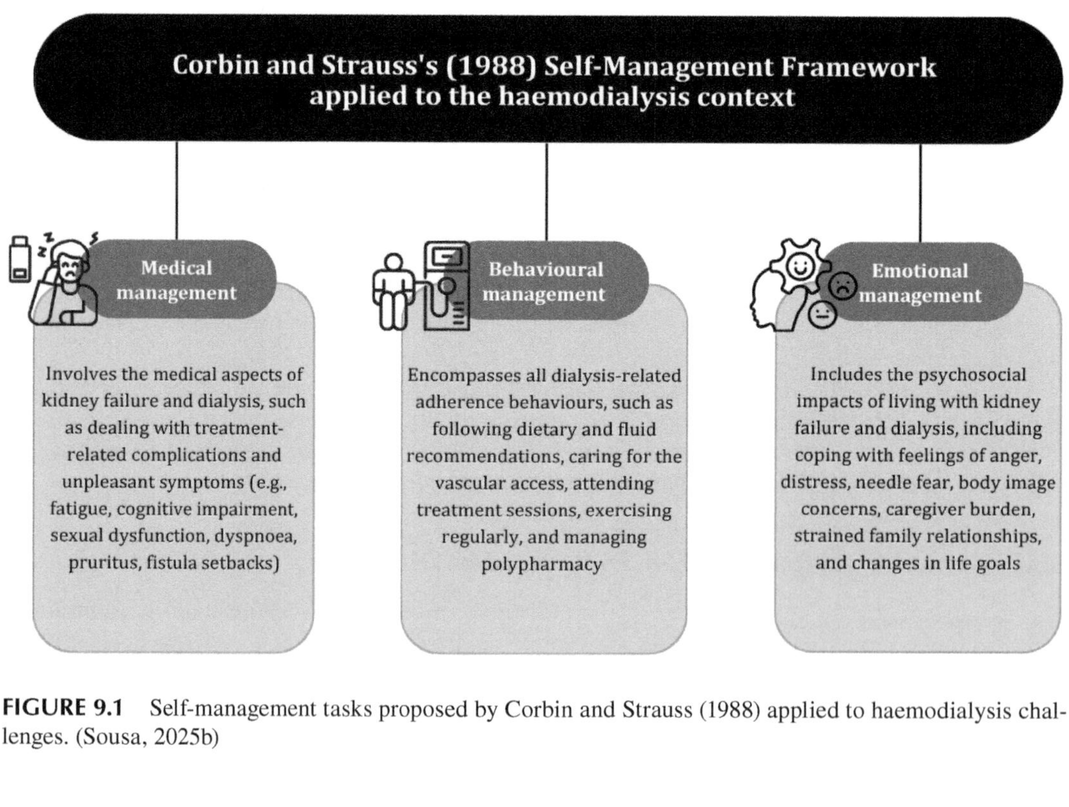

FIGURE 9.1 Self-management tasks proposed by Corbin and Strauss (1988) applied to haemodialysis challenges. (Sousa, 2025b)

chronic illnesses progress through three main phases: crisis, chronic, and terminal (Rolland, 1987). The crisis phase refers to the symptomatic period before diagnosis and the initial adjustment to dialysis; the chronic phase encompasses the ongoing experience of long-term treatment and is characterized by a period of clinical stability followed by gradual health decline during which treatment becomes physically and emotionally demanding (Jablonski, 2004); and, finally, the terminal phase that involves the recognition of impending death and, subsequently, the mourning process experienced by family members (Rolland, 1987, 2005, 2019).

Figure 9.2 illustrates the kidney failure trajectory following Jablonski's (2004) adaptation of Rolland's (1987) Family Systems Illness Model.

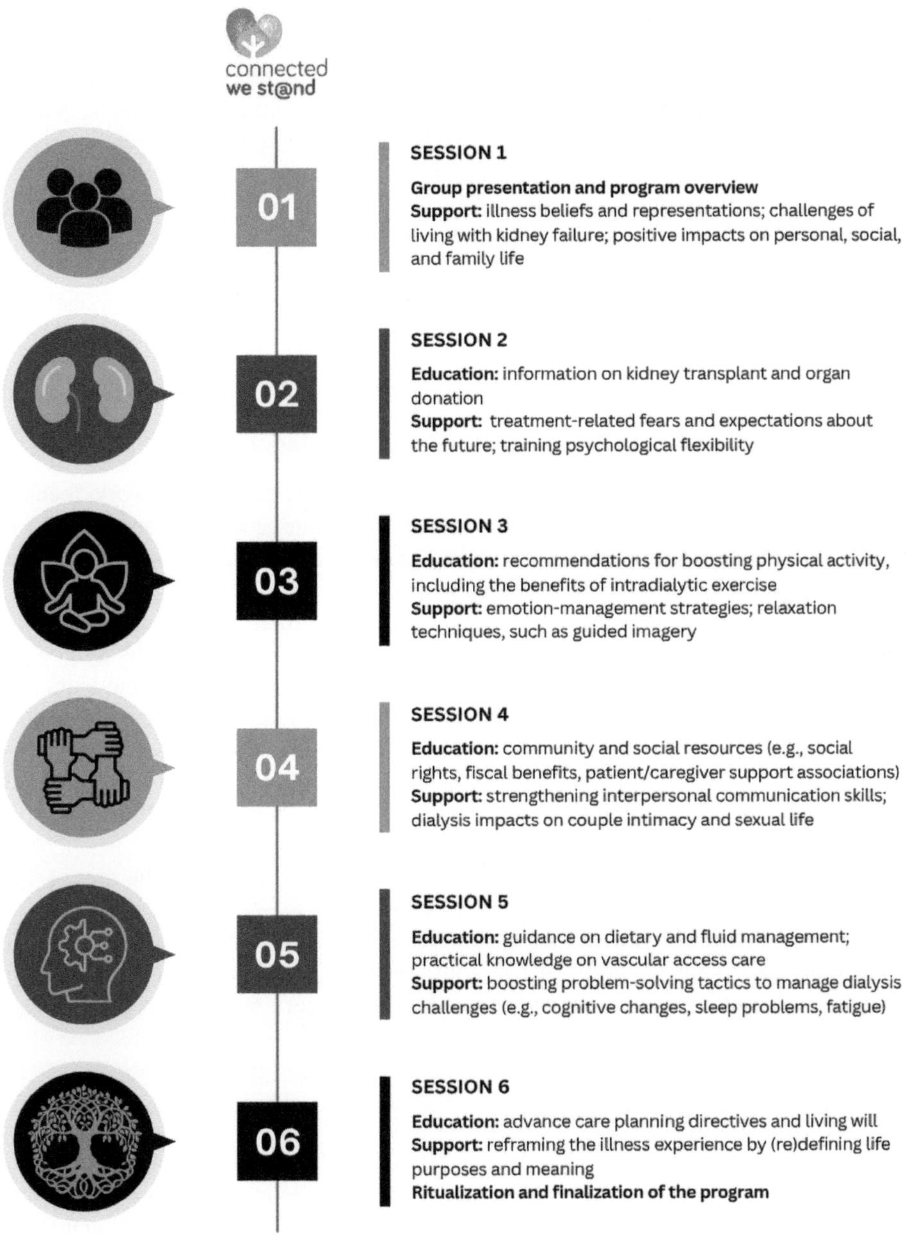

FIGURE 9.2 The kidney failure trajectory according to Jablonski's (2004) adaptation of Rolland's (1987) Family Systems Illness Model. (Sousa, 2025b)

The next point of this *Chapter* specifies the medical, behavioural, and emotional management challenges faced by people living (and/or caring for a significant other) with kidney failure and haemodialysis treatments.

Medical Management of Haemodialysis-Related Complications

The first task of Corbin and Strauss's (1988) Self-Management Framework refers to the strategies individuals use to manage the physical effects of prolonged treatment. Haemodialysis-related complications are caused by multiple factors, including suboptimal adherence to medical recommendations, accumulation of uraemic toxins, electrolyte imbalances, polypharmacy side effects, chronic inflammation, and the clinical burden of comorbidities such as diabetes and cardiovascular disease (Siriwardana et al., 2020). In this context, effective medical management requires patients to monitor biological indicators (e.g., blood pressure, interdialytic weight, blood glucose levels) and manage several treatment-related symptoms, including fatigue, muscle cramps, pruritus, sexual problems, and cognitive impairment (Fletcher et al., 2022). As these adverse effects often occur in clusters, people on haemodialysis face a significant symptom burden that can disrupt their ability to engage fully in personal, social, professional, and family life, as well as pursue their broader life goals (Kalantar-Zadeh et al., 2022; Levin et al., 2024; Moskovitch et al., 2020).

These challenges also affect family caregivers, who play a vital role in supporting symptom monitoring and management, with many reporting heightened psychological, physical, and practical distress as a result of the ongoing demands of haemodialysis caregiving in their daily routines (Sousa et al., 2022a, 2024b).

Behavioural Management and Treatment Adherence in Haemodialysis

The second task of Corbin and Strauss's (1988) Self-Management Framework focuses on the changes individuals implement to effectively manage the challenges of chronic illness, including adopting new health behaviours (and/or modifying existing ones) to improve physical and mental health outcomes.

In haemodialysis, behavioural management is closely linked to treatment adherence, i.e., the extent to which patients' behaviour aligns with the medical recommendations agreed upon with renal care professionals (Murali et al., 2019; Sabaté, 2003). Key adherence behaviours involve following strict dietary and fluid restrictions, attending dialysis sessions as prescribed, maintaining an exercise routine, caring for the vascular access, and managing complex medication regimens (Murali et al., 2019). Family caregivers' support is crucial to motivate and assist the cared-for person in adhering to and maintaining these behaviours (Gilbertson et al., 2019; Hoang et al., 2022; Sousa et al., 2019).

Table 9.1 summarizes haemodialysis-specific adherence behaviours and the main self-management challenges they entail for patients and their caregivers.

It is noteworthy that treatment adherence in haemodialysis is critical to preventing complications and maximizing patient quality of life and survival; yet, nonadherence is widespread and currently acknowledged as a major global public health concern (GBD Chronic Kidney Disease Collaboration, 2020).

Emotional Management in Haemodialysis

The third self-management task in Corbin and Strauss's (1988) Self-Management Framework – emotional management – refers to how individuals cope with the psychosocial stressors of chronic illness. In kidney failure, this task encompasses all efforts to address the emotional (e.g., frustration, uncertainty), cognitive (e.g., confusion, memory problems), and perceptual (e.g., beliefs about treatment efficacy, expectations regarding kidney transplantation) responses to the demands of

TABLE 9.1
Adherence Behaviours in Haemodialysis

Adherence behaviour	Description
Dialysis attendance	Haemodialysis demands strict attendance to a rigid schedule of treatment sessions – typically three times a week, each lasting about four hours – which can be disrupted by long travel times, limited access to dialysis centres, and often high transportation costs. These challenges can significantly interfere with work, finances, social life, and family commitments, ultimately compromising patient/caregiver quality of life (Chenitz et al., 2014).
Regular exercise	Reduced physical activity is common in people on haemodialysis and is associated with a greater risk of depression, muscle weakness, changes in blood pressure, and premature death (Bündchen et al., 2021). Low motivation, poor family/social support, and the presence of clinical symptoms (e.g., hypotension, fatigue) make it difficult for this population to enrol and/or maintain an exercise routine (Baker et al., 2022).
Dietary and fluid restrictions	Patients must follow a complex and restrictive diet that is low in potassium, phosphorus, sodium, and fluids; these restraints require constant meal planning and self-discipline, frequently exacerbating frustration, social isolation, and leading to family tension (Ikizler et al., 2020; Sousa et al., 2021, 2022a). Caregivers also struggle to understand or help manage nutritional recommendations, especially if missing adequate information or guidance (Sousa et al., 2022a). Nonadherence may require extending the duration of each dialysis session or increasing the number of sessions per week, raising the risk of adverse health outcomes in this population (Daugirdas et al., 2006).
Vascular access care	Proper maintenance of the vascular access, most commonly the arteriovenous fistula (AVF), is pivotal to ensuring dialysis efficacy but can be physically and emotionally draining due to needle fear, pain, visible disfigurement of the arm, and lack of patient/caregiver skills to handle fistula setbacks, like haemorrhages and persistent infections (Sousa et al., 2017, 2022b).
Polypharmacy intake	People on haemodialysis often take a large number of medications daily, raising the risk of polypharmacy, side effects, and nonadherence. Managing complex medication regimens can be overwhelming, especially without clear instructions or caregiver support (Sousa et al., 2022a).

treatments. In haemodialysis, managing difficult emotions is particularly challenging, as patients often experience cycles of intermittent clinical depression and/or anxiety that may undermine treatment adherence and exacerbate physical symptoms (Cukor et al., 2008, 2021; Jablonski, 2004). Over time, the demands of this kidney replacement therapy can place significant pressure on patient–family relationships, giving rise to interpersonal tensions and intensifying caregiver distress and burden (Jablonski, 2004; Moore et al., 2020; Paschou et al., 2018).

SELF-MANAGEMENT INTERVENTIONS IN HAEMODIALYSIS

Self-management interventions are a core component of interdisciplinary renal rehabilitation (Sousa et al., 2024a, 2025a). As multifaceted programmes, such interventions are generally designed to strengthen patients' and caregivers' confidence and skills in managing the complex emotional, behavioural, and cognitive challenges inherent in living with a chronic condition (Lin and Wood, 2013).

In the renal literature, cumulative evidence has shown that timely education and psychosocial support can help patients to cope with the requirements of haemodialysis, promoting treatment adherence, improving clinical and laboratory indicators, such as blood pressure, interdialytic weight, and serum markers, and alleviating symptoms like fatigue, pain, and psychological distress (Bernier-Jean et al., 2021; Griva et al., 2018; Lin and Hwang, 2020; Yangöz et al., 2021). Nonetheless, the positive outcomes of patient-centred programmes in nephrology tend to be modest and short-lived, with numerous studies reporting low intervention adherence and high dropout rates (Bonner et al., 2014; Hudson et al., 2017). A key weakness of these interventions lies in the minimal involvement of family caregivers, whose informational and supportive needs are often neglected (Gilbertson et al., 2019; McGuigan et al., 2024; Tong et al., 2008). The traditional focus on the individual receiving treatments overlooks that sustained behavioural change is more likely to occur within the context of close interpersonal relationships, thereby underestimating the vital role that family support plays in helping individuals navigate the complexities of kidney therapies (Browne et al., 2020; Bonner et al., 2014; Narva et al., 2016; Sousa et al., 2019). Notably, although caregiver-oriented interventions are scarce, recent reviews have highlighted their consistent benefits in reducing caregiver burden and improving quality of life (Bártolo et al., 2022; Hovadick et al., 2021; McGuigan et al., 2024). Yet, the promises of dyadic-based approaches remain largely unexplored, and limited evidence exists on their feasibility and acceptability in haemodialysis (Sousa et al., 2024a, 2025a).

Another significant limitation is the lack of understanding regarding this population's preferences, expectations, and needs – knowledge that is essential for guiding the design and implementation of tailored disease management programmes (Sousa et al., 2023). In this regard, priority-setting guidelines in nephrology have already highlighted a mismatch between the needs and preferences of people with kidney failure and their family caregivers, and the research priorities of investigators and dialysis providers (Tong et al., 2015, 2017, 2018). More specifically, whilst healthcare professionals tend to prioritize the optimization of clinical outcomes, patients and caregivers favour initiatives aimed at refining the management of physical symptoms and psychosocial stressors (Tong et al., 2015, 2017, 2018). This misalignment has led to the proliferation of interventions that tend to neglect important dialysis-related health behaviours, principally physical activity and vascular access care (Sousa et al., 2022a, 2022b, 2023). To address these gaps, there is an urgent need to involve patients and caregivers in the process of (co)designing disease management activities by identifying their expectations, preferences, and assistance priorities, thus making these interventions more aligned with their lived experiences and more likely to endorse meaningful and sustained engagement (Sousa et al., 2023). Notwithstanding, some logistical barriers may still hinder patient/caregiver participation and retention in such initiatives, specifically the geographic distance and travel costs to the intervention site, scheduling conflicts with dialysis treatments and/or other life responsibilities, and the need to juggle (or assist a person dealing with) unpleasant symptoms during intervention sessions (Chan et al., 2016; Sousa et al., 2023). These limitations indicate a clear need for further research to develop alternative, more accessible interventions that are both viable for this population and easier to implement and replicate within routine clinical practice in often overstretched dialysis centres (Sousa et al., 2024a, 2025a).

The Potential of Online Interventions

Internet-mediated approaches have emerged as a promising avenue to help overcome long-standing barriers to participation in self-management programmes for individuals undergoing haemodialysis and their families. In this context, online interventions offer greater flexibility, reduced logistical demands and costs, and the likelihood of facilitating dyadic participation (i.e., involving both the patient and their caregiver in conjoint self-management activities) in interdisciplinary practices, especially in the post-COVID-19 pandemic context (Sousa et al., 2024a, 2025a).

Despite these advantages, very few programmes specifically designed for this population are currently available or published. While existing early-stage trials have yielded encouraging findings regarding the feasibility, acceptability, and effectiveness of online interventions in alleviating psychological distress (Chan et al., 2016; Hernandez et al., 2018; Hudson et al., 2016, 2017; Jakubowski et al., 2020; Nadort et al., 2022), these initiatives have adopted a patient-centred approach and did not involve family caregivers. Moreover, insufficient attention has been paid to crucial self-management domains, mainly in terms of disease/treatment-related knowledge, and coping with haemodialysis medical, behavioural, and emotional demands.

Overall, more work is needed to investigate the potential of online, interdisciplinary, and family-inclusive interventions capable of addressing the complex and multifaceted challenges faced by people on haemodialysis and their caregivers.

Next, this *Chapter* describes the steps taken to design, implement, and test the 'Connected We St@nd' programme, an evidence-informed, interdisciplinary, Internet-mediated disease management intervention purposely developed with and for people on haemodialysis and their family caregivers, with the possibility of being offered as a dyadic-based intervention.

DESIGNING AND IMPLEMENTING THE 'CONNECTED WE ST@ND' PROGRAMME

The development of the 'Connected We St@nd' programme followed a stepwise approach, integrating four sequential stages: (i) qualitative interviews with diverse stakeholders (patients, family caregivers, and dialysis professionals) exploring the lived experiences, unmet needs, preferences, and expectations of this population regarding disease management; (ii) a comprehensive literature review on the preferences of people on haemodialysis and family caregivers for Internet-mediated interventions; (iii) identification of theory-based intervention strategies; and (iv) collaborative input from a multidisciplinary team of healthcare professionals and researchers with expertise in nephrology and chronic illness management (Sousa et al., 2024a, 2025a).

Findings from the qualitative interviews highlighted that both patients and caregivers needed more information about the disease and its treatment (e.g., the causes of kidney failure, dialysis procedures, dietary and fluid recommendations, fistula care). Participants also expressed a need for easier access to community resources (e.g., home support services, information about social rights), along with better support in addressing psychosocial adjustment challenges. These included psychological distress, caregiver burden, coping with physical symptoms, strained marital and family relationships, and uncertainty about future treatment pathways, namely concerns and expectations related to kidney transplantation (Sousa et al., 2023, 2024a, 2025a). In turn, dialysis professionals expressed their beliefs about the value of strengthening self-management interventions in haemodialysis, particularly for fostering positive communication and mutual support between patients and their families (Sousa et al., 2023). However, some concerns were raised about the organizational challenges of implementing such programmes in renal care settings. One major issue is the limited availability of potential participants, as both patients and their caregivers often have little free time due to the inflexible schedule of dialysis sessions and the associated caregiving responsibilities. Additional challenges include travel difficulties to the intervention site, scheduling conflicts with the intervention facilitators, and, at times, a lack of motivation or reluctance on the part of patients and caregivers to engage in initiatives led by dialysis centres (Sousa et al., 2023, 2025a; Sousa, 2025b).

Combined, the literature review and empirical data underscored the importance of integrating both educational and psychosocial support components, with materials delivered via accessible and appealing multimedia formats such as videos and downloadable booklets for future reference; direct interaction with healthcare professionals via videoconferencing was also identified as a valued aspect for enhancing participants' engagement in the programme (Coumoundouros et al., 2023; Donald et al., 2019; Schiffer et al., 2021).

Following these insights, the theoretical foundations of the intervention programme were primarily informed by the (previously described) Corbin and Strauss's Self-Management Framework (1988) and shaped by Lorig and Holman's (2003) self-management competencies, namely problem-solving,

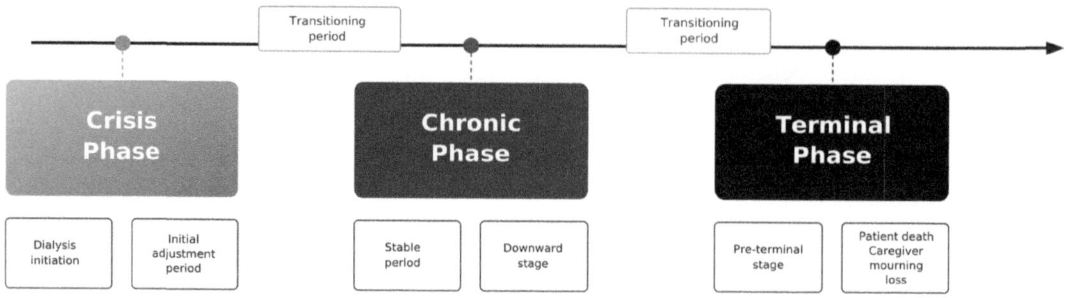

FIGURE 9.3 The 'Connected we St@nd' intervention programme. (Sousa, 2025b; Sousa et al., 2024a, 2025c)

decision-making, resource utilization, collaboration with healthcare providers, action planning, and the enhancement of self-efficacy.

Guided by these frameworks, a multidisciplinary team of experts in nephrology, dialysis nursing, health psychology, health education, renal nutrition, physical exercise, and social work collaboratively prepared the programme's content (Sousa et al., 2024a, 2025a).

Programme Content and Implementation

The 'Connected We St@nd' programme adopts an interdisciplinary, dyad-oriented, and hybrid (asynchronous/synchronous) delivery model. It comprises six weekly sessions that combine asynchronous educational modules with synchronous group-based psychosocial support sessions conducted via videoconference. The educational component includes a series of expert-led videos (of approximately 20 minutes each) that address fundamental aspects of kidney failure, including knowledge on dialysis-related health behaviours (e.g., nutritional recommendations, physical activity) and available community resources (e.g., social rights, information on patient/caregiver support associations). This content was complemented by downloadable booklets, renal-friendly recipes, and relaxation audio guides. In the psychosocial support component, each session was planned to last approximately 120 minutes and facilitated by two trained health psychologists; this part of the programme aimed to enhance communication skills, emotional regulation tactics, problem-solving strategies, adaptive coping, and sense of meaning and purpose (Sousa et al., 2024a, 2025a).

The 'Connected We St@nd' programme was hosted on a dedicated digital platform (http://www.togetherwestand.pt), which allowed registered participants secure access to all asynchronous materials and synchronous sessions. This platform also provided opportunities for participants to submit anonymous questions to healthcare experts. The intervention was designed to accommodate the dyadic nature of haemodialysis self-management, with content applicable and meaningful to both patients and caregivers, allowing flexibility in individual or conjoint participation (Sousa et al., 2024a, 2025a).

Figure 9.3 presents the sequential sessions of the 'Connected We St@nd' programme.

TESTING THE 'CONNECTED WE ST@ND' PROGRAMME

A pilot feasibility study was conducted with 26 participants – 16 patients and 10 family caregivers, including four patient-caregiver dyads (couples) – to evaluate the feasibility, acceptability, and impacts of the intervention programme (Sousa et al., 2024a), followed by a secondary exploratory analysis of its preliminary clinical effectiveness (Sousa et al., 2025a). Main conclusions are explained below.

Feasibility and Acceptability

Feasibility metrics included eligibility, consent, retention, completion, and intervention adherence rates, while the acceptability of the 'Connected We St@nd' programme was evaluated through focus group interviews (FGIs) conducted two weeks post-intervention (Sousa et al., 2024a).

In terms of feasibility, the findings indicated excellent consent, retention, and completion rates (all above 90%), along with high eligibility (77.5%) and strong adherence to the psychosocial support sessions (69%), surpassing benchmarks reported in previous face-to-face and digital interventions for this population (Hernandez et al., 2018; Hudson et al., 2017; Jakubowski et al., 2020).

As for acceptability, semi-inductive thematic analysis – guided by the Theoretical Framework of Acceptability (Sekhon et al., 2017) – showed that participants consistently expressed positive attitudes towards the programme (Sousa et al., 2024a). Key facilitators of intervention acceptability included the perception of meaningful peer interactions, positive guidance from health psychologists during support sessions, the relevance and coherence of the programme's content and materials, the flexibility of the asynchronous component, and user confidence in the digital platform used to implement the intervention, with no reported accessibility issues. Patients and caregivers also appreciated the synchronous group support sessions as an opportunity to share experiences and build connections with people from diverse and geographically distant kidney care settings, defining the group sessions as useful, insightful, and well-organized (Sousa et al., 2024a).

Altogether, these results provide evidence of the programme's feasibility and acceptability among the target population.

Positive Impacts and Clinical Effectiveness

The impacts of completing the 'Connected We St@nd' programme for individuals undergoing haemodialysis and family caregivers were examined using both qualitative and quantitative methods (Sousa et al., 2024a, 2025a). In the FGIs, participants described the intervention as both informative and emotionally supportive. More specifically, findings suggested that the intervention helped to enhance patient/caregiver understanding of kidney replacement therapies, improve their ability to manage difficult emotions, and strengthen communication with dialysis staff and close family members, including within marital relationships (Sousa et al., 2024a). Following the programme, both patients and caregivers reported increased confidence in making treatment-related decisions and handling the challenges of dialysis and caregiving, stating a better understanding of dietary restrictions and the management of treatment-related complications (both inter- and intradialytic). Family caregivers also felt more prepared to support the cared-for person during periods of clinical instability or psychological distress, while still maintaining other family routines and responsibilities (Sousa et al., 2024a). Additionally, the intervention appeared to foster a more balanced and less fatalistic view of haemodialysis and its impacts on daily life. This contributed to the demystification of this kidney therapy and encouraged greater psychological flexibility and acceptance, helping participants feel that the demands of haemodialysis or caregiving can be managed and/or overcome (Sousa et al., 2024a).

To complement qualitative findings, a quantitative secondary analysis examined the clinical relevance of the 'Connected We St@nd' programme through pre- and post-intervention assessments of subjective well-being (i.e., positive and negative affect), psychological distress, purpose in life, health-related quality of life, patient treatment adherence, and caregiver burden (Sousa et al., 2025a). Statistical analysis combined nonparametric tests, effect sizes, and reliable change indices to assess the clinical significance of pre- and post-intervention changes.

The results showed that, among adults on haemodialysis, large effect sizes were observed for improvements in positive affect, purpose in life, and two dimensions of quality of life, particularly psychological health and environmental quality, with a medium effect size in overall quality of life. For caregivers, large effects were obtained for increases in positive affect, psychological health,

TABLE 9.2
Main features of the Connected We St@nd' Online Programme

The 'Connected We St@nd' Intervention Programme

Mode of delivery	Online
Format	Asynchronous educational modules + synchronous psychological support sessions
Duration	Six weeks
Structure	Weekly asynchronous educational videos (~20 minutes) paired with 120-minute synchronous group support
Facilitators	Educational videos: different healthcare professionals with experience in dialysis (e.g., Fistula Nurse Specialist, Renal Nutritionist, Nephrologist, Social Worker) Psychological support: 2 Clinical Health Psychologists
Target population	Individuals on haemodialysis, family caregivers, or patient–caregiver dyads
Intervention focus	Health education + psychosocial skills training
Core topics covered	Dialysis processes, lifestyle/behavioural change and treatment adherence, symptom management, emotional regulation, positive communication, problem-solving, purpose in life
Feasibility and acceptability	Feasible and acceptable with satisfactory intervention adherence
Participant feedback	Enhanced self-efficacy and communication within the triad patients/caregivers/dialysis providers, reduced dialysis-related stigma, improved confidence in making treatment-related decisions, accessible and user-friendly digital platform
Preliminary outcomes	Improved psychological health, subjective well-being, overall quality of life, and purpose in life
Attendance challenges	Online format may reduce intervention adherence barriers and organizational constraints; poor digital health literacy in haemodialysis may difficult widespread programme implementation
Future endeavours	Plans for a large-scale trial

Source: Adapted from Sousa et al. (2025c).

quality of social relationships, and overall quality of life, along with reductions in subjective caregiver burden. Psychological health – a dimension of the World Health Organisation Quality of Life questionnaire (WHOQOL-BREF) that encompasses emotional well-being, self-esteem, and cognitive functioning – showed the highest proportion of patients and caregivers with reliable clinical changes at post-intervention (Sousa et al., 2025a).

As a whole, these findings showed that participation in the 'Connected We St@nd' programme yielded important benefits and clinically meaningful improvements across multiple psychosocial domains for both patients and family caregivers, suggesting that this intervention shows promise in promoting effective renal disease management. Table 9.2 recaps the main features of the 'Connected We St@nd' online programme.

FINE-TUNING THE 'CONNECTED WE ST@ND' PROGRAMME: 'LESSONS LEARNED' AND FUTURE DIRECTIONS

This *Chapter* relies on the main findings from the first implementation of the 'Connected We St@nd' programme, involving a sample of 16 adults undergoing haemodialysis and 10 family caregivers, including four dyads (i.e., couples who participated conjointly in the sessions). While the methodological limitations of this early-phase trial are outlined in more detail in two recently published scientific articles (cf. Sousa et al., 2024a, 2025a), some practical and implementation-related caveats are worth discussing to guide the refinement of the intervention programme and inform its potential dissemination and integration into routine nephrology care.

First, perfecting the monitoring of participant engagement with the asynchronous component is a critical next step, since the digital platform created to deliver the intervention did not allow for the tracking of video views or materials downloads, thereby limiting the capacity to assess intervention adherence and fidelity more robustly and objectively. As a result, engagement with the educational part of the programme was assessed through self-reports, which may not accurately reflect actual usage (Sousa et al., 2024a, 2025a). Although synchronous sessions were used to review and consolidate content from the educational modules, future implementations of the 'Connected We St@nd' programme should prioritize the use of platforms with built-in tracking features to ensure accurate assessment of exposure and engagement.

Second, the acceptability of the programme was assessed solely from the participants' perspective, without incorporating the perspectives of healthcare professionals involved in its delivery. In this sense, understanding the positive and negative experiences of intervention facilitators is of utmost importance for better grasping the viability and sustainability of implementing this type of intervention in real-world nephrology settings, as well as for enhancing the clinical utility of the programme internationally (Sousa et al., 2024a, 2025a).

Third, during the FGIs, some participants expressed the need for more time to delve deeper into topics such as the impact of kidney disease on sexuality, travel planning during dialysis, and the role of palliative care in nephrology, suggesting that a nephrologist should be present in one of the synchronous sessions to address medical concerns more directly. Even though accommodating these additions may require extending the number of sessions, these are important considerations for forthcoming uses of the programme (Sousa et al., 2024a, 2025a).

Fourth, participants expressed high satisfaction with the digital platform used to deliver the intervention. However, this aspect was assessed qualitatively and without the use of standardized scales. Future uses of the 'Connected We St@nd' programme should therefore include usability measures (System Usability Scale; Lewis, 2018) to ensure the digital tools meet established user experience standards (Sousa et al., 2024a, 2025a).

Finally, while the online format of the 'Connected We St@nd' programme offers several strengths – including innovation, feasibility in the pilot phase, and potential scalability – it is not without its limitations. It is noteworthy that digital literacy remains a significant concern in this clinical population, as many patients and caregivers may have limited familiarity with technology-assisted tools or feel insecure about using them for health-related purposes (Jain and Green, 2016; Schrauben et al., 2021). Factors such as older age, lower education levels, and socioeconomic disadvantage may further restrict digital access or confidence, potentially affecting programme engagement and adherence (Jain and Green, 2016; Schrauben et al., 2021).

CONCLUSIONS

The 'Connected We St@nd' programme addresses longstanding gaps in kidney care by integrating evidence-informed, interdisciplinary psychosocial and educational components, engaging both patients and family caregivers, and allowing the intervention to be completed as a dyadic activity according to participants' preferences. Its online delivery mode helps mitigate common barriers to intervention adherence and retention in face-to-face practices, making it particularly suitable for integration into routine practice, especially in the post-pandemic context. Still, additional research efforts are needed (and encouraged) to develop and test user-friendly digital tools to try to maximize the reach of online interventions as a useful resource for successful disease management in haemodialysis. Bearing this in mind, plans are currently underway to pursue a large clinical trial of the 'Connected We St@nd' programme to, in the due course, encourage its widespread use.

ACKNOWLEDGEMENTS

This work was supported by FEDER, through COMPETE2020-Programa Operacional Competitividade e Internacionalização (POCI) and by National Funds (OE), through FCT/MCTES, under the grant number POCI-01-0145-FEDER-030228. Additionally, Helena Sousa had a Doctoral Grant (https://doi.org/10.54499/2020.04821.BD) financed by FCT (Fundação para a Ciência e Tecnologia) through FSE (Fundo Social Europeu).

REFERENCES

Baker, L.A., March, D.S., Wilkinson, T.J., et al. (2022) 'Clinical practice guideline exercise and lifestyle in chronic kidney disease', *BMC Nephrology*, 23(1), p. 75. https://doi.org/10.1186/s12882-021-02618-1

Barlow, J., Wright, C., Sheasby, J., Turner, A. and Hainsworth, J. (2002) 'Self-management approaches for people with chronic conditions: A review', *Patient Education and Counseling*, 48(2), pp. 177–187. https://doi.org/10.1016/s0738-3991(02)00032-0

Bártolo, A., Sousa, H., Ribeiro, O. and Figueiredo, D. (2022) 'Effectiveness of psychosocial interventions on the burden and quality of life of informal caregivers of hemodialysis patients: A systematic review', *Disability and Rehabilitation*, 44(26), pp. 8176–8187. https://doi.org/10.1080/09638288.2021.2013961

Bernier-Jean, A., Wong, G., Saglimbene, V., et al. (2021) 'Dietary potassium intake and all-cause mortality in adults treated with hemodialysis', *Clinical Journal of the American Society of Nephrology*, 16(12), pp. 1851–1861. https://doi.org/10.2215/CJN.08360621

Bonner, A., Havas, K., Douglas, C., Thepha, T., Bennett, P., and Clark, R. (2014) 'Self-management programmes in stages 1-4 chronic kidney disease: A literature review', *Journal of Renal Care*, 40(3), pp. 194–204. https://doi.org/10.1111/jorc.12058

Browne, T., Swoboda, A., Ephraim, P.L., et al. (2020) 'Engaging patients and family members to design and implement patient-centered kidney disease research', *Research Involvement and Engagement*, 6(1), p. 66. https://doi.org/10.1186/s40900-020-00237-y

Buemi, M., Bruno, A., Cordova, F., et al. (2020) 'Negative emotions in end-stage renal disease: Are anxiety symptoms related to levels of circulating catecholamines?, *Current Psychology*, 39, pp. 729–735. https://doi.org/10.1007/s12144-018-9796-8

Bündchen, D.C., Sousa, H., Afreixo, V., et al. (2021) 'Intradialytic exercise in end-stage renal disease: An umbrella review of systematic reviews and/or meta-analytical studies', *Clinical Rehabilitation*, 35(6), pp. 812–828. https://doi.org/10.1177/0269215520986784

Chan, R., Dear, B.F., Titov, N., Chow, J. and Suranyi, M. (2016) 'Examining internet-delivered cognitive behaviour therapy for patients with chronic kidney disease on haemodialysis: A feasibility open trial', *Journal of Psychosomatic Research*, 89, pp. 78–84. https://doi.org/10.1016/j.jpsychores.2016.08.012

Chenitz, K.B., Fernando, M. and Shea, J.A. (2014) 'In-center hemodialysis attendance: Patient perceptions of risks, barriers, and recommendations', *Hemodialysis International*, 18(2), pp. 364–373. https://doi.org/10.1111/hdi.12139

Corbin, J.M. and Strauss, A. (1988) *Unending work and care: Managing chronic illness at home*. San Francisco: Jossey-Bass.

Coumoundouros, C., El Arab, R.A., Farrand, P., et al. (2023) 'Potential implementers' perspectives on the development and implementation of an e-mental health intervention for caregivers of adults with chronic kidney disease: Qualitative interview study', *JMIR Human Factors*, 10, p. e51461. https://doi.org/10.2196/51461

Cukor, D., Cohen, S.D. and Kimmel, P.L. (2021) 'Coping with chronic illness: The challenge of patients with renal disease', in Cukor, D., Cohen, S.D. and Kimmel, P.L. (eds.) *Psychosocial aspects of chronic kidney disease: Exploring the impact of CKD, dialysis, and transplantation on patients*. Cambridge, MA: Elsevier Academic Press, pp. 9–25. https://doi.org/10.1016/B978-0-12-817080-9.00002-6

Cukor, D., Coplan, J., Brown, C., Peterson, R.A. and Kimmel, P.L. (2008) 'Course of depression and anxiety diagnosis in patients treated with hemodialysis: A 16-month follow-up', *Clinical Journal of the American Society of Nephrology*, 3(6), pp. 1752–1758. https://doi.org/10.2215/CJN.01120308

Daugirdas, J.T., Blake, P. and Ing, T.S. (eds.) (2006). *The handbook of dialysis*. 4th edn. Philadelphia: Lippincott Williams & Wilkins. https://doi.org/10.1002/dat.20141

Donald, M., Beanlands, H., Straus, S., et al. (2019) 'Identifying needs for self-management interventions for adults with CKD and their caregivers: A qualitative study', *American Journal of Kidney Diseases*, 74(4), pp. 474–482. https://doi.org/10.1053/j.ajkd.2019.02.006

Fletcher, B.R., Damery, S., Aiyegbusi, O.L., et al. (2022) 'Symptom burden and health-related quality of life in chronic kidney disease: A global systematic review and meta-analysis', *PLOS Medicine*, 19(4), p. e1003954. https://doi.org/10.1371/journal.pmed.1003954

GBD Chronic Kidney Disease Collaboration. (2020) 'Global, regional, and national burden of chronic kidney disease, 1990–2017: A systematic analysis for the Global Burden of Disease Study 2017', *The Lancet*, 395(10225), pp. 709–733. https://doi.org/10.1016/S0140-6736(20)30045-3

Gilbertson, E.L., Krishnasamy, R., Foote, C., Kennard, A.L., Jardine, M.J. and Gray, N.A. (2019) 'Burden of care and quality of life among caregivers for adults receiving maintenance dialysis: A systematic review', *American Journal of Kidney Diseases*, 73(3), pp. 332–343. https://doi.org/10.1053/j.ajkd.2018.09.006

Griva, K., Nandakumar, M., Ng, J.H., et al. (2018) 'Hemodialysis self-management intervention randomized trial (HED-SMART): A practical low-intensity intervention to improve adherence and clinical markers in patients receiving hemodialysis', *American Journal of Kidney Diseases*, 71(3), pp. 371–381. https://doi.org/10.1053/j.ajkd.2017.09.014

Hernandez, R., Burrows, B., Wilund, K., et al. (2018) 'Feasibility of an internet-based positive psychological intervention for hemodialysis patients with symptoms of depression', *Social Work in Health Care*, 57(10), pp. 864–879. https://doi.org/10.1080/00981389.2018.1523268

Himmelfarb, J., Vanholder, R., Mehrotra, R. and Tonelli, M. (2020) 'The current and future landscape of dialysis', *Nature Reviews Nephrology*, 16(10), pp. 573–585. https://doi.org/10.1038/s41581-020-0315-4

Hoang, V.L., Green, T. and Bonner, A. (2018) 'Informal caregivers' experiences of caring for people receiving dialysis: A mixed-methods systematic review', *Journal of Renal Care*, 44(2), pp. 82–95. https://doi.org/10.1111/jorc.12235

Hoang, V.L., Green, T. and Bonner, A. (2022) 'Examining social support, psychological status and health-related quality of life in people receiving haemodialysis', *Journal of Renal Care*, 48(2), pp. 102–111. https://doi.org/10.1111/jorc.12380

Hovadick, A.C., Jardim, V.R., Paúl, C., Pagano, A., Reis, I. and Torres, H. (2021) 'Interventions to improve the well-being of family caregivers of patients on hemodialysis and peritoneal dialysis: A systematic review', *PeerJ*, 9, p. e11713. https://doi.org/10.7717/peerj.11713

Hudson, J.L., Moss-Morris, R., Game, D., et al. (2016) 'Improving distress in dialysis (iDiD): A feasibility two-arm parallel randomized controlled trial of an online cognitive behavioral therapy intervention with and without therapist-led telephone support for psychological distress in patients undergoing haemodialysis', *BMJ Open*, 6(4), p. e011286. https://doi.org/10.1136/bmjopen-2016-011286

Hudson, J.L., Moss-Morris, R., Norton, S., et al. (2017) 'Tailored online cognitive behavioral therapy with or without therapist support calls to target psychological distress in adults receiving haemodialysis: A feasibility randomized controlled trial', *Journal of Psychosomatic Research*, 102, pp. 61–70. https://doi.org/10.1016/j.jpsychores.2017.09.009

Ikizler, T.A., Burrowes, J.D., Byham-Gray, L.D., et al. (2020) 'KDOQI clinical practice guideline for nutrition in CKD: 2020 update', *American Journal of Kidney Diseases*, 76(3 Suppl 1), pp. S1–S107. https://doi.org/10.1053/j.ajkd.2020.05.006

Jablonski, A., 2004. 'The illness trajectory of end-stage renal disease dialysis patients', *Research and Theory for Nursing Practice*, 18(1), pp. 51–72. https://doi.org/10.1891/rtnp.18.1.51.28053~

Jain, D. and Green, J.A. (2016) 'Health literacy in kidney disease: Review of the literature and implications for clinical practice', *World Journal of Nephrology*, 5(2), pp. 147–151. https://doi.org/10.5527/wjn.v5.i2.147

Jakubowski, K.P., Jhamb, M., Yabes, J., et al. (2020) 'Technology-assisted cognitive-behavioral therapy intervention for end-stage renal disease', *Translational Behavioral Medicine*, 10(3), pp. 657–663. https://doi.org/10.1093/tbm/ibz077

Kalantar-Zadeh, K., Lockwood, M.B., Rhee, C.M., et al. (2022) 'Patient-centred approaches for the management of unpleasant symptoms in kidney disease', *Nature Reviews Nephrology*, 18(3), pp. 185–198. https://doi.org/10.1038/s41581-021-00518-z

Kidney Disease: Improving Global Outcomes Chronic Kidney Disease Guideline Development Work Group Members. (2013) 'Evaluation and management of chronic kidney disease: Synopsis of the kidney disease: Improving global outcomes 2012 clinical practice guideline', *Annals of Internal Medicine*, 158(11), pp. 825–830. https://doi.org/10.7326/0003-4819-158-11-201306040-00007

Kovesdy, C.P. (2022) 'Epidemiology of chronic kidney disease: An update 2022', *Kidney International Supplements*, 12(1), pp. 7–11. https://doi.org/10.1016/j.kisu.2021.11.003

Levin, A., Ahmed, S.B., Carrero, J.J., et al. (2024) 'Executive summary of the KDIGO 2024 clinical practice guideline for the evaluation and management of chronic kidney disease: Known Knowns and Known unknowns', *Kidney International*, 105(4), pp. 684–701. https://doi.org/10.1016/j.kint.2023.10.016

Lewis, J.R. (2018). 'The system usability scale: Past, present, and future'. *International Journal of Human–Computer Interaction*, 34(7), pp. 577–590. https://doi.org/10.1080/10447318.2018.1455307

Li, P.K., Chan, G.C., Chen, J., et al. (2021) 'Tackling dialysis burden around the world: A global challenge', *Kidney Diseases (Basel)*, 7(3), pp. 167–175. https://doi.org/10.1159/000515541

Lin, C.C. and Hwang, S.J. (2020) 'Patient-centered self-management in patients with chronic kidney disease: Challenges and implications', *International Journal of Environmental Research and Public Health*, 17(24), p. 9443. https://doi.org/10.3390/ijerph17249443

Lin, C.E. and Wood, J.J. (2013) 'Self-management interventions', in Volkmar, F.R. (ed.) *Encyclopedia of autism spectrum disorders*. New York: Springer, pp. 2735–2743. https://doi.org/10.1007/978-1-4419-1698-3_481

Lok, C.E., Huber, T.S., Lee, T., et al. (2020) 'KDOQI clinical practice guideline for vascular access: 2019 update', *American Journal of Kidney Diseases*, 75(4 Suppl 2), pp. S1–S164. https://doi.org/10.1053/j.ajkd.2019.12.001

Lorig, K.R. and Holman, H. (2003) 'Self-management education: History, definition, outcomes, and mechanisms', *Annals of Behavioral Medicine*, 26(1), pp. 1–7. https://doi.org/10.1207/S15324796ABM2601_01

McGuigan, K., Laurente, G., Christie, A., et al. (2024) 'Effectiveness of interventions for informal caregivers of people with end-stage chronic illness: A systematic review', *Systematic Reviews*, 13(1), p. 245. https://doi.org/10.1186/s13643-024-02641-x

Moore, C., Skevington, S., Wearden, A. and Mitra, S. (2020) 'Impact of dialysis on the dyadic relationship between male patients and their female partners', *Qualitative Health Research*, 30(3), pp. 380–390. https://doi.org/10.1177/1049732319869908

Moskovitch, J.T., Mount, P.F. and Davies, M.R.P. (2020) 'Changes in symptom burden in dialysis patients assessed using a symptom-reporting questionnaire in clinic', *Journal of Palliative Care*, 35(1), pp. 59–65. https://doi.org/10.1177/0825859719827315

Murali, K.M., Mullan, J., Roodenrys, S., Hassan, H.C., Lambert, K. and Lonergan, M. (2019) 'Strategies to improve dietary, fluid, dialysis or medication adherence in patients with end stage kidney disease on dialysis: A systematic review and meta-analysis of randomized intervention trials', *PLoS One*, 14(1), p. e0211479. https://doi.org/10.1371/journal.pone.0211479

Nadort, E., Schouten, R.W., Boeschoten, R.E., et al. (2022) 'Internet-based treatment for depressive symptoms in hemodialysis patients: A cluster randomized controlled trial', *General Hospital Psychiatry*, 75, pp. 46–53. https://doi.org/10.1016/j.genhosppsych.2022.01.008

Narva, A.S., Norton, J.M. and Boulware, L.E. (2016) 'Educating patients about CKD: The path to self-management and patient-centered care', *Clinical Journal of the American Society of Nephrology*, 11(4), pp. 694–703. https://doi.org/10.2215/CJN.07680715

Paschou, A., Damigos, D., Skapinakis, P. and Siamopoulos, K. (2018) 'The relationship between burden and depression in spouses of chronic kidney disease patients', *Depression Research and Treatment*, 2018, p. 8694168. https://doi.org/10.1155/2018/8694168

Rolland, J.S. (1987) 'Family systems and chronic illness: A typological model', *Journal of Psychotherapy and the Family*, 3(3), pp. 143–168. https://doi.org/10.1300/J287v03n03_10

Rolland, J.S. (2005) 'Cancer and the family: An integrative model', *Cancer*, 104(11), pp. 2584–2595. https://doi.org/10.1002/cncr.21489

Rolland, J.S. (2019) 'The family, chronic illness, and disability: An integrated practice model', in Fiese, B.H., Celano, M., Deater-Deckard, K., Jouriles, E.N. and Whisman, M.A. (eds.) *APA handbook of contemporary family psychology: Applications and broad impact of family psychology*. Washington, DC: American Psychological Association, pp. 85–102. https://doi.org/10.1037/0000100-006

Sabaté, E. (ed.) (2003) *Adherence to long-term therapies: Evidence for action*. Geneva: World Health Organization.

Schiffer, L., Gertges, R., Nöhre, M., et al. (2021) 'Use and preferences regarding internet-based health care delivery in patients with chronic kidney disease', *BMC Medical Informatics and Decision Making*, 21(1), p. 34. https://doi.org/10.1186/s12911-020-01375-9

Schrauben, S.J., Appel, L., Rivera, E., et al. (2021) 'Mobile health (mHealth) technology: Assessment of availability, acceptability, and use in CKD', *American Journal of Kidney Diseases*, 77(6), pp. 941–950. https://doi.org/10.1053/j.ajkd.2020.10.013

Sekhon, M., Cartwright, M. and Francis, J.J. (2017) 'Acceptability of healthcare interventions: An overview of reviews and development of a theoretical framework', *BMC Health Services Research*, 17(1), p. 88. https://doi.org/10.1186/s12913-017-2031-8

Siriwardana, A.N., Hoffman, A.T., Brennan, F.P., Li, K. and Brown, M.A. (2020) 'Impact of renal supportive care on symptom burden in dialysis patients: A prospective observational cohort study', *Journal of Pain and Symptom Management*, 60(4), pp. 725–736. https://doi.org/10.1016/j.jpainsymman.2020.04.030

Sousa, C.N., Marujo, P., Teles, P., Lira, M.N. and Novais, M.E. (2017) 'Self-care on hemodialysis: Behaviors with the arteriovenous fistula', *Therapeutic Apheresis and Dialysis*, 21(2), pp. 195–199. https://doi.org/10.1111/1744-9987.12522

Sousa, H. (2025b) *We-Disease: Promoting psychosocial adjustment and adherence in end-stage renal disease through a family-based intervention* [doctoral thesis]. Aveiro: University of Aveiro.

Sousa, H., Bártolo, A., Ribeiro, O. and Figueiredo, D. (2022b) 'A family-centred perspective on the arteriovenous fistula in end-stage renal disease: Findings from dyadic interviews', *Scandinavian Journal of Caring Sciences*, 36(2), pp. 426–438. https://doi.org/10.1111/scs.13055

Sousa, H., Ribeiro, O., Bártolo, A., et al. (2024a) 'The `Connected we st@nd´ programme: A feasibility pilot study of an online self-management intervention for adults on in-centre haemodialysis and family caregivers', *British Journal of Health Psychology*, 29(3), pp. 589–608. https://doi.org/10.1111/bjhp.12715

Sousa, H., Ribeiro, O., Bártolo, A., et al. (2025a) 'Clinical relevance of an online self-management intervention in haemodialysis: A secondary data analysis of the connected we st@nd programme', *Journal of Renal Care*, 51(1), p. e70012. https://doi.org/10.1111/jorc.70012

Sousa, H., Ribeiro, O., Christensen, A.J. and Figueiredo, D. (2022a) 'Caring for parents with end-stage renal disease: What do adult children face and how do they cope?, *Journal of Clinical Nursing*, 31(23–24), pp. 3454–3463. https://doi.org/10.1111/jocn.16172

Sousa, H., Ribeiro, O., Christensen, A.J. and Figueiredo, D. (2023) 'Designing family-based interventions in kidney failure: The perspectives of the triad patients on haemodialysis/family caregivers/healthcare professionals', *British Journal of Health Psychology*, 28(3), pp. 672–689. https://doi.org/10.1111/bjhp.12647

Sousa, H., Ribeiro, O. and Figueiredo, D. (2021) 'End-stage renal disease is not yours, is not mine, is OURS: Exploring couples lived experiences through dyadic interviews', *Hemodialysis International*, 25(3), pp. 313–322. https://doi.org/10.1111/hdi.12929

Sousa, H., Ribeiro, O. and Figueiredo, D. (2024b) 'The hemodialysis distress thermometer for caregivers (HD-DT-C): Development and testing of the psychometric properties of a new tool for screening psychological distress among family caregivers of adults on hemodialysis', *Quality of Life Research*, 33(6), pp. 1513–1526. https://doi.org/10.1007/s11136-024-03627-x

Sousa, H., Ribeiro, O. and Figueiredo, D. (2025c) 'Strengthening renal psychology in Portuguese dialysis centres: The implementation of evidence-informed psychological practices', *Portuguese Kidney Journal*, 39(2), pp. 84–93. https://doi.org/10.71749/pkj.83

Sousa, H., Ribeiro, O., Paúl, C., et al. (2019) 'Social support and treatment adherence in patients with end-stage renal disease: A systematic review', *Seminars in Dialysis*, 32(6), pp. 562–574. https://doi.org/10.1111/sdi.12831

Stall, N.M., Campbell, A., Reddy, M. and Rochon, P.A. (2019) 'Words matter: The language of family caregiving', *Journal of the American Geriatrics Society*, 67(10), pp. 2008–2010. https://doi.org/10.1111/jgs.15988

Tong, A., Crowe, S., Chando, S., et al. (2015) 'Research priorities in CKD: Report of a national workshop conducted in Australia', *American Journal of Kidney Diseases*, 66(2), pp. 212–222. https://doi.org/10.1053/j.ajkd.2015.02.341

Tong, A., Manns, B., Hemmelgarn, B., et al. (2017) 'Establishing core outcome domains in hemodialysis: Report of the standardized outcomes in nephrology-hemodialysis (SONG-HD) consensus workshop', *American Journal of Kidney Diseases*, 69(1), pp. 97–107. https://doi.org/10.1053/j.ajkd.2016.05.022

Tong, A., Manns, B., Wang, A.Y.M., et al. (2018) 'Implementing core outcomes in kidney disease: Report of the standardized outcomes in nephrology (SONG) implementation workshop', *Kidney International*, 94(6), pp. 1053–1068. https://doi.org/10.1016/j.kint.2018.08.018

Tong, A., Sainsbury, P. and Craig, J.C. (2008) 'Support interventions for caregivers of people with chronic kidney disease: A systematic review', *Nephrology Dialysis Transplantation*, 23(12), pp. 3960–3965. https://doi.org/10.1093/ndt/gfn415

Torreggiani, M., Piccoli, G.B., Moio, M.R., et al. (2023) 'Choice of the dialysis modality: Practical considerations', *Journal of Clinical Medicine*, 12(9), p. 3328. https://doi.org/10.3390/jcm12093328

Yangöz, ŞT., Özer, Z. and Boz, İ (2021) 'Comparison of the effect of educational and self-management interventions on adherence to treatment in hemodialysis patients: A systematic review and meta-analysis of randomized controlled trials', *International Journal of Clinical Practice*, 75(5), p. e13842. https://doi.org/10.1111/ijcp.13842

10 Shaping Independence
Self-Management in Arthrogryposis Multiplex Congenita through Shared Stories

Noémi Dahan-Oliel, Sarah Cachecho, Vasiliki B Darsaklis, Megan Jaclyn Sions, Klaus Dieterich, Kristen Donlevie, Maureen Donohoe, Alicja Fąfara, Mona Hoy, Claire Huzar, Francis Lacombe, Valentina Maestri, Carolina Navalòn, Ani Samargian, Kristin Schewe Loxley, Véronique Thellier, Misha Walker, Lena Wekre Lande, and Lisa Wagner

INTRODUCTION

Arthrogryposis multiplex congenita, or AMC, is a group of rare diseases affecting one in 3000–4300 live births (Lowry et al., 2010). AMC is defined by the presence of joint contractures in two or more different body parts, affecting the upper limbs, lower limbs, spine, and/or jaw (Dahan-Oliel et al., 2019; Elfassy et al., 2023). Causes include genetic and environmental factors in addition to abnormalities during fetal development (Dahan-Oliel et al., 2019). Individuals with AMC have limited joint movements, with or without muscle weakness, in the involved body areas. Other body systems may also be affected, such as the central nervous, cardiac, respiratory, or gastrointestinal systems (Dahan-Oliel et al., 2019). Depending on the extent of joint contractures, individuals with AMC may present with difficulties in activities of daily living, mobility and participation in various areas of life (e.g., social and physical activities, work, household activities), and this may be exacerbated by the presence of pain (Amor et al., 2011; Cirillo et al., 2019; Hyer et al., 2021). The overall goal of rehabilitation for this population is to promote function and autonomy in the areas that are meaningful to children, youth and adults with AMC.

Starting rehabilitation in the first year of life is important to minimize joint contractures and maximize development and autonomy (Dahan-Oliel et al., 2025). Surgical interventions are also often warranted to promote better joint range of motion and alignment (Hansen-Jaumard et al., 2020; Wagner et al., 2019). Since AMC is a lifelong condition, functional and rehabilitation needs will evolve over time (Wagner et al., 2019). As AMC is rare, it may be difficult for rehabilitation practitioners to develop an expertise with this population, especially in healthcare settings where clinicians may encounter only a few clients with AMC throughout their careers (Elfassy et al., 2020). Individuals and families with AMC often have to seek out expertise in larger health centers with a team dedicated to AMC, access to which may be difficult depending on the geographical area. As individuals with AMC transition to the adult health care system, rehabilitation services tend to significantly decrease (Elfassy et al., 2020). However, it remains important for individuals with AMC to continue leading an active lifestyle to maintain health and function (Altiok et al., 2019; Dai et al., 2018; Wagner et al., 2019).

With these considerations in mind, individuals with AMC and their families must take charge of their condition, become experts and learn to manage their health daily. Health interventions

DOI: 10.1201/9781003599074-11

Self-management

Individual	Family	Community	Health care system
▶ Personal Factors ▶ Goals	▶ Preferences ▶ Socio-economic factors ▶ Caregiver health	▶ Social support ▶ Availability of ressources ▶ Finacial support	▶ Availability of resources ▶ Patient-provider relationship

Areas for intervention : Clinic/rehabilitation visits Home excercise program Orthotic use Assistive devices Pain management Exercise/fitness

HEALTH OUTCOMES : Joint movement and muscle strength **Motor development** Participation in areas of life (self-care, school, work, leisure) **Cardiovascular health** Quality of life

FIGURE 10.1 Factors to consider for self-management in AMC rehabilitation to maximize health outcomes.

that encourage self-management can empower individuals to actively care for themselves, ultimately improving health outcomes over the long-term (Abrahams et al., 2019). This chapter discusses self-management in rehabilitation for individuals with AMC across the lifespan, gathering the perspectives of clinicians and people with lived experience. Specifically, this chapter is authored by occupational, physical and speech therapists, physiatrists, orthopedic surgeons, adults with AMC and caregivers of children with AMC from 10 countries in North and South America, Europe and Asia.

The goal of this chapter is to provide tools and support for people with AMC, rehabilitation specialists, health care practitioners and the AMC community to better guide self-management as a lifelong skill for a healthy lifestyle. Self-management encompasses different approaches and brings together multiple players to ensure its long-term integration and success. Collaboration between the individual, the family and the healthcare providers ensures interventions are tailored to the individual/family's needs, preferences, personal, and social factors (Modi et al., 2012; Sadler et al., 2014). Availability of resources and community services may also impact self-management behaviors and should be considered. Figure 10.1 illustrates the core concepts and factors that need to be considered for self-management in AMC. This chapter will discuss how self-management is integrated in the rehabilitation of individuals with AMC across the lifespan- from infancy to school age children, adolescents, and adults to the aging population), including interventions related to orthotic use and pain management, physical activities, and psychosocial well-being. Finally, the role of AMC support groups in self-management will be discussed.

REHABILITATION AND SELF-MANAGEMENT IN INFANCY AND TODDLERHOOD

Babies born with AMC can present very differently at birth, depending on their underlying condition and the extent of their joint contractures (Dahan-Oliel et al., 2019). Typically, in AMC, contractures are the most severe at birth and may improve significantly over time with the appropriate healthcare interventions (Kowalczyk and Felus, 2016). Caregivers may be aware of their child's diagnosis in half of pregnancies, while the other half will only find out after birth (Dahan-Oliel et al., 2019). Caring for an infant with AMC can be overwhelming for caregivers and families as many may face a diagnostic odyssey to find out their child's condition adding a layer of fear, uncertainty or guilt for the caregivers (Elekanachi et al., 2024). Furthermore, caregivers have to learn about a new condition and how to navigate the healthcare system while juggling their other roles (Elekanachi et al., 2024).

Children with AMC require a family-centered multidisciplinary approach for their care, and the rehabilitation team is an important player in the first years of life (Wagner et al., 2019).

Through conservative rehabilitation approaches, infants with AMC can significantly improve their joint mobility, given the appropriate interventions are put in place (Dahan-Oliel et al., 2025). During infancy, rehabilitation interventions aim at minimizing joint contractures and maximizing the baby's development, through a daily home exercise program carried out by the family and with regular follow-ups with the rehabilitation team once or twice per month (Binkiewicz-Glinska et al., 2013; Dahan-Oliel et al., 2025). Interventions include gentle stretching of the contracted joints, encouraging active movements of available muscle groups, use of orthotics for the upper and/or lower limbs, serial casting, positioning and stimulating developmental milestones (Dahan-Oliel et al., 2025; Wagner et al., 2019). Rehabilitation professionals are among the first to intervene with babies with AMC and their family, so their role in setting the stage for successful self-management is essential. In the infancy and toddler stages, self-management refers to the caregiver's management of their child's healthcare and rehabilitation needs. Here, we describe self-management principles to consider for families of infants and toddlers with AMC, including early intervention/home exercise programs, use of orthotics and adaptive equipment, and peri-operative rehabilitation. Consideration of personal factors promotes a holistic approach to care and empowers caregivers to be involved in the management of their child's condition.

Early Intervention, Setting the Stage for a Successful Collaboration

A collaborative relationship between the caregivers and the rehabilitation providers, based on trust and communication, fosters a positive environment for realistic and meaningful goals. By involving the caregivers in decision-making and taking into consideration their unique realities and socio-demographic context, rehabilitation providers can adapt their intervention approaches to maximize adherence and compliance to the proposed treatments (Sadler et al., 2014). In infancy, adherence and compliance with the rehabilitation interventions, whether during in-person visits, home exercise programs or for orthotic use, are very important to maximize the child's functional outcomes. Therefore, to maximize "buy-in" and compliance from families, education must be provided regarding rehabilitation interventions, why they are being performed and how they can impact their child's progress. Different approaches can be used to facilitate the learning and integration of the recommended interventions. The home exercise program must be demonstrated and practiced with the caregivers, and reviewed regularly (e.g., how to stretch, how often, how long, how to put on an orthosis and important precautions, how to position the child for play, how to stimulate movements, etc.) (Dahan-Oliel et al., 2025). This approach helps build caregiver's confidence in their ability to carry out a home program and ensures that it is done effectively and safely at home. Other media can be used to ensure compliance with the home program. For example, written information in addition to visual support such as videos or pictures taken during rehabilitation treatment can be useful for families to consult when needed. In addition, brainstorming with the caregivers on how to effectively integrate those interventions into their daily routine, while minimizing the burden, is more likely to ensure adherence and compliance with the home program. For example, stretching exercises may be done during diaper changes, while playing with the baby or during bathtime, depending on what is more realistic for the caregiver. Rehabilitation interventions continue to be important and may shift in terms of goals and priorities after the first year of life. Rehabilitation interventions begin to diversify as the child grows, and it is important to revisit rehabilitation goals to ensure that the needs, priorities and preferences of the child and their families are being met. Joint contractures continue to be monitored, and interventions previously mentioned continue throughout growth (i.e., stretching, strengthening, orthotics). In addition, interventions to stimulate developmental milestones become more predominant, such as encouraging rolling, sitting, scooting or crawling, and standing. As the child begins to explore their environment, hand function is also stimulated to work on reaching, grasp and release, bilateral hand skills, and hand to mouth activities, leading up to self-feeding and other activities of daily living (Wagner et al., 2019).

To encourage the child to develop their skills and gain independence in play, mobility, and activities of daily living, they should be stimulated and encouraged to perform those activities themselves, as much as possible. Through trial and exploration, a child can develop their own ways of doing things and find their own compensatory strategies to be able to perform a given activity. For example, a child who does not have sufficient active elbow flexion to bring their hand to the mouth will learn to use an external surface as a support to assist in moving their arm passively. To achieve that, a child must be given the time, space and opportunity to practice.

Use of Orthotics and Adaptive Equipment

Depending on the child's needs and abilities, the use of adaptive equipment may be introduced in the first few years of life (e.g., stander, walker, wheelchair, adapted utensils for self-feeding). When considering the use of adaptive equipment, discussion and collaboration between the rehabilitation team and the family will help decide on the importance, the need, and the choice of such equipment, to maximize their acceptance and use by the child and the family. The child and caregivers must be involved in decision-making regarding proposed equipment to ensure that aspects of accessibility, feasibility and ease of use in different contexts are considered (Dahan-Oliel et al., 2025). Orthotics are also an essential part of rehabilitation management in AMC. Upper and lower extremity orthotics are introduced in infancy to provide a stretch to contracted joints and promote functional positioning. As they grow into toddlerhood, orthotics are revised to accommodate for growth and can be used to promote function. Caregivers' feedback on orthotics, such as proper fit, comfort, and ease of use, is imperative to ensure orthotics are used consistently.

Family Engagement in a Perioperative Context

A child with AMC may undergo several orthopedic surgeries early in life (Hansen-Jaumard et al., 2020), and rehabilitation can maximize outcomes post-surgery. After orthopedic surgery, rehabilitation interventions can include exercises and orthotic use with the goals to promote an active return or improvement of function. Rehabilitation interventions aim to reduce pain, improve range of motion, strength and mobility and optimize function in daily activities (Cachecho et al., 2024). In the absence of these rehabilitation interventions and adequate follow-up, surgical outcomes are suboptimal. Pre-operative education in this context helps prepare families to know what to expect post-operatively and engages the child and their family to be active participants in the post-operative process.

Considering Personal Factors for a Holistic Approach

Since caregivers are pivotal at managing their child's healthcare and rehabilitation needs, several factors should be considered to promote adherence to self-management and compliance with rehabilitation treatment. Factors such as the family's social situation (i.e., presence or absence of a support system), their socioeconomic situation, and the caregivers' health (physical, emotional and psychological) may affect self-management (Sadler et al., 2014). Therefore, the approaches and the expectations toward self-management may need to be adapted and revisited over time. Frequent check-ins with the family may be needed to ensure the home exercise program is well understood and carried out. This can be done through more frequent visits in rehabilitation if the family situation permits, or through virtual appointments which have become more common practice in the past few years (Gagnon et al., 2020). Rehabilitation practitioners must consider the psychosocial impact of caring for a child with AMC and the burden it can have on families (Elekanachi et al., 2024). Therefore, early referral to appropriate resources within the healthcare system (e.g., social work, psychology), and in the community (e.g., community programs, financial support) is important to ensure families are well supported in their journey (Almasri et al., 2018). Meeting other families with children with AMC through support groups (e.g., in-person meetings, social media, virtual groups) is extremely valuable to share experiences, provide mutual support, and break the feeling of isolation some families may feel (Steen et al., 2017). To better understand the primordial role support groups, play in self-management of AMC throughout the lifespan, refer to the section dedicated to the topic later in this chapter.

As children with AMC grow and transition from infancy into the school-age years, the focus of rehabilitation and self-management evolves to support increasing autonomy, participation in daily routines, and engagement in educational and social environments—laying the foundation for more active involvement in decisions related to orthotic use, physical activity, pain management, and psychosocial well-being. The following reflection from a caregiver of a child with AMC underscores the importance of evolving self-management through childhood: "As a caregiver to my 5-year-old daughter with AMC, self-management means helping her learn to try before saying she can't do something. It's about encouraging her to see that she doesn't have to be like everyone else to be capable and valuable. Every day, we work on helping her understand that her uniqueness is a strength, and that with a little creativity, determination, and the use of adaptive aids, she can do just as much as anyone else. It's important to us that she feels accepted for who she is and knows there's always a place for her."

REHABILITATION AND SELF-MANAGEMENT IN SCHOOL-AGED CHILDREN

During the school years, the concept of self-management evolves from a predominantly caregiver-centered approach in infancy to a family-centered approach as children develop increased autonomy. School-aged children are broadening their perspectives to include school environments, increasing understanding of peer relationships and determining their individual preferences for participation. Instead of the continual therapy approaches that support early intervention in the infant years, with increased life demands, therapy transitions to more episodic care that is more goal oriented on specific tasks. Here we will discuss self-management principles, including collaborative relationships for input, the approaches to care and community engagement.

Collaborative Relationships

Our healthcare decision-making, compliance, and expectations now include a more vocal input from the growing school age child. The health care professional has the knowledge of body structure and function and assistive equipment, while the school age child has the lived experience and the spirit and spunk of determination. They have goals in mind for increased independence that may or may not coincide with caregivers and healthcare professionals. Together, collaborative outside-the-box thinking leads to increased functional independence in chosen activities. Health care professionals have options for more tendon transfer surgeries as the school- aged child has the ability to be more compliant with restrictions and follow protocols. Understanding and taking more ownership of their bodies, the school- aged child gives input to surgical decision-making interventions. As school-aged children can now express their concerns for their future, they are able to share firsthand their pain experience and the impact on their daily routine, as well as potential concerns for the future.

Self- management through a multidisciplinary team approach, where the child and their family are not just recipients of care but provide input and advocate for their needs and help establish goals, is a must. Collaboration is paramount as each member can share their perspectives, their philosophies, their insight on the goals and expectations for care. Healthcare professionals provide tools and opportunities; the growing child can assume more responsibility for their own range of motion and orthotic wearing; caregivers help provide a home environment where the child has the opportunity to try new tasks, practice tasks for proficiency and then efficiency, and gain self-efficacy. Establishing relationships is key to navigating the needs and opinions of each member of the team.

Approaches to Care

As the school-age child leaves the home, the need for increased independence in mobility, in activities of daily living and in life activities become paramount. Health care professionals have a responsibility to facilitate maximum independence and participation. Utilizing a client- and family-centered approach, the healthcare professional develops an individualized treatment plan that is guided by the patient's goals and informed by their personal values and perspective. Often, the team approaches independence in mobility or activities of daily living as an "either/or" approach when perhaps a "both/and" approach is best. Let's take a closer look. For mobility, the school age child encounters more diverse terrains that require varying speeds of movement, and typically more endurance than ever before. Typically, we address mobility in terms of ambulation only by looking at alternative methods as "failure." However, people without AMC may drive their cars or take a subway to the grocery store, use an elevator to ascend a few flights of stairs and may use an escalator when tired. Perhaps self-management can promote more positive attitudes and increased advocacy for normalizing adapted mobility in the AMC population as it is in the non-AMC population. Energy conservation principles also emerge during this period, as children may be able to walk independently, but to save energy and increase productivity in school, they may choose to use a wheelchair instead. Also learning self-awareness is another crucial principle during this stage. Indeed, the person with AMC starts to learn to be in tune with what their body needs, to ask for help, and to be able to self-advocate.

As a mother of a six-year-old with AMC shared: "Self-management for my 6 year-old means being able to advocate for her own needs throughout the day, such as assistance with getting her braces and shoes on and off, requesting her wheelchair for long distances when she is tired or anticipates she might not make it back to the starting location without it, and recognizing when she needs some Tylenol to take the edge off the pain so that she can focus in class. It means knowing what the day will look like and planning ahead to ensure maximal participation and enjoyment. For example, if going to a park later with friends, then maybe the morning is spent at the table doing arts and crafts to rest her feet, so that she has the ability to play without issue."

That same "both/and approach" can be seen within the area of participation. Should we provide assistive equipment to assist with independence or does that burden them with another piece of equipment? Health care professionals need to help with the experience of completing activities of daily living. Many times, introducing assistive equipment allows the child the ability to further understand how to complete a task, and then once the concept is understood, the child with AMC can progress, as they are able, past the initial use of assistive equipment. Self-management allows the health care professionals to introduce approaches and engages the school age child's intuitive mind to bring the task into fruition in their own style.

Engagement with Community

Community is now the lived environment for the school age child. From visiting friends' homes, to school, to community activities, the school age child with AMC wants to engage. Hearing information just from their healthcare professional in a therapeutic environment is not always the best avenue for knowledge sharing. Active engagement with school-aged children needs to meet them where they are. Technology can be a great advantage for the school age child with AMC. Virtual resources provide lived experiences of how to put socks on and off, hold a lunch tray, and put your hair in a ponytail. The team should embrace these resources as good starting points to pursuing independence. Telehealth options can expand delivery of services to assist with activity and participation in the community, in addition to other types of rehabilitation therapies (Gagnon et al., 2021). Engagement with community enables transition from functional independence in mobility and activities of daily living of early school age to the promotion of a healthy, active lifestyle in the teenage/adolescence school age years by promoting community-based engagement, e.g., gym memberships versus constant physical or occupational therapy sessions. Engagement in the community can be with peers, as well as with individuals with AMC. The rise of 3D printers has brought both options for designs for assistive equipment but also fostered collaboration with peers through knowledge sharing. For example, schools can team up 3D classes with students needing adaptations, creating public awareness about AMC and increasing access to adaptive strategies and promoting self-advocacy through technology and inclusive environments. Self-management within the community can mean engagement and learning FOR the school age child with AMC but also advocacy and knowledge sharing FROM the child with AMC.

The transition from school-aged childhood to adolescence marks a critical period in which rehabilitation and self-management approaches must be recalibrated to address the increasing complexity of developmental, functional, and psychosocial demands—supporting individuals with AMC in assuming greater agency over independent living, educational and vocational training and community engagement.

REHABILITATION, PHYSICAL ACTIVITY, AND SELF-MANAGEMENT THROUGH ADOLESCENCE

As individuals with AMC reach adolescence, rehabilitation interventions should start addressing needs and concerns regarding transition to adulthood. This period involves many changes in the lives of individuals with AMC, such as starting college or university, working, moving away from the family home to independent living, managing transportation, finances, and health needs. These changes can bring in new challenges to autonomy and participation, which have been voiced as concerns by youth with AMC (Elfassy et al., 2020) and their caregivers (Elekanachi et al., 2024). Identifying transition goals and working toward them should be done in collaboration between the healthcare professional (e.g., social worker, occupational therapist), the young adult with AMC, and their caregiver when appropriate. In their article on quality of life in youth with AMC, Altiok et al. (2019) identified areas to consider in preparing for the transition to adulthood. These areas include patient education, screening for and management of obesity, mental health, need for assistive devices and tools, architectural and community barriers, and transportation needs and vocational training.

Self-management Strategies and Tips

To accompany young adults in their transition to adulthood, self-management habits should be introduced during their early adolescence in order to empower them to take charge of their own health while relying less and less on their caregiver, when possible. Strategies are adjusted according to the youth's preferences and abilities. Some may not achieve independence in all areas and may always require assistance from another person. It becomes important to teach the youth to self-advocate and ask for help when needed (Wagner et al., 2019). This may be challenging for some who may be reluctant to ask for help, therefore it is important to normalize this early in the rehabilitation process. Table 10.1 describes different strategies that can be used by young adults to manage different areas of their life as they transition to adulthood. First and foremost, knowledge and education about their own condition is key, not only for them to understand their physical needs, but to give them the tools to explain their condition to others and advocate for themselves (Elekanachi et al., 2024; Elfassy et al., 2020). Throughout growth, giving children and youth the opportunity to practice activity skills, to try adaptive equipment and to problem solve through trial and error will also help build self-confidence and gradually increase their participation and independence in various activities (Dahan-Oliel et al., 2025; Wagner et al., 2019). Transitions may be emotionally challenging and bring stress or anxiety.

TABLE 10.1
Self-Management Strategies for Adolescents with AMC to Prepare for Adulthood

Areas	Strategies
Medical and Physical Self-Management	Understand your type of arthrogryposis and how it affects your body
	Track medical and rehabilitation appointments using a calendar or reminder app
	Learn to manage medications independently and communicate their pain experience effectively for optimizing pain management
	Stick to a regular exercise routine as recommended by your care team to maintain mobility and function
	Understand adult healthcare services you can access
Daily Living Skills and Adaptations	Use assistive tools for dressing, grooming, eating, writing, etc., to maximize and optimize capacities and skills
	Practice independent living skills—start small and build confidence
	Problem-solve with others strategies for overcoming physical or environmental barriers within the home and community (e.g., school)
Emotional and Social Self-Management	Participate in hobbies and interests that boost self-esteem
	Talk to someone about stress, anxiety, or sadness—consider therapy if needed
	Connect with peers who understand your experience (online or in-person groups)
	Engage in a group sport/adapted sport
Communication and Advocacy	Ask questions and speak up during medical appointments; voice your goals
	Practice explaining your condition to teachers, coaches, or employers
	Understand your rights and how to ask for accommodations
	Obtain and maintain contacts of various professionals with knowledge and expertise in disability-related questions and rights of people with disabilities (e.g., accountant, lawyer, notary).
Educational and Vocational Planning	Use individualized education plan and office for students with disability to access school accommodations
	Plan for post-school goals like college, vocational training, or work with your support team.
	Explore careers that fit your interests and abilities—start early!

Not only should youth learn how and where to find the needed support, part of the emotional self-management process is to also learn how to recognize those signs of stress or anxiety. Quote from an adult with AMC *"Realizing what triggers made me feel worse and what resources I found that made me feel better, helped to then adhere to those resources that helped me and made me feel better."*

Supports and Resources

Transition also involves navigating new environments, such as school and work. Issues with accessibility may emerge; accommodations and adaptations may be required. Although youth are encouraged to seek out resources and advocate for themselves, the support of individuals with the knowledge and expertise on how to navigate those resources remains very important. These may include occupational therapists, social workers, or school counselors, who can assist in planning for school and work goals. It can also include professionals, such as lawyers or accountants, with knowledge of disability-related questions who can provide support in other matters (e.g., financial, rights of people with disabilities).

Finally, as individuals transition out of their pediatric healthcare system and into the adult healthcare system, access to medical and rehabilitation services becomes more limited and may be used on a "as needed" basis only (Wagner et al., 2019). In order to be equipped for such a shift and to ensure continuity in care, adolescents with AMC and their family should be guided toward appropriate adult resources. For example, infographics were created by people with AMC for people with AMC and for medical professionals to provide knowledge and awareness to promote successful interactions when seeking healthcare as adults (Arthrogryposis Multiplex Congenita Support, Inc., n.d.) This may involve direct referral to specific services, or written lists of specialists or centers. There is a lack of evidence in the literature on transition of adolescents with AMC to adulthood. Understanding transition needs of youth and young adults with AMC and identifying effective transition and self-management programs for youth with AMC should include mixed-methods and a participatory research approach to empower youth with AMC as they transition out of pediatric care and toward adulthood. Research on self-management and transition programs in other rare diseases, such as osteogenesis imperfecta (Carrier et al., 2018; Michalovic et al., 2020), has been done and offers promising avenues to address this gap.

As individuals with AMC transition from adolescence into adulthood, rehabilitation, and self-management approaches must shift to support full participation in adult roles and responsibilities, with an emphasis on long-term maintenance of function, independence in health-related decision-making, and sustained engagement in areas such as employment, relationships, orthotic and pain management, physical activity, and psychosocial well-being.

REHABILITATION, PHYSICAL ACTIVITY, AND SELF-MANAGEMENT THROUGH ADULTHOOD

Adulthood revolves around taking responsibility for all aspects of life, including education, work, family, and leisure. For adults with AMC, this includes increased responsibility to manage one's own health condition. Many adults with AMC report a level of quality of life equivalent to the average population, while a higher proportion have a graduate degree compared to the average US population (Nouraei et al., 2017). Almost half of the adult population live with a partner and many adults struggle with pain in their joints and muscles (Nouraei et al., 2017). Physical activity and intermittent rehabilitation as needed is important for adults with AMC to maintain their physical function and independence (Wagner et al., 2019). Despite ongoing medical needs, people with rare conditions, such as AMC, often transition from a childhood under the care of well-versed medical professionals, to an adulthood healthcare system with unfamiliar clinicians requiring increased self-management and leading to the need to explain their medical condition and justify necessary resources to promote ongoing well-being (Gibson et al., 2015; Song et al., 2020; Wallis, 2007). Adults with AMC have been known to employ a range of strategies to communicate their health needs to medical providers and to enhance self-management of their condition; this includes utilizing peer support groups, providing medical professionals with infographics on AMC, and turning to sports as a means of ongoing physical rehabilitation.

A retrospective review on 43 adults with AMC indicated that types of disability varied by genotype (Dai et al., 2018). Overall, participants reported the well-known signs of AMC including joint stiffness, deformities, and muscle weakness. In addition, participants were found to require interventions for technical aids, as well as other less visible disorders that could contribute to severe participation restriction, particularly pain and psychological problems such as anxiety, fatigue, difficulty in sexual life, altered self-esteem, and feelings of solitude. Severe respiratory disorders were infrequent and were linked to *PIEZO2* mutations. In Amyoplasia, difficulties in walking were more frequently reported and due to skeletal problems and not to respiratory impairments as in *PIEZO2*. Although functional independence was diminished in Amyoplasia compared to other AMC types, respiratory and swallowing capacities were affected in other AMC types and not in Amyoplasia. These findings indicate the importance of multidisciplinary management and genomic testing for accurate and timely diagnosis (Dieterich et al., 2019). Additionally, understanding hereditary patterns through genetic testing and counseling is a cornerstone of informed family planning, empowering individuals and couples to make choices grounded in knowledge about inherited health risks, carrier status, and reproductive options (Kristoffersson and Johansson-Soller, 2024). Understanding inheritance patterns enables prospective parents to assess recurrence risks and reproductive options rooted in their own genetic profiles (Arduç et al., 2025). Given the complexity of AMC, it's essential to advocate for access to genetic specialists, such as certified genetic counselors and medical geneticists, as well as specialty sonographers. Skilled sonographers can detect early signs such as fetal akinesia, joint contractures, and atypical limb positioning on ultrasound—sometimes visible in the second trimester—and help guide timing for diagnostic procedures like chorionic villus sampling or amniocentesis (Arduç et al., 2025).

In the context of AMC, discussions around family planning and sexuality are deeply interconnected: understanding one's genetic risk through carrier screening and inheritance patterns not only informs reproductive decisions, but also shapes the ways individuals with AMC perceive and express their sexual identity and reproductive autonomy. Research on physical disabilities highlights a persistent stereotype: many people assume that individuals with disabilities are without sexual interest or desire. These misconceptions can leave people with disabilities overlooked in conversations about intimacy, relationships, and reproductive autonomy despite their shared desires for connection, romantic partnership, and parenthood (Anderson and Kitchin, 2000).

Sexuality should be approached in a timely and appropriate manner for each individual, taking into account their level of openness, cultural background, and personal development. Sexuality is a fundamental aspect of self-management and rehabilitation, contributing to overall well-being, identity, and quality of life for individuals with disabilities, including those with AMC. Although there is a paucity of research on sexuality in AMC specifically, parallels can be drawn from other populations. A mixed-methods systematic review on health literacy in young people with cerebral palsy identified information gaps in topics such as aging with cerebral palsy, sexuality, and navigating intimate relationships (Ding et al., 2024). A study on the sexual experiences of women with cerebral palsy reported a lack of accessible exam tables, hospital staff unfamiliar with physical disabilities, and assumptions that women with cerebral palsy are not sexually active (Gray et al., 2021). Prior work has identified barriers to sexual health care as well as to accessing sexual and reproductive health services for people with disabilities, including medical professionals' lack of knowledge and awareness and structural barriers such as medical facilities lacking accessible equipment (Ganle et al., 2020; Rowen et al., 2015). Building capacity and development of self-efficacy may assist with the identification of needs. Parents, partners, and persons with AMC should be provided with age-appropriate information about sexuality that includes specific information with respect to AMC. Addressing sexuality in individuals with AMC involves recognizing their unique physical needs and promoting confidence and autonomy. Open communication is essential, fostering trust and comfort when discussing desires, boundaries, and limitations. Principles of energy conservation can help manage fatigue, allowing individuals to engage in sexual activity without becoming overly exhausted. Positioning aids and adaptive equipment can enhance comfort, reduce pain, and support creative exploration, making intimacy more accessible and enjoyable. Emphasizing fun and exploration encourages positive experiences, while maintaining respect for the individual's preferences and boundaries is crucial. Ultimately, a supportive, inclusive approach promotes sexual well-being and empowerment.

Due to the wide spectrum of physical function among the AMC population, opportunities to be physically active or participate in physical activities vary largely from person to person (Wagner et al., 2019). As a result, rehabilitation should be person-centered and tailored to fit each individual. However, pain, fatigue, and a lack of adult rehabilitation services may result in many not having the option to continue physical rehabilitation (Nouraei et al., 2017). Given the complexity of receiving specialized medical care after transitioning from integrated pediatric care into the adult healthcare system, it is unsurprising that many adults with AMC become lost in the medical system. The role and importance of physical and occupational rehabilitation becomes crucial, as these are often the only *treatments* that adults receive besides ongoing surgeries (Colver et al., 2020; Odling et al., 2020; Wallis, 2007; Wan et al., 2019). Developing monitored and adapted physical activity programs, as well as an inclusive leisure activity, can provide both physical and emotional benefits. The clinical benefits of practicing physical activity and sports among people with disabilities include improvements in affective well-being, reduced levels of anxiety and depression, better self-confidence, and higher belief in one's capabilities (Shephard, 1991).

Participation in sports is associated with positive outcomes, like having the opportunity for social interaction and genuine enjoyment. Sports provide a space to connect with others and experience a sense of belonging. Disabled adults describe a feeling of freedom and purpose and that sports present an opportunity to battle stereotypes about disability (Aitchison et al., 2022).

For adults with AMC who have undergone many surgical interventions throughout their lifetimes, the ongoing practice of physical activity has proven to be one of the most effective long-term chronic treatments triggered by a yearning for improved self-management and physical and emotional self-care (Figure 10.2).

Up until this point, few studies have investigated the lived experiences of adults with AMC. More recently, AMC experts have turned their focus to the ongoing needs of adults with AMC with the goal of enhancing self-management of the condition throughout the lifespan (Dai et al., 2018; Wagner et al., 2019). Adults with AMC develop a myriad of compensatory and adaptive strategies

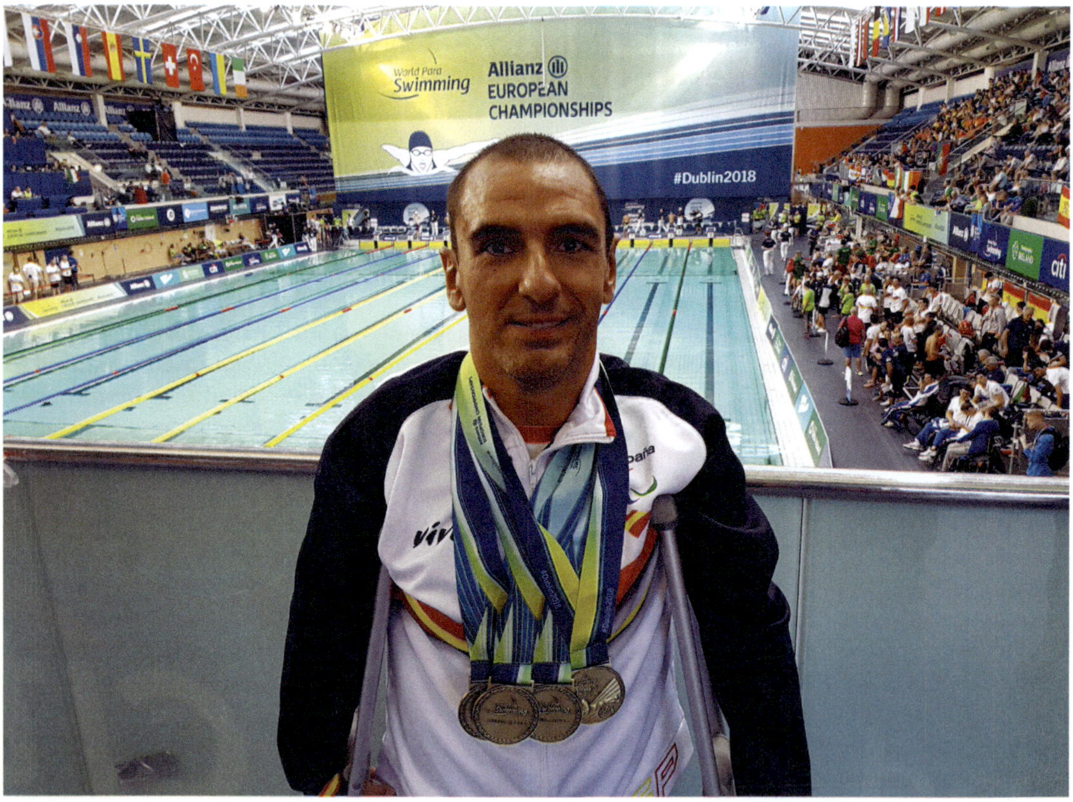

FIGURE 10.2 Miguel Angel Tajuelo, paralympic swimmer with AMC from Spain, competing at Europeo Dublín 2018.

to manage their condition and maintain engagement in meaningful activities; future studies should include participatory research to gain perspectives from those with lived experience on the best methods for effective self-management of AMC throughout adulthood.

IS IT POSSIBLE TO DELAY THE AGING PROCESS IN AMC? SELF-MANAGEMENT TO PROMOTE HEALTH

Aging is defined as the accumulation of degenerative changes in an individual over time (Bowen and Atwood, 2004), and in humans, it is understood as a multidimensional process involving physical, social, and psychological transformations. A distinction is often made between the universal aging process that affects all people and "probabilistic ageing," which encompasses changes that may occur in some individuals but not in others. From this perspective, a congenital disability such as AMC can be viewed as a contributor to a form of probabilistic aging, where the effects of aging may emerge earlier or with greater intensity than in the general population. While significant medical and functional changes are commonly associated with individuals over the age of 70, research shows that people with disabilities often experience similar age-related complications 20–25 years earlier. Aging involves degenerative changes across multiple organ systems—including the musculoskeletal, respiratory, cardiovascular, and nervous systems—which progressively reduce the functional reserves of these organs. For individuals born with a disability like AMC, reserve capacities in one or more organ systems may already be compromised from birth, making them more susceptible to additional strains and functional decline as they age.

In this context, two important health principles should be prioritized to promote longevity and quality of life in people with AMC: enhancing the reserve capacity of vital organs before deterioration begins and actively preventing the progressive loss of function.

For instance, bone health is a significant concern. Although bone mass typically decreases with age—contributing to osteopenia and osteoporosis—people with AMC may experience reduced bone mineral density (BMD) at an earlier age. A French retrospective study (mean age 33 years) reported that individuals with AMC had BMD values at the femoral neck and total hip approximately 1 to 1.2 standard deviations below normal, with nearly half having experienced at least one fracture and 86% showing insufficient vitamin D levels (Romand et al., 2024). These findings underscore the importance of early assessment using dual-energy X-ray absorptiometry (DXA) and timely intervention through vitamin D supplementation, especially in those with a history of falls or fractures. Similarly, muscle health is another area where early decline is common. Biological aging naturally leads to reductions in muscle strength, mass, oxygen uptake, and joint flexibility due to changes such as decreased collagen production, tendon shortening, and increased fibrosis. In individuals with AMC, these changes are compounded by congenital characteristics such as joint contractures, muscle underdevelopment, fibrosis, and neuromuscular anomalies—including motor neuron dysfunction and connective tissue abnormalities. As a result, individuals with AMC begin life with altered and often diminished muscle function, which makes them particularly vulnerable to sarcopenia—the age-related loss of muscle mass and strength. To counteract these effects, regular physiotherapy and consistent physical activity are essential throughout life to help preserve mobility and maintain functional independence for as long as possible.

This brings into focus the concept of *successful aging*, often defined as "adding life to years," emphasizing that the quality of life is as important as its duration. While there is no single agreed-upon definition, successful aging generally includes the absence of chronic disease and the maintenance of good physical, cognitive, and social functioning into later life. In AMC, successful aging must be understood within the context of lifelong disability and unique health challenges. A scoping review of adult AMC patients (Cachecho et al., 2021) found that, despite substantial physical limitations, many individuals reported psychosocial health—including emotional well-being and social functioning—on par with the general population. However, chronic fatigue and pain were common and closely linked to decreased well-being and elevated emotional stress. A powerful illustration of successful aging in AMC is offered through a case study (Riemer and Steen, 2013) that followed a woman with Amyoplasia—the most common form of AMC—who lived to age 93. Over her lifetime, she underwent 21 surgeries and experienced a slow decline in muscle strength, initially in her legs and later in her arms. Still, she retained independence, worked for 32 years, and walked unaided until age 37. Interestingly, her musculoskeletal pain diminished with age, although other age-related health issues gradually emerged. Her story demonstrates that even with severe physical limitations, individuals with AMC can live long, fulfilling lives characterized by resilience, effective coping strategies, and strong personal motivation. This case also underscores the importance of individualized care, including treatment plans that accommodate gradual strength decline and avoid overtraining in adulthood.

Aging with AMC, therefore, involves a dynamic interplay between typical age-related changes, the congenital nature and etiology of AMC, and the accumulated effects of living with a lifelong disability. Awareness of how these factors interact is essential for designing effective long-term care strategies. With close follow-up, informed decision-making, and early interventions, it is possible to delay functional loss and promote sustained health and well-being. Rehabilitation is central to this process. To fully realize its potential social, economic, and health benefits, rehabilitation must be timely, of high quality, and accessible. Ideally, it should begin as soon as a health concern is identified and continue alongside other medical care throughout the individual's life. Such an approach not only supports physical functioning but also enhances psychological well-being, making it possible for individuals with AMC to age with dignity, independence, and an improved quality of life.

LIFELONG APPROACHES TO REHABILITATION

Key components of a comprehensive, lifelong approach to rehabilitation and self-management in individuals with AMC include the use of orthotics, effective pain management strategies, and participation in support groups tailored to the AMC community. Together, these elements play a vital role in promoting functional independence, enhancing quality of life, and fostering a sense of empowerment. This section explores how each of these supports contribute to long-term well-being and how they can be integrated into a sustainable care plan across the lifespan.

Orthotics and Their Importance to Function and Mobility

Upper and lower extremity orthotics play a key role in the treatment of arthrogryposis multiplex congenita (AMC) from birth through adulthood. These devices serve as lifelong tools that enable participation, promote autonomy, and support the vital mind-body connection. Effective communication and a clear understanding of the individual's goals in childhood, adolescence, or adulthood are essential to the successful use of orthotics. Treatment adherence is deeply linked to these personal goals, and the same style of orthosis may serve entirely different functions at different stages of life. This is why education must begin early. Families need to understand the nature of their child's impairments and activity limitations and learn how to adapt these understandings as their child grows. Likewise, children must gradually learn how to work with their limitations in various contexts: at home, at school, with friends, and during personal care. Through this process, orthotics, physiotherapy, mobility aids such as wheelchairs or walking canes, and assistive devices become familiar tools and are instruments of independence. The patient and their family are the epicenter of this care model. Without informed, active participation, even the most well-designed orthosis may fall short of its potential. Orthoses must be highly individualized, continuously reassessed, and carefully fitted by clinicians with both technical expertise and a deep understanding of the person's holistic needs, including their medical, emotional, and social context. Orthotic decisions—particularly for the lower limbs—must also be coordinated with surgical planning and tailored to specific mobility goals, including walking, standing, or independent wheelchair use. This section follows the evolving story of orthotic care

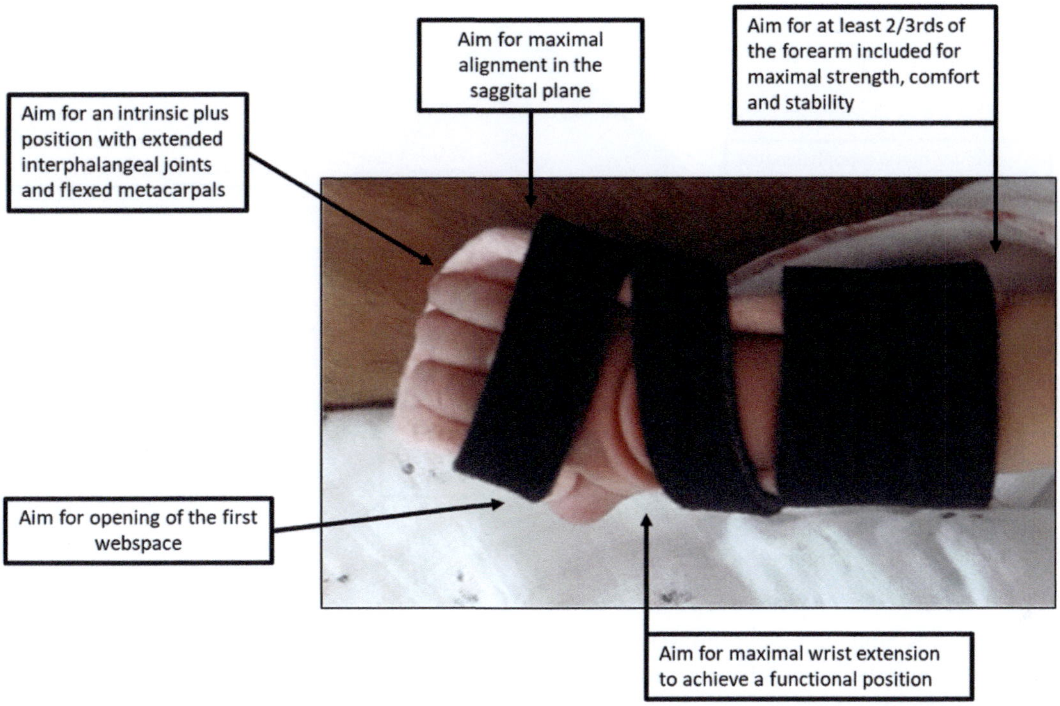

FIGURE 10.3 Landmarks for a night orthosis in Amyoplasia to promote optimal joint alignment.

across the lifespan, offering a deeper understanding of how to promote self-management and participation from infancy through adulthood.

An Evolving Journey in AMC

The journey begins at birth, where infants with AMC often present with visible limitations in joint range of motion, muscle imbalances, and skin tension. From the earliest moments, interventions such as static orthoses are introduced to correct or accommodate joint limitations and to gently encourage functional movement patterns. These orthoses, custom-made for each tiny limb, work to restore the balance between opposing muscles and gradually improve range of motion in both directions of movement (Figure 10.3). For some families, these devices are changed as often as every one to two weeks during the infant's first months, a routine that becomes part of the rhythm of early life. Each adjustment brings new possibilities—a slightly straighter wrist, a better-positioned knee, or a more responsive elbow. These small gains form the building blocks of future independence.

As infants with AMC grow into toddlers, their curiosity and desire to explore push them into action. Despite their physical limitations, they begin to find ways to interact with their environment using unique compensation strategies that reflect both their creativity and their bodies' innate adaptability. Often, children will discover new ways to roll, scoot, or manipulate objects, even if they cannot follow typical developmental pathways. Differences in muscle strength between agonist and antagonist muscle groups result in movement patterns that may seem unusual but serve a very real purpose for that child. It's during this time that orthoses take on a more dynamic role. Functional orthoses (Figure 10.4), sometimes equipped to assist with grasping or tool use, become part of daily life—not just therapeutic devices, but tools of exploration. Children may wear custom-designed splints that help them hold a crayon or feed themselves, gradually building the confidence and physical ability to participate in age-appropriate activities. Posturing with orthoses is frequently combined with treatment sessions that include active assistance and muscle stimulation. Therapists

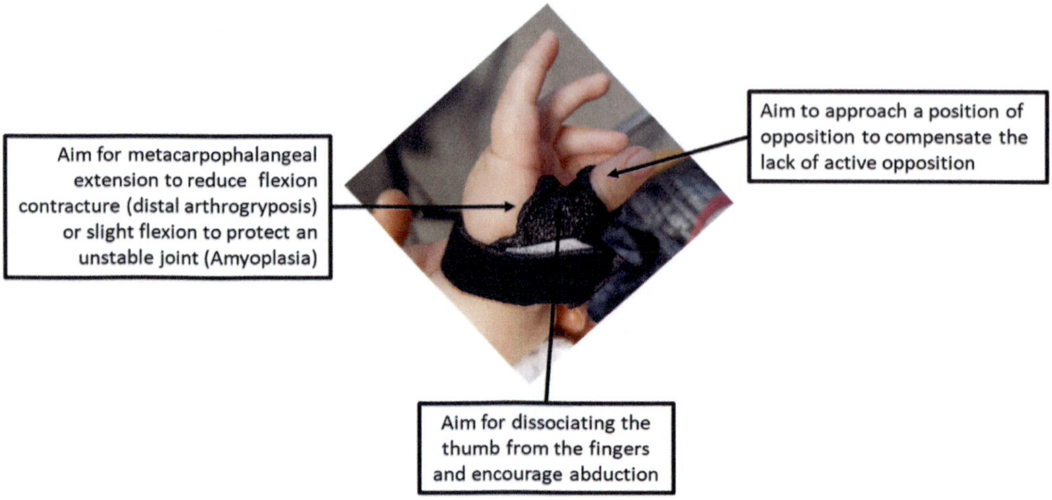

FIGURE 10.4 Use of orthosis to promote functional prehension pattern.

and caregivers guide the child through movements they cannot perform alone. For instance, some movements may be impossible against gravity but can be achievable with support. In doing so, children learn to activate specific muscle groups and create new motor pathways. This early stage of motor learning is both delicate and critical. It is a period where success depends on continuous adaptation of the child and of the care team. For example, gains in flexibility and muscle balance must be vigilantly preserved as the child grows, because bone growth introduces new challenges. As bones lengthen, the alignment between muscle groups shifts, and the risk of overstretching weak muscles becomes real. Functional improvements achieved in infancy can easily be lost without regular monitoring and maintenance. Night orthoses remain essential during this time, helping to preserve the gains made during the day and guarding against joint contractures during rest.

Over time, surgical interventions may become part of the treatment journey. These are considered not as failures of therapy but as another tool to support function. Procedures such as carpal wedge osteotomies to align the wrist or posterior elbow releases to enhance flexion are weighed carefully against the child's current capabilities and future goals. The aim is always to preserve or improve function, never to force conformity to a "normal" template. For children with clubfeet, a modified Ponseti method remains the gold standard, with careful attention to the duration of casting to achieve correction without compromising the knee or hip. Likewise, in cases of congenital vertical talus, a reverse Ponseti technique followed by surgical fixation is often used to reposition the navicular bone. Post-operative care may include casting and eventually orthoses such as AFOs or KAFOs to support the knees and maintain the corrected alignment. Each intervention must be tailored to the child's capacity for standing or walking, always balancing the need for mobility with the preservation of muscle and joint health. Yet, caution is just as important as intervention. For example, promoting knee flexion too aggressively in children with certain types of AMC may inadvertently result in tibial deformities like anterolateral bowing. In these cases, the well-intended use of orthotics or casts can paradoxically lead to a loss of knee extension and ultimately hinder standing or walking. This is why precision in application—particularly bending the knee according to the correct joint axis—is non-negotiable. Poor alignment can cause more harm than good, leading to stiffness, instability, or secondary deformities that compound the primary condition.

As children with AMC grow into adolescence and adulthood, their needs change, but the core principles of care remain. Orthotics, which played such a prominent role in early development, may be used less frequently in adulthood, sometimes even abandoned altogether. Yet, many adults with AMC continue to experience pain and functional challenges that could benefit from thoughtful orthotic support. Lightweight designs, including neoprene braces or supportive resting splints, can provide joint stability without restricting movement. This is especially important for adults who need to maintain independence in self-care, including the ability to put on and remove their orthoses without assistance. Customized orthopedic footwear may also be necessary, and again, the emphasis shifts toward comfort, usability, and maintaining walking efficiency without creating new physical burdens. Throughout this lifelong journey, the role of orthotics remains fundamentally about enabling participation—supporting each individual's ability to engage in daily life, develop autonomy, and adapt to their body's changing needs. Whether used to stabilize a hypermobile thumb in a child learning to use a fork, or to reduce pain in an adult working at a desk job, orthotics must always be part of a bigger picture: one that considers the full human experience of living with AMC.

Pain Management

Pain is defined by the International Association for the Study of Pain (IASP) as an unpleasant sensory and emotional experience associated with or resembling that associated with actual or potential tissue damage (Raja et al., 2020). Key principles regarding pain are provided in Figure 10.5 (Raja et al., 2020). Spencer et al. (2010) suggested pain is not an issue for children with AMC. But, in 2018, during the 3rd International Symposium on Arthrogryposis, persons with AMC and their caregivers suggested pain was a critical factor in functional independence and community participation (Sions et al., 2022). In support, Sions et al. (2022) found 71% of adolescents and 89% of adults with AMC reported mild-to-moderate pain, as evaluated with seven-day average pain intensity rating, with 50% of adolescents and 90% of adults reporting multisite pain, as evaluated with pain body diagrams (Sions et al., 2022). Nouraei et al. (2017) similarly reported that 75% of adults with AMC have regular joint and/or muscle pain. Sions et al. (2022) reported greater seven-day pain intensity, more painful locations, and worse coping were associated with reduced functional mobility among adolescents and adults with AMC. Cachecho et al. (2021) reported pain as a key factor in mental health, social relationships, and quality-of-life. Altogether, evidence suggests that individuals living with AMC should be empowered to discuss with their healthcare team their pain intensity, location, functional impact, and pain-related thoughts and behaviors, to assist with developing an individualized and effective pain management plan.

Lack of pain reporting is impacted by individuals' past experiences and culture. For example, adults with AMC may not report pain because they perceive pain as 'a normal part of life' (Peacock and Patel, 2008), given pain started in childhood. Individuals who have experienced medical provider dismissal of their pain complaints may fail to report subsequent pain complaints. Cultures may view questioning of medical providers, which is necessary for shared decision-making for effective pain management, to be disrespectful. But, because pain is a personal experience, open and honest dialogue between individuals and their healthcare team about what pain management strategies are or are not working is critical. Communication challenges help explain suboptimal pain management. Lack of pain vocabulary for

1. Pain is a personal experience to be respected.
2. Past pain experiences shape future pain perceptions.
3. Pain is subjective, but measurement can be objective.
4. Pain assessment should be multi-dimensional.

FIGURE 10.5 Key pain principles.

pain reporting can lead to under- and misdiagnosis, as well as under- and over-medicating (O'Donnell and Rosen, 2014). Increased reliance on non-verbal pain behaviors, e.g., flinching when a body part is touched, grabbing a body part (Raja et al., 2020), and caregiver reporting of behavioral changes may be necessary when someone is unable to effectively communicate their pain.

Pain may be acute, localized, and purpose driven. For example, after a fracture or an orthopedic procedure, pain may remind the individual to take it easy, allowing for tissue healing. In the early healing phase, frequent pain reporting is recommended to ensure pain complaints are adequately addressed, facilitating trust between the individual, their caregivers, and the healthcare team and reducing risks of negative long-term consequences from acute pain (Gan, 2017).

Conversely, chronic pain, which persists or recurs for longer than three months (Treede et al., 2019), may outlive its protective purpose, be difficult to localize, and fluctuate with or without known triggers. Chronic pain may persist because the underlying medical condition cannot be successfully treated or despite 'successful' management of a condition, which may be explained by the biopsychosocial complexity of chronic pain (Perrot et al., 2019). With chronic pain, multi-faceted interventions may be more effective than singular interventions, such as pain medication (e.g., acetaminophen, ibuprofen) alone (Table 10.3). Further, interventions may need to address thoughts and behaviors for effective pain management, as well as biological causes of the individual's pain (e.g., bony malalignment, tissue stretch, nerve injury). Figures 10.6 and 10.7 and Tables 10.2–10.7 indicate various pain management strategies.

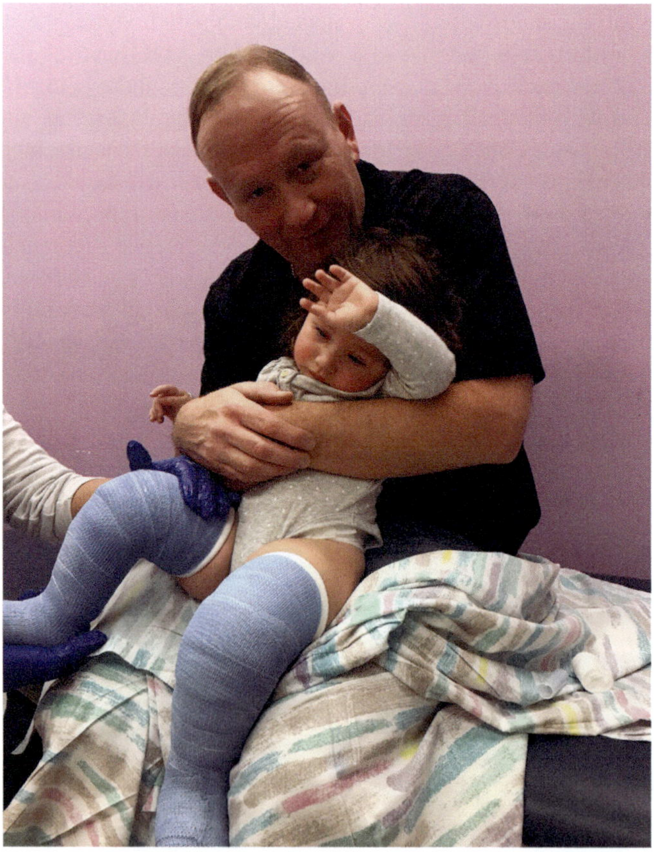

FIGURE 10.6 Post-operatively, use a combination of strategies for pain management, including pillows for supporting the body and surgical region, casts to protect the surgical site and promote tissue healing, and distraction techniques, such as watching videos or playing games on a tablet.

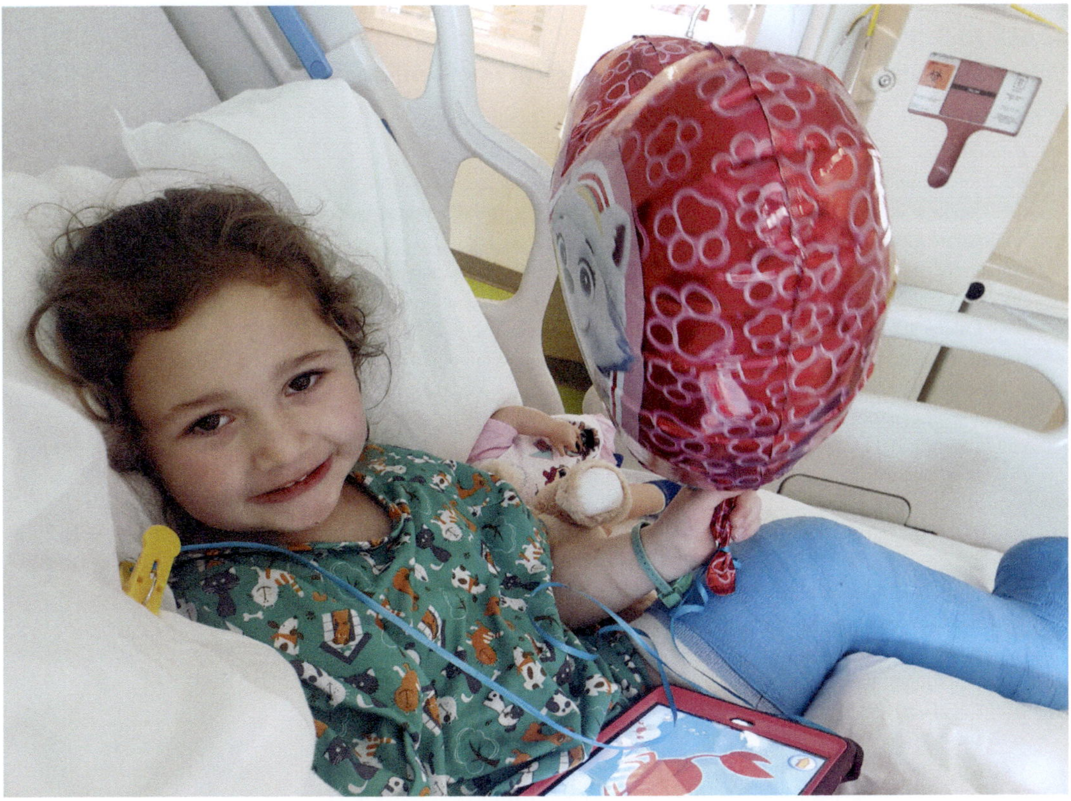

FIGURE 10.7 During uncomfortable or painful procedures, such as serial casting for clubfoot management, educate, and encourage the caregiver to hold young children.

TABLE 10.2
Pain Management Strategies—Understand Pain, Recovery Trajectories, and Mitigate Distress

In General	Acute Pain	Chronic Pain
• Structured education on the concept of pain and pain management strategies (Dahan-Oliel et al., 2025) • When possible, select providers with shorter medical appointment wait times (Liddy et al., 2017)	• Minimize the number of painful procedures performed in newborns (Committee on Fetus and Newborn and Section on Anesthesiology and Pain Medicine 2016) • Establish a pain management plan with the medical team before procedures (Frizzell et al., 2017) • Preoperatively, plan for post-operative social support • Seek out child-friendly medical environments (Chumpitazi et al., 2022) • 'Medical play' (Chumpitazi et al., 2022) • Avoid restraining children for medical procedures (Friedrichsdorf and Goubert, 2020) • Ask the medical team questions regarding what to expect post-operatively, including medication needs, length of stay, and realistic goals for pain control (Chou et al., 2016)	• Getting back to prior activities (e.g., daily school attendance, social life, recreational activities) (Friedrichsdorf and Goubert, 2020) • Optimistic expectation of improvement (Beasley et al., 2017) • Sufficient sleep (Afolalu et al., 2018; Valrie et al., 2013) • For adults: Oregan Pain Guidance modules (https://www.oregonpainguidance.org/paineducationtoolkit/)

TABLE 10.3
Pain Management Strategies—Pharmacological Interventions

In General	Acute Pain	Chronic Pain
• Consult your medical providers prior to starting any new medication to ensure it is safe and appropriate given comorbidities, concurrent medications, and allergies (Chou et al., 2016) • Avoid medication as the sole pain management strategy • Medication type should match the type of pain experienced, (Schug and Stannard, 2011) • With new medication use, promptly report any suspected side effects to your medical provider • Caregivers of children should receive education on pain assessment and appropriate administration of pain medications (Chou et al., 2016) • Patients and caregivers should receive education on tapering medications from the medical team	• In infants and children, topical agents can be effective for local pain control, e.g., blood draws, stitches (Chumpitazi et al., 2022; Hall and Anand, 2014) • Children: over-the-counter pain medications (e.g., acetaminophen, ibuprofen) can be used for mild-to-moderate pain and in conjunction with other strategies for moderate to severe pain (Trottier et al., 2022) • Hospitalized children ≥6 years old and adults with adequate cognitive function and post-operative pain may benefit from patient-controlled analgesia (PCA) for pain medication delivery • Advocate for acute pain assessment and immediate management. • Surgical, site-specific pain mitigating techniques (Chou et al., 2016) • Acetaminophen, non-steroidal anti-inflammatories, and Gabapentinoids as post-operative pain management options (Chou et al., 2016) • Access to pain specialists (Chou et al., 2016)	• Medications that may be prescribed include acetaminophen, non-steroidal anti-inflammatories, antidepressants, Gabapentinoids, skeletal muscle relaxants, benzodiazepines, opioids, and topical agents (e.g., lidocaine) (American Society of Anesthesiologists Task Force on Chronic Pain, 2010)

THERAPEUTIC EDUCATION PROGRAM: THE FRENCH EXPERIENCE

Individuals living with rare diseases like AMC often encounter significant health disparities, including limited access to accurate information, specialist care, and community resources. These barriers can be especially daunting in early life when families are overwhelmed with navigating complex medical systems while also learning how to manage daily challenges. Therapeutic

TABLE 10.4
Pain Management Strategies—Thermal, Electrical Stimulation, and Vibration

In General	Acute Pain	Chronic Pain
• Cold therapy (e.g., ice pack applied for 10–20 minutes) (Malanga et al., 2015) • Heat therapy (e.g., heat wrap applied for 15–20 minutes) (Malanga et al., 2015; Trubalski et al., 2025) • Children: vibration devices (Chumpitazi et al., 2022; Merino-Lobato et al., 2023) • Adults : Transcutaneous electrical stimulation (TENS) (Johnson et al., 2022)	• Cold therapy (Chou et al., 2016) • TENS helps reduce acute post-operative medication use (Bjordal et al., 2003)	• Heat therapy may be preferred over cold therapy for chronic pain self-management, but this is a personal preference

TABLE 10.5
Pain Management Strategies—Positioning and Supportive Devices

In General	Acute Pain	Chronic Pain
• Pillows (Figure 10.6), supportive orthotics, wheelchairs, and orthoses (braces) may help to support the body and limbs in optimal positions • Clinicians may offer low-profile, external support options, like athletic taping, in conjunction with other pain management techniques	• Immobilization with casts (Figure 10.6), or orthoses • Use of a removable orthosis • Use limb elevation • Newborns: skin-to-skin contact with a caregiver and facilitated tucking (i.e., gently placing in fetal position) (Hall and Anand, 2014) • Educate caregivers of infants and children in holding techniques (Figure 10.7) (Sri Rahyanti et al., 2017)	• Find a variety of comfortable positions, both upright and while lying down • When sitting for prolonged periods, consider a mobile seat cushion that allows a little bit of wiggle. Ensure feet are supported to minimize back stress. • For individuals who do not routinely wear orthoses (braces), temporary use may provide external support, reducing pain associated with muscle overuse or prolonged tissue stress

Education Programs (TEPs) have emerged as a powerful tool to address these gaps—offering structured, evidence-based approaches to foster awareness, build knowledge, and promote long-term self-management. In France, TEPs are regulated by regional health authorities and require health professionals and expert patients to undergo specific training and certification before implementing these programs. The focus is not just on delivering information but on empowering individuals and families to become active participants in their own care.

People with AMC typically begin intensive rehabilitation and orthopedic interventions from birth, meaning families are introduced to hands-on, daily management very early in their journey. Recognizing that medical interventions alone are not sufficient, the team in Grenoble developed a targeted TEP for people with AMC that addresses not only physical needs but also the psychological, social, and educational aspects of living with the condition. The development of this program was not straightforward—it began with a thorough needs assessment involving children, adults, and

TABLE 10.6
Pain Management Strategies—Energy Conservation, Physical Activity, and Movement

In General	Acute Pain	Chronic Pain
• Consult healthcare team prior to starting a new physical activity program (Bull et al., 2020) • Assistive devices for self-care (Cachecho et al., 2024) • Embrace the mindset of "it is okay to ask for help" and "supportive devices mitigate pain" • Consider aquatic (i.e., pool-based) exercise • Therapist-generated home stretching program • Mind-body exercise, e.g., yoga (Brown et al., 2017; Majeed et al., 2018)	• Work with your medical provider to determine guidelines for exercising in the presence of pain (e.g., number of repetitions, maximum pain level). • Range-of-motion and strengthening exercises after tissue healing post-acute injury (e.g. fracture)	• Avoid the 'Boom-and-Bust' cycle of activity, where one pushes beyond their limitations (i.e., Boom) and then has an extended period of recovery (i.e., Bust) (Andrews et al., 2012) • Use activity pacing as a pain management strategy, incorporating planned periods of rest and activity (e.g., exercise) with the goal of maintaining or increasing engagement in activities (Barakou et al., 2023) • Consider alternative mobility (e.g., wheelchair, scooter) for longer distances to allow participation in preferred activities

TABLE 10.7
Pain Management Strategies—Distraction and Mental Strategies

In General	Acute Pain	Chronic Pain
• Guided imagery, relaxation and breathing techniques, listening to music, watching videos (Figure 10.6), participating in interactive games or activities, and singing (American Academy of Pediatrics, 2001; Chumpitazi et al., 2022; Hartling et al., 2013) • Progressive muscle relaxation (i.e., purposeful tension of muscles followed by conscious deliberate release of muscle tension) (Conrad and Roth, 2007; Muhammad Khir et al., 2024; Rainforth et al., 2007) • Mitigating caregiver anxiety, distress, and unnecessary overly protective behaviors (Law et al., 2019)	• Infants: massage, breastfeeding, and non-nutritive sucking (Hall and Anand, 2014) • Virtual reality (Huang et al., 2022; Mallari et al., 2019) • Focus on the positive aspects of medical procedures (e.g., walking better) • Follow painful procedures with something pleasant to reduce pain perception and pain memories • Being offered choices regarding preferred coping style (Rokke and Lall, 1992)	• Use 'Temptation Bundling', i.e., do a preferred activity while doing a non-preferred activity • Supportive psychotherapy, group therapy or counseling, peer-to-peer support, relaxation training, cognitive behavioral therapy, biofeedback, and graded motor imagery (American Society of Anesthesiologists, 2010; Dahan-Oliel et al., 2025; Elekanachi et al., 2024; Ramsey et al., 2017)

their families to understand their real-world challenges. This collaborative inquiry revealed several recurring themes: limited access to medical knowledge about AMC, difficulty managing chronic pain and fatigue, the psychological toll of living with a visible condition, and anxieties about aging with AMC. These insights shaped the creation of tailored workshops, specifically adapted for different age groups—from infants and toddlers to adolescents and adults—each designed to support participants at their respective life stages (Table 10.8).

The workshops reflect the lived realities of AMC and promote hands-on learning and dialogue. For children, topics such as "How to move my body" and "I sleep with my splints" are approached in age-appropriate, engaging formats. Adolescents and adults explore more complex issues, including managing fatigue, navigating the emotional landscape of illness, and preparing for the future. A notable strength of the TEP structure is the time and space it creates for open discussion—something not always feasible in busy clinical appointments. In a group setting, participants can speak openly, share strategies, and validate one another's experiences. This atmosphere of shared learning fosters not only knowledge acquisition but also emotional growth and community building. As one parent expressed after attending a session for toddlers, "It did me a lot of good to see that we are not alone." Another participant, a young girl with AMC, appreciated how the complexity of the condition was presented in a way she could understand: "It was informative and clear." And for an adult with distal arthrogryposis, the experience provided both education

TABLE 10.8
Examples of Topics Covered in Therapeutic Education Programs

Children	Adults
How to speak about my arthrogryposis	How to talk about my arthrogryposis
How to move my body	Pain
I sleep with my splints	Fatigue
With proper positioning and aids, I do things on my own.	Aging

and emotional uplift: "I learned more about my illness. I met new people, and it boosted my spirits." These testimonials highlight how TEPs go beyond the delivery of medical facts to foster a sense of belonging, normalize the challenges of living with AMC, and support the development of lifelong self-advocacy skills. By offering a structured space where knowledge meets empathy, TEPs enable participants to define and pursue their own health goals. Whether it's learning how to communicate about their condition, building practical routines, or understanding how to manage future changes related to aging, individuals are equipped to navigate their health journeys with greater confidence.

While therapeutic education programs focus on structured learning led by professionals, support groups offer a complementary dimension of care through peer connection. Both serve critical roles, yet they differ in focus and format. TEPs are designed to build concrete self-management skills through targeted instruction and workshops rooted in best clinical practices. Support groups, on the other hand, center around the emotional strength of shared lived experience. They offer a safe space where individuals and families can connect informally, exchange stories, and draw mutual encouragement. The Grenoble team recognized that these approaches are not mutually exclusive but rather mutually reinforcing. When used together, TEPs and support groups create a holistic framework that addresses both the intellectual and emotional needs of individuals with AMC. Therapeutic education provides the "how" of managing life with a rare condition, while peer support affirms the "why," reminding individuals they are not alone on this journey. Similar to TEPs, support groups also play valuable roles in supporting individuals with chronic illnesses, but they differ in focus and structure. TEPs are designed to enhance patients' self-management skills through structured, evidence-based education led by healthcare professionals. In contrast, support groups emphasize the power of shared experiences, offering a space where individuals can connect, share personal stories, and provide mutual encouragement. Importantly, both approaches complement each other: management education equips patients with the tools to take control of their health, while shared experiences in a group setting reinforce emotional resilience and a sense of community.

AMC SUPPORT GROUPS

For individuals with AMC and their families, navigating the complexities of a rare congenital condition can feel isolating and overwhelming particularly in the absence of visible, everyday support systems. In this context, AMC support groups (Table 10.9) play an invaluable role. They serve as a bridge between clinical care and lived experience, addressing both the emotional and practical challenges of living with AMC across the lifespan (Steen et al., 2017). These groups are more than just social networks; they are communities of shared understanding, practical knowledge, and mutual empowerment. Their websites often serve as rich repositories of information offering up-to-date educational resources on AMC management, as well as practical guidance on living with the condition. Beyond digital platforms, support groups create opportunities for connection through in-person conferences, regional gatherings, and virtual meet-ups, allowing individuals and families to form meaningful relationships with others who share similar journeys.

One of the most profound contributions of AMC support groups is the emotional and psychological support they provide. Whether a family is facing a new diagnosis or confronting ongoing life challenges, support groups offer a safe space where individuals of all ages can connect, share, and feel seen. This sense of belonging can be transformative. For many families, especially in the early stages after diagnosis, the emotional burden can include grief, anxiety, fear, and frustration. Meeting others who have walked the same path offers comfort and validation. Shared experiences help normalize feelings and offer perspective, making it easier to cope with the psychological demands of the condition (Elekanachi et al., 2024). As individuals and families exchange their stories, they discover coping strategies to manage stress, navigate setbacks, and celebrate milestones such as a child learning to feed themselves or an adult advocating for workplace accommodations (Dahan-Oliel et al., 2025).

TABLE 10.9
List of AMC Support Groups and Organizations

Support Group	Country	Website	Social Media
Interessengemeinschaft Arthrogryposis (IGA) e.V	Austria Germany Switzerland	https://arthrogryposis.de	www.facebook.com/arthrogryposis.de
Fundación AMC Colombia	Colombia		www.facebook.com/fundacionamccolombia www.youtube.com/@fundacionamccolombia8183
Landsforeningen for arm/bendefekte og AMC	Denmark	www.arm-bendefekte-amc.dk	https://www.facebook.com/groups/120965148828/
European Alliance for Arthrogryposis	Europe	www.arthrogryposis-alliance.eu	
Alliance Arthrogrypose	France	www.arthrogrypose.fr	www.facebook.com/Alliance.Arthrogrypose/
The Arthrogryposis Association of Ireland	Ireland	www.arthrogryposis.ie	https://www.facebook.com/groups/274462052571245/
Fundación Mexicana de Artrogriposis	Mexico		www.facebook.com/fundacionamcmx/ www.instagram.com/fundacionamcmx/
Spierziekten Nederland	Netherland	www.spierziekten.nl/overzicht/arthrogryposis-multiplex-congenita	https://www.facebook.com/Spierziekten-Nederland-107697852587742 http://www.youtube.com/user/spierziekten
The Arthrogryposis Group of New Zealand	New Zealand	https://tangz.org.nz	https://www.facebook.com/groups/160498894062982/
AMC-Foreningen	Norway	www.amc-foreningen.no/Foreningen/	https://facebook.com/amcforeningen https://instagram.com/amc.foreningen/
Asociación Artrogriposis Múltiple Congénita España	Spain	https://artrogriposis.org	www.facebook.com/ArtrogriposisEspana/ www.instagram.com/artrogriposis.espana/ https://www.youtube.com/@artrogriposisespana
AMC-föreningen i Sverige	Sweden	https:// amcforeningen.se	https://www.facebook.com/groups/281357121940797/ www.instagram.com/amcforeningen/
The Arthrogryposis Group (TAG)	United Kingdom	https://arthrogryposis.co.uk	https://www.facebook.com/arthrogryposis.co.uk https://www.instagram.com/the_arthrogryposis_group_uk/
AMC Support, Inc. (AMCSI)	United States	https://amcsupport.org	https://www.facebook.com/AMCSUPPORT/ https://www.instagram.com/amcsupport/

In addition to emotional support, AMC support groups provide a valuable platform for information exchange. They offer not just medical facts but also lived knowledge including strategies that families and individuals have developed through trial, error, and adaptation. This may include tips for improving participation in daily activities like dressing, feeding, or using assistive technology, as well as creative solutions for increasing mobility or participating in leisure activities. Shared strategies for managing symptoms such as fatigue, chronic pain, or limited range of motion also help individuals optimize their function in daily life. These insights often extend far beyond what is discussed in a clinical setting and serve as a powerful form of peer education that is practical, personalized, and deeply relatable.

Support groups also play a crucial role in helping families navigate complex healthcare systems. Their collective knowledge of specialist centers, clinicians experienced in AMC, and rehabilitation services across regions make them an essential resource for locating and accessing high-quality care. They can also assist in identifying available funding opportunities, both public and private, for medical treatment, equipment, or home modifications. These supports can be especially critical when insurance coverage is limited or absent. Many support groups employ or work closely with specialized social workers who help guide families through bureaucratic systems. This may include help with applications for disability recognition, government grants, or mobility aids, as well as assistance with housing and vehicle adaptations. Some organizations even broker collaboration agreements with external partners, offering access to legal advisors, psychologists, in-home therapy providers, and adapted sport or recreation centers. In doing so, they become a hub that connects families to a multidisciplinary ecosystem of support services designed to promote independence and quality of life.

Another key function of support groups is empowerment, particularly in fostering self-advocacy. By witnessing how others overcome challenges and assert their rights, individuals with AMC are encouraged to take ownership of their health and their lives. Over time, the confidence and resilience gained through peer support can translate into self-directed action: setting personal goals, seeking out resources, and standing up for their needs in school, the workplace, and healthcare settings. This process is especially vital during transitional periods, such as adolescence to adulthood, when individuals are learning to advocate for themselves in more independent roles. The guidance offered by support groups can make these transitions more manageable and less intimidating, equipping individuals with the language, strategies, and community backing needed to navigate them successfully. Ultimately, AMC support groups serve as a lifelong companion to individuals and families—supporting not only their immediate needs but also their long-term development and resilience. By addressing the emotional, practical, and systemic challenges associated with AMC, these groups help people build meaningful lives filled with connection, purpose, and self-determination. In the continuum of care for AMC, support groups are not ancillary—they are essential, anchoring individuals within a broader community of support and advocacy that evolves with them at every stage of life.

CONCLUSION

Self-management is a critical component of care for individuals with AMC, not only as a general life skill but as an essential strategy for navigating the condition across the lifespan. The complexity and evolving needs associated with AMC require a dynamic and individualized approach to rehabilitation, which remains a constant yet adaptable support system from infancy through adulthood. Rehabilitation professionals are uniquely positioned to foster self-management by equipping individuals and families with the knowledge, skills, and confidence needed to manage daily challenges and promote long-term well-being. Importantly, the role of peers and community support, particularly through AMC-specific support groups, cannot be understated. These networks offer emotional, informational, and practical support that reinforces professional interventions and empowers individuals to take an active role in their care. Together, these elements underscore the value of a collaborative, lifespan-oriented approach to self-management and rehabilitation in AMC.

ACKNOWLEDGMENTS

We acknowledge the contribution of caregivers, partners and persons with AMC in sharing excerpts reflecting self-management through their lens. We also acknowledge the expertise of the various international multidisciplinary teams who contributed their invaluable experiences to shape the knowledge shared in this chapter.

Dr. Dahan-Oliel is supported by a clinical research scholar award from the Fonds de recherche du Québec (#329833, 2024-2027).

REFERENCES

Abrahams, N., Gilson, L., Levitt, N.S. and Dave, J.A. (2019) 'Factors that influence patient empowerment in inpatient chronic care: Early thoughts on a diabetes care intervention in South Africa', *BMC Endocrine Disorders*, 19(1), p. 133. doi:10.1186/s12902-019-0465-1.

Afolalu, E.F., Ramlee, F. and Tang, N.K.Y. (2018) 'Effects of sleep changes on pain-related health outcomes in the general population: A systematic review of longitudinal studies with exploratory meta-analysis', *Sleep Medicine Reviews*, 39, pp. 82–97. doi:10.1016/j.smrv.2017.08.001.

Aitchison, B., Rushton, A., Martin, P., Barr, M., Soundy, A. and Heneghan, N. (2022) 'The experiences and perceived health benefits of individuals with a disability participating in sport: A systematic review and narrative analysis', *Disability and Health Journal*, 15(1). doi:10.1016/j.dhjo.2021.101164.

Almasri, N.A., An, M. and Palisano, R.J. (2018) 'Parents' perception of receiving family-centered care for their children with physical disabilities: A meta-analysis', *Physical & Occupational Therapy in Pediatrics*, 38(4), pp. 427–443. doi:10.1080/01942638.2017.1337664.

Altiok, H., Flanagan, A., Krzak, J.J. and Hassani, S. (2019) 'Quality of life, satisfaction with life, and functional mobility of young adults with arthrogryposis after leaving pediatric care', *American Journal of Medical Genetics Part C: Seminars in Medical Genetics*, 181(3), pp. 461–468. doi:10.1002/ajmg.c.31717.

American Academy of Pediatrics, Committee on Psychosocial Aspects of Child and Family Health and Task Force on Pain in Infants, Children, and Adolescents. (2001) 'The assessment and management of acute pain in infants, children, and adolescents', *Pediatrics*, 108(3), pp. 793–797. doi:10.1542/peds.108.3.793.

American Society of Anesthesiologists Task Force on Chronic Pain Management and American Society of Regional Anesthesia and Pain Medicine. (2010) 'Practice guidelines for chronic pain management: An updated report', *Anesthesiology*, 112(4), pp. 810–833. doi:10.1097/ALN.0b013e3181c43103.

Amor, C.J., Spaeth, M.C., Chafey, D.H. and Gogola, G.R. (2011) 'Use of the pediatric outcomes data collection instrument to evaluate functional outcomes in arthrogryposis', *Journal of Pediatric Orthopaedics*, 31(3), pp. 293–296. doi:10.1097/BPO.0b013e31820cad93.

Anderson, P. and Kitchin, R. (2000) 'Disability, space and sexuality: Access to family planning services', *Social Science & Medicine*, 51(8), pp. 1163–1173. doi:10.1016/S0277-9536(00)00019-8.

Andrews, N.E., Strong, J. and Meredith, P.J. (2012) 'Activity pacing, avoidance, endurance, and associations with patient functioning in chronic pain: A systematic review and meta-analysis', *Archives of Physical Medicine and Rehabilitation*, 93(11), pp. 2109–2121.e7. doi:10.1016/j.apmr.2012.05.029.

Arduç, A., De Vries, J.I.P., Tan-Sindhunata, M.B., Waisfisz, Q., Pajkrt, E. and Linskens, I.H. (2025). Perinatal genetic diagnostic yield in a population of fetuses with the phenotype arthrogryposis multiplex congenita: A cohort study 2007-2021. *European Journal of Human Genetics*. Advance online publication. doi:10.1038/s41431-025-01848-3.

Arthrogryposis Multiplex Congenita Support, Inc. (n.d.) *Occupational Therapy*. Available at: https://amcsupport.org/occupational-therapy/ (Accessed: 30 July 2025).

Barakou, I., et al. (2023) 'Self-regulation of effort for a better health-related quality of life: A multidimensional activity pacing model for chronic pain and fatigue management', *Annals of Medicine*, 55(2), p. 2270688. doi:10.1080/07853890.2023.2270688.

Beasley, M.J., Ferguson-Jones, E.A. and Macfarlane, G.J. (2017) 'Treatment expectations but not preference affect outcome in a trial of CBT and exercise for pain', *Canadian Journal of Pain*, 1(1), pp. 161–170. doi:10.1080/24740527.2017.1384297.

Binkiewicz-Glinska, A., Sobierajska-Rek, A., Bakula, S., Wierzba, J., Drewek, K., Kowalski, I.M. and Zaborowska-Sapeta, K. (2013) 'Arthrogryposis in infancy, multidisciplinary approach: Case report', *BMC Pediatrics*, 13, p. 184. doi:10.1186/1471-2431-13-184.

Bjordal, J.M., Johnson, M.I. and Ljunggreen, A.E. (2003) 'Transcutaneous electrical nerve stimulation (TENS) can reduce postoperative analgesic consumption: A meta-analysis with assessment of optimal treatment parameters for postoperative pain', *European Journal of Pain*, 7(2), pp. 181–188. doi:10.1016/S1090-3801(02)00098-8.

Bowen, R.L. and Atwood, C.S. (2004) 'Living and dying for sex: A theory of aging based on the modulation of cell cycle signaling by reproductive hormones', *Gerontology*, 50(5), pp. 265–290. doi:10.1159/000079125.

Brown, M.L., Rojas, E. and Gouda, S. (2017) 'A mind-body approach to pediatric pain management', *Children (Basel)*, 4(6), p. 50. doi:10.3390/children4060050.

Bull, F.C., et al. (2020) 'World Health Organization 2020 guidelines on physical activity and sedentary behaviour', *British Journal of Sports Medicine*, 54(24), pp. 1451–1462. doi:10.1136/bjsports-2020-102955.

Cachecho, S., Boruff, J., Wong, T., Lacombe, F. and Dahan-Oliel, N. (2021) 'Psychosocial wellbeing among children and adults with arthrogryposis: A scoping review', *Health and Quality of Life Outcomes*, 19(1), p. 263. doi:10.1186/s12955-021-01896-5.

Cachecho, S., Fąfara, A., Lacombe, F., Bussières, A. and Dahan-Oliel, N. (2024) 'Current rehabilitation practice for the evaluation and treatment of children with arthrogryposis: An international survey', *Disability and Rehabilitation*, 46(1), pp. 96–104. doi:10.1080/09638288.2022.2161644.

Carrier, J.I., Siedlikowski, M., Chougui, K., Plourde, S.A., Mercier, C., Thevasagayam, G., Lafrance, M., Wong, T., Bilodeau, C., Michalovic, A., Thorstad, K., Rauch, F. and Tsimicalis, A. (2018) 'A best practice initiative to optimize transfer of young adults with osteogenesis imperfecta from child to adult healthcare services', *Clinical Nurse Specialist*, 32(6), pp. 323–335. doi:10.1097/NUR.0000000000000407

Chou, R., Gordon, D.B., de Leon-Casasola, O.A., Rosenberg, J.M., Bickler, S., Brennan, T., Carter, T., Cassidy, C.L., Chittenden, E.H., Degenhardt, E., Griffith, S., Manworren, R., McCarberg, B., Montgomery, R., Murphy, J., Perkal, M.F., Suresh, S., Sluka, K., Strassels, S. and Thirlby, R. (2016) 'Management of postoperative pain: A clinical practice guideline from the American Pain Society, the American Society of Regional Anesthesia and Pain Medicine, and the American Society of Anesthesiologists' Committee on Regional Anesthesia, Executive Committee, and Administrative Council', *Journal of Pain*, 17(2), pp. 131–157.

Chumpitazi, C.E., Chang, C. and Atanelov, Z. (2022) 'Managing acute pain in children presenting to the emergency department without opioids', *JACEP Open*, 3(2), p. e12664. doi:10.1002/emp2.12664.

Cirillo, A., Collins, J., Sawatzky, B., Hamdy, R. and Dahan-Oliel, N. (2019) 'Pain among children and adults living with arthrogryposis multiplex congenita: A scoping review', *American Journal of Medical Genetics Part C: Seminars in Medical Genetics*, 181(3), pp. 436–453. doi:10.1002/ajmg.c.31725.

Colver, A., Rapley, T., Parr, J., McConachie, H., Davey-Pearce, G., Le Couteur, A., McDonagh, J., Bennett, C., Maniatopoulos, G., Pearce, M., Reape, D., Chater, N., Gleeson, H. and Vale, L. (2020) 'Facilitating transition of young people with long-term health conditions from children's to adults' healthcare services—implications of a 5-year research programme', *Clinical Medicine*, 20(1), pp. 4–80.

Committee on Fetus and Newborn and Section on Anesthesiology and Pain Medicine. (2016) 'Prevention And management of procedural pain in the neonate: An update', *Pediatrics*, 137(2), p. e20154271. doi:10.1542/peds.2015-4271.

Conrad, A. and Roth, W.T. (2007) 'Muscle relaxation therapy for anxiety disorders: It works but how?', *Journal of Anxiety Disorders*, 21(3), pp. 243–264. doi:10.1016/j.janxdis.2006.08.001.

Dahan-Oliel, N., Cachecho, S., Araujo, C., Fąfara, A., Lacombe, F., Samargian, A., Costa, C., Donohoe, M., Flanagan, A., Kowalczyk, B., Krakie, C., Wagner, L., Navalón, C., Pacey, V., Steen, U., Walker, M., Wong, T. and Bussières, A. (2025) 'Consensus-based recommendations for the rehabilitation of children with arthrogryposis multiplex congenita: An integrated knowledge translation approach', *Orphanet Journal of Rare Diseases*, 20(1), p. 168. doi:10.1186/s13023-025-03671-x.

Dahan-Oliel, N., Cachecho, S., Barnes, D., Bedard, T., Davison, A.M., Dieterich, K., Hall, J.G., et al. (2019) 'International multidisciplinary collaboration toward an annotated definition of arthrogryposis multiplex congenita', *American Journal of Medical Genetics Part C: Seminars in Medical Genetics*, 181(3), pp. 288–299.

Dahan-Oliel, N., van Bosse, H.J.P., Bedard, T., Darsaklis, V.B., Hall, J.G. and Hamdy, R.C. (2019) 'Research platform for children with arthrogryposis multiplex congenita: Findings from the pilot registry', *American Journal of Medical Genetics Part C: Seminars in Medical Genetics*, 181(3), pp. 427–435. doi:10.1002/ajmg.c.31724.

Dai, S., Dieterich, K., Jaeger, M., Wuyam, B., Jouk, P.S. and Perennou, D. (2018) 'Disability in adults with arthrogryposis is severe, partly invisible, and varies by genotype', *Neurology*, 90(18), pp. e1596–e1604. doi:10.1212/wnl.0000000000005418.

Dieterich, K., Le Tanno, P., Kimber, E., Jouk, P.S., Hall, J. and Giampietro, P. (2019) 'The diagnostic workup in a patient with AMC: Overview of the clinical evaluation and paraclinical analyses with review of the literature', *American Journal of Medical Genetics Part C: Seminars in Medical Genetics*, 181(3), pp. 337–344. doi:10.1002/ajmg.c.31730.

Ding, J.Y., Cleary, S.L. and Morgan, P.E. (2024) 'Health literacy in adolescents and young adults with cerebral palsy: A mixed methods systematic review', *Disability and Rehabilitation*, 46(24), pp. 5717–5729. doi:10.1080/09638288.2024.2311879.

Elekanachi, R.U., Lajoie, A., Tavukcu, S., Snider, L.M. and Dahan-Oliel, N. (2024) 'The experience of caregiving for children with rare musculoskeletal conditions: A qualitative study in arthrogryposis multiplex congenita', *Orphanet Journal of Rare Diseases*, 19(1), p. 235. doi:10.1186/s13023-024-03224-8.

Elfassy, C., Darsaklis, V.B., Snider, L., Gagnon, C., Hamdy, R. and Dahan-Oliel, N. (2020) 'Rehabilitation needs of youth with arthrogryposis multiplex congenita: Perspectives from key stakeholders', *Disability and Rehabilitation*, 42(16), pp. 2318–2324. doi:10.1080/09638288.2018.1559364.

Elfassy, C., Wagner, L., Higgins, J., Montpetit, K., Snider, L. and Dahan-Oliel, N. (2023) 'Stakeholder engagement in the development of an upper extremity outcome measure for children with rare musculoskeletal conditions', *Research Involvement and Engagement*, 9(1), p. 64. doi:10.1186/s40900-023-00479-6.

Friedrichsdorf, S.J. and Goubert, L. (2020) 'Pediatric pain treatment and prevention for hospitalized children', *Pain Reports*, 5(1), p. e804. doi:10.1097/PR9.0000000000000804.

Frizzell, K.H., Cavanaugh, P.K. and Herman, M.J. (2017) 'Pediatric perioperative pain management', *Orthopedic Clinics of North America*, 48(4), pp. 467–480. doi:10.1016/j.ocl.2017.06.007.

Gagnon, M., Collins, J., Elfassy, C., Merlo, G.M., Marsh, J., Sawatzky, B. and Dahan-Oliel, N. (2020) 'A telerehabilitation intervention for youths with arthrogryposis multiplex congenita: Protocol for a pilot study', *JMIR Research Protocols*, 9(6), p. e18688.

Gagnon, M., Marino Merlo, G., Yap, R., Collins, J., Elfassy, C., Sawatzky, B., Marsh, J., Hamdy, R., Veilleux, L.N. and Dahan-Oliel, N. (2021) 'Using telerehabilitation to deliver a home exercise program to youth with arthrogryposis: Single cohort pilot study', *Journal of Medical Internet Research*, 23(7), p. e27064. doi:10.2196/27064.

Gan, T.J. (2017) 'Poorly controlled postoperative pain: Prevalence, consequences, and prevention', *Journal of Pain Research*, 10, pp. 2287–2298. doi:10.2147/JPR.S144066.

Ganle, J., Baatiema, K., Quansah, L. and Danso-Appiah, R. (2020) 'Barriers facing persons with disability in accessing sexual and reproductive health services in sub-Saharan Africa: A systematic review', *PLoS One*, 15(10), p. e0238585. doi:10.1371/journal.pone.0238585.

Gibson, W., Gourdin, D. and Krouse, H. (2015) 'Asthma self-management goals, beliefs and behaviors of urban African American adolescents prior to transitioning to adult health care', *Journal of Pediatric Nursing*, 30(6), pp. 53–61. doi:10.1016/j.pedn.2015.06.012.

Gray, S.H., Byrne, R., Christensen, S., Williams, D., Wylie, M., Fowler, E., Gaebler-Spira, D., Marciniak, C. and Glader, L. (2021) 'Women with cerebral palsy: A qualitative study about their experiences with sexual and reproductive health education and services', *Journal of Pediatric Rehabilitation Medicine*, 14(2), pp. 285–293. doi:10.3233/PRM-210020.

Hall, R.W. and Anand, K.J.S. (2014) 'Pain management in newborns', *Clinics in Perinatology*, 41(4), pp. 895–924. doi:10.1016/j.clp.2014.08.010.

Hansen-Jaumard, D., Elfassy, C., Montpetit, K., Ghalimah, B., Hamdy, R. and Dahan-Oliel, N. (2020) 'A review of the orthopedic interventions and functional outcomes among a cohort of 114 children with arthrogryposis multiplex congenita', *Journal of Pediatric Rehabilitation Medicine*, 13(3), pp. 263–271. doi:10.3233/PRM-190657.

Hartling, L., Shaik, M.S., Tjosvold, L., Leicht, R., Liang, Y., Kumar, M. and Klassen, T.P. (2013) 'Music to reduce pain and distress in the pediatric emergency department: A randomized clinical trial', *JAMA Pediatrics*, 167(9), pp. 826–835. doi:10.1001/jamapediatrics.2013.200.

Huang, Q., Li, X., Wang, X., Zhu, M., Chen, J., He, L., Zhang, J. and Zhou, Y. (2022) 'Using virtual reality exposure therapy in pain management: A systematic review and meta-analysis of randomized controlled trials', *Value in Health*, 25(2), pp. 288–301. doi:10.1016/j.jval.2021.04.1285.

Hyer, L.C., Carson, L.T., Carpenter, A.M. and Westberry, D.E. (2021) 'Patient-reported outcome measurement information system (PROMIS) scores in pediatric patients with arthrogryposis', *Journal of Pediatric Orthopaedics*, 41(9), pp. e727–e732. doi:10.1097/BPO.0000000000001933.

Johnson, M.I., et al. (2022) 'Efficacy and safety of transcutaneous electrical nerve stimulation (TENS) for acute and chronic pain in adults: A systematic review and meta-analysis of 381 studies (the meta-TENS study)', *BMJ Open*, 12(2), p. e051073. doi:10.1136/bmjopen-2021-051073.

Jones, C.M.P., Swadron, S.P., Babineau, J., McCabe, T., Bhandari, M. and Guyatt, G.H. (2024) 'Opioids for acute musculoskeletal pain: A systematic review with meta-analysis', *Drugs*, 84(3), pp. 305–317. doi:10.1007/s40265-024-01999-5.

Kowalczyk, B. and Feluś, J. (2016) 'Arthrogryposis: An update on clinical aspects, etiology, And treatment strategies', *Archives of Medical Science*, 12(1), pp. 10–24. doi: 10.5114/aoms.2016.57578

Kristoffersson, U. and Johansson-Soller, M. (2024) 'Pregnancy planning and genetic testing: Exploring advantages, and challenges', *Genes (Basel)*, 15(9), p. 1205. doi:10.3390/genes15091205.

Law, E., et al. (2019) 'Psychological interventions for parents of children and adolescents with chronic illness', *Cochrane Database of Systematic Reviews*, 3(6), p. CD009660. doi:10.1002/14651858.CD009660.pub4.

Liddy, C., et al. (2017) 'Patient perspectives on wait times and the impact on their life: A waiting room survey in a chronic pain clinic', *Scandinavian Journal of Pain*, 17(1), pp. 53–57. doi:10.1016/j.sjpain.2017.07.015.

Lowry, R.B., Sibbald, B., Bedard, T. and Hall, J.G. (2010) 'Prevalence of multiple congenital contractures including arthrogryposis multiplex congenita in Alberta, Canada, and a strategy for classification and coding', *Birth Defects Research Part A: Clinical and Molecular Teratology*, 88(12), pp. 1057–1061. doi:10.1002/bdra.20738.

Majeed, M.H., Ali, A.A. and Sudak, D.M. (2018) 'Mindfulness-based interventions for chronic pain: Evidence and applications', *Asian Journal of Psychiatry*, 32, pp. 79–83. doi:10.1016/j.ajp.2017.11.025.

Malanga, G.A., Yan, N. and Stark, J. (2015) 'Mechanisms and efficacy of heat and cold therapies for musculoskeletal injury', *Postgraduate Medicine*, 127(1), pp. 57–65. doi:10.1080/00325481.2015.992719.

Mallari, B., et al. (2019) 'Virtual reality as an analgesic for acute and chronic pain in adults: A systematic review and meta-analysis', *Journal of Pain Research*, 12, pp. 2053–2085. doi:10.2147/JPR.S200498.

Merino-Lobato, C., et al. (2023) 'Virtual reality vs. Buzzy®. Efficacy in pain and anxiety management during pediatric venipuncture. Systematic review and meta-analysis', *Journal of Pediatric Nursing*, 73, pp. 22–33. doi:10.1016/j.pedn.2023.08.014.

Michalovic, A., Anderson, C., Thorstad, K., Rauch, F. and Tsimicalis, A. (2020) 'Exploring the perceived self-management needs of young adults with osteogenesis imperfecta', *Clinical Nurse Specialist*, 34(3), pp. 99–106. doi:10.1097/NUR.0000000000000517.

Modi, A.C., Pai, A.L., Hommel, K.A., Hood, K.K., Cortina, S., Hilliard, M.E., Guilfoyle, S.M., Gray, W.N. and Drotar, D. (2012) 'Pediatric self-management: A framework for research, practice, and policy', *Pediatrics*, 129(2), pp. e473–e485. doi:10.1542/peds.2011-1635.

Muhammad Khir, S., et al. (2024) 'Efficacy of progressive muscle relaxation in adults for stress, anxiety, and depression: A systematic review', *Psychology Research and Behavior Management*, 17, pp. 345–365. doi:10.2147/PRBM.S437277.

Nouraei, H., Sawatzky, B., MacGillivray, M. and Hall, J. (2017) 'Long-term functional and mobility outcomes for individuals with arthrogryposis multiplex congenita', *American Journal of Medical Genetics Part A*, 173(5), pp. 1270–1278.

O'Donnell, F.T. and Rosen, K.R. (2014) 'Pediatric pain management: A review', *Mo Med*, 111(3), pp. 231–237.

Odling, M., Jonsson, M., Janson, C., Melén, E., Bergstrom, A. and Kull, I. (2020) 'Lost in transition from pediatric to adult healthcare? Experiences of young adults with severe asthma', *Journal of Asthma*, 57(10), pp. 1119–1127.

Peacock, S. and Patel, S. (2008) 'Cultural influences on pain', *Reviews in Pain*, 1(2), pp. 6–9. doi:10.1177/204946370800100203.

Perrot, S., Cohen, M., Barke, A., Korwisi, B., Rief, W. and Treede, R.D. (2019) 'The IASP classification of chronic pain for ICD-11: Chronic secondary musculoskeletal pain', *Pain*, 160(1), pp. 77–82. doi:10.1097/j.pain.0000000000001389.

Rainforth, M.V., et al. (2007) 'Stress reduction programs in patients with elevated blood pressure: A systematic review and meta-analysis', *Current Hypertension Reports*, 9(6), pp. 520–528. doi:10.1007/s11906-007-0094-3.

Raja, S.N., Carr, D.B., Cohen, M., Finnerup, N.B., Flor, H., Gibson, S., Keefe, F.J., Mogil, J.S., Ringkamp, M., Sluka, K.A., Song, X.J., Stevens, B., Sullivan, M.D., Tutelman, P.R., Ushida, T. and Vader, K. (2020) 'The revised international association for the study of pain definition of pain: Concepts, challenges, and compromises', *Pain*, 161(9), pp. 1976–1982. doi:10.1097/j.pain.0000000000001939

Ramsey, L.H., Karlson, C.W. and Collier, A.B. (2017) 'Mirror therapy for phantom limb pain in a 7-year-old male with osteosarcoma', *Journal of Pain and Symptom Management*, 53(6), pp. e5–e7. doi:10.1016/j.jpainsymman.2017.02.003.

Riemer, G. and Steen, U. (2013) 'Amyoplasia: A case report of an old woman', *Disability and Rehabilitation*, 35(11), pp. 950–958. doi:10.3109/09638288.2012.717577.

Rokke, P.D. and Lall, R. (1992) 'The role of choice in enhancing tolerance to acute pain', *Cognitive Therapy and Research*, 16(1), pp. 53–65. doi:10.1007/bf01172956.

Romand, X., Gastaldi, R., Pérennou, D., Baillet, A. and Dieterich, K. (2024) 'Bone mineral density in adults with arthrogryposis multiplex congenita: A retrospective cohort analysis', *Scientific Reports*, 14(1), p. 8206. doi:10.1038/s41598-024-58083-x.

Rowen, T., Stein, S. and Tepper, S. (2015) 'Sexual health care for people with physical disabilities', *The Journal of Sexual Medicine*, 12(3), pp. 584–589. doi:10.1111/jsm.12810.

Sadler, E., Wolfe, C.D. and McKevitt, C. (2014) 'Lay and health care professional understandings of self-management: A systematic review and narrative synthesis', *SAGE Open Medicine*, 2, p. 2050312114544493. doi:10.1177/2050312114544493.

Schug, S.A. and Stannard, K. (2011) *Mechanisms of vascular disease: A reference book for vascular specialists*. Adelaide: University of Adelaide Press.

Shephard, R.J. (1991) 'Benefits of sport and physical activity for the disabled: Implications for the individual and for society', *Scandinavian Journal of Rehabilitation Medicine*, 23(2), pp. 51–59. https://pubmed.ncbi.nlm.nih.gov/1832786/

Sions, J.M., Donohoe, M., Beisheim-Ryan, E.H., Pohlig, R.T., Shank, T.M. and Nichols, L.R. (2022) 'Characterizing pain among adolescents and young adults with arthrogryposis multiplex congenita', *Pediatric Physical Therapy*, 34(3), pp. 288–295. doi:10.1097/PEP.0000000000000913.

Song, H., Dennis, S., Levesque, J. and Harris, M. (2020) 'What do consumers with chronic conditions expect from their interactions with general practitioners? A qualitative study of Australian consumer and provider perspectives', *Health Expectations*, 23(3), 707–716.

Spencer, H.T., Bowen, R.E., Caputo, K., Green, T.A. and Lawrence, J.F. (2010) 'Bone mineral density and functional measures in patients with arthrogryposis', *Journal of Pediatric Orthopedics*, 30(5), pp. 514–518. doi:10.1097/BPO.0b013e3181df6185.

Sri Rahyanti, N.M., Nurhaeni, N. and Wanda, D. (2017) 'Could a certain sitting position reduce the pain experienced by a child? The benefits of parental holding and an upright position', *Comprehensive Child and Adolescent Nursing*, 40(supl), pp. 8–13. doi:10.1080/24694193.2017.1386965.

Steen, U., Christensen, E. and Samargian, A. (2017) 'Adults living with amyoplasia: Function, psychosocial aspects, and the benefit of AMC support groups', *Journal of Pediatric Orthopedics*, 37(Suppl 1), pp. S31–S32. doi:10.1097/BPO.0000000000001003.

Treede, R.D., Rief, W., Barke, A., Aziz, Q., Bennett, M.I., Benoliel, R., Cohen, M., Evers, S., Finnerup, N.B., First, M.B., Giamberardino, M.A., Kaasa, S., Korwisi, B., Kosek, E., Lavand'homme, P., Nicholas, M., Perrot, S., Scholz, J., Schug, S., Smith, B.H., Svensson, P., Vlaeyen, J.W.S. and Wang, S.J. (2019) 'Chronic pain as a symptom or a disease: The IASP classification of chronic pain for the International Classification of Diseases (ICD-11)', *Pain*, 160(1), pp. 19–27. doi:10.1097/j.pain.0000000000001384.

Trottier, E.D., Ali, S., Bhatt, M., Cheng, A., Gravel, J., Harrison, D., Joubert, G., Lemyre, B., Paes, B. and Yaskina, M. (2022) 'Best practices in pain assessment and management for children', *Paediatrics & Child Health*, 27(7), pp. 429–448. doi:10.1093/pch/pxac048

Trubalski, M., Nowak, J., Zieliński, T., Kowalczyk, A. and Majewska, K. (2025) 'Harnessing the heat: A comprehensive review of heat therapy's role in managing lumbar pain', *Wiadomosci Lekarskie*, 78(3), pp. 615–620. doi:10.36740/WLek/202481.

Valrie, C.R., Gil, K.M., Redding-Lallinger, R. and Daeschner, C.W. (2013) 'A systematic review of sleep in pediatric pain populations', *Journal of Developmental & Behavioral Pediatrics*, 34(2), pp. 120–128. doi:10.1097/DBP.0b013e31827d5848.

Wagner, L.V., Cherry, J.S., Sawatzky, B.J., Fąfara, A., Elfassy, C., Eriksson, M., Montpetit, K., Bucci, T. and Donohoe, M. (2019) 'Rehabilitation across the lifespan for individuals with arthrogryposis', *American Journal of Medical Genetics Part C: Seminars in Medical Genetics*, 181(3), pp. 385–392. doi:10.1002/ajmg.c.31729.

Wallis, C. (2007) 'Transition of care in children with chronic disease', *British Medical Journal*, 334(7606), pp. 1231–1232. doi:10.1136/bmj.39232.425197.BE.

Wan, H., Carey, K., D'Silva, A., Kasparian, N. and Farrar, M. (2019) 'Getting ready for the adult world": How adults with spinal muscular atrophy perceive and experience healthcare, transition and well-being', *Orphanet Journal of Rare Diseases*, 14(74), pp. 1–13. doi:10.1186/s13023-019-1052-2.

11 From Service Encounters to Simulation and Knowledge Translation

Pathways to Self-Management in Aphasia

Emna Fakhfakh and Carole Anglade

INTRODUCTION

Aphasia is an acquired language disorder most commonly caused by stroke, though it may also arise from traumatic brain injury, tumours, or progressive neurological diseases (Chapey, 2008). It affects the ability to produce and comprehend spoken and written language, while leaving intelligence and memory intact. Epidemiological estimates suggest that approximately one third of stroke survivors will experience some form of aphasia in the acute phase (Engelter et al., 2006), and that between one fifth and one quarter live with chronic aphasia years after onset (Plowman et al., 2012). In Canada alone, tens of thousands of individuals are currently living with aphasia (Heart and Stroke Foundation of Canada, 2017). Beyond its prevalence, aphasia is significant because of its persistence: recovery is often partial, and many individuals must adapt to long-term changes in communication.

The consequences of aphasia extend far beyond language impairment. Studies consistently show reduced quality of life, increased social isolation, and elevated risk of depression among people with aphasia (Cruice et al., 2003; Hilari & Byng, 2009; Northcott et al., 2016a). Many report difficulties maintaining employment, managing finances, or sustaining relationships. Aphasia alters not only communication but also self-concept and identity (Shadden, 2005). Partners and families are deeply affected, as communication challenges can disrupt roles and relationships (Pound et al., 2018).

Participation restrictions are particularly visible in community interactions. Everyday activities such as ordering food in a café, purchasing groceries, or managing administrative tasks may become daunting (Dalemans et al., 2008; Worrall et al., 2007). These activities allow individuals to live independently, to enact social roles, and to feel integrated into their communities (Dalemans et al., 2008, 2010a; Northcott et al., 2016b). When participation is restricted, autonomy and wellbeing suffer. The World Health Organization's International Classification of Functioning, Disability and Health (ICF) provides a useful framework for understanding this dynamic, emphasising that disability is the result of interactions between impairments, activities, participation, and environmental factors (WHO, 2011). Aphasia exemplifies this model: while the impairment is linguistic, the impact is most visible in activities and participation, and the environment can either mitigate or exacerbate difficulties.

Over the past decades, rehabilitation has increasingly recognised that successful intervention must address participation as well as impairment (Kagan et al., 2008; Simmons-Mackie, 2001). Speech–language pathologists traditionally focused on linguistic recovery, but contemporary approaches integrate functional communication, social participation, and quality of life as central

DOI: 10.1201/9781003599074-12

outcomes (Chapey et al., 2000; Kagan & Simmons-Mackie, 2007). This shift aligns with broader movements in rehabilitation towards patient-centred care and empowerment. Within this evolution, the concept of self-management has gained prominence (Jones et al., 2013; Kendall et al., 2007). Originating in the context of chronic conditions such as diabetes or arthritis (Barlow et al., 2002), self-management refers to the ability of individuals to take an active role in managing symptoms, treatment, lifestyle changes, and the psychological and social consequences of illness. Self-management programmes typically include skill development, problem-solving, decision-making, and the use of resources.

Applied to aphasia, self-management involves more than learning language strategies. It encompasses the ways in which people adapt to communication challenges in daily life, how they maintain participation despite barriers, and how they make informed decisions about rehabilitation and social engagement. Yet, despite its relevance, self-management in aphasia remains underexplored in both research and clinical practice. Speech–language pathologists themselves have emphasised that supporting self-management "has to be the way of the future" for aphasia rehabilitation, even if current approaches and service structures are not yet fully aligned with this vision (Nichol et al., 2023). One reason may be that language difficulties obscure the forms of competence that people display. Another is that traditional rehabilitation models often frame autonomy in terms of linguistic ability alone.

For people with aphasia, however, self-management can happen in subtle but powerful ways. While traditional therapy may focus on structured exercises within the clinic, much of the patients' activities occur outside, in the everyday encounters where communication, environment, and identity intersect. Some people with aphasia can navigate grocery stores, cafés, and service counters by mobilising gestures, pointing, facial expressions, and contextual cues (Anglade et al., 2019, 2021). These micro-interactions are seldom documented in clinical trials, yet they are critical to everyday autonomy.

This chapter draws on more than ten years of qualitative and participatory research to highlight the lived expertise of people with aphasia in managing community service encounters. This line of work began with the doctoral studies of the second author, who in 2015 initiated for her doctoral thesis the recruitment of people living with chronic aphasia in order to explore how they managed their condition in everyday interactions outside the home. Building on this foundation, we begin by presenting empirical findings that document how individuals with moderate-to-severe aphasia accomplish transactions despite linguistic limitations, and how these successful experiences contribute to confidence and independence. We then describe how these insights informed the development of immersive simulation technologies designed to recreate service encounters in rehabilitation settings, offering opportunities for graded, feedback-rich practice that prepares individuals for real-life situations. Finally, we turn to the ethical dimension of knowledge translation, exploring how access to information in aphasia-friendly formats is itself a condition for autonomy and informed choice.

By integrating empirical evidence, technological innovation, and knowledge translation, the chapter contributes to current discussions of self-management in rehabilitation. It argues that the everyday competencies displayed by people with aphasia in navigating service encounters constitute a form of self-management that is often unrecognised in clinical discourse. Supporting these competencies—through accessible environments, realistic training tools, and equitable access to information—offers a practical and grounded approach to rehabilitation that values autonomy and participation.

EMPIRICAL FINDINGS: LIVED EXPERTISE IN SERVICE ENCOUNTERS

Understanding how people with aphasia manage everyday service encounters requires close attention to the details of interaction. These are moments where independence and communication intersect in ways that are highly consequential for daily life. Buying food, paying bills, or ordering a coffee are not trivial routines; they are among the practical activities that define autonomy and participation. Yet, for people with aphasia, these interactions can be challenging precisely because they involve fast-paced exchanges, unfamiliar interlocutors, and the need for verbal precision. Our research programme sought to capture what happens in these moments, not in simulated role-plays, but in the ordinary venues where people shop, order, and ask for services.

Methodological Approach

The first set of studies was conducted in Montréal, Canada, with six adults living with moderate-to-severe post-stroke aphasia (Anglade et al., 2019). These studies formed part of the second author's doctoral research, carried out under the supervision of Professors Croteau and Le Dorze. Recruitment criteria were deliberately inclusive: participants varied in severity, years post-onset, and prior community engagement. What united them was the willingness to carry out everyday errands while being observed. Rather than imposing artificial tasks, participants selected venues that were meaningful in their own routines: a neighbourhood grocery store, a café they frequented, or a municipal counter. Interactions were video-recorded, with ethical approval and the consent of both participants and clerks.

The methodological choice to focus on naturally occurring interactions was important. Role-play or structured tasks can simplify the complexity of everyday life, whereas real interactions capture the contingencies that matter: background noise, waiting customers, unexpected questions, or clerks who had never met the person before. Using the lens of conversation analysis (CA), we examined how exchanges were organised turn by turn, focusing not only on speech but also on gestures, gaze, body orientation, and the use of environmental resources.

In total, twenty interactions were recorded and transcribed. The second study analysed 59 request sequences across these encounters that displayed formulation difficulty (Anglade et al., 2021). This analysis shed light on how multimodal resources were deployed, and how clerks responded. Both studies shared the same orientation: to document competence-in-interaction, rather than deficit.

Structure of Service Encounters

A robust finding across settings was that transactions followed a stable four-phase structure: readiness, item, price, and closure. Across these phases, people with aphasia combined speech, gesture, and environmental cues to initiate interactions, identify desired items, negotiate payment, and bring transactions to a close. While difficulties were most visible in item identification and price understanding, mutual understanding was usually achieved through the use of multimodal resources and the collaboration of clerks.

Multimodality and Competence-In-Interaction

The second study examined 59 request sequences produced by people with aphasia during service encounters, focusing on those that displayed formulation difficulties (Anglade et al., 2021). Rather than treating these moments as communicative breakdowns, the analysis considered them as opportunities to observe how interactional competence was enacted. People with aphasia did not abandon their efforts when speech was insufficient; instead, they mobilised additional resources. These included gestures, gaze direction, body positioning, and the use of contextual cues available in the environment.

Equally important was the active role of clerks. In many sequences, clerks responded to incomplete or ambiguous requests by offering candidate understandings, sometimes repeating or reformulating, other times pointing to possible items.

The outcome across all cases was that requests were ultimately understood. This finding highlights that communicative success in service encounters does not depend solely on fluent verbal production or linguistic abilities. It is achieved through the dynamic alignment of multimodal strategies deployed by the person with aphasia and the responsive behaviours of the clerk. In this sense, self-management in aphasia can be seen not as an individual act alone but as a collaborative process distributed across interlocutors and their shared environment.

Links to International Research and Theory

These findings resonate with a body of work emphasising that people with aphasia communicate better than they speak (Goodwin, 2004; Kagan, 1998). The notion of "competence despite impairment" challenges deficit models and supports the idea of resilience and adaptation. Research by Dalemans and colleagues on participation also highlights the role of environment and social support in enabling everyday activities (Dalemans et al., 2008, 2010b). Our studies add empirical detail to these frameworks by showing how micro-level strategies combine with structural features such as price displays to shape autonomy.

The analysis also aligns with the World Health Organization's International Classification of Functioning (ICF), which conceptualises disability as the interaction between impairment, activity, and participation, mediated by environmental and personal factors (WHO, 2011). Service encounters provide a microcosm where these dimensions intersect. They illustrate that successful participation cannot be reduced to impairment scores but must be understood in relation to environment and interaction.

Implications for Rehabilitation

From a rehabilitation perspective, these empirical findings suggest that therapy should go beyond language recovery to include interactional competence and environmental adaptation. Rather than rehearsing isolated scripts, clinicians can help patients explore the main phases of transactions and encourage the use of multimodal resources—speech, gesture, writing, or technology. Confidence-building is key: experiencing successful transactions, even with difficulty, reinforces the belief that participation is possible. Rehabilitation can also extend its scope by collaborating with businesses to promote communication-friendly practices, such as clear price displays or pictorial menus.

Ultimately, these empirical studies show that self-management in aphasia is already happening. People with aphasia are not waiting passively for recovery; they are managing their lives every time they buy bread, order coffee, or pay for services. Their lived expertise deserves recognition and integration into rehabilitation models.

TECHNOLOGICAL INNOVATION: IMMERSIVE SIMULATION AS A BRIDGE BETWEEN CLINIC AND COMMUNITY

Preparing people with aphasia for participation in everyday encounters poses a major challenge for rehabilitation. Clinics are controlled environments: predictable, safe, and relatively quiet. Community interactions are the opposite: noisy, unpredictable, and often fast-paced. Traditional methods of preparing patients, such as rehearsing dialogues or engaging in role-play with a clinician, provide important opportunities for practice but fail to capture these contingencies. A patient might practise the phrase "I would like a coffee, please" in therapy, only to be confronted in real life with a clerk who speaks quickly, who offers unexpected choices, or who asks an unrelated question. The difficulty is not only linguistic but situational. It is precisely this gap between clinical rehearsal and everyday reality that motivated the development of immersive simulation.

The initial idea for such a project came from Eve Nadeau, a speech–language pathologist with more than 20 years of experience in rehabilitation with people living with aphasia, who experienced such a gap in her daily clinical practice. Building on her insight, our team sought to design environments where people with aphasia could safely practise the kinds of interactions they encounter every day, while still being exposed to the contingencies that make those encounters challenging. Virtual reality (VR) offered a promising medium. Unlike printed scripts or tabletop exercises, VR could recreate spatial orientation, body positioning, background noise, and the presence of other customers. It could also allow the repetition of scenarios under varied conditions, enabling users to test strategies multiple times. Importantly, such immersive environments also hold potential for better generalisation of therapy gains to everyday life, by more closely approximating the ecological and interactional demands of real-world encounters, although empirical evidence for this generalisation remains limited in stroke or aphasia rehabilitation (Laver et al., 2017; Marshall et al., 2018). Recent work in other domains similarly suggests that immersive and customisable VR scenarios can support metacognitive reflection and the transfer of skills into daily practice, provided that environments are realistic and meaningful (Hansa & Hansen, 2025; Lowell & Tagare, 2023). The design process was explicitly collaborative, inspired by Design Thinking (Altman et al., 2018). Rather than beginning with ready-made prototypes, our first step was to work with people with aphasia and clinicians to identify what a future simulation should address. We conducted individual interviews with five people living with aphasia and four speech–language pathologists to gather their views on everyday interactions—particularly service encounters—and to better understand both the obstacles they encountered and the facilitators that supported successful participation. Building on these interviews, participants were then invited to join two mixed focus groups, each bringing together people with aphasia and clinicians. Across two sessions per group, participants discussed the challenges they faced and the goals they wanted to achieve, and they worked together to outline the foundations of two possible simulations that could support these objectives in the future. The analysis of the interviews and focus groups was carried out in collaboration with graduate students Esther Kagayano and Emna Fakhfakh (first author), whose contributions were central to identifying themes and structuring the findings.

In this way, the simulation project began not with technology but with the lived experiences of those most affected. The discussions generated ideas for scenarios that could one day replicate the structure of real service encounters and provide opportunities for practice. Grocery stores, restaurants, and specialised shops were frequently mentioned as priorities, since they are central to daily autonomy. These settings were consistently described in terms that aligned with the four-phase sequence identified in our empirical studies: readiness, item selection, price understanding, and closure.

Although the virtual prototypes are still in development, the principles of design are already emerging from this participatory groundwork. Participants stressed the need for scenarios that do not simply present static choices but guide users through the sequential structure of real encounters. They imagined situations where the environment would include background noise or waiting customers, and where clerks could respond in different ways—sometimes welcoming, sometimes showing impatience—thus reflecting the variability of community life. These discussions provided the blueprint for scenarios that, once developed, could allow people with aphasia to practise under controlled variation, repeating interactions with different challenges, and learning how to manage breakdowns without the social pressure of a real queue.

This co-design process itself reflects a philosophy of self-management, already endorsed by others with people living with aphasia (Kulnik et al., 2019). By identifying the goals that matter to them, articulating the barriers they face, and envisioning the kinds of support they would find useful, people with aphasia positioned themselves not as passive recipients of rehabilitation but as active agents shaping the conditions of their participation. Future simulations, grounded in their lived experience, are intended not to prescribe fixed strategies but to provide flexible spaces where users can trial, adapt, and evaluate approaches for themselves. In this sense, the participatory groundwork is not only a step toward new technology but also an illustration of self-management in action: people with aphasia taking the lead in defining how rehabilitation can better support their everyday autonomy.

KNOWLEDGE TRANSLATION: ACCESS TO INFORMATION AS AUTONOMY

Self-management in rehabilitation requires not only the capacity to use strategies in daily life but also the ability to make informed decisions. This second dimension presupposes access to relevant information in a form that can be understood and discussed by the person concerned. In aphasia, this requirement is rarely met. Research findings are typically communicated in technical language, through academic journals or professional training, which are inaccessible to most people with language impairments. Without adapted knowledge translation (KT), people with aphasia remain dependent on clinicians to mediate information for them, limiting their opportunities to participate actively in choices about rehabilitation and everyday life.

The Mots-Croisés project was designed to address this gap. The initiative originated with the Quebec Association of People with Aphasia (AQPA), which in 2022 was marking its 40th anniversary. The association approached two researchers to collaborate on a series of events that would bring research findings directly to people with aphasia and their families. The project was co-led by AQPA and these researchers, with Professor Anna Zumbansen (University of Ottawa) serving as principal investigator, alongside the last author of this chapter. The guiding principle was that people with aphasia are not only participants in research but also its rightful addressees. If rehabilitation is to foster self-management, then evidence must be made available in formats that allow people to interrogate, interpret, and apply it themselves.

Methodological approach

The series consisted of eight conferences held during 2022, all in French, the main language used by the aphasic members at AQPA. Each presentation was pre-recorded on video, with the researcher speaking directly to the camera. Subtitles were added to every video, ensuring that participants could rely on written support alongside the spoken message. To maximise accessibility, videos were made available online two weeks before each event, allowing participants to watch them at their own pace, to stop and replay sections, or to view them with family members. This preparation stage was crucial: it meant that people came to the live event already familiar with the content and ready to engage in discussion.

The events themselves were held in AQPA's Montréal facilities, which were fully accessible and already familiar to members. Each session followed the same format. First, the pre-recorded video was projected for the group. Immediately afterwards, the presenting researcher was available in person for a live question period. Finally, the event concluded with a shared meal, providing an informal setting for further exchanges between participants, families, and researchers.

The content of the presentations was prepared in close collaboration with AQPA staff. Slides were simplified, technical vocabulary was avoided, and pictograms and images were used to reinforce key points. The pace of delivery was intentionally slowed, and each video was structured around a small number of main ideas rather than dense argumentation. In this way, accessibility was embedded in the design, rather than added afterwards.

Participation and Engagement

Attendance was strong. Across the first four events, 274 people participated, including 89 individuals living with aphasia. Family members, researchers and volunteers comprised the remainder. The composition of the audience reflected AQPA's community base: people with chronic aphasia of varying severity, attending with spouses or relatives, and accustomed to the association's activities.

Participation during the question periods was a notable outcome. To our surprise, 44% of all questions came directly from people with aphasia themselves. This proportion is significant, as it suggests that the adapted format did more than make the content comprehensible: it created conditions for people with aphasia to intervene as active participants. The questions were varied. Some sought clarification about the research methods or findings. Some participants used the space to share personal experiences that resonated with the evidence presented, while others contributed in creative ways, including composing short poems that captured their reflections.

This high rate of participation challenges assumptions that people with aphasia are unlikely to engage with research directly. It demonstrates that, given accessible formats and supportive contexts, they not only understand the material but also take an interest in debating and contextualising it. The presence of families added another dimension: spouses often asked questions about implications for their own roles, and discussions between relatives and people with aphasia continued during the informal meals.

In one of the *Mots-Croisés* sessions, a participant asked a question about bilingualism and aphasia. What began as a request for clarification developed into a substantive exchange with the presenting researcher. The discussion led to an invitation for the participant to contribute as a patient-partner in the researcher's university teaching, sharing his experience and perspectives on bilingualism with future speech–language pathologists. This outcome illustrates another dimension of self-management: accessible knowledge does not only enable people with aphasia to make informed choices for themselves, it can also create opportunities for them to take on new roles as contributors of knowledge. By positioning their lived expertise as a resource for education and professional training, initiatives like *Mots-Croisés* extend self-management beyond the individual to participation in shaping the rehabilitation field itself.

Implications for Self-Management

The *Mots-Croisés* project highlights several mechanisms by which knowledge translation supports self-management. First, access to research in an aphasia-friendly format enables people with aphasia to act as informed partners in their own rehabilitation. They can evaluate whether findings are relevant, raise questions with clinicians, and decide whether to try new strategies. Second, the opportunity to ask questions publicly positions people with aphasia as legitimate consumers of evidence. This role is not symbolic; it alters the dynamics of rehabilitation by validating that their perspective matters. Third, family members, by attending and engaging with the material, are better equipped to support joint decision-making in everyday life.

From an analytic standpoint, the project also demonstrates the feasibility of adapting dissemination without major resources. The key features—pre-recorded subtitled videos, simplified slides, slower pace, and allocated discussion time—were achievable within the means of a community association and a small team of researchers. The result was a format that facilitated genuine engagement.

The role of AQPA was critical. As initiator and co-organiser, the association ensured that the topics addressed corresponded to the concerns of members. It also provided the trusted environment in which participation could flourish. This underlines that KT for self-management is not only a technical question of format but also a relational process, dependent on collaboration between researchers and community organisations.

CONCLUSIONS, IMPLICATIONS AND FUTURE DIRECTIONS

Taken together, the empirical studies, the immersive simulation project, and the knowledge translation initiative presented in this chapter demonstrate that self-management in aphasia is not simply a matter of practising language exercises. It emerges at the intersection of individual strategies, supportive environments, and accessible information.

From a clinical perspective, one of the most direct implications is the need to integrate everyday service encounters into therapy. Speech–language pathologists can use the four-phase structure identified in our studies as a practical framework. By rehearsing readiness, item selection, price understanding, and closure, therapy can target not only linguistic forms but also the sequential organisation of interaction. For instance, a clinician might practise greeting behaviours that establish readiness, encourage patients to experiment with gestures during item requests, or simulate price statement when no visual display is available. These practices normalise multimodality and reduce the stigma that patients sometimes feel when relying on gesture or writing. They also allow individuals to leave therapy with strategies that map directly onto the tasks they face outside. Documenting outcomes in terms of confidence and frequency of independent transactions could complement traditional impairment measures, shifting evaluation towards participation goals.

At the level of service delivery, the findings highlight the central role of environmental accessibility. The success of transactions was strongly influenced by factors such as whether prices were displayed, whether items could be pointed to, or whether card payment was accepted. These are not linguistic variables but design features of the environment. Rehabilitation services could expand their remit to include advocacy for communication-friendly venues. Mapping local businesses that already provide accessible conditions, creating "aphasia-friendly" accreditation schemes, or offering clerk training are feasible, low-cost interventions that could have disproportionate impact. Partner training, a well-established approach in rehabilitation, could be extended to service staff, providing short modules on strategies such as waiting, offering candidate understandings, and showing items. These small adjustments align with universal design principles and benefit not only people with aphasia but also other groups with communication or cognitive difficulties. Such efforts are beginning to take shape internationally, often led by community organisations responding to the needs of their members. To see websites related to these initiatives on communication access training in the UK, Australia, the USA, and Québec, Canada, see references (Communication Access, n.d., UK; Scope, n.d.; Australia; Aphasia Access, n.d., USA; and Artère, 2022, Québec, Canada).

For research, several directions emerge. One concerns the extension of observational studies beyond shops and cafés to other public services. Transport systems, healthcare settings, and municipal offices present different challenges, often involving more complex documents, security procedures, or multi-step transactions. Go-along studies, where researchers accompany participants on their daily journeys, are particularly promising for capturing the flow of participation across environments. Such methods can reveal how barriers accumulate across a single outing, for example when difficulties in reading a bus timetable are compounded by challenges in asking for assistance at a counter. By documenting these cumulative experiences, research can better inform systemic interventions.

Doctoral work currently underway, including that of Emna Fakhfakh, is beginning to map the broader structural facilitators and barriers within community services and how to better target them in rehabilitation. These strands collectively suggest that a full understanding of participation requires attention not only to the person with aphasia but also to their networks and the institutions they engage with.

Another research avenue is the evaluation of immersive simulation. Comparative trials could assess whether practising in VR translates into measurable improvements in real-world participation compared to traditional role-play. Outcome measures might include not only linguistic performance but also the number of independent outings, self-reported confidence, and satisfaction with participation. Implementation research is also needed to determine how such technologies can be integrated into routine rehabilitation services, given constraints of cost, training, and infrastructure.

In a broader sense, these implications suggest a reframing of self-management. In conditions such as diabetes or chronic obstructive pulmonary disease, self-management is often conceptualised as the ability of individuals to monitor symptoms, adhere to medication, and adjust behaviours. In aphasia, the equivalent lies not in biological monitoring but in communicative participation: the ability to manage interactions, navigate environments, and make informed choices. This requires a distributed perspective where autonomy is understood as emerging from the alignment of personal strategies, partner behaviours, and environmental affordances. Rehabilitation that acknowledges this complexity is better equipped to support genuine participation. The conceptual model of self-management proposed by Van de Velde et al. (2019) directly supports the framework of this chapter, as it integrates person-centred attributes (active participation, responsibility, coping strategies), person–environment-oriented attributes (access to information, partnership with clinicians, social support), and synthesis attributes (medical, role, and emotional management). Our reflection does not aim to broaden this model, but rather to illustrate and operationalise it in the field of aphasia. In this context, certain attributes take on a particular meaning: coping strategies include the multimodal management of interactions in varied communicative environments, while access to information requires linguistic and visual adaptations that enable autonomous understanding. Aphasia thus emerges as a privileged ground for showing how self-management is concretely embodied in daily life, in articulation with the individual, their environment, and their social network.

In summary, the future of self-management in aphasia rehabilitation lies in integrating interactional competence into therapy, promoting environmental accessibility through community partnerships, and embedding accessible knowledge dissemination into research and practice. These steps will ensure that people with aphasia are not merely recipients of care but active managers of their participation in everyday life.

REFERENCES

Altman, M., Huang, T. T., & Breland, J. Y. (2018). Design thinking in health care. *Preventing Chronic Disease, 15*, E117.

Anglade, C., Le Dorze, G., & Croteau, C. (2019). Service encounter interactions of people living with moderate-to-severe post-stroke aphasia in their community. *Aphasiology, 33*(9), 1061–1082. https://doi.org/10.1080/02687038.2018.1532068

Anglade, C., Le Dorze, G., & Croteau, C. (2021). How clerks understand the requests of people living with aphasia in service encounters. *Clinical Linguistics & Phonetics, 35*(1), 84–99.

Aphasia Access. (n.d.). Communication Access. *Aphasia Access.* https://www.aphasiaaccess.org/communication-access/

Artère. (2022). Guide théorique du projet ACCES – Accessibilité communicationnelle des commerces de proximité. *Université Laval.* https://acces.atemi.dev/wp-content/uploads/2022/11/Guide-theorique.pdf

Barlow, J., Wright, C., Sheasby, J., Turner, A., & Hainsworth, J. (2002). Self-management approaches for people with chronic conditions: A review. *Patient Education and Counseling, 48*(2), 177–187.

Chapey, R. (Ed.). (2008). *Language Intervention Strategies in Aphasia and Related Neurogenic Communication Disorders* (5th ed.). Lippincott Williams & Wilkins.

Chapey, R., Duchan, J. F., Elman, R. J., Garcia, L. J., Kagan, A., Lyon, J. G., & Simmons Mackie, N. (2000). Life participation approach to aphasia: A statement of values for the future. *The ASHA Leader, 5*(3), 4–6. https://doi.org/10.1044/leader.FTR.05032000.4

Communication Access UK. (n.d.). About Communication Access UK. *Communication Access UK.* https://communication-access.co.uk/about

Cruice, M., Worrall, L., Hickson, L., & Murison, R. (2003). Finding a focus for quality of life with aphasia: Social and emotional health, and psychological well-being. *Aphasiology, 17*(4), 333–362. https://doi.org/10.1080/02687030244000707

Dalemans, R., De Witte, L., Beurskens, A., Van Den Heuvel, W., & Wade, D. (2010a). An investigation into the social participation of stroke survivors with aphasia. *Disability and Rehabilitation, 32*(20), 1678–1685. https://doi.org/10.3109/09638281003649938

Dalemans, R., De Witte, L., Wade, D., & Van den Heuvel, W. (2008). A description of social participation in working-age persons with aphasia: A review of the literature. *Aphasiology, 22*(10), 1071–1091.

Dalemans, R., De Witte, L., Wade, D., & van den Heuvel, W. (2010b). Social participation through the eyes of people with aphasia. *International Journal of Language & Communication Disorders, 45*(5), 537–550. https://doi.org/10.3109/13682820903223633

Engelter, S. T., Gostynski, M., Papa, S., Frei, M., Born, C., Ajdacic-Gross, V., Gutzwiller, F., & Lyrer, P. A. (2006). Epidemiology of aphasia attributable to first ischemic stroke: Incidence, severity, fluency, etiology, and thrombolysis. *Stroke, 37*(6), 1379–1384.

Goodwin, C. (2004). A competent speaker who can't speak: The social life of aphasia. *Journal of Linguistic Anthropology*, *14*(2), 151–170. https://doi.org/10.1525/jlin.2004.14.2.151

Hansa, J., & Hansen, H. (2026). User-centered qualitative evaluation of a fully immersive, head-mounted virtual reality application prototype to facilitate real-life transfer in voice therapy. *International Journal of Speech-Language Pathology*, *28*(2), 303–315.

Heart and Stroke Foundation of Canada. (2017). *Stroke Report*. https://www.heartandstroke.ca/-/media/pdf-files/canada/stroke-report/strokereport2017en.ashx

Hilari, K., & Byng, S. (2009). Health-related quality of life in people with severe aphasia. *International Journal of Language & Communication Disorders*, *44*(2), 193–205.

Jones, F., Livingstone, E., & Hawkes, L. (2013). Getting the balance between encouragement and taking over'—Reflections on using a new stroke self-management programme. *Physiotherapy Research International*, *18*(2), 91–99.

Kagan, A. (1998). Supported conversation for adults with aphasia: Methods and resources for training conversation partners. *Aphasiology*, *12*(9), 816–830. https://doi.org/10.1080/02687039808249575

Kagan, A., & Simmons-Mackie, N. (2007). Beginning with the end: Outcome-driven assessment and intervention with life participation in mind. *Topics in Language Disorders*, *27*(4), 309–317. https://doi.org/10.1097/01.TLD.0000299885.39488.bf

Kagan, A., Simmons-Mackie, N., Rowland, A., Huijbregts, M., Shumway, E., McEwen, S., Threats, T., & Sharp, S. (2008). Counting what counts: A framework for capturing real-life outcomes of aphasia intervention. *Aphasiology*, *22*(3), 258–280.

Kendall, E., Catalano, T., Kuipers, P., Posner, N., Buys, N., & Charker, J. (2007). Recovery following stroke: The role of self-management education. *Social Science & Medicine*, *64*(3), 735–746.

Kulnik, S. T., Pöstges, H., Townsend, R., Micklethwaite, P., & Jones, F. (2019). A gift from experience: Co-production and co-design in stroke and self-management. *Design for Health*, *3*(1), 98–118. https://doi.org/10.1080/24735132.2019.1577524

Laver, K. E., Lange, B., George, S., Deutsch, J. E., Saposnik, G., & Crotty, M. (2017). Virtual reality for stroke rehabilitation. *Cochrane Database of Systematic Reviews*, *2017*(11), CD008349. https://doi.org/10.1002/14651858.CD008349.pub4

Lowell, V. L., & Tagare, D. (2023). Authentic learning and fidelity in virtual reality learning experiences for self-efficacy and transfer. *Computers & Education: X Reality*, *2*, 100017.

Marshall, J., Devane, N., Edmonds, L., Talbot, R., Wilson, S., Woolf, C., & Zwart, N. (2018). Delivering word retrieval therapies for people with aphasia in a virtual communication environment. *Aphasiology*, *32*(9), 1054–1074. https://doi.org/10.1080/02687038.2018.1488237

Nichol, L., Rodriguez, A. D., Pitt, R., Wallace, S. J., & Hill, A. J. (2023). "Self-management has to be the way of the future": Exploring the perspectives of speech-language pathologists who work with people with aphasia. *International Journal of Speech-Language Pathology*, *25*(2), 327–341

Northcott, S., Marshall, J., & Hilari, K. (2016b). What factors predict who will have a strong social network following a stroke? *Journal of Speech, Language, and Hearing Research*, *59*(4), 772–783.

Northcott, S., Moss, B., Harrison, K., & Hilari, K. (2016a). A systematic review of the impact of stroke and aphasia on quality of life. *Aphasiology*, *30*(11), 1321–1341. https://doi.org/10.1080/02687038.2016.1182223

Plowman, E., Hentz, B., & Ellis, C. (2012). Post-stroke aphasia prognosis: A review of patient-related and stroke-related factors. *Journal of Evaluation in Clinical Practice*, *18*(3), 689–694.

Pound, C., Parr, S., Lindsay, J., & Woolf, C. (2018). *Beyond Aphasia: Therapies for Living With Communication Disability*. Routledge.

Scope. (n.d.). Communication Accessibility. *Scope Australia*. Retrieved from https://www.communication-hub.com.au/CommunicationHub/Communication_Hub/Supporting-communication/Communication_accessibility.aspx (Accessed August 31, 2025).

Shadden, B. (2005). Aphasia as identity theft: Theory and practice. *Aphasiology*, *19*(3–5), 211–223.

Simmons-Mackie, N. (2001). Social approaches to aphasia intervention. In: *Language Intervention Strategies in Aphasia and Related Neurogenic Communication Disorders* (pp. 246–268). Lippincott Williams & Wilkins.

Van de Velde, D., De Zutter, F., Satink, T., Costa, U., Janquart, S., Senn, D., & De Vriendt, P. (2019). Delineating the concept of self-management in chronic conditions: A concept analysis. *BMJ Open*, *9*(7), e027775.

WHO. (2011). *World Report on Disability*. UN World Health Organisation.

Worrall, L., Rose, T., Howe, T., McKenna, K., & Hickson, L. (2007). Developing an evidence-base for accessibility for people with aphasia. *Aphasiology*, *21*(1), 124–136.

12 Finding the Path of Self-Management in Multiple Sclerosis
From Insight to Future

Chungyi Chiu, Mojtaba Khaliji, and Md Refat Uz Zaman Sajib

MULTIPLE SCLEROSIS EPIDEMIOLOGY

Globally, 2.8 million people live with multiple sclerosis (MS), which is 30% higher than in 2013 (Khan and Hashim 2025; Marcus 2022; Walton *et al.* 2020). In the US, about one million people live with MS. Females are two to three times more likely to have MS than males (Hittle *et al.* 2023). The onset age typically ranges from 20 to 30 years, and additionally, the recent trend shows that the prevalence shifts to older ages, with a peak age of 60 (Portaccio *et al.* 2024). The racial ratio per 1,000 people is approximately 4 White (non-Hispanic), 3 Black (non-Hispanic), 2 other races, and 1.5 Hispanic/Latino (Hittle *et al.* 2023). MS is a chronic autoimmune neurodegenerative disease and a major cause of neurological disability in young adults (Portaccio *et al.* 2024). An aberrant autoimmune attack leads to neuroinflammation, which subsequently causes demyelination and axonal damage, resulting in lesions within the central nervous system. Diagnosis follows the 2017 McDonald criteria, supported by brain magnetic resonance imaging (MRI) and a lumbar puncture (spinal tap). When the brain and spinal cord are affected by MS, neural transmission is damaged, resulting in a range of neurological symptoms (Khan and Hashim 2025; Marcus 2022; Walton *et al.* 2020).

Common symptoms include eye pain, vision loss (optic neuritis), weakness in sensation in the body, balance difficulty, tingling, numbness, pain, clumsiness when walking, cognitive impairments (e.g., difficulties in concentration, multitasking, thinking, or learning, or difficulties with memory or judgment), bladder control issues, physical and/or mental fatigue, mood change, and depression and anxiety (Khan and Hashim 2025; Marcus 2022; Walton *et al.* 2020). These symptoms may occur unexpectedly and randomly (relapse), but are followed by periods of improvement (remission); this is relapsing-remitting MS. By contrast, when these symptoms worsen over time, it is progressive MS. People with relapsing-remitting MS may gradually develop secondary progressive MS (Khan and Hashim 2025; Marcus 2022; Walton *et al.* 2020). Recent evidence of progression independent of relapse activity (PIRA) considers MS a continuum progression where relapsing and progressive features variably coexist from the earliest stages of the disease (Portaccio *et al.* 2024).

MULTIPLE SCLEROSIS TREATMENT AND RECOMMENDATION

Although there is no cure for MS, several classes of disease-modifying therapies (DMT), such as interferons, glatiramer, teriflunomide, S1P receptor modulators, fumarates, cladribine, and several types of monoclonal antibodies, can decrease MS relapses by approximately 29–68% (McGinley *et al.* 2021; National Institute of Neurological Disorders and Stroke 2025). The side effects of DMT include infection, injection site reactions, low heart rate, and autoimmune thyroid disease (McGinley *et al.* 2021; National Institute of Neurological Disorders and Stroke 2025). Due to MS

DOI: 10.1201/9781003599074-13

symptoms, declining health and function can further develop comorbidities, such as hypertension, hyperlipidemia, functional cardiovascular disease, ischemic heart disease, cerebrovascular disease, and peripheral vascular disease, diabetes, autoimmune thyroid and miscellaneous autoimmune conditions, migraine, lung and skin conditions, depression, anxiety, and other psychiatric disorders (Salter *et al.* 2024). These comorbidities increase the MS activity, including relapse activity, disability worsening, or any new lesions on MRI (Salter *et al.* 2024).

Besides medical treatment, the most common recommendation from medical professionals is lifestyle modification, which effectively addresses many common MS symptoms, comorbidities, and disability progression, including less fatigue, better sleep, reduced pain, improved mood and disease management, and better information processing speed (Strober *et al.* 2018; Wills and Probst 2022). Recommended behaviors include: avoiding cigarette smoking; engaging in regular physical activity (aerobic and resistance, safety-tailored); adopting a Mediterranean-style dietary pattern (more vegetables, fruits, legumes, whole grains, nuts and seeds, olive oil, and fish; less fried foods, butter/cheese, red and processed meats, and sweets); maintaining social engagement; and pursuing cognitively stimulating activities (e.g., reading, creative writing, drawing, puzzles or music, learning a new language). Implementing these behaviors depends on effective self-management (task-specific self-efficacy, goal-setting, action planning, monitoring, and coping strategies) (Katz Sand *et al.* 2023; National Multiple Sclerosis Society 2025; Strober *et al.* 2018; Wills and Probst 2022).

A systematic review of 57 existing self-management programs, encompassing physical activity, fatigue, dietary, stress/coping, emotional, symptom, and medical management, as well as lifestyle and wellbeing programs, holds promise for managing MS and its sequelae (Wills and Probst 2022). With other systematic reviews of self-management interventions for MS, self-management can be effective to improve health, function, knowledge, adherence to treatment, and quality of life physically, psychologically, and socially (Kidd *et al.* 2017; Rae-Grant *et al.* 2011; Yamaguchi and Yatsushiro 2019). However, it is warranted that various study heterogeneities limit the overall effects, suggesting that more self-management approaches with rigorous examination are needed (Wills and Probst 2022). Additionally, due to constellations of MS co-existing symptoms, comorbidities, and disabilities, applying multicomponent, multimodal delivery of self-management approaches is recommended (Wills and Probst 2022).

Moreover, living with MS is costly, driven by treatment of MS and comorbidities, employment loss, and caregiving needs. In the United States, the average annual per-person cost is $88,487, and the total societal burden is $85.4 billion (Bebo *et al.* 2022). Of this total, direct medical costs (disease-modifying therapies, medications for comorbid conditions, hospital/outpatient care, and equipment such as canes or wheelchairs) account for $63.3 billion; indirect costs (missed work and early retirement) for $21.0 billion; and nonmedical costs (informal caregiving and home/vehicle modifications) for $1.1 billion (Bebo *et al.* 2022). Because many cost drivers are tied to symptom burden and functional limitations, lifestyle modification through self-management may offer a cost-conscious way to improve outcomes and, potentially, reduce utilization.

SELF-MANAGEMENT DEFINITION AND STRATEGIES

Researchers have defined self-management. Lorig (1993, p. 11), a leading researcher in self-management, defined self-management as "learning and practicing the skills necessary to carry on an active and emotionally satisfying life in the face of a chronic condition." Richard and Shea (2011, p. 261) explained self-management as "the ability of the individual, in conjunction with family, community, and healthcare professionals, to manage symptoms, treatments, lifestyle changes, and psychosocial, cultural, and spiritual consequences of health conditions." Engaging in self-management will help patients be active in controlling their chronic condition and reclaiming a meaningful life (Lorig 2003; Richard and Shea 2011; Thorne *et al.* 2003).

Corbin and Strauss (1988) considered self-management, including three key tasks: (1) *medical management of the condition*, such as taking medication as prescribed, adhering to a special diet, or using an inhaler; (2) *maintaining, changing, and creating new meaningful behaviors or life roles*, for example, an individual with walking difficulties who adopted an equipment to keep walking or modifying a bicycle to bike; (3) *dealing with and managing the emotional reactions* to *the impacts of living with a chronic condition*, such as frustration, anger, fear, stress, and depression. Lorig and Holman (2003) proposed five core self-management skills. *First, problem-solving skills*, these include problem definition, generation of possible solutions, such as the solicitation of suggestions from friends and healthcare professionals, solution implementation, and evaluation of results. *Second, decision-making*, patients need to have the needed knowledge (enough, valid, appropriate information) to make day-to-day decisions in responding to changes in symptoms or health conditions. *Third, finding and utilizing resources*, it is important to be aware that many patients receive pamphlets of resources, but they do not know how to use them. Furthermore, it is essential to find multiple resources simultaneously for optimal results. *Fourth, forming active partnerships with healthcare providers,* it is essential for people with chronic, progressive conditions such as MS. It is worth noting that US healthcare policy has increasingly emphasized patient empowerment and increased responsibility of self-management. Table 12.1 summarizes this trend, showing how successive laws have progressively shifted greater responsibility to patients. The *Patient Self-Determination Act* (1990) laid an early foundation for patient empowerment by requiring healthcare institutions to inform individuals of their rights to make care decisions, including the use of advance directives (Patient Self-Determination Act 1990). The *Health Information Technology for Economic and Clinical Health* (HITECH) Act (HITECH Act, 2009) built on this by promoting the adoption of electronic health records and patient portals, thereby improving access to health information and supporting self-monitoring (Blumenthal 2010). The *Affordable Care Act* (ACA 2010) further advanced the agenda through the creation of the Patient-Centered Outcomes Research Institute (PCORI), expansion of preventive services, and promotion of patient-centered medical homes and accountable care organizations that integrate self-management planning (Patient Protection and

TABLE 12.1
U.S. Health Policies Emphasizing Patient Empowerment and Self-Management

Act/Provision (Year)	Key Features/Purpose	How It Supports Empowerment/Self-Management
Patient Self-Determination Act (PSDA 1990)	Required healthcare facilities to inform patients of rights regarding treatment decisions	Advanced patient autonomy and responsibility in decision-making, particularly via advance directives (Patient Self-Determination Act 1990).
Health Information Technology for Economic and Clinical Health (HITECH) Act (2009)	Promoted adoption and "meaningful use" of electronic health records (EHRs)	Enabled widespread use of patient portals and access to health data, enhancing transparency and self-monitoring (Blumenthal 2010).
Patient Protection and Affordable Care Act (ACA 2010)	Comprehensive reform, expanding coverage, regulating insurers, and enhancing care models	Created the Patient-Centered Outcomes Research Institute (PCORI), expanded no-cost preventive services, and supported patient-centered medical homes and accountable care organizations with self-management planning (Patient Protection and Affordable Care Act 2010; Selby *et al.* 2012).
Medicare Chronic Care Management (CCM) Provisions (2015)	Reimbursed providers for managing patients with multiple chronic conditions between visits	Incentivized care planning, goal-setting, and ongoing support for self-management in chronic conditions (CMS 2015).
21st Century Cures Act	Accelerated medical research and strengthened health IT interoperability	Prohibited "information blocking" and enhanced patients' rights to access and share electronic health information, aiding active engagement in self-management (Adler-Milstein and Pfeifer 2017).

Affordable Care Act 2010; Selby *et al.* 2012). More recently, *Medicare Chronic Care Management* provisions have incentivized ongoing self-management support for people with multiple chronic conditions (CMS 2015), while the 21st Century Cures Act (2016) strengthened patients' rights to access and share their electronic health data by requiring interoperability and prohibiting information blocking (Adler-Milstein and Pfeifer 2017).

Fifth, taking action, this is more about learning how to change a behavior or implement solutions. Factors to perform behavior change successfully are high task-specific self-efficacy, attainable steps, measurable short-term and long-term practical goals, being time-bound (e.g., 10 minutes per term, 3 times a day, for the next 14 days), and being related to individual values (e.g., being responsible for personal and family health and wellness).

SELF-MANAGEMENT EXPERIENCE AND NEEDS AMONG PEOPLE WITH MS

Unexpected and varying MS symptoms and functional impairments could demand people with MS to manage MS daily and make several behavior changes to mitigate symptom severity and disability impact (Knaster *et al.* 2011). The uncertainty of disease progression can heighten stress and depression, which in turn may worsen MS and make long-term adaptation more difficult. Motivation for sustained self-management often arises from a sense of necessity, positive experiences with coping strategies, and support from healthcare providers, family, friends, and peers (Knaster *et al.* 2011). These factors reinforce self-efficacy, a central determinant of effective self-management (Bandura 1977). Important coping skills include accessing reliable information, adhering to medical treatment, monitoring and preventing symptoms, and mobilizing social support. People with MS consistently emphasize that self-management interventions should be motivating, tailored to individual needs and disease stage (including technology-based options), and provide accessible resources (Knaster *et al.* 2011). Systematic reviews echo these recommendations, highlighting essential strategies such as knowledge acquisition, self-monitoring, problem-solving, goal-setting, skill development, identifying personal strengths, and rehearsing learned skills (Lorig *et al.* 2001; Warsi *et al.* 2004).

When exploring the self-management tools needed by people with MS, Chiu's team found that many people with MS used the Internet to diligently seek and evaluate information; however, fatigue or cognitive issues quickly tire them. Also, they are vigilant about misinformation online, and some of their healthcare providers discourage them from searching online. It is worth noting that people with MS journaled many things, including what they have learned about symptom triggers and behavioral consequences (e.g., too tight scheduling, excessive exercise, stress), while tracking the time and duration of occurrence of old and new symptoms. Their notes helped them remember questions to ask their healthcare providers and assisted them in adjusting their medical treatment. It is worth noting again that one consistent piece of advice from MS healthcare providers to people with MS, regardless of their MS variation and progression, is a healthy lifestyle (e.g., exercise, diet, emotional regulation, sleep hygiene, and taking vitamin D). However, due to the chronic nature of this disease, self-management for people with MS extends beyond the individual effort of monitoring symptoms, adhering to their treatment plans, and maintaining rehabilitation practices, which are deeply influenced by their surrounding ecosystem of family, clinicians, healthcare systems, and societal policies (Figure 12.1). Each of these dimensions, personal, family, clinical, system, and policy, interplays with the others, presenting an interdependent care experience rather than separate modules. Despite this interconnectedness, MS care often remains fragmented, with gaps in communication, inconsistent support, and uneven access to resources, leaving people with MS and their caregivers to bear much of the responsibility for integration.

It is critical for people with MS to find sustainable strategies and receive support to maintain their self-management needs over time. With the increasing popularity, acceptance, and even basic awareness of digital health technologies (e.g., mobile applications, patient portals) that integrate artificial intelligence (AI), it is imperative to examine and forecast how AI can help people with MS manage and maintain their health.

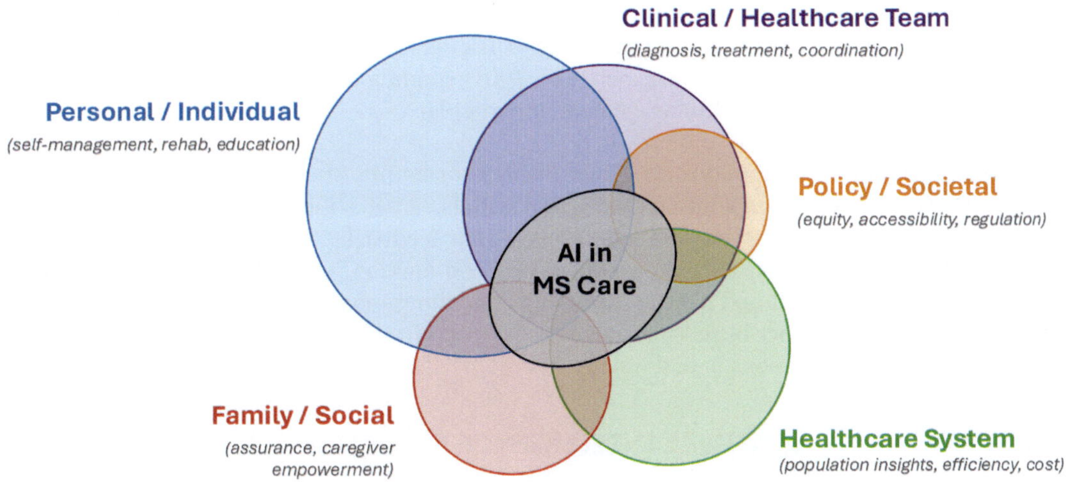

FIGURE 12.1 Multidimensional self-management in comprehensive MS self-management.

DIGITAL HEALTH AND AI IN SELF-MANAGEMENT FOR PEOPLE WITH MS

Digital health technologies provide an opportunity to address this fragmentation by connecting efforts across these dimensions. In this context, the concept of *digital health-seeking behavior* (DHSB), the processes by which individuals seek, appraise, utilize, decide on, and act upon health information and services, offers a behavioral framework to understand how people with MS and caregivers already engage with digital tools in navigating their care. Consequently, AI can act as a connective force in the MS care scenario, strengthening these behaviors and bridging the dimensions of MS care. Being on the overlapping porch of personal habits, family reassurance, clinical expertise, system efficiency, and policy oversight, AI has the potential to transform self-management from a set of isolated tasks into a seamless, adaptive, and patient-centered ecosystem.

ARTIFICIAL INTELLIGENCE (AI)

Definition. AI broadly refers to computational systems capable of performing tasks traditionally requiring human intelligence, such as learning, reasoning, pattern recognition, and adaptive decision-making (Russell and Norvig 2021). Within healthcare, AI encompasses both symbolic systems (e.g., rule-based reasoning, ontologies) and statistical/machine learning systems (e.g., predictive modeling, neural networks).

Taxonomy. A useful taxonomy of AI in healthcare can be organized along five axes:

1. Learning paradigm – supervised learning (prediction from labeled data), unsupervised learning (clustering, dimensionality reduction), reinforcement learning (dynamic adaptation), and self-/semi-supervised methods for large-scale unannotated data (LeCun 2022).
2. Techniques – natural language processing (NLP), computer vision (CV), digital phenotyping, time-series forecasting, recommender systems, and uncertainty quantification (Russell and Norvig 2021).
3. Architecture – from shallow models (logistic regression, decision trees) to advanced deep learning (convolutional neural networks [CNNs], transformers, graph neural networks [GNNs]).
4. Data modalities – structured data (electronic health records [EHRs], unstructured clinical text, sensor/wearable data, speech, and patient-reported outcomes [PROs]).

5. Theoretical grounding – behavioral frameworks such as COM-B (Capability, Opportunity, Motivation-Behavior) (Michie *et al.* 2011), self-efficacy theory (Bandura 1977), or the Chronic Care Model (CCM) (Wagner *et al.* 2001), guiding how AI integrates into healthcare in general and into self-management in particular.

AI systems can be conceptualized as having either (or both) of two major functions: *observation/monitoring* (tracking symptoms, physiological signals, or behavioral patterns via sensors, apps, or clinical records) and *intervention/control* (providing feedback, recommendations, or actions designed to influence patient behavior, clinical decision-making, or healthcare resource allocation) (LeCun 2022; Russell and Norvig 2021). By combining monitoring and feedback loops, AI becomes an adaptive partner in self-management, learning from patient, system, and environment data and tailoring interventions in real time.

APPLICATIONS OF ARTIFICIAL INTELLIGENCE IN MS SELF-MANAGEMENT

The contributions of AI systems to self-management can be mapped across the five self-management dimensions (Figure 12.1) elaborated in the previous section. In the following sections, we will examine some of these contributions along each dimension, based on the findings from recent research and literature.

Personal/Individual Dimension: From Reactive Coping to Proactive Mastery

The personal/individual dimension of MS care intersects with the full range of daily living challenges imposed by the disease. At this level, self-management encompasses medical management (e.g., symptom tracking, medication adherence, and rehabilitation practices), role and daily life management (balancing work, family, and physical independence), emotional management (coping with uncertainty, fatigue, and mood fluctuations), decision-making management (navigating treatment options and knowing when to escalate care), and social and resource management (drawing on digital tools, health literacy, and available support). For people with MS, the continuity of these tasks is more critical than in the case of otherwise healthy individuals managing general health behaviors, since people with MS continuously face the unpredictable consequences of the illness on goals, activities, and sense of self (Bodenheimer *et al.* 2002; Corbin and Strauss 1988; Lorig 1993; Lorig and Holman 2003). Within this context, self-efficacy emerges as a key determinant of success; yet self-management is also shaped by digital literacy, emotional resilience, and access to facilitative resources. The personal dimension is thus the most immediate but also the most vulnerable to disruptions by symptoms and interruptions, where digital health-seeking behavior (DHSB) – particularly the domains of seeking, appraising, and acting – plays a central role in sustaining everyday self-management (Kontos *et al.* 2014; Stellefson *et al.* 2011).

Self-management at the individual level has traditionally been reactive, with people with MS adjusting only after symptoms such as fatigue or relapse have escalated. Recent AI applications shift this trajectory toward *proactive mastery,* where individuals can anticipate problems, regulate daily routines, and strengthen self-efficacy. Reviews highlight rapid progress in digital phenotyping, relapse prediction, and personalized coaching, demonstrating AI's capacity to reinforce medical, role/daily life, and emotional self-management (De Brouwer *et al.* 2024; dos Santos *et al.* 2024; Naji *et al.* 2023; Pilehvari *et al.* 2024). Table 12.2 summarizes some of the applications of AI to this dimension of self-management.

Wearable-based fatigue prediction enables people with MS to anticipate dips in energy, rest proactively, and avoid sudden crashes, thereby reducing anxiety and reinforcing daily pacing strategies. Patients often describe feeling more in control of their condition, and their actions include resting earlier, conserving energy, and preventing symptom exacerbations (Moebus *et al.* 2024). Here, the digital health-seeking behavior (DHSB) domains of appraising, deciding, and acting are central, as people with MS must interpret sensor outputs, adjust pacing and rest accordingly, and follow through with

TABLE 12.2
Applications of AI to the Personal/Individual Dimension

Application	AI Characteristics	Impact on Self-Management	Perception and Affect	Self-Management Action	Self-Management Aspect(s)	DHSB Domain(s)
Wearable/PROs for symptom tracking and fatigue prediction (Moebus *et al.* 2024)	*Supervised learning* (Generalized Additive Models [GAMs], e.g., random forest [RF] and support-vector machine [SVM])	Improves self-monitoring	More aware, felt more in control	Pace activity, rest proactively, prevent flare-ups.	**Medical** (symptom monitoring, treatment adjustment), **Decision-making** (identifying when to modify activity).	**Appraise** (interpret sensor data), **Decide** (adjust pacing/rest), **Act** (change routine for symptom control).
Relapse dashboards using PRO data (Brown *et al.* 2020; Chalkou *et al.* 2021; Zhao *et al.* 2020)	*Supervised* + *semi-supervised models, ensemble learning*	Increases awareness of early changes	Certain, decisive (*early recognition reduces uncertainty*)	Call neurologist earlier, adjust plans, seek timely care.	**Medical** (relapse detection), **Decision-making** (recognizing when to seek professional help).	**Seek** (receive prediction info), **Appraise** (evaluate relapse risk), **Act** (seek care early).
Motivational feedback (Hors-Fraile *et al.* 2018; Kazemi *et al.* 2022)	*Conversational natural language processing (NLP) models* (transformers, rule-based chatbots)	Builds self-efficacy	More certain, decisive in planning	Take medications consistently, follow exercise plans.	**Emotional** (coping with uncertainty, enhancing confidence), **Medical** (sustaining adherence).	**Utilize** (apply chatbot feedback), **Decide** (commit to behavior), **Act** (adhere to plan).
Daily guidance (Forman *et al.* 2019; Lei *et al.* 2012; Nahum-Shani *et al.* 2016)	*Reinforcement learning* (RL) with *policy networks*	Supports daily decision-making	Relieved of decision fatigue and uncertainty and more secure	Structure daily routines, conserve energy, avoid exacerbations.	**Role/daily life** (pacing, energy balancing), **Decision-making** (planning daily routines).	**Appraise** (weigh RL guidance), **Decide** (choose daily strategy), **Act** (follow structured routine).

changes in daily activity. These systems are commonly built using *supervised learning* approaches such as *random forests (RFs)* and *convolutional neural networks* (*CNNs)* trained on accelerometer and smartphone sensor data (Dini *et al.* 2025; dos Santos *et al.* 2024; Moebus *et al.* 2024).

Predictive dashboards that communicate relapse risk similarly provide reassurance and decisiveness. People with MS using such tools report greater certainty about when to contact their neurologist, which strengthens medical and decision-making dimensions of self-management (Brown *et al.* 2020; Chalkou *et al.* 2021; Zhao *et al.* 2020). This application activates the digital health-seeking behavior (DHSB) domains of seeking, appraising, and acting, where people with MS seek prediction information, evaluate relapse risks, and act by contacting clinicians or modifying their plans. Technically, these dashboards are underpinned by *supervised learning models*. Early systems often relied on *logistic regression* and *Cox regression models* to predict relapses or disability progression (Brown *et al.* 2020). More advanced prognostic dashboards employ *cause-specific Cox models* and *competing risks survival analysis* to generate individualized relapse probabilities (Chalkou *et al.* 2021). Recent work demonstrates the advantages of *ensemble methods*, such as *random forests* and *gradient boosting (XGBoost)*, as well as *neural networks*, which are particularly effective in managing incomplete or noisy patient-reported outcomes and high-dimensional clinical data (Zhao *et al.* 2020).

Conversational AI has emerged as an important tool for adherence and motivation. Chatbots and recommender systems that deliver tailored reminders and encouragement have been shown to increase self-efficacy and support patients in sustaining health routines (Hors-Fraile *et al.* 2018). In people with MS specifically, smartphone-based continuous care models have improved both treatment adherence and self-efficacy, highlighting the potential of digital conversational support to reinforce daily self-management (Kazemi *et al.* 2022). In this context, the digital health-seeking (DHSB) domains of utilizing, deciding, and acting are most salient, as people with MS apply chatbot feedback, decide to commit to behavioral changes, and act by adhering to medication or exercise regimens. These systems are implemented using *natural language processing (NLP)* methods, ranging from *rule-based dialogue engines* to recommender-driven conversation flows, with emerging work exploring more advanced *transformer-based language models* for personalized motivational support.

Finally, *reinforcement learning (RL)* has been introduced to provide adaptive daily guidance. By recommending when to rest and when to remain active, reinforcement learning-based systems reduce the stress of constant decision-making, leaving people with MS feeling relieved and secure in their routines (Forman *et al.* 2019). Daily guidance interventions engage the digital health-seeking behavior (DHSB) domains of appraising, deciding, and acting, with people with MS weighing adaptive recommendations, selecting strategies for structuring routines, and implementing these into practice. These interventions employ *policy-network approaches to sequential decision-making*, which balance exploration and exploitation to optimize activity recommendations in real time (Lei *et al.* 2012; Nahum-Shani *et al.* 2016).

Clinical/Healthcare Team Dimension: From Passive Recipient to Active Partner

The clinical dimension of self-management in MS encompasses the roles and relationships of healthcare providers, including neurologists, rehabilitation specialists, nurses, and primary care practitioners. Within this dimension, effective self-management is shaped by clinicians' ability to interpret and synthesize diverse patient-reported and clinical data, provide individualized guidance, and communicate effectively with patients. Clinical care in MS is inherently complex, as disease trajectories are heterogeneous, relapses occur unpredictably, and treatment responses vary across individuals (Miller and Leary 2007; Ontaneda *et al.* 2017). Accordingly, high-quality care depends not only on clinical expertise but also on sustained patient–clinician engagement, shared decision-making, and trust throughout the continuum of care. As digital health technologies increasingly integrate sources such as electronic health records (EHRs), imaging, and patient diaries into clinical workflows, the clinical dimension serves as a bridge between individual-level practices and system-level organization, thereby shaping the sustainability and direction of self-management (Marziniak *et al.* 2018; Tea *et al.* 2024; Ziemssen and Haase 2021).

The clinical dimension of self-management has often positioned people with MS as recipients of care rather than active participants. However, AI is beginning to shift this dynamic by enabling more personalized risk prediction, treatment tailoring, and decision support. Such innovations enhance patient–clinician dialogue and foster a greater sense of partnership and ownership in care. Recent studies highlight how predictive modeling and imaging AI systems are reshaping clinical decision-making, while natural language processing tools applied to clinical notes and conversational systems are reducing barriers to shared planning (De Brouwer *et al.* 2024; Sheikhalishahi *et al.* 2019; Yousef *et al.* 2024). Table 12.3 provides a summary of the contributions of AI to this dimension of self-management.

TABLE 12.3
Applications of AI to the Clinician/Healthcare Team Dimension

Application	AI Characteristics	Impact on Self-Management	Perception and Affect	Self-Management Action	Self-Management Aspect(s)	DHSB Domain(s)
Predictive models for individualized relapse and progression risks (De Brouwer *et al.* 2024; Yousef *et al.* 2024; Zhao *et al.* 2020)	*Supervised learning* (logistic regression, gradient boosting, tabular transformers) trained on EHRs and PROs	Provides objective grounding for care plans	Informed, reassured about objective risk assessments	Commit to agreed plan, participate in shared decisions.	**Decision-making** (informed discussion, shared planning with clinicians), **Medical** (relapse/progression monitoring, treatment tailoring, adherence to the treatment plan), **Resource** (navigating treatment options).	**Seek** (receive clinician's input), **Appraise** (interpret personalized risk data), **Decide** (align with shared plan).
Imaging AI for lesion detection and monitoring (Kamraoui *et al.* 2022; Umirzakova *et al.* 2025)	*Deep learning (CNNs)* for lesion segmentation and longitudinal MRI tracking	Enhances tailored care through objective imaging insights	Assured (*tailored therapies improve motivation/adherence*)	Adhere more consistently to treatment.	**Medical** (individualized, treatment, adherence to the treatment plan).	**Utilize** (apply tailored recommendations), **Decide** (accept or modify therapy), **Act** (follow treatment regimen).
Extract EDSS/functional scores (Chase *et al.* 2017; Yang *et al.* 2022)	*NLP* (Naïve Bayes classification, CNNs)	Facilitates assessment and goal setting	Supported (*reduced documentation burden, more dialogue*)	Engage more actively in visit dialogue, goal setting.	**Decision-making** (engagement), **Resource** (efficient encounters with the healthcare team).	**Appraise** (evaluate disability/functional data), **Decide** (adjust life planning), **Act** (implement long-term changes).
Decision aids and comparative effectiveness tools (Elwyn *et al.* 2016; Salas-Vega *et al.* 2015)	*Supervised learning models (*CNNs for image processing, multi-modal deep neural networks, ensemble methods)	Supports shared decision-making	Ownership of decision (*shared decision-making strengthens engagement*)	Weigh risk/benefits, align behavior with chosen therapy.	**Decision-making** (weighing), **Medical** (alignment with and adherence to the treatment plan).	**Appraise** (compare treatment options), **Decide** (select preferred therapy), **Act** (adhere to chosen treatment).

Predictive models that generate individualized relapse and progression risks help people with MS feel reassured that their care plans are grounded in objective data, encouraging commitment to monitoring and treatment regimens (De Brouwer *et al.* 2024; Yousef *et al.* 2024; Zhao *et al.* 2020). Here, the digital health-seeking behavior (DHSB) domains of seeking, appraising, and deciding are central, as people with MS seek clinician input, appraise individualized risk information, and decide collaboratively on treatment and monitoring plans. These predictions are generated using *supervised learning algorithms,* including *logistic regression, gradient boosting machines (GBMs),* and *transformer-based models* trained on combinations of electronic health records (EHRs) and patient-reported outcomes (PROs).

Imaging AI further advances personalization. By linking MRI lesion profiles to treatment decisions, people with MS gain reassurance that their care is tailored to their condition, which can enhance adherence – especially when imaging insights aid lesion monitoring and progression assessment (Kamraoui *et al.* 2022; Umirzakova *et al.* 2025). This capability primarily activates the digital health-seeking behavior (DHSB) domains of utilizing, deciding, and acting, as people with MS incorporate imaging-informed recommendations, make choices aligned with their clinical status, and consistently adhere to prescribed regimens. These applications rely heavily on *deep learning architectures* such as *convolutional neural networks (CNNs)* trained on longitudinal MRI data (Kamraoui *et al.* 2022; Umirzakova *et al.* 2025).

Clinical natural language processing (NLP) also supports partnership by reducing documentation burdens. Automated extraction of disability measures such as the Expanded Disability Status Scale (EDSS) from unstructured notes frees clinicians to engage more in dialogue, which patients perceive as increased support (Chase *et al.* 2017; Yang *et al.* 2022). In this context, the digital health-seeking behavior (DHSB) domains of appraising, deciding, and acting are activated, as people with MS evaluate disability and functional information, decide how to adjust life planning, and act by implementing long-term changes. These capabilities are achieved using *Naïve Bayes classifiers* and *convolutional neural networks (CNNs),* which can infer structured outcomes from clinical text with minimal labeled data (Chase *et al.* 2017; Yang *et al.* 2022).

Finally, decision aids that present therapeutic options side-by-side help people with MS to strengthen their sense of ownership over treatment choices, thereby reducing decisional anxiety and enhancing commitment to care (Elwyn *et al.* 2016). Comparative effectiveness tools engage the digital health-seeking behavior (DHSB) domains of appraising, deciding, and acting, with people with MS comparing treatment options, deciding on their preferred therapy, and acting by following the chosen regimen. Emerging approaches are underpinned by *supervised learning models* that integrate data from electronic health records (EHRs), imaging, and laboratory tests to generate treatment comparisons (Salas-Vega *et al.* 2015). By translating these complex data streams into accessible option-by-option comparisons, such systems hold promises for advancing shared decision-making in MS.

Healthcare System Dimension: From Bureaucratic Burden to Supported Navigation

The healthcare system dimension encompasses the organizational and institutional frameworks that structure MS care, including hospitals, rehabilitation centers, public health infrastructures, and insurance schemes. These structures are primarily oriented toward efficiency, equity, and sustainability at the population level rather than individualized care (Nolte and McKee 2008; WHO 2016). For people with MS, such system-level arrangements directly shape access to specialized services, continuity of care, affordability, and availability of rehabilitation resources (Kleij *et al.* 2017). Persistent challenges – including limited clinical capacity, geographic disparities, and financial constraints – remain decisive factors influencing the degree of self-management support that patients receive (Abbasi Dashtaki *et al.* n.d.; Heppner *et al.* 2025; McGinley *et al.* 2024). These systemic barriers affect both individual and clinical outcomes, as interruptions in service delivery can compromise long-term autonomy. Thus, the healthcare system acts simultaneously as an enabler and a limiter of self-management, setting the structural boundaries within which personal, family, and clinical efforts unfold (Corbin and Strauss 1988; Glasgow *et al.* 2005).

At the healthcare system level, self-management is often undermined by bureaucratic complexity and fragmented pathways. People with MS frequently struggle with referral delays, uncoordinated services, and inconsistent follow-up. AI is helping to reduce this burden by orchestrating care pathways, predicting readmissions, and ensuring continuity across institutions. Reviews of system-level AI stress its potential to transform healthcare into a proactive, supportive infrastructure that reinforces resource and role/daily life management (Miotto *et al.* 2018; Rajkomar *et al.* 2019; Shickel *et al.* 2018). Table 12.4 presents some of the contributions of AI to the Healthcare System dimension of self-management.

TABLE 12.4
Applications of AI to the Healthcare System Dimension

Application	AI Characteristics	Impact on Self-Management	Perception and Affect	Self-Management Action	Self-Management Aspect(s)	DHSB Domain(s)
Automated referrals and follow-up coordination (Rajkomar *et al.* 2019; Shickel *et al.* 2018; Woodcock 2022)	*Supervised ensembles* (e.g., GBMs) and *RL hybrids* with *policy networks* for dynamic scheduling	Streamlines care pathways and reduces system delays	Relieved (*reduced friction and increased satisfaction*)	Attend timely appointments, maintain continuity of care, engage more consistently in rehabilitation	**Resource** (navigation and access to services), **Role/daily life** (reduced logistical burden).	**Seek** (find referral info), **Appraise** (assess service relevance), **Act** (attend coordinated care).
Readmission prediction for proactive outreach (Carter *et al.* 2018; Rajkomar *et al.* 2019; Yu and Xie 2020)	*Supervised ensembles* (GBM, logistic regression, RF) using hospital EHRs	Enables proactive contact and continuity of care	Cared for (*patients flagged, follow-up coordinated*)	Engage with follow-up care, report symptoms promptly	**Resource** (reducing burden).	**Utilize** (accept automated referral), **Act** (follow referral steps).
Multi-site training for inclusive MS AI apps (Rieke *et al.* 2020; Sheller *et al.* 2020; Yang *et al.* 2019)	*Federated learning (FL)* using *federated transformers*	Improves inclusivity and generalizability of AI models	Reassured (*privacy preserved, robust diverse models built*)	Trust recommendations, use apps consistently	**Resource** (equitable access), **Decision-making** (trust).	**Appraise** (trust services), **Decide** (adopt/reject apps), **Utilize** (use apps).
Post-deployment monitoring (FDA 2021; Finlayson *et al.* 2021)	*Post-hoc calibration* + *drift detection frameworks*	Maintains long-term trust and safety of AI tools	Secure and safe (*trust in AI tools grows*)	Continue using AI-guided apps with confidence	**Decision-making** (confidence), **Resource** (trustworthy systems).	**Appraise** (trust services), **Decide** (adopt/reject apps), **Utilize** (use apps).

AI is increasingly applied to streamline referrals and follow-up scheduling, reducing fragmentation and supporting continuity of care (Rajkomar *et al.* 2019; Shickel *et al.* 2018). For people with MS, coordinated referrals and automated follow-ups have the potential to lessen the burden of navigating complex care systems, thereby conserving emotional and physical energy. Automated self-scheduling, for instance, has been associated with increased patient satisfaction and reduced effort in managing appointments (Woodcock 2022). This application activates the digital health-seeking behavior (DHSB) domains of seeking, appraising, and acting, where people with MS locate referral information, evaluate the relevance of services, and act by attending coordinated care without delays. These functions are typically achieved through *supervised ensembles* such as *Gradient Boosting Machines (GBMs)* and *reinforcement learning (RL) hybrids* that employ *policy networks* for dynamic scheduling.

Readmission prediction offers a model of proactive support. While MS-specific data on patient-reported reassurance when contacted early are limited, broader evidence shows that patients who perceive attentive and engaged care – where providers listen carefully – are significantly less likely to be readmitted and report greater understanding and confidence during care transitions (Carter *et al.* 2018). In this context, the digital health-seeking behavior (DHSB) domains of utilizing and acting are most salient: People with MS utilize hospital outreach by accepting automated follow-up contacts and act by reporting symptoms earlier and engaging in coordinated care. These systems typically employ *supervised ensemble models* – including *logistic regression, gradient boosting machines (GBMs), and random forests* – trained on hospital electronic health records (EHRs) to flag readmission risk and enable timely outreach (Rajkomar *et al.* 2019; Yu and Xie 2020).

Federated learning (FL) reassures people with MS that AI models reflect diverse populations, not just local cohorts. This inclusivity enhances trust and encourages consistent app use (Rieke *et al.* 2020; Sheller *et al.* 2020; Yang *et al.* 2019). This approach engages the digital health-seeking behavior (DHSB) domains of appraising, deciding, and utilizing, as people with MS appraise the trustworthiness of federated systems, decide whether to adopt or reject apps, and utilize them consistently once reassured. Technically, federated learning uses *federated transformers* and *distributed optimization* to train models across institutions without exchanging raw data.

Finally, people with MS feel more secure when reassured that AI tools remain accurate over time. Post-deployment monitoring infrastructures employ techniques such as calibration, drift detection, and uncertainty quantification to preserve confidence in model outputs (FDA 2021; Finlayson *et al.* 2021). These trustworthiness frameworks ensure that deployed models remain valid and safe. Post-deployment monitoring involves the digital health-seeking behavior (DHSB) domains of appraising, deciding, and utilizing, where people with MS evaluate the reliability of AI tools, decide whether to adopt or continue using them, and utilize AI-guided apps with sustained confidence.

Family/Social Dimension: From Isolation to Shared Responsibility

The family and social dimension highlights the interpersonal and communal contexts that shape the self-management practices of people with MS. Family members, caregivers, and friends frequently provide essential support, ranging from emotional reassurance and advocacy during medical consultations to assistance with medication management, mobility, and daily routines (Bogosian *et al.* 2009; Grytten and Måseide 2006; Pakenham and Cox 2018). While such involvement enhances patient safety and autonomy, it can also generate caregiver strain, disrupt family dynamics, and compromise caregiver well-being (McKeown *et al.* 2004). Yet, these supports are often uneven, and when caregiver burden is high or social connections are weak, patient agency may be undermined. Emerging AI applications – such as caregiver stress detection, recommender systems, and peer-matching – are beginning to redistribute responsibility and strengthen networks of support. Although most current evidence comes from dementia research, reviews suggest substantial potential for adapting these approaches to MS self-management (Borna *et al.* 2024; Meiland *et al.* 2017). Table 12.5 shows some of the applications of AI to the Family/Social dimension of self-management.

Stress-detection systems provide caregivers with resources before burnout occurs, leaving people with MS feeling less guilty and more confident in their support network, which translates into steadier adherence (Borna *et al.* 2024; Meiland *et al.* 2017). Here, the digital health-seeking behavior (DHSB) domains of seeking, appraising, and acting are salient, since families seek support tools, appraise stress indicators, and act by adjusting caregiving strategies to ensure sustainability. These systems rely on *supervised affect detection* models and *lightweight language models* trained on voice diaries and text (Borna *et al.* 2024). While this has not been implemented in the context of MS, peer-matching platforms can reduce loneliness by connecting peers to peers with similar experiences. Patients feel understood and less alone, which strengthens resilience and coping (Naslund *et al.* 2016). Peer-connection platforms involve the digital health-seeking behavior (DHSB) domains of seeking, appraising, and acting, with people with MS seeking peers, appraising their credibility, and acting by engaging in support groups and adopting coping strategies. Technically, these systems leverage *graph neural networks (GNNs)* with *fairness constraints* to match individuals safely. An example of such algorithms can be found in Liu et al. (2023).

TABLE 12.5
Applications of AI to the Family/Social Dimension

Application	AI Characteristics	Impact on Self-Management	Perception and Affect	Self-Management Action	Self-Management Aspect(s)	DHSB Domain(s)
Caregiver stress detection (Borna *et al.* 2024; Meiland *et al.* 2017)	*Supervised affect detection models* (speech/text), *lightweight language models* (voice diaries, caregiver notes)	Provides resources before burnout, sustaining caregiving capacity	Less guilty, more secure (*burnout reduces, consistent caregiving*)	Families monitor stress, adjust caregiving strategies, sustain long-term support	**Emotional** (reduced guilt, stronger confidence), **Resource** (sustainable caregiving).	**Seek** (access caregiver support tools), **Appraise** (interpret stress signals), **Act** (adjust caregiving strategies).
Peer-connection (Liu *et al.* 2023; Naslund *et al.* 2016)	*Graph neural networks (GNNs)* with fairness-aware post-processing	Expands social support networks	Understood, less alone (*social support and resilience*)	Engage socially, adopt coping strategies from peers	**Social** (expanding peer support), **Emotional** (building coping strategies and resilience).	**Seek** (connect with peers), **Appraise** (evaluate peer credibility), **Act** (join support groups).
Loneliness detection systems (Badal *et al.* 2024; Doryab *et al.* 2019; Yamada *et al.* 2021)	*Natural language processing (NLP) on interview speech; passive sensing* (smartphone, wearables), *affect detection + recommender algorithms*	Identifies early signals of isolation, enables proactive interventions	Connected, resilient (*reduced loneliness results in resilience*)	Seek support interventions, utilize suggested coping activities, act to strengthen social ties	**Emotional** (coping with loneliness, identity adaptation), **Social** (sustaining relationships).	**Seek** (find interventions for loneliness), **Utilize** (practice coping skills), **Act** (maintain social ties).

Additionally, loneliness detection systems intervene when early signals of isolation appear, leaving the person feeling more connected and resilient. It should be noted that the evidence for such systems comes from the literature on older adults and is yet to be transferred to MS research. These approaches combine affect detection models with recommender algorithms to suggest social contacts or activities. For example, Yamada et al. (2021) demonstrated that acoustic and linguistic markers in speech can reveal loneliness, while Badal et al. (2024) showed that natural language processing (NLP) applied to interview transcripts predicts loneliness risk. Similarly, Doryab et al. (2019) used passive smartphone sensing to identify behavioral patterns linked to loneliness, illustrating how AI can both detect indicators of loneliness and inform timely interventions. These systems activate the digital health-seeking behavior (DHSB) domains of seeking, utilizing, and acting, as people with MS seek interventions for loneliness, utilize coping strategies, and act by maintaining and strengthening social ties.

Policy/Societal Dimension: From Skepticism to Trust and Inclusion

The policy/societal dimension constitutes the overarching framework within which all other domains of MS care are embedded. Policy decisions shape access to healthcare services, reimbursement for pharmacological and digital interventions, standards of equity in care provision, and the regulatory safeguards governing data privacy and protection (OECD 2023; WHO 2021). At the same time, societal attitudes strongly influence the visibility of MS as a chronic condition, mediating levels of stigma, inclusivity, and public awareness (Corrigan *et al.* 2014). Structural barriers such as the digital divide, fragmented insurance coverage, and burdensome regulation reverberate across families, clinical encounters, and health systems, ultimately shaping the quality of life of people with MS (Marrie *et al.* 2022; Mizell 2024; Moghavem *et al.* 2024). As such, this dimension highlights the necessity of aligning self-management strategies with broader commitments to equity, ethics, and public health, thereby extending beyond purely clinical or individual initiatives.

At the policy and societal level, supportive frameworks determine whether AI becomes a trusted ally in self-management or remains fragmented and inequitable. Without regulatory assurance, fairness safeguards, and scaling models, people with MS risk skepticism and exclusion. Reviews emphasize that transparency, safety, and equity are prerequisites for adoption (FDA 2021; Hersh *et al.* 2023; Laurson-Doube *et al.* 2024). Regulatory frameworks such as FDA Software as Medical Device (SaMD) guidelines instill confidence that AI tools are safe and validated, encouraging adoption (FDA 2021). These are operationalized through *audit pipelines* and *model card generators*. By establishing these frameworks, AI moves from skepticism toward becoming an inclusive and reliable societal resource. Here, the digital health-seeking behavior (DHSB) domains of appraising and deciding are central, since people with MS judge the trustworthiness of AI systems and decide whether to accept or reject their use. Table 12.6 presents some of the contributions made by AI to the Policy/Societal dimension of self-management.

Fairness audits reassure people with MS that systems are inclusive. Patients feel represented when tools undergo bias detection and subgroup testing, motivating sustained use (Mehrabi *et al.* 2021; Rajkomar *et al.* 2019). These safeguards employ *counterfactual analysis, disparity metrics,* and *federated governance frameworks.* This use case involves the digital health-seeking behavior (DHSB) domains of seeking and utilizing, as people with MS seek out inclusive platforms and utilize AI-enabled resources with reassurance of equitable access. Additionally, scaling frameworks ensure consistency. People with MS feel confident when AI interventions are available across home and clinical settings, reducing fragmentation (Michie *et al.* 2011; Wagner *et al.* 2001). These rely on *implementation science models* such as the Capability, Opportunity, Motivation-Behavior model (COM-B) (Michie *et al.* 2011), and the Chronic Care Model (CCM) (Wagner *et al.* 2001). Scaling frameworks primarily engage the digital health-seeking behavior (DHSB) domains of utilizing and acting, as people with MS adopt standardized systems and sustain long-term use across diverse care

TABLE 12.6
Applications of AI to the Policy/Societal Dimension

Application	AI Characteristics	Impact on Self-Management	Perception and Affect	Self-Management Action	Self-Management Aspect(s)	DHSB Domain(s)
FDA SaMD compliance (FDA 2021)	*Audit pipelines* and *model card generators*	Builds trust	Confident in safety (*trust in AI tools grows*)	Adopt and consistently use AI-enabled apps	**Resource** (trustworthy systems), **Decision-making** (confidence in technology).	**Appraise** (judge system trustworthiness), **Decide** (accept/reject use).
Equity and fairness (Mehrabi *et al.* 2021; Rajkomar *et al.* 2019)	*Fairness audits* using *counterfactuals, disparity metrics, FL governance*	Ensures equitable access	Reassured of inclusion (*bias reduced, equity improved*)	Continue engaging with AI tools across groups	**Resource** (equitable access), **Social** (reducing disparities).	**Seek** (access inclusive platforms), **Utilize** (utilize AI-enabled resources).
Scaling (Michie *et al.* 2011; Wagner *et al.* 2001)	*Implementation science frameworks for scaling AI*	Creates infrastructures for scalability	Confident in consistency (*AI interventions standardized and scaled*)	Rely on AI tools across settings and over time	**Resource** (scalable systems), **Medical** (consistent access to interventions).	**Utilize** (adopt standardized systems), **Act** (sustain long-term use).

settings. It should be noted that these are not AI-related theories; rather, they provide theoretical frameworks within which AI methods should be implemented.

Challenges, Considerations, and Future Directions

Despite progress, research remains biased toward supervised learning and motor-focused outcomes, particularly gait, fatigue, and fall risk (Dini *et al.* 2025). Cognitive, emotional, and social applications – where methodologies like self-supervised learning, conversational natural language processing (NLP), and graph-based models could offer significant impact – are underexplored (Amin *et al.* 2024). At the clinical interface, imaging convolutional neural networks (CNNs) and electronic health record (EHR)-based gradient boosting models dominate, while patient-reported outcomes (PROs) are seldom integrated, reducing opportunities for patient-centered dialogue (Amin *et al.* 2024). Similarly, caregiver and family recommender AI, though promising, remain underused in MS when compared to dementia. At the system level, federated learning is advancing, but trust labs for calibration and drift detection remain underdeveloped (Amin *et al.* 2024; FDA 2021). Without robust monitoring, patients may lose confidence in deployed tools. Policy frameworks also remain high-income-centric, with limited global applicability.

The next wave of AI for MS self-management must diversify methods, broaden outcomes, and align more closely with the lived realities of people with MS. Some future directions could include:

- Expanding beyond overused supervised deep networks for motor outcomes toward self-supervised, multimodal, and reinforcement learning (RL) approaches for cognition, mood, and social support.
- Integrating patient-reported outcomes (PROs) and patient voices alongside imaging and electronic health record (EHR) data for richer, patient-centered AI.

- Investing in caregiver- and family-centered AI, leveraging recommender systems and affect detection tailored to MS.
- Operationalizing trustworthy AI through explainable architectures, calibration methods, and fairness audits.
- Building equitable governance frameworks, ensuring that federated and deployed models serve diverse populations across health systems.

CONCLUSION

People with MS continue to face complex self-management challenges across personal, clinical, and community contexts. As noted by Mesko *et al.* (2025), the evolution of patient empowerment – driven by digital health and AI – suggests a shift from paternalistic models toward equal-level partnerships, grounded in agency, resources, and supportive context. Building on this, future care for MS should aim to develop mutual-learning ecosystems, where individuals and AI systems co-adapt and co-support within everyday life and healthcare environments. We hope this chapter serves as a guide – offering both structure and inspiration – for advancing empowered, equitable self-management in MS and similar chronic conditions.

REFERENCES

Abbasi Dashtaki, S.A.D., Majdinasab, N.M., Ghanbari, S.G., and Moradi Kalboland, M.M.K., n.d. The relationship between self-care ability and health-promoting behaviors of patients with multiple sclerosis. *Jundishapur Journal of Chronic Disease Care*, 13 (4), e140345.

Adler-Milstein, J., and Pfeifer, E., 2017. Information blocking: Is it occurring and what policy strategies can address it?. *The Milbank Quarterly*, 95 (1), 117–135. https://doi.org/10.1111/1468-0009.12241

Amin, M., Martínez-Heras, E., Ontaneda, D., and Prados Carrasco, F., 2024. Artificial intelligence and multiple sclerosis. *Current Neurology and Neuroscience Reports*, 24 (8), 233–243.

Badal, V.D., Reinen, J.M., Twamley, E.W., Lee, E.E., Fellows, R.P., Bilal, E., and Depp, C.A., 2024. Investigating acoustic and psycholinguistic predictors of cognitive impairment in older adults: Modeling study. *JMIR Aging*, 7, e54655.

Bandura, A., 1977. Self-efficacy: Toward a unifying theory of behavioral change. *Psychological Review*, 84 (2), 191.

Bebo, B., Cintina, I., LaRocca, N., Ritter, L., Talente, B., Hartung, D., Ngorsuraches, S., Wallin, M., and Yang, G., 2022. The economic burden of multiple sclerosis in the United States: Estimate of direct and indirect costs. *Neurology*, 98 (18), e1810–e1817.

Blumenthal, D., 2010. Launching HITECH. *The New England Journal of Medicine*, 362 (5), 382–385. https://doi.org/10.1056/NEJMp0912825

Bodenheimer, T., Lorig, K., Holman, H., and Grumbach, K., 2002. Patient self-management of chronic disease in primary care. *Jama*, 288 (19), 2469–2475.

Bogosian, A., Moss-Morris, R., Yardley, L., and Dennison, L., 2009. Experiences of partners of people in the early stages of multiple sclerosis. *Multiple Sclerosis Journal*, 15 (7), 876–884.

Borna, S., Maniaci, M.J., Haider, C.R., Gomez-Cabello, C.A., Pressman, S.M., Haider, S.A., Demaerschalk, B.M., Cowart, J.B., and Forte, A.J., 2024. Artificial intelligence support for informal patient caregivers: A systematic review. *Bioengineering*, 11 (5), 483–500. https://doi.org/10.3390/bioengineering11050483

Brown, F.S., Glasmacher, S.A., Kearns, P.K., MacDougall, N., Hunt, D., Connick, P., and Chandran, S., 2020. Systematic review of prediction models in relapsing remitting multiple sclerosis. *PLoS One*, 15 (5), e0233575.

Carter, J., Ward, C., Wexler, D., and Donelan, K., 2018. The association between patient experience factors and likelihood of 30-day readmission: A prospective cohort study. *BMJ Quality & Safety*, 27 (9), 683.

Centers for Medicare & Medicaid Services (CMS), 2015. *Chronic care management services*. Available at: https://www.cms.gov/medicare/medicare-fee-for-service-payment/physicianfeedbackprogram/chronic-care-management (Accessed: 28 September 2025).

Chalkou, K., Steyerberg, E., Bossuyt, P., Subramaniam, S., Benkert, P., Kuhle, J., Disanto, G., Kappos, L., Zecca, C., and Egger, M., 2021. Development, validation and clinical usefulness of a prognostic model for relapse in relapsing-remitting multiple sclerosis. *Diagnostic and Prognostic Research*, 5 (1), 17.

Chase, H.S., Mitrani, L.R., Lu, G.G., and Fulgieri, D.J., 2017. Early recognition of multiple sclerosis using natural language processing of the electronic health record. *BMC Medical Informatics and Decision Making*, 17 (1), 24.

Corbin, J.M., and Strauss, A., 1988. *Unending work and care: Managing chronic illness at home*. Jossey-bass.

Corrigan, P.W., Druss, B.G., and Perlick, D.A., 2014. The impact of mental illness stigma on seeking and participating in mental health care. *Psychological Science in the Public Interest*, 15 (2), 37–70.

De Brouwer, E., Becker, T., Werthen-Brabants, L., Dewulf, P., Iliadis, D., Dekeyser, C., Laureys, G., Van Wijmeersch, B., Popescu, V., and Dhaene, T., 2024. Machine-learning-based prediction of disability progression in multiple sclerosis: An observational, international, multi-center study. *PLOS Digital Health*, 3 (7), e0000533.

Dini, M., Comi, G., and Leocani, L., 2025. Digital remote monitoring of people with multiple sclerosis. *Frontiers in Immunology*, 16, 1514813.

Doryab, A., Villalba, D.K., Chikersal, P., Dutcher, J.M., Tumminia, M., Liu, X., Cohen, S., Creswell, K., Mankoff, J., Creswell, J.D., and Dey, A.K., 2019. Identifying behavioral phenotypes of loneliness and social isolation with passive sensing: Statistical analysis, data mining and machine learning of smartphone and fitbit data. *JMIR Mhealth Uhealth*, 7 (7), e13209.

dos Santos, M.P., Heckler, W.F., Bavaresco, R.S., and Barbosa, J.L.V., 2024. Machine learning applied to digital phenotyping: A systematic literature review and taxonomy. *Computers in Human Behavior*, 161, 108422.

Elwyn, G., Frosch, D.L., and Kobrin, S., 2016. Implementing shared decision-making: Consider all the consequences. *Implementation Science*, 11 (1), 114.

Finlayson, S.G., Subbaswamy, A., Singh, K., Bowers, J., Kupke, A., Zittrain, J., Kohane Isaac, S., and Saria, S., 2021. The clinician and dataset shift in artificial intelligence. *New England Journal of Medicine*, 385 (3), 283–286.

Forman, E.M., Kerrigan, S.G., Butryn, M.L., Juarascio, A.S., Manasse, S.M., Ontañón, S., Dallal, D.H., Crochiere, R.J., and Moskow, D., 2019. Can the artificial intelligence technique of reinforcement learning use continuously-monitored digital data to optimize treatment for weight loss? *Journal of Behavioral Medicine*, 42 (2), 276–290.

Glasgow, R.E., Wagner, E.H., Schaefer, J., Mahoney, L.D., Reid, R.J., and Greene, S.M., 2005. Development and validation of the patient assessment of chronic illness care (PACIC). *Medical Care*, 43 (5), 436–444.

Grytten, N., and Måseide, P., 2006. 'When i am together with them i feel more ill.' The stigma of multiple sclerosis experienced in social relationships. *Chronic Illness*, 2 (3), 195–208.

Health Information Technology for Economic and Clinical Health Act of 2009, Pub. L. No. 111-5, § Title XIII, 123 Stat. 226 (2009).

Heppner, J.W., Choma, A., Otto, T., and Collins, E., 2025. Financial assistance value for equitable access to specialty medications for adults with multiple sclerosis using health system pharmacy services. *International Journal of MS Care*, 27 (Q1), 50–55.

Hersh, C.M., Morrow, S.A., Williams, M.J., Amezcua, L., Halper, J., and Wandersee, K., 2023. Diversity, equity, and inclusion in the multiple sclerosis community: A call to action. *International Journal of MS Care*, 25 (5), 199–205.

Hittle, M., Culpepper, W.J., Langer-Gould, A., Marrie, R.A., Cutter, G.R., Kaye, W.E., Wagner, L., Topol, B., LaRocca, N.G., and Nelson, L.M., 2023. Population-based estimates for the prevalence of multiple sclerosis in the United States by race, ethnicity, age, sex, and geographic region. *JAMA Neurology*, 80 (7), 693–701.

Hors-Fraile, S., Schneider, F., Fernandez-Luque, L., Luna-Perejon, F., Civit, A., Spachos, D., Bamidis, P., and de Vries, H., 2018. Tailoring motivational health messages for smoking cessation using an mHealth recommender system integrated with an electronic health record: A study protocol. *BMC Public Health*, 18 (1), 698.

Kamraoui, R.A., Mansencal, B., Manjon, J.V., and Coupé, P., 2022. Longitudinal detection of new MS lesions using deep learning. *Frontiers in Neuroimaging*, 1, 948235.

Katz Sand, I., Levy, S., Fitzgerald, K., Sorets, T., and Sumowski, J.F., 2023. Mediterranean diet is linked to less objective disability in multiple sclerosis. *Multiple Sclerosis Journal*, 29 (2), 248–260.

Kazemi, S.M., Rakhshan, M., Rivaz, M., and Izadi, S., 2022. The effects of continuous care model using a smartphone application on adherence to treatment and self-efficacy among patients with multiple sclerosis. *BMC Medical Informatics and Decision Making*, 22 (1), 53.

Khan, G., and Hashim, M.J., 2025. Epidemiology of multiple sclerosis: Global, regional, national and sub-national-level estimates and future projections. *Journal of Epidemiology and Global Health*, 15 (1), 21.

Kidd, T., Carey, N., Mold, F., Westwood, S., Miklaucich, M., Konstantara, E., Sterr, A., and Cooke, D., 2017. A systematic review of the effectiveness of self-management interventions in people with multiple sclerosis at improving depression, anxiety and quality of life. *PloS One*, 12 (10), e0185931.

Kleij, K.-S., Tangermann, U., Amelung, V.E., and Krauth, C., 2017. Patients' preferences for primary health care – A systematic literature review of discrete choice experiments. *BMC Health Services Research*, 17 (1), 476.

Knaster, E.S., Yorkston, K.M., Johnson, K., McMullen, K.A., and Ehde, D.M., 2011. Perspectives on self-management in multiple sclerosis. *American Journal of Speech-Language Pathology*, 13 (3), 146–152.

Kontos, E., Blake, K.D., Chou, W.-Y.S., and Prestin, A., 2014. Predictors of eHealth usage: Insights on the digital divide from the health information national trends survey 2012. *Journal of Medical Internet Research*, 16 (7), e172.

Laurson-Doube, J., Helme, A., Nonino, F., Piggott, T., Rijke, N., and Saylor, D., 2024. WHO considers multiple sclerosis treatments essential. *The Lancet Neurology*, 23 (2), 140.

LeCun, Y., 2022. A path towards autonomous machine intelligence version 0.9. 2, 2022-06-27. *Open Review*, 62 (1), 1–62.

Lei, H., Nahum-Shani, I., Lynch, K., Oslin, D., and Murphy, S.A., 2012. A "SMART" design for building individualized treatment sequences. *Annual Review of Clinical Psychology*, 8, 21–48.

Liu, Y., Fang, A., Moriarty, G., Kraut, R., and Zhu, H., 2023. *Agent-based simulation for online mental health matching*. arXiv preprint arXiv:2303.11272.

Lorig, K., 1993. Self-management of chronic illness: A model for the future. *Generations: Journal of the American Society on Aging*, 17 (3), 11–14.

Lorig, K., 2003. Self-management education: More than a nice extra. *Medical Care*, 41 (6), 699–701.

Lorig, K., Sobel, D., Ritter, P., Laurent, D., and Hobbs, M., 2001. Effect of a self-management program on patients with chronic disease. *Effective Clinical Practice*, 4 (6), 256–262.

Lorig, K.R., and Holman, H.R., 2003. Self-management education: History, definition, outcomes, and mechanisms. *Annals of Behavioral Medicine*, 26 (1), 1–7.

Marcus, R., 2022. What is multiple sclerosis? *Jama*, 328 (20), 2078–2078.

Marrie, R.A., Kosowan, L., Cutter, G., Fox, R., and Salter, A., 2022. Disparities in telehealth care in multiple sclerosis. *Neurology Clinical Practice*, 12 (3), 223–233.

Marziniak, M., Brichetto, G., Feys, P., Meyding-Lamadé, U., Vernon, K., and Meuth, S.G., 2018. The use of digital and remote communication technologies as a tool for multiple sclerosis management: Narrative review. *JMIR Rehabilitation and Assistive Technologies*, 5 (1), e7805.

McGinley, M.P., Goldschmidt, C.H., and Rae-Grant, A.D., 2021. Diagnosis and treatment of multiple sclerosis: A review. *Jama*, 325 (8), 765–779.

McGinley, M.P., Harvey, T., Lopez, R., Ontaneda, D., and Buchalter, R.B., 2024. Geographic disparities in access to neurologists and multiple sclerosis care in the United States. *Neurology*, 102 (2), e207916.

McKeown, L.P., Porter-Armstrong, A.P., and Baxter, G.D., 2004. Caregivers of people with multiple sclerosis: Experiences of support. *Multiple Sclerosis Journal*, 10 (2), 219–230.

Mehrabi, N., Morstatter, F., Saxena, N., Lerman, K., and Galstyan, A., 2021. A survey on bias and fairness in machine learning. *ACM Computing Surveys*, 54 (6), Article 115.

Meiland, F., Innes, A., Mountain, G., Robinson, L., van der Roest, H., García-Casal, J.A., Gove, D., Thyrian, J.R., Evans, S., Dröes, R.-M., Kelly, F., Kurz, A., Casey, D., Szcześniak, D., Dening, T., Craven, M.P., Span, M., Felzmann, H., Tsolaki, M., and Franco-Martin, M., 2017. Technologies to support community-dwelling persons with dementia: A position paper on issues regarding development, usability, effectiveness and cost-effectiveness, deployment, and ethics. *JMIR Rehabilitation and Assistive Technologies*, 4 (1), e1.

Mesko, B., deBronkart, D., Dhunnoo, P., Arvai, N., Katonai, G., and Riggare, S., 2025. The evolution of patient empowerment and its impact on health care's future. *Journal of Medical Internet Research*, 27, e60562.

Michie, S., van Stralen, M.M., and West, R., 2011. The behaviour change wheel: A new method for characterising and designing behaviour change interventions. *Implementation Science*, 6, 42.

Miller, D.H., and Leary, S.M., 2007. Primary-progressive multiple sclerosis. *The Lancet Neurology*, 6 (10), 903–912.

Miotto, R., Wang, F., Wang, S., Jiang, X., and Dudley, J.T., 2018. Deep learning for healthcare: Review, opportunities and challenges. *Briefings in Bioinformatics*, 19 (6), 1236–1246.

Mizell, R., 2024. The impact of insurance restrictions in newly diagnosed individuals with multiple sclerosis. *International Journal of MS Care*, 26 (1), 17–21.

Moebus, M., Gashi, S., Hilty, M., Oldrati, P., and Holz, C., 2024. Meaningful digital biomarkers derived from wearable sensors to predict daily fatigue in multiple sclerosis patients and healthy controls. *iScience*, 27 (2), 108953.

Moghavem, N., Castañeda, G.R., Chatfield, A.J., and Amezcua, L., 2024. The impact of medical insurance on health care access and quality for people with multiple sclerosis in the United States: A scoping review. *Multiple Sclerosis Journal*, 30 (3), 299–307.

Nahum-Shani, I., Smith, S.N., Spring, B.J., Collins, L.M., Witkiewitz, K., Tewari, A., and Murphy, S.A., 2016. Just-in-time adaptive interventions (JITAIs) in mobile health: Key components and design principles for ongoing health behavior support. *Annals of Behavioral Medicine*, *52*(6), 446–462. https://doi.org/10.1007/s12160-016-9830-8.

Naji, Y., Mahdaoui, M., Klevor, R., Kissani, N., and Raymond, K., 2023. Artificial intelligence and multiple sclerosis: Up-to-date review. *Cureus*, 15 (9), e45863.

Naslund, J.A., Aschbrenner, K.A., Marsch, L.A., and Bartels, S.J., 2016. The future of mental health care: Peer-to-peer support and social media. *Epidemiology and Psychiatric Sciences*, 25 (2), 113–122.

National Institute of Neurological Disorders and Stroke, 2025. *Multiple Sclerosis [online].* Available at: https://www.ninds.nih.gov/health-information/disorders/multiple-sclerosis

National Multiple Sclerosis Society, 2025. *Cognitive health in multiple sclerosis [online].* Available at: https://www.nationalmssociety.org/managing-ms/living-with-ms/cognitive-health#:~:text=Reading,or%20to%20play%20an%20instrument

Nolte, E., and McKee, M., 2008. *EBOOK: Caring for people with chronic conditions: A health system perspective.* Maidenhead: McGraw-Hill Education.

Ontaneda, D., Thompson, A.J., Fox, R.J., and Cohen, J.A., 2017. Progressive multiple sclerosis: Prospects for disease therapy, repair, and restoration of function. *The Lancet*, 389 (10076), 1357–1366.

Organisation for Economic Co-operation and Development (OECD), 2023. *Health at a glance 2023: OECD indicators.* Paris: OECD Publishing.

Pakenham, K.I., and Cox, S., 2018. Effects of benefit finding, social support and caregiving on youth adjustment in a parental illness context. *Journal of Child and Family Studies*, 27 (8), 2491–2506.

Patient Protection and Affordable Care Act, Pub. L. No. 111-148, 124 Stat. 119 (2010).

Patient Self-Determination Act, Pub. L. No. 101-508, 104 Stat. 1388 (1990).

Pilehvari, S., Morgan, Y., and Peng, W., 2024. An analytical review on the use of artificial intelligence and machine learning in diagnosis, prediction, and risk factor analysis of multiple sclerosis. *Multiple Sclerosis and Related Disorders*, 89, 105761.

Portaccio, E., Magyari, M., Havrdova, E.K., Ruet, A., Brochet, B., Scalfari, A., Di Filippo, M., Tur, C., Montalban, X., and Amato, M.P., 2024. Multiple sclerosis: Emerging epidemiological trends and redefining the clinical course. *The Lancet Regional Health–Europe*, 44, 100997.

Rae-Grant, A.D., Turner, A.P., Sloan, A., Miller, D., Hunziker, J., and Haselkorn, J.K., 2011. Self-management in neurological disorders: Systematic review of the literature and potential interventions in multiple sclerosis care. *Journal of Rehabilitation Research & Development*, 48 (9), 1087–1100.

Rajkomar, A., Dean, J., and Kohane, I., 2019. Machine learning in medicine. *New England Journal of Medicine*, 380 (14), 1347–1358.

Richard, A.A., and Shea, K., 2011. Delineation of self-care and associated concepts. *Journal of Nursing Scholarship*, 43 (3), 255–264.

Rieke, N., Hancox, J., Li, W., Milletarì, F., Roth, H.R., Albarqouni, S., Bakas, S., Galtier, M.N., Landman, B.A., Maier-Hein, K., Ourselin, S., Sheller, M., Summers, R.M., Trask, A., Xu, D., Baust, M., and Cardoso, M.J., 2020. The future of digital health with federated learning. *NPJ Digital Medicine*, 3 (1), 119.

Russell, S.J., and Norvig, P., 2021. *Artificial intelligence: A modern approach* (Global Edition 4e). Harlow: Pearson.

Salas-Vega, S., Haimann, A., and Mossialos, E., 2015. Big data and health care: Challenges and opportunities for coordinated policy development in the EU. *Health Systems & Reform*, 1 (4), 285–300.

Salter, A., Lancia, S., Kowalec, K., Fitzgerald, K.C., and Marrie, R.A., 2024. Comorbidity and disease activity in multiple sclerosis. *JAMA Neurology*, 81 (11), 1170–1177.

Selby, J.V., Beal, A.C., and Frank, L., 2012. The patient-centered outcomes research institute (PCORI) national priorities for research and initial research agenda. *JAMA*, 307(15), 1583–1584. https://doi.org/10.1001/jama.2012.500

Sheikhalishahi, S., Miotto, R., Dudley, J.T., Lavelli, A., Rinaldi, F., and Osmani, V., 2019. Natural language processing of clinical notes on chronic diseases: Systematic review. *JMIR Medical Informatics*, 7 (2), e12239.

Sheller, M.J., Edwards, B., Reina, G.A., Martin, J., Pati, S., Kotrotsou, A., Milchenko, M., Xu, W., Marcus, D., Colen, R.R., and Bakas, S., 2020. Federated learning in medicine: Facilitating multi-institutional collaborations without sharing patient data. *Scientific Reports*, 10 (1), 12598.

Shickel, B., Tighe, P.J., Bihorac, A., and Rashidi, P., 2018. deep EHR: A survey of recent advances in deep learning techniques for electronic health record (EHR) analysis. *IEEE Journal of Biomedical and Health Informatics*, 22 (5), 1589–1604.

Stellefson, M., Hanik, B., Chaney, B., Chaney, D., Tennant, B., and Chavarria, E.A., 2011. eHealth literacy among college students: A systematic review with implications for eHealth education. *Journal of Medical Internet Research*, 13 (4), e102.

Strober, L.B., Becker, A., and Randolph, J.J., 2018. Role of positive lifestyle activities on mood, cognition, well-being, and disease characteristics in multiple sclerosis. *Applied Neuropsychology: Adult*, 25 (4), 304–311.

Tea, F., Groh, A.M., Lacey, C., and Fakolade, A., 2024. A scoping review assessing the usability of digital health technologies targeting people with multiple sclerosis. *NPJ Digital Medicine*, 7 (1), 168.

Thorne, S., Paterson, B., and Russell, C., 2003. The structure of everyday self-care decision making in chronic illness. *Qualitative Health Research*, 13 (10), 1337–1352.

U. S. Food and Drug Administration (FDA), 2021. *Artificial Intelligence/Machine learning (AI/ML)-based software as a medical device (SaMD) action plan.* Silver Spring, MD: U.S. Food and Drug Administration.

Umirzakova, S., Shakhnoza, M., Sevara, M., and Whangbo, T.K., 2025. Deep learning for multiple sclerosis lesion classification and stratification using MRI. *Computers in Biology and Medicine*, 192, 110078.

Wagner, E.H., Austin, B.T., Davis, C., Hindmarsh, M., Schaefer, J., and Bonomi, A., 2001. Improving chronic illness care: Translating evidence into action. *Health Affairs*, 20 (6), 64–78.

Walton, C., King, R., Rechtman, L., Kaye, W., Leray, E., Marrie, R.A., Robertson, N., La Rocca, N., Uitdehaag, B., and van Der Mei, I., 2020. Rising prevalence of multiple sclerosis worldwide: Insights from the Atlas of MS. *Multiple Sclerosis Journal*, 26 (14), 1816–1821.

Warsi, A., Wang, P.S., LaValley, M.P., Avorn, J., and Solomon, D.H., 2004. Self-management education programs in chronic disease: A systematic review and methodological critique of the literature. *Archives of Internal Medicine*, 164 (15), 1641–1649.

Wills, O.C., and Probst, Y.C., 2022. Understanding lifestyle self-management regimens that improve the life quality of people living with multiple sclerosis: A systematic review and meta-analysis. *Health and Quality of Life Outcomes*, 20 (1), 153.

Woodcock, E.W., 2022. Barriers to and facilitators of automated patient self-scheduling for health care organizations: Scoping review. *Journal of Medical Internet Research*, 24 (1), e28323.

World Health Organization (WHO), 2016. *Framework on integrated, people-centred health services: Report by the secretariat (A69/39).* Geneva: World Health Organization.

World Health Organization (WHO), 2021. *Global strategy on digital health 2020–2025.* Geneva: World Health Organization.

Yamada, Y., Shinkawa, K., Nemoto, M., and Arai, T., 2021. Automatic assessment of loneliness in older adults using speech analysis on responses to daily life questions. *Frontiers in Psychiatry*, 12, Article 712684.

Yamaguchi, S., and Yatsushiro, R., 2019. Significance and potential of self-management research for HTLV-1 associated myelopathy: Review of self-management for people with multiple sclerosis. *Journal of Rural Medicine*, 14 (1), 7–25.

Yang, Q., Li, X., Ding, X., Xu, F., and Ling, Z., 2022. Deep learning-based speech analysis for Alzheimer's disease detection: A literature review. *Alzheimer's Research & Therapy*, 14 (1), 186.

Yang, Q., Liu, Y., Chen, T., and Tong, Y., 2019. Federated machine learning: Concept and applications. *ACM Transactions on Intelligent Systems and Technology*, 10 (2), Article 12.

Yousef, H., Malagurski Tortei, B., and Castiglione, F., 2024. Predicting multiple sclerosis disease progression and outcomes with machine learning and MRI-based biomarkers: A review. *Journal of Neurology*, 271 (10), 6543–6572.

Yu, K., and Xie, X., 2020. Predicting hospital readmission: A joint ensemble-learning model. *IEEE Journal of Biomedical and Health Informatics*, 24 (2), 447–456.

Zhao, Y., Wang, T., Bove, R., Cree, B., Henry, R., Lokhande, H., Polgar-Turcsanyi, M., Anderson, M., Bakshi, R., and Weiner, H.L., 2020. Ensemble learning predicts multiple sclerosis disease course in the SUMMIT study. *NPJ Digital Medicine*, 3 (1), 135.

Ziemssen, T., and Haase, R., 2021. Digital innovation in multiple sclerosis management. *Brain Sciences*, 12 (1), 40.

Section II

Lived Experiences of Self-Management

13 Self-Management in Visual Impairment Rehabilitation

Yong Yang and Buxin Han

INTRODUCTION

Visual impairment, especially blindness, is a severe disability. It not only presents various etiologies and degrees of severity, but also can arise at any stage of life. Therefore, the impact of visual impairment on individuals is complex. This complexity leads to differences among individuals with visual impairment, and brings significant challenges to related research. As an individual with congenital visual impairment and a researcher in the mental health of individuals with visual impairment, I encountered the challenges due to this complexity and the scarcity of research while preparing this manuscript. During the writing process, I will endeavor to overcome these challenges and hope to facilitate a better understanding of visual impairment, individuals with visual impairment, and relevant knowledge about rehabilitation among readers.

I have congenital retinitis pigmentosa. In the early stages, aside from night blindness, color blindness, and the inability to discern subtle facial expressions, my visual impairment had a relatively minor impact on my studies and daily life. However, as my visual impairment progressively worsened, its effects became more pronounced, significantly challenging both my learning and everyday life. I found it increasingly difficult to see the content on the blackboard during classes and had to resort to using a magnifying glass to read books. I also relied on screen-reading software to operate computers and, eventually, began using a white cane. These experiences have deeply influenced my personal and professional life. Since 2006, I have been working and living alongside individuals with visual impairment, which has given me a broader perspective on the challenges we collectively face. My wife is also a person with congenital visual impairment. In 2018, I earned my master's degree in psychology, and currently, I am a Ph.D. candidate in psychology. Given the limited research and the complex nature of visual impairment, I would like to share my personal experiences and research findings on self-management in visual impairment rehabilitation. Rehabilitation is a multifaceted process that encompasses medical, psychological, and other aspects. Therefore, I will focus primarily on medical and psychological rehabilitation.

According to the World Health Organization (2019), at least 2.2 billion people worldwide are visually impaired or blind, including 123.7 million people with moderate or severe distance vision impairment or blindness. In fact, the causes for the visual impairment and blindness are extremely diverse. At the same time, their impacts are also complex and varied. Based on whether the causes are linked to the optic neural pathways, Begeer et al. (2014) divide visual impairment into ocular-plus blindness and ocular blindness. Based on the time of onset, visual impairment can further be divided into congenital visual impairment and acquired visual impairment. It's important to note that the concept of visual impairment is broad and inclusive. In addition to the classification mentioned above, it also includes blindness, light perception, and low vision. However, regardless of the type of visual impairment, it has serious consequences for the individual across the life course and has influences far beyond vision itself.

DOI: 10.1201/9781003599074-15

IMPACT OF VISUAL IMPAIRMENT ON PERCEPTION AND COGNITION

Visual impairment, especially blindness, is a severe disability. Its impact on perception, cognition, and other abilities is also complex and multifaceted, encompassing both positive and negative aspects.

Self-experience

As mentioned above, initially, the impact of visual impairment on me was mainly in terms of color perception and night blindness. Through saturation and brightness, I could distinguish colors, but it was difficult for me to name them accurately. For colors that are similar to each other, I could not differentiate them. At night, I mainly rely on my residual vision, hearing, touch, and sense of obstacles to navigate. As my visual impairment worsened, I also began to use a white cane. In special situations or at certain times, I also rely on my sense of smell to make judgments about my surroundings. Currently, when outdoors, especially in unfamiliar areas, it is difficult for me to form a cognitive map, which involves developing spatial awareness and memory of the surroundings. In social interactions, initially, I was not able to perceive subtle facial expressions, such as eye contact. Now, my visual impairment has progressed to the point where I can barely discern facial expressions and body language at all. My ability to perceive others' emotions has progressively transitioned from a reliance on residual vision and auditory cues to an almost exclusive dependence on hearing.

I have never been able to perceive micro-expressions, but this does not mean that I do not understand them. In fact, I can comprehend them through reading or descriptions from others. However, this mode of understanding also imposes limitations. Since I cannot perceive them visually, it is difficult for me to form a concrete mental image of a particular micro-expression (for example, a gaze). The impact of this visual absence extends far beyond this. For instance, when I recall an image of a smiling face in my mind, I can more easily feel the joy associated with it. In contrast, when I am asked to imagine a tender, affectionate gaze in my mind, not only do I lack an image of such a gaze, but I also struggle to experience the emotions conveyed by it. This is also true for individuals with congenital total blindness; they similarly find it difficult to form visual-based mental representations. A review study has shown that blind individuals have difficulty simulating emotional expressions (Valente et al. 2018).

Related Studies

Visual impairment significantly affects perception across various domains. Research on Gestalt perception has shown that children with cerebral visual impairment perform worse than those with normal sight, while children with ocular visual impairment fall between two groups (van der Zee et al. 2019). Infants with congenital blindness have weaker integration abilities of tactile and auditory information compared to infants with normal sight (Gori et al. 2021). However, individuals with visual impairment often develop enhanced abilities in other sensory modalities. For example, Alibegović et al. (2018) found that children with visual impairment had a better developed tactile perception compared to children with normal sight, and that there was a significant difference in two-point discrimination and stereognosis between two groups. This compensatory mechanism extends to social perception as well. Although individuals with visual impairment may struggle to detect subtle emotional states, they can rely on residual vision, hearing, touch, smell, or even their sense of obstacles to compensate (Qiu et al. 2020). In the domain of speech perception, visually impaired children face challenges due to the lack of visual models of speech movements, which negatively affects their speech sound discrimination (Brouwer et al. 2024; Brouwer and Gordon-Pershey 2021).

However, it is interesting to note that blind children often outperform their sighted peers in verbal working memory (Withagen et al. 2013). Finally, in terms of motion perception, individuals with cerebral visual impairment (CVI) exhibit deficits in motion perception (Pamir et al. 2021). Other sensory modalities (e.g., auditory and tactile) could influence the motion perception of individuals with visual impairment. For example, the reliance of individuals with congenital visual impairment on other sensory modalities could lead to the changes in motor representations associated with movement performed by others (Imbiriba et al. 2013).

Visual impairment influences cognition. A meta-analysis has shown that there is a bidirectional relationship between vision and cognition (Vu et al. 2021). A longitudinal study further found that visual impairment increased the risk of cognitive function impairment (Cao et al. 2023). Spatial cognition and theory of mind, as important cognitive abilities, are crucial for the mobility and social interaction of individuals with visual impairment, but these abilities are also negatively affected by visual impairment. Visual deprivation has a negative impact on the development of spatial ability. Visual impairment, especially congenital visual impairment, seriously hinders the development of spatial cognition, although other senses can play a certain degree of compensatory role (Bollini et al. 2023; Gori et al. 2021; Morelli et al. 2020). In fact, Bollini et al. (2023) found that the extent of the impact of visual impairment on spatial cognition varied depending on the severity of the visual impairment. Specifically, the visual spatial cognition of children with low vision is affected, but their auditory spatial cognition remains relatively intact. This suggests that the residual vision in low-vision children may still provide some degree of calibration, helping them to show comparable performance to sighted children in auditory conditions. In contrast, children with complete blindness are affected not only in visual spatial cognition but also in auditory spatial cognition. The complete absence of visual input impacts the development of the external spatial frame, which in turn affects their performance in auditory conditions.

Congenital visual impairment hinders theory of mind development in children and may even lead to deficits in theory of mind in adulthood. Mutual gaze, nonverbal referential communication (joint attention), and the observation of emotional states can contribute to theory of mind development. However, these are huge challenges for people with visual impairment. Visual impairment negatively influences theory of mind development. Research has shown that the development of first-order false belief in children with visual impairment is delayed (Brambring and Asbrock 2010; Green et al. 2004; Mcalpine and Moore 1995; Minter et al. 1998; Roch-Levecq 2006). However, research on adults with congenital visual impairment has shown that they and peers with normal sight recruit the same neural network for theory of mind processing (Bedny et al. 2009). Electroencephalographic studies on perspective-taking in adults with congenital blindness further showed the coexistence of deficits and compensatory mechanisms (Papageorgiou et al. 2020). This point is also supported by relevant studies. Language of children with visual impairment is correlated with theory of mind (Bartoli et al. 2019; Green et al. 2004; Pijnacker et al. 2012). Roch-Levecq (2006) also found that the visual acuity of children with visual impairment was significantly correlated with scores in theory of mind tasks. Additionally, other sensory modalities, including audition and olfaction, also play a compensatory role in social assessments among blind individuals, further highlighting the complexity of sensory interactions in theory of mind development (Sorokowska et al. 2018).

MEDICAL REHABILITATION: MULTISENSORY INTERVENTION STRATEGIES

Given the profound impact of visual impairment on perception and cognition, fostering the development of relevant abilities in individuals with visual impairments has become a critical component of the socialization process. In this process, making full use of residual vision and other senses is a core rehabilitation strategy and should be emphasized.

Gestalt Perception Ability Training

Gestalt perception is crucial for cognitive development. Research indicated that gestalt perception contributed to reasoning and problem-solving (Hong et al. 2021). However, van der Zee et al. (2019) found that children with visual impairments more often performed weakly than age-matched controls. Therefore, it is necessary to leverage residual vision and other senses to promote the development of gestalt perception. According to the principles of Gestalt perception, targeted training can be conducted through the following methods:

Part-to-Whole Integration Training. In rehabilitation training and daily life, a methodology involving the sequential presentation of partial information from images or objects is employed. This approach guides individuals with visual impairments to utilize their residual vision and tactile to incrementally construct a comprehensive visual or tactile mental representation. By doing so, it reinforces their capacity for information integration, which in turn fosters the development of higher-order cognitive functions such as reasoning and problem-solving.

Training in Categorization and Inductive Reasoning. By leveraging multi-sensory channels such as residual vision, touch, and hearing, this approach helps individuals with visual impairments compare the characteristic differences of various objects, categorize them, and ultimately promote concept formation.

Improvement in Speech Perception

Children with visual impairments face significant challenges in speech and language development, particularly in the areas of phonological awareness, speech perception, and speech production (Brouwer et al. 2024; Brouwer and Gordon-Pershey 2021; Georgiou 2020). These challenges may affect their early literacy and communication skills. A multi-sensory intervention strategy is required.

Residual Vision Assistance. Brouwer and Gordon-Pershey (2021) argued that the lack of access to visual models of speech movements could be a key factor in speech sound discrimination and speech sound production delays or deficits. Leveraging their residual vision, children with visual impairments can observe a speaker's lip patterns and facial expressions, which facilitates a greater understanding and more accurate imitation of speech. This capacity for visually-assisted speech comprehension and imitation not only contributes to more effective learning of speech production and discrimination but also enhances phonological awareness and fosters speech perception.

Enhancing Role of Haptics. In a Braille reading task, individuals with early blindness exhibited stronger functional connectivity in key brain regions associated with language and memory compared to those with late blindness (Ankeeta et al. 2021). This enhanced functional connectivity suggests that early tactile training and Braille education can effectively leverage brain plasticity to promote the development of language and memory skills. Tactile training can include speech perception training (e.g., perception of vocal cord vibrations and lip movements), tactile memory training (e.g., learning Braille letters and words, tactile memory exercises), as well as comprehensive language training (e.g., Braille reading).

Utilizing Auditory Strengths. Visually impaired children significantly outperform sighted children in auditory and verbal memory tasks, especially in working memory tasks involving language processing (Withagen et al. 2013). This auditory advantage establishes a vital basis for speech development and should be maximized. First, auditory discrimination training enhances children's sensitivity to different speech sounds, particularly to similar ones. Second, conducting auditory memory retelling training helps children with visual impairments better process and remember linguistic information. Finally, encourage children with visual impairments to express themselves actively and create a rich and diverse language environment for them, including activities like listening to stories, and communicating with their parents and other children.

Cultivation of Spatial Cognition and Navigation Skills

Vision plays a crucial role in the development of spatial cognition. Visual impairment significantly impairs this ability (Bollini et al. 2023; Morelli et al. 2020; Zou and Zhou 2023). Nevertheless, evidence from both case studies and experimental research demonstrates that multi-sensory information, including auditory, tactile, and olfactory information, is of critical importance to the spatial cognition and navigation of individuals with visual impairments (Ferah 2025; Morelli et al. 2020; Papadopoulos et al. 2018). Therefore, the full utilization of residual vision and non-visual senses is essential for the spatial cognitive rehabilitation of individuals with visual impairments.

Residual Vision. Children with low vision have impaired visual spatial cognition, while children with complete blindness have impaired visual and auditory spatial cognition (Bollini et al. 2023). Better navigation performance is associated with higher visual acuity in individuals with visual impairments (Zou and Zhou 2023). Parents should help children with visual impairments develop their visual-spatial cognition and multi-sensory spatial cognitive integration skills. For example, locating or grasping objects can effectively train the visual-spatial cognitive abilities of children with visual impairments. Combining residual vision with hearing and touch can help these children better perceive space, exercise multi-sensory spatial cognitive integration, and promote the development of spatial cognition. Adults with visual impairments can utilize their residual vision to perceive their surroundings, identify key landmarks, and orient themselves in space.

Non-visual Senses. A case study showed that auditory and tactile training improved spatial localization and cognition in the visually impaired child (Morelli et al. 2020). Hearing, touch, and smell are also important senses for spatial orientation and navigation in adults with visual impairments (Ferah 2025). For children with visual impairments, training in auditory discrimination—such as identifying different sounds and their directions—haptic perception of an object's position and spatial relationships, and olfactory recognition of various scents, collectively enhances their spatial orientation and spatial cognition. For adults with visual impairments, spatial orientation and navigation are significantly enhanced by auditory perception of environmental sounds, tactile detection of obstacles and street edges, and olfactory discrimination of ambient smells.

Promoting Theory of Mind Development

Theory of mind development involves the interaction between visual and linguistic experience (Bedny and Saxe 2012). Initially, vision is dominant. With the development of verbal skills, language is increasingly important. Individuals with visual impairments rely more on hearing in social interactions (Sorokowska et al. 2018). Therefore, utilizing residual vision, hearing, and language can promote theory of mind development.

Utilizing Residual Vision. The visual acuity of children with visual impairments is significantly correlated with scores in theory of mind tasks (Roch-Levecq 2006). Infants' observation of others' behaviors, maternal language, and the development of their own language jointly promote theory of mind development (Ruffman 2023). Consequently, individuals with visual impairments can leverage their residual vision for the observation of others' facial expressions and physical gestures, thereby understanding others' emotions and intentions. Moreover, through the application of a modified "Three Mountains Task" paradigm, they can train their visual perspective-taking ability and overcome the cognitive limitations of egocentrism.

Auditory and Language Reinforcement. Visually impaired children's language is positively correlated with theory of mind (Bartoli et al. 2019; Pijnacker et al. 2012). The link between language and cognition begins to emerge in three-month-old infants, and this link promotes cognitive development and extends beyond infants' initial cognitive capacities (Perszyk and Waxman 2018). Adults with visual impairments rely more on auditory cues for social perception (Sorokowska et al. 2018). Consequently, in interactions with visually impaired individuals, the use of mental state language (e.g., describing others' feelings, thoughts) can promote their theory of mind development. Moreover, reading literary works is an effective way to enhance theory of mind. In terms of hearing, visually impaired individuals can judge others' emotions through intonation and tone of voice.

Rehabilitation Advice Based on Personal Experience

Based on the research, this chapter explores how to utilize residual vision and non-visual senses to promote the development of perception, speech, spatial cognition, and theory of mind. Subsequently, based on my personal experience, this chapter will further elaborate on the relevant perspectives.

Residual vision is crucial for the perceptual and cognitive development of individuals with visual impairments. It was only as I gained a deeper understanding of visual impairment that I gradually recognized its importance. It is my hope that individuals with visual impairments and the relevant parties will fully appreciate the role of residual vision and utilize it in a rational and scientific manner. Drawing on personal experience, this chapter explores the topic from three perspectives. First, the relevant parties should help visually impaired children make the most of residual vision to promote cognitive development and enhance social adaptation skills. Second, in the process of utilizing residual vision, individuals with visual impairments can make use of assistive devices, such as optical magnifiers and electronic visual aids. Finally, individuals with visual impairments should protect their residual vision by balancing work and rest. At the same time, they should learn to use screen reader software as early as possible. Screen readers can not only reduce reliance on electronic visual aids but also effectively support learning and work. For example, after using an electronic visual aid for an extended period during the postgraduate entrance exam, I experienced blurred vision and severe visual fatigue once the test was over.

Second, multisensory integration can compensate for visual impairments. The information conveyed by vision is multidimensional and rich, while non-visual senses find it more difficult to provide information of equivalent richness. Therefore, individuals with visual impairments must rely on multisensory integration to complete daily life tasks. Multisensory integration is a crucial ability for them to cope with the challenges of life. When navigating independently, I rely on my residual vision, hearing, touch, and smell. One night in the first year of my PhD, I made my first solo trip back to the dormitory from the office. A journey that should have taken 20 minutes ended up taking over 40 minutes because I got lost. Getting lost made me very anxious. The fear of being discovered and embarrassed made me even more nervous. This made it difficult for me to effectively use hearing and touch for spatial orientation. Subsequently, I quickly adjusted my emotions and conducted spatial localization through Multisensory integration. First, I used my hearing to identify the sound of traffic, confirming that the road outside campus was to my right. Then, I proceeded in the opposite direction, using my touch to locate distinctive landmarks. After locating the uneven ground through the tactile in my feet, I continued to move forward and touched the holly with my hands. These distinctive markers helped me find my bearings, allowing me to return to the dormitory smoothly.

Finally, in terms of language, I also have some points to make. First, the inability to see phonetic symbols increases the difficulty of learning the pronunciation of English words. When I can see the phonetic symbols, I can quickly learn the pronunciation of words. At present, I can only learn through repeated listening, combined with the application of pronunciation rules. Therefore, parents of children with visual impairments should help their children master pronunciation as early as possible to promote language development. Second, when the intonation does not match the emotional content conveyed by the words, I find it difficult to accurately infer others' emotions. At this time, proactive communication can eliminate misunderstandings. This, in turn, leads to a better understanding and inference of others' mental states. Finally, visual impairment also affects my emotional perception. For example, although I can literally understand the emotional message conveyed by an affectionate gaze, the emotional experience it evokes within me is relatively weak. For example, when I hear about or see the unfortunate experiences of individuals with disabilities, I feel a stronger sadness. Therefore, in social situations, individuals with visual impairments should be aware of their emotions in a timely manner and avoid letting their visual impairment experiences affect them.

IMPACT OF VISUAL IMPAIRMENT ON MENTAL HEALTH

Self-Experience

Due to the uniqueness of my eye condition, I had never studied or lived with members of the visually impaired community before graduating from university, nor had I truly accepted my own identity as a visually impaired person. To break free from the potential negative impacts of visual impairment, I consistently strived to study and worked. When others pointed fingers at me or talked about my visual impairment, I would suppress my negative emotions and force myself to hold back from showing vulnerability. However, when this suppression exceeded the limit I could bear, I would also lose control of my emotions, get into arguments with people, and even lash out physically in a moment of impulse.

Actually, the non-acceptance of my visual impairment left me confused when it came to career choices. My parents, first teachers, and friends all encouraged me to change my fate through education, so I made great efforts to pursue higher education. After graduating from college, my visual impairment led to repeated setbacks in my job hunting, making it difficult for me to find a suitable job. After a period of struggle, I began to live and work with visually impaired individuals. During this process, I met my wife, who is also visually impaired. When interacting with them, I noticed that despite their visual impairment, they could face life proactively and effectively. I also inadvertently began to accept my own identity as a visually impaired person. After getting married, my wife and I made a joint decision that I would pursue a postgraduate degree in psychology to better assist the visually impaired community. Under the meticulous guidance of my supervisor, I clarified my research direction and have been focusing on the mental health of visually impaired individuals.

Related Studies

Individuals with visual impairments face more severe mental health problems. Sims et al. (2018) argued that youth with visual impairments were at increased risk for mental illnesses and general mental health concerns. A systematic review and meta-analysis showed that the overall pooled prevalence of depression or dysthymia among visually impaired children or adolescents was 14% (Bakhla et al. 2023). Two Longitudinal studies from China also found that visual impairment significantly predicted depression and anxiety (Yao et al. 2024; Zhao et al. 2022).

It is crucial to study the factors that promote the mental health of individuals with visual impairments for psychological rehabilitation. Zapata and Pearlstein (2022) found that lower disability self-worth was significantly associated with higher depression and anxiety in individuals with visual impairments. Additionally, social isolation, perceived support, and experiences of adverse events are independently associated with visually impaired individuals' depressive symptoms (Brunes and

Heir 2020). Kurtović and Ivančić (2019) argued that optimism, pessimism, self-esteem, and social functioning should be focused on to prevent depression in rehabilitation practices of individuals with visual impairments.

PSYCHOLOGICAL REHABILITATION: AN INTERVENTION BASED ON THE FIVE DIMENSIONS

Rehabilitation encompasses medical rehabilitation and psychological rehabilitation. Traditional rehabilitation services overly focus on providing material assistance and skills training, while neglecting the emotional, psychological, identity, and social belonging needs of visually impaired individuals (Watermeyer and Botha 2025). This neglect is detrimental to comprehensive rehabilitation, especially psychological rehabilitation. Based on cultural differences, Kirmayer (2007) categorized the self into egocentric self, sociocentric self, ecocentric self, and cosmocentric self. Based on traditional Chinese culture, Han and Kong (2025) proposed the Four-fold Self Theory, including individual, social, natural, and cosmic levels.

In the practice of psychological rehabilitation, how visually impaired individuals properly handle the relationships between visual impairment and the self, others, and the world—thereby effectively coping with various challenges, improving their own mental health, exploring the meaning of life, and realizing self-worth—is undoubtedly a highly profound and pressing issue that urgently requires exploration. Based on the aforementioned discussions, personal experiences, and my empirical research, five dimensions (self-compassion, forgiveness, gratitude, attachment, and spirituality) are selected. Based on these dimensions, I will discuss their current research status and my own experience, with the aim of providing beneficial guidance for visually impaired individuals on their journey of psychological rehabilitation.

SELF-COMPASSION

Self-compassion, which can be understood as compassion for the experience of suffering turned inward, is a productive way of approaching distressing thoughts and emotions (Neff 2023). It engenders mental and physical well-being. Davies et al. (2021) found that self-compassion and shame mediated the relationship between adverse interpersonal experiences and self-esteem for individuals with intellectual disabilities. A longitudinal study with autistic individuals also showed that there were negative correlations between self-compassion and subsequent anxiety/depression (Galvin et al. 2024). These findings have also been verified in relevant studies involving individuals without disabilities. Self-compassion mediates the link between childhood maltreatment and psychopathology (Lassri and Gewirtz-Meydan 2022), and between childhood maltreatment and depression (Tao et al. 2021). Additionally, a few meta-analyses showed that self-compassion was negatively associated with psychological distress (Baxter and Sirois 2025; Marsh et al. 2018), and positively associated with physical health and health behavior (Phillips and Hine 2021). Finally, self-compassion contributes to compassion for others (Lalor and Khoshfetrat 2024) and reduces aggression (Guan et al. 2024). In summary, self-compassion can help us better cope with the challenges of life, enhance our mental health and improve our quality of life. Whether in facing personal suffering or in our interactions with others, self-compassion can play a positive role.

Self-compassion is not just a fixed personality trait, it is a skill that can be learned and practiced (Neff 2023). Neff thinks that self-compassion includes three domains and six elements—how people emotionally respond to suffering (with kindness or judgment), how they cognitively understand their predicament (as part of the human experience or as isolating), and how they pay attention to suffering (in a mindful or overly identified manner). According to the domains and elements, mindfulness practice, Diary of Self-Critical and Self-Compassionate Thoughts, and Compassionate letter writing are effective interventions (Arimitsu 2016; Gilbert and Procter 2006; Neff 2023).

Mindfulness practice. Mindfulness practices focus on enhancing awareness of the present moment through practices such as mindful breathing, body scans, and mindful eating. It helps individuals to develop a non-judgmental attitude towards their own experiences, thereby facilitating more effective observation and management of their cognitive and affective processes. The enhancement of this ability, in turn, promotes the development of self-compassion. Taking mindfulness breathing as an example, it is a simple and effective method of mindfulness practice. Its core lies in helping practitioners cultivate awareness of the present moment by focusing on the process of breathing. During the practice, when thoughts and other sensations arise, practitioners simply need to perceive their presence, avoid self-judgment, and then gently redirect their attention back to breathing.

Diary of self-critical and self-compassionate thoughts. The diary of Self-Critical and Self-Compassionate Thoughts is a tool for recording and reflecting on self-critical and self-compassionate thoughts. When using it, first record the situations that trigger self-criticism or self-compassion, then describe the corresponding thoughts and feelings in detail. By comparing the impact of these two thought patterns on emotions and behaviors, we ultimately explore how to respond to future challenges with greater self-compassion.

Self-compassion writing. Self-compassion writing is a method of expressing kindness and understanding toward oneself through writing, in order to enhance one's level of self-compassion. Its purpose is to guide individuals to experience the three core components of self-compassion through writing—mindfulness (focusing on present-moment feelings), common humanity (recognizing that life challenges are part of being human), and self-kindness (actively showing concern for our own distress). Based on previous research findings, we provide two templates for writing to support effective practice.

Self-compassion related to body (Gracias and Stutts 2024). The text consists of four parts. First, you should write what happened, your thoughts and feelings. Second, you should write a message to yourself about accepting any "flaws" (e.g., I accept my body despite, etc.). Third, you should write a message to yourself focusing on your body's functions, purpose, and its strengths (e.g., I appreciate that my body allows me to, etc.). Finally, you should write a message to yourself expressing kindness and love toward your body (e.g., I will treat my body with kindness, etc.).

Self-compassion related to adverse experience (Wang et al. 2024). The text consists of three parts. The first focuses on mindfulness of self-compassion. You should write down your thoughts and feelings about the adverse event that you have experienced. The second focuses on self-kindness. After Imagining that a close friend were to experience a similar event, you write down your concern to him/her. The third focuses on common humanity). You should write down other people in your life and the similar events.

Forgiveness

Forgiveness is an affective, cognitive, and behavioral phenomenon in which negative reactions toward one's offender are reduced, not by denying one's right to such reactions but by viewing the offender with compassion, benevolence, and love (Vismaya et al. 2024). Meta-analyses have demonstrated that forgiveness interventions promote mental well-being (Akhtar and Barlow 2018); additionally, forgiveness is positively correlated with physical health (Lee and Enright 2019). Byra et al. (2020) further found that forgiveness was positively correlated with the acceptance of disability.

Enright's process model and REACH model are two important and effective interventions in promoting forgiveness (Akhtar and Barlow 2018; Vismaya et al. 2024). Although Enright's process model is more effective than REACH model, the latter relies more on self-direction. Therefore, the two models are introduced.

Enright's process model includes four stages. The first is the uncovering stage. Individuals acknowledge and confront their pain, anger, or hurt caused by others, as well as identify their defense mechanisms. The second is the decision stage. Individuals commit to forgive. The third is the work stage. Individuals engage in cognitive and emotional work to reframe their perspective on the offense. The fourth is the deepening stage. Individuals focus on finding new meaning in life.

REACH model includes five steps, which are recall, empathy, altruistic, commit, and hold. The first step is to recall thoughts, feelings, and behaviors associated with the hurt as much as possible. The second step is to develop empathy for the offender. The third is to perform altruistic acts of forgiveness. The fourth step is to make a commitment to forgive. The fifth step is to hold onto forgiveness in times of difficulty.

Although forgiveness can reduce victims' negative reactions, it is not essential to the healing process. The level and frequency of abuse can affect the effectiveness of forgiveness (Cowden et al. 2019; Lahav et al. 2019). Forgiveness mediates the association between relational dependence and stronger intentions to return to the abusive partner (Crapolicchio et al. 2021). Hence, forgiveness can increase the risk of repeated abuse. Finally, forgiveness is a right of the victim, never an obligation, as well as not equating to reconciliation.

Gratitude

Gratitude is a general state of appreciation and thankfulness for the personal benefit individuals perceive that they have received from others (Kirca et al. 2023). The meta-analyses demonstrate that gratitude interventions can significantly enhance mental health, as evidenced by increased life satisfaction, positive emotions, and happiness, as well as a reduction in symptoms of anxiety and depression (Diniz et al. 2023; Kirca et al. 2023). Moreover, gratitude is also very important for individuals with disabilities. Research showed that gratitude of individuals with physical disabilities could predict their optimism (Lestari and Fajar 2020).

Tolcher et al. (2024) argued that gratitude journaling had a more significant positive impact on well-being and affective functioning, Compared with the other two gratitude interventions (reflection and app prompted reflection). According to the study by Hartanto et al. (2023), we should write a gratitude journal following the instructions below:

There are many things in our lives, both large and small, that we might be grateful for. Think back over the past day and write down in detail three things that you are grateful for today. Furthermore, please elaborate on why you feel grateful and provide contextual information where necessary.

For individuals with disabilities, gratitude can also be an extremely complex issue. Individuals with disabilities who had access to paid personal assistants often felt more comfortable and in control of their lives, while those who relied on the goodwill of others often experienced a considerable amount of shame and frustration in relation to their ongoing needs (Galvin 2004). Specifically, paid care allows them to express their gratitude through economic compensation, and this form of gratitude is healthy and does not have a negative impact on their mental health. In contrast, unpaid care, due to the lack of economic compensation, turns gratitude into a psychological burden, which has an adverse effect on the mental health of individuals with disabilities.

Attachment

Attachment develops in childhood based upon child–caregiver interactions, specifically how successful the infant is in their proximity-seeking behavior in times of threat (Hirst et al. 2019). Attachment anxiety and attachment avoidance are the two primary dimensions of insecure attachment (Hirst et al. 2019; Zheng et al. 2020). Individuals with attachment anxiety are characterized by a fear of being abandoned or rejected by others and tend to employ hyperactivating emotion-regulation strategies. In contrast, individuals with attachment avoidance are characterized by a tendency to avoid emotional closeness with others and typically use deactivating emotion-regulation strategies.

Meta-analyses have revealed that anxious attachment and avoidant attachment are negatively correlated with forgiveness (Hirst et al. 2019), self - compassion (Huang and Wu 2025), and interpersonal trust (Bao et al. 2022), while they are positively correlated with depression (Zheng et al. 2020). Another meta-analysis has shown that parents' insecure attachment is positively correlated with child maltreatment, indicating that parents with insecure attachment are more likely to have a tendency to abuse their children (Lo et al. 2019).

Although few attempts have been made to develop interventions to promote attachment security, existing studies provide some insights. A meta-analysis has revealed that Paternal and maternal sensitivity is correlated with child attachment security (Madigan et al. 2024). Another meta-analysis has shown that the maltreated infants are significantly more likely to have an insecure attachment than the controls (Baer and Martinez 2006). Hence, the key insights are as follows:

First, an attachment figure needs to be sensitive to the emotions and needs of an individual with visual impairment and provides appropriate and timely responses.

Second, an attachment figure should provide emotional support to an individual with visual impairment, encourage him/her to express his/her feelings, and offer positive feedback.

Third, an attachment figure should avoid maltreating an individual with visual impairment.

Finally, an individual with visual impairment should establish positive interactive relationships with his/her peers.

Spirituality

Spirituality is the dynamic dimension of human life that relates to the way individuals experience, express and seek meaning, purpose and transcendence, and the way they connect to the moment, to self, to others, to nature, to the significant and the sacred (Timmins et al. 2023). A meta-analysis of longitudinal studies showed that religion or spirituality had a positive effect on mental health (Garssen et al. 2021). Another meta-analysis revealed that the counseling and spiritual care program could significantly reduce the anxiety levels of patients with chronic diseases and improve their quality of life, treatment, and recovery processes (Salari et al. 2023). Spirituality is a source of strength for individuals with disabilities to cope with difficulties. Older people with intellectual disability seek and receive solace from religious and spiritual practices, especially when they are lonely, in poor health, distressed, or bereaved (Timmins et al. 2023). Mugeere et al. (2020) argued that religiosity and spirituality gave individuals with disabilities the strength to keep going and understand the events in their lives when they were swimming against the tide of challenges.

Despite the relative scarcity of research on how to foster spiritual development, the existing studies still offer many valuable insights. Hajinejad et al. (2019) argued that insight in personal belief, spiritual socialization, and peace of mind could promote spirituality among the older adults. A meta-analysis has further shown that secular mindfulness programs can enhance spirituality, and this enhancement persists even after the program has ended (Landau and Jones 2021).

Spirituality and religion may be important factors in facilitating adjustment and wellness for individuals with disabilities. However, according to the study by Hodge and Reynolds (2019), individuals with disabilities could experience a decline in their religious faith and participation, especially when they question God or feel disappointed due to their disabilities.

Rehabilitation Advice Based on Personal Experience

Visual impairment brings us many additional difficulties and challenges. As the widely circulated proverb goes: "When God closes a door for you, he will surely open a window for you." For individuals with visual impairments, finding that open window may be difficult. However, a good mental state is the key to overcoming challenges. It illuminates the path forward like a bright lamp, giving us strength and courage. In the earlier parts, the research status of the five dimensions—self-compassion, forgiveness, gratitude, attachment, and spirituality—has been discussed. Next, I will share my own experiences. I hope this can help you understand my psychological journey from the door to the window and provide you with more insights.

Self-Compassion

Congenital visual impairment is like an invisible giant hand that clings to me tightly, never leaving my side. It is also like that vulnerable and helpless "child" deep in my heart—often sorrowful, robbing me of peace. Since I left the small mountain village where I was born and raised to pursue my studies, and later became a doctoral student in psychology, I have been striving to break free from its restraints, yet I have never succeeded. Until one day, it suddenly dawned on me: I have long been integrated with it. It is a part of my life. I am it, and it is me.

When I hear someone say that I am "blind," this "child" inside me becomes incredibly vulnerable in an instant, feeling sad and upset, and may even fly into a rage. He makes me cry silently and also makes me explode with anger, even to the point of hitting someone. At that moment, I have no idea whether these feelings of pain, anger, and helplessness belong to him or to me. But as time goes by, I begin to understand that these feelings are both his and mine. They are a part of my life, the weakest and most genuine part of myself deep inside.

I also truly regard him as my own child, loving him, understanding him, encouraging him, supporting him, and tolerating him with all my heart, and giving him the space and time to grow. In this process, I gradually learn to reconcile with him, accept his existence, and even begin to be grateful for him. Because he allows me to understand myself more profoundly and makes me stronger.

One night, I was crossing the street alone. When I accidentally bumped into someone, the person turned around and shouted angrily, "Are you blind or something?!" I calmly replied, "Sorry, I really am blind." After saying that, my eyes filled with tears and I felt mixed emotions. At that moment, I suddenly realized that the "child" who once felt vulnerable and helpless because of his blindness had slowly grown up and become strong. I had learned to face other people's misunderstandings and accusations without being easily swayed by my emotions. I knew that I had begun to accept my own imperfections and had learned to reconcile with myself.

Forgiveness and Gratitude

Compared with people without disabilities, we may encounter more misunderstandings, discrimination, and even abuse. If we hold onto resentment, it is like a whirlpool that traps us in an inescapable cycle and pulls us deeper into it. Forgiveness is not a sign of weakness, but a wisdom of life and a sublimation of the soul. It is not for those who have hurt us, but for ourselves. It enables us to break free from the whirlpool of resentment, ground ourselves in the present, and live well.

I have told myself many times that I should forgive those who hurt me. Yet a voice inside me always questions why I should forgive. So I then tell myself not to forgive, but to take revenge. But another voice soon follows, asking what difference there will be between me and them after taking revenge. I sink deeper into pain and confusion. Countless struggles amid this confusion have made me realize that I need to step back and view all the people and things around me from a higher perspective. It's like standing atop a tall building—everything below seems so tiny, with adults looking like infants, while the distant scenery stretches endlessly. In fact, aren't those setbacks just a faint splash of color in the painting of my life?

It was not until that moment of realizing this that I finally came to my senses, suddenly understanding why visually impaired performers paid no mind to children's teasing. Looking back on the past, when I was a child, I once joined a group of friends in making fun of visually impaired performers. We shouted "blind" loudly at them and even mimicked the way they walked. Yet they remained unperturbed, continuing to focus wholeheartedly on their performances without distraction. Perhaps, in their eyes, we were just ignorant, innocent children. The memory made me truly understand why we should allow others' ignorance and narrow-mindedness to turn into shackles that bind us. We should instead ground ourselves in the present and focus on our own affairs—just as those performers did, choosing to rise above trivial hurt and hold fast to what matters most in their lives.

In our daily lives, others often lend us a helping hand. These acts of assistance help us extricate ourselves from difficult situations, endow us with the strength to confront the future head-on, and make us feel love and hope. When we encounter discrimination, the help from others can also alleviate the negative impact caused by discrimination to a certain extent. Frankly speaking, such help can sometimes leave us with a sense of helplessness, especially when we have no way to repay it.

In fact, I have received help from many people. Among them were teachers, classmates, strangers, and even individuals with visual impairments. After graduating from college, I once fell into a difficult situation: I couldn't find a job and had to live a wandering life alone in Beijing. Just when I was at my most helpless, a person with blindness took me in and patiently taught me the skills of traditional Chinese medicine massage. His help allowed me to barely gain a foothold in this city. Before he passed away, he told me, "You have the ability to do more things that are meaningful—things that matter more to our community." This experience not only enabled me to master a skill but also helped me understand the significance of helping others. Later, I encountered my beloved supervisor, Buxin Han. It was he who opened the door to psychology for me and guided me onto this path filled with exploration and discovery. The phrase he bestowed upon me—"Do one's duty, give one's best, and never give up"—is like a beacon of light that illuminates my way forward at all times and motivates me to keep moving ahead. This saying from my mentor has also become my family motto; it has integrated into my life, serving as my courage when facing difficulties, my wisdom when making choices, and my humility when achieving success.

During the seven years I spent pursuing my doctoral degree, I endured immense pressure. Yet, it was the pieces of help I had received in the past—like beacons of light—that illuminated my path forward, allowing me to see hope amid hardships and find direction when I felt lost. I deeply understand that it is precisely this warm assistance that has shaped me into the person I am today. I often quietly tell myself that I must repay their kindness of recognizing my potential. However, fate is cruel: that person with blindness has passed away. Every time I think about being unable to repay his kindness, my heart is filled with endless sorrow.

Attachment and Spirituality

Compared with other groups of individuals with disabilities, individuals with visual impairments tend to rely more on the help of others. Therefore, good interpersonal relationships are of vital importance to us. In fact, interpersonal relationships are extremely closely related to our attachment styles. Individuals with visual impairments who have a secure attachment style are often able to build a stronger sense of security and more easily develop healthy and stable interpersonal relationships. This sense of security not only makes us more confident when interacting with others, but also provides emotional comfort and psychological support when we face difficulties and challenges, helping us better cope with various situations in life.

I have established a secure attachment with my father. When he was alive, he sincerely told me on several occasions that if his eyes could be transplanted to me, he would do so without hesitation. Similarly, my wife has also built this precious attachment bond with her father. However, fate is unpredictable. During my pursuit of a doctoral degree, our fathers passed away one after another, plunging my wife and me into profound grief at the same time.

Secure attachment undoubtedly plays a crucial role in our lives. It endows us with the courage and strength to face life's challenges. It is precisely this solid emotional foundation that helps us get through the difficult times in life. Nevertheless, the passing of our loved ones still leaves us with profound emotional trauma. After my father passed away, for as long as three years, I couldn't even conjure up his face in my mind. This feeling was as if I had never had a father.

Spirituality holds profound significance for us. It enables us to gain a deep understanding of the meaning of life. Conversely, the exploration of life's meaning also motivates us to pay attention to and nurture our own spirituality.

For me, the meaning of life lies in contributing something meaningful to the visually impaired community. Specifically, it means dedicating myself to promoting our mental health and advancing our engagement in psychological counseling and education work. This life purpose has sustained me in the past decade or so, no matter what challenges I have faced. As the meaning of life becomes increasingly clear, my spirituality has also continued to grow. I suddenly feel that my inner self is more peaceful, and I have more wisdom to face various challenges in life.

Fate has bestowed upon the visually impaired community a life of great heaviness. Yet this heaviness is not unendurable. Visual impairment gives us the chance to feel more of the love in the world, and also allows us to more profoundly perceive the cruelty of human nature. The former endows us with the courage to face life's harsh realities head-on, while the latter grants us the wisdom to transcend suffering.

How can we transform this heavy life into a source of human wealth and wisdom—one that nourishes people's souls, alleviates suffering in the world, and brings happiness and peace? This is perhaps the shared mission that our community bears. May each of us, guided by this mission, find our own life's compass, let our lives shine with a unique radiance amid challenges, leave our footprints in the progress of human civilization, and add a touch of warmth and hope to this world.

REFERENCES

Akhtar, S., & Barlow, J. (2018). Forgiveness therapy for the promotion of mental well-being: A systematic review and meta-analysis. Trauma, Violence, & Abuse, 19(1), 107–122.

Alibegović, D. R., Teskeredžić, A., & Kudumović, A. (2018). Differences in tactile perception in children with and without visual impairment. Human: Journal for Interdisciplinary Studies, 8(2), 65–70.

Ankeeta, A., Saxena, R., Kumaran, S. S., Dwivedi, S. N., Jagannathan, N. R., & Narang, V. (2021). Evaluation of memory and language network in children and adolescents with visual impairment: A combined functional connectivity and voxel-based morphometry study. Neuro-Ophthalmology, 45(3), 147–161.

Arimitsu, K. (2016). The effects of a program to enhance self-compassion in Japanese individuals: A randomized controlled pilot study. The Journal of Positive Psychology, 11(6), 559–571.

Baer, J. C., & Martinez, C. D. (2006). Child maltreatment and insecure attachment: A meta-analysis. Journal of Reproductive and Infant Psychology, 24(3), 187–197.

Bakhla, A. K., Pallavi, P., Kisku, R. R., Goyal, N., Kumar, A., & Prasad, K. (2023). Prevalence of depression in visually impaired children and adolescents: A systematic review and meta-analysis. Indian Journal of Psychiatry, 65(4), 396–403.

Bao, X., Li, S., Zhang, Y., Tang, Q., & Chen, X. (2022). Different effects of anxiety and avoidance dimensions of attachment on interpersonal trust: A multilevel meta-analysis. Journal of Social and Personal Relationships, 39(7), 2069–2093.

Bartoli, G., Bulgarelli, D., & Molina, P. (2019). Theory of mind development in children with visual impairment: The contribution of the adapted comprehensive test ToM storybooks. Journal of Autism and Developmental Disorders, 49(9), 3494–3503. https://doi.org/10.1007/s10803-019-04064-3

Baxter, R., & Sirois, F. M. (2025). Self-compassion and psychological distress in chronic illness: A meta-analysis. British Journal of Health Psychology, 30(1), e12761.

Bedny, M., Pascual-Leone, A., & Saxe, R. R. (2009). Growing up blind does not change the neural bases of theory of mind. Proceedings of the National Academy of Sciences, 106(27), 11312–11317. https://doi.org/10.1073/pnas.0900010106

Bedny, M., & Saxe, R. (2012). Insights into the origins of knowledge from the cognitive neuroscience of blindness. Cognitive Neuropsychology, 29(1–2), 56–84.

Begeer, S., Dik, M., Voor De Wind, M. J., Asbrock, D., Brambring, M., & Kef, S. (2014). A new look at theory of mind in children with ocular and ocular-plus congenital blindness. Journal of Visual Impairment & Blindness, 108(1), 17–27.

Bollini, A., Cocchi, E., Salvagno, V., & Gori, M. (2023). The causal role of vision in the development of spatial coordinates: Evidence from visually impaired children. Journal of Experimental Psychology: Human Perception and Performance, 49(7), 1042–1052.

Brambring, M., & Asbrock, D. (2010). Validity of false belief tasks in blind children. Journal of Autism and Developmental Disorders, 40(12), 1471–1484. https://doi.org/10.1007/s10803-010-1002-2

Brouwer, K., & Gordon-Pershey, M. (2021). The relationship between speech perception and speech production in children with visual impairments. Journal of Visual Impairment & Blindness, 115, 251–257.

Brouwer, K. K., Gordon-Pershey, M., & Stransky, M. (2024). Speech, language, and literacy in children with visual impairments: The national survey of children's health. Communication Disorders Quarterly, 45(4), 263–269.

Brunes, A., & Heir, T. (2020). Social interactions, experiences with adverse life events and depressive symptoms in individuals with visual impairment: A cross-sectional study. BMC Psychiatry, 20(1), 224.

Byra, S., Mróz, J., & Kaleta, K. (2020). Forgiveness and acceptance of disability in people with traumatic spinal cord injury—the mediating role of disability appraisal. A cross-sectional study. Spinal Cord, 58(12), 1317–1324.

Cao, K., Hao, J., & Wang, N. L. (2023). Visual impairment as a risk factor of cognitive function impairment a six-year cohort study. European Journal of Ophthalmology, 33(6), 2146–2153.

Cowden, R. G., Worthington, E. L. Jr, Griffin, B. J., & Garthe, R. C. (2019). Forgiveness moderates relations between psychological abuse and indicators of psychological distress among women in romantic relationships. South African Journal of Science, 115(11–12), 95–101.

Crapolicchio, E., Regalia, C., Bernardo, G. A. D., & Cinquegrana, V. (2021). The role of relational dependence, forgiveness and hope on the intention to return with an abusive partner. Journal of Social and Personal Relationships, 38(9), 2474–2493.

Davies, L., Randle-Phillips, C., Russell, A., & Delaney, C. (2021). The relationship between adverse interpersonal experiences and self-esteem in people with intellectual disabilities: The role of shame, self-compassion and social support. Journal of Applied Research in Intellectual Disabilities, 34(4), 1037–1047.

Diniz, G., Korkes, L., Tristão, L. S., Pelegrini, R., Bellodi, P. L., & Bernardo, W. M. (2023). The effects of gratitude interventions: A systematic review and meta-analysis. Einstein (São Paulo), 21, eRW0371.

Ferah, B. (2025). Spatial inferences of visually impaired individuals concerning wayfinding: A case study of Istanbul's Kadikoy area. Journal of Transport Geography, 123, 104100.

Galvin, J., Howes, A., & Richards, G. (2024). Longitudinal associations between autistic traits, self-compassion, anxiety and depression in autistic and non-autistic adults without intellectual disability. Journal of Autism and Developmental Disorders, 54(12), 4571–4583.

Galvin, R. (2004). Challenging the need for gratitude: Comparisons between paid and unpaid care for disabled people. Journal of Sociology, 40(2), 137–155.

Garssen, B., Visser, A., & Pool, G. (2021). Does spirituality or religion positively affect mental health? Meta-analysis of longitudinal studies. The International Journal for the Psychology of Religion, 31(1), 4–20.

Georgiou, G. P. (2020). Speech perception in visually impaired individuals might be diminished as a consequence of monomodal cue acquisition. Medical Hypotheses, 143, 110088.

Gilbert, P., & Procter, S. (2006). Compassionate mind training for people with high shame and self-criticism: Overview and pilot study of a group therapy approach. Clinical Psychology & Psychotherapy: An International Journal of Theory & Practice, 13(6), 353–379.

Gori, M., Campus, C., Signorini, S., Rivara, E., & Bremner, A. J. (2021). Multisensory spatial perception in visually impaired infants. Current Biology, 31(22), 5093–5101.

Gracias, K. R., & Stutts, L. A. (2024). The impact of compassion writing interventions on body dissatisfaction, self-compassion, and fat phobia. Mindfulness, 15(7), 1793–1802.

Green, S., Pring, L., & Swettenham, J. (2004). An investigation of first-order false belief understanding of children with congenital profound visual impairment. British Journal of Developmental Psychology, 22(1), 1–17. https://doi.org/10.1348/026151004772901087

Guan, F., Zhan, C., Li, S., Tong, S., & Peng, K. (2024). Effects of self-compassion on aggression and its psychological mechanism through perceived stress. BMC Psychology, 12(1), 1–12.
Hajinejad, F., Ebrahimi, E., de Jong, A., & Ravanipour, M. (2019). Factors promoting Iranian older adults' spirituality: A qualitative content analysis. BMC Geriatrics, 19(1), 132.
Han, B. X., & Kong, Q. Y. (2025). 艺术文化的心理疗愈功能——重评失调的认知 [The psychological healing function of art and culture—A re-appraisal of disordered cognition]. Journal of Nanjing Normal University (Social Science Edition)/南京师大学报(社会科学版), 2025(1), 58–67.
Hartanto, A., Kaur, M., Kasturiratna, K. S., Quek, F. Y., & Majeed, N. M. (2023). A critical examination of the effectiveness of gratitude intervention on well-being outcomes: A within-person experimental daily diary approach. The Journal of Positive Psychology, 18(6), 942–957.
Hirst, S. L., Hepper, E. G., & Tenenbaum, H. R. (2019). Attachment dimensions and forgiveness of others: A meta-analysis. Journal of Social and Personal Relationships, 36(11–12), 3960–3985.
Hodge, D. R., & Reynolds, C. (2019). Spirituality among people with disabilities: A nationally representative study of spiritual and religious profiles. Health & Social Work, 44(2), 75–86.
Hong, J. C., Hwang, M. Y., Chen, M. S., & Tai, K. H. (2021). Explorative and exploitative learning affected by extraneous cognitive load and gameplay anxiety in a gestalt perception game. Journal of Educational Computing Research, 59(2), 209–229.
Huang, M., & Wu, E. Z. (2025). The associations between self-compassion and adult attachment: A meta-analysis. Journal of Social and Personal Relationships, 42(2), 681–713.
Imbiriba, L. A., Russo, M. M., de Oliveira, L. A. S., Fontana, A. P., Rodrigues, E. D. C., Garcia, M. A. C., & Vargas, C. D. (2013). Perspective–taking in blindness: Electrophysiological evidence of altered action representations. Journal of Neurophysiology, 109(2), 405–414.
Kirca, A., M. Malouff, J., & Meynadier, J. (2023). The effect of expressed gratitude interventions on psychological wellbeing: A meta-analysis of randomised controlled studies. International Journal of Applied Positive Psychology, 8(1), 63–86.
Kirmayer, L. J. (2007). Psychotherapy and the cultural concept of the person. Transcultural Psychiatry, 44(2), 232–257.
Kurtović, A., & Ivančić, H. (2019). Predictors of depression and life satisfaction in visually impaired people. Disability and Rehabilitation, 41(9), 1012–1023.
Lahav, Y., Renshaw, K. D., & Solomon, Z. (2019). Domestic abuse and forgiveness among military spouses. Journal of Aggression, Maltreatment & Trauma, 28(2), 243–260.
Lalor, J., & Khoshfetrat, A. (2024). An examination of the association between mindfulness and compassion for others in psychotherapists: A mediating role of self-compassion. Counselling and Psychotherapy Research, 24(3), 1006–1013.
Landau, S. D., & Jones, F. W. (2021). Finding the spiritual in the secular: A meta-analysis of changes in spirituality following secular mindfulness-based programs. Mindfulness, 12(7), 1567–1581.
Lassri, D., & Gewirtz-Meydan, A. (2022). Self-compassion moderates the mediating effect of self-criticism in the link between childhood maltreatment and psychopathology. Journal of Interpersonal Violence, 37(23–24), NP21699–NP21722.
Lee, Y. R., & Enright, R. D. (2019). A meta-analysis of the association between forgiveness of others and physical health. Psychology & Health, 34(5), 626–643.
Lestari, R., & Fajar, M. (2020). Gratitude, self-esteem and optimism in people with physical disabilities. Prizren Social Science Journal, 4(2), 14–21.
Lo, C. K., Chan, K. L., & Ip, P. (2019). Insecure adult attachment and child maltreatment: A meta-analysis. Trauma, Violence, & Abuse, 20(5), 706–719.
Madigan, S., Deneault, A. A., Duschinsky, R., Bakermans-Kranenburg, M. J., Schuengel, C., van IJzendoorn, M. H., & Verhage, M. L. (2024). Maternal and paternal sensitivity: Key determinants of child attachment security examined through meta-analysis. Psychological Bulletin, 150(7), 839.
Marsh, I. C., Chan, S. W., & MacBeth, A. (2018). Self-compassion and psychological distress in adolescents – A meta-analysis. Mindfulness, 9, 1011–1027.
Mcalpine, L. M., & Moore, C. L. (1995). The development of social understanding in children with visual impairments. Journal of Visual Impairment and Blindness, 89(4), 349–358. https://doi.org/10.1177/0145482X9508900408
Minter, M., Hobson, R. P., & Bishop, M. (1998). Congenital visual impairment and "theory of mind. British Journal of Developmental Psychology, 16(2), 183–196. https://doi.org/10.1111/j.2044-835X.1998.tb00918.x
Morelli, F., Aprile, G., Cappagli, G., Luparia, A., Decortes, F., Gori, M., & Signorini, S. (2020). A multidimensional, multisensory and comprehensive rehabilitation intervention to improve spatial functioning in the visually impaired child: A community case study. Frontiers in Neuroscience, 14, 768.

Mugeere, A. B., Omona, J., State, A. E., & Shakespeare, T. (2020). "Oh God! Why did you let me have this disability?": Religion, spirituality and disability in three African countries. Journal of Disability and Religion, 24(1), 64–81.

Neff, K. D. (2023). Self-compassion: Theory, method, research, and intervention. Annual Review of Psychology, 74(1), 193–218.

Pamir, Z., Bauer, C. M., Bailin, E. S., Bex, P. J., Somers, D. C., & Merabet, L. B. (2021). Neural correlates associated with impaired global motion perception in cerebral visual impairment (CVI). NeuroImage: Clinical, 32, 102821.

Papadopoulos, K., Barouti, M., & Koustriava, E. (2018). Differences in spatial knowledge of individuals with blindness when using audiotactile maps, using tactile maps, and walking. Exceptional Children, 84(3), 330–343.

Papageorgiou, C. C., Kouroupetroglou, G. T., Stachtea, X. P., Papageorgiou, P. C., Mavromatos, A. K., Chrousos, G. P., Logothetis, N. K., & Tsaltas, E. (2020). Perspective-taking in blindness: An event-related brain potentials study with the continuous wavelet transform. IEEE Access, 8, 76657–76670. http://doi.org/10.1109/ACCESS.2020.2990095

Perszyk, D. R., & Waxman, S. R. (2018). Linking language and cognition in infancy. Annual Review of Psychology, 69(1), 231–250.

Phillips, W. J., & Hine, D. W. (2021). Self-compassion, physical health, and health behaviour: A meta-analysis. Health Psychology Review, 15(1), 113–139.

Pijnacker, J., Vervloed, M. P. J., & Steenbergen, B. (2012). Pragmatic abilities in children with congenital visual impairment: An exploration of non-literal language and advanced theory of mind understanding. Journal of Autism and Developmental Disorders, 42(11), 2440–2449. https://doi.org/10.1007/s10803-012-1500-5

Qiu, S., An, P., Hu, J., Han, T., & Rauterberg, M. (2020). Understanding visually impaired people's experiences of social signal perception in face-to-face communication. Universal Access in the Information Society, 19, 873–890.

Roch-Levecq, A. C. (2006). Production of basic emotions by children with congenital blindness: Evidence for the embodiment of theory of mind. British Journal of Developmental Psychology, 24(3), 507–528. https://doi.org/10.1348/026151005X50663

Ruffman, T. (2023). Belief it or not: How children construct a theory of mind. Child Development Perspectives, 17(2), 1. https://doi.org/10.1111/cdep.12483

Salari, N., Kazeminia, M., Abdi, A., Abdolmaleki, A., Abdoli, N., Mohammadi, M., & Shohaimi, S. (2023). Effects of counselling and spiritual care program on anxiety in patients with chronic diseases: A systematic review and meta-analysis. Current Psychology, 42(12), 9943–9952.

Sims, S. V., Dreyzehner, J. K., DeCarlo, D. K., & Lombardo, T. (2018). Mental health needs of blind and visually impaired youth and their families. Journal of the American Academy of Child & Adolescent Psychiatry, 57(10), S96.

Sorokowska, A., Oleszkiewicz, A., & Sorokowski, P. (2018). A compensatory effect on mate selection? Importance of auditory, olfactory, and tactile cues in partner choice among blind and sighted individuals. Archives of Sexual Behavior, 47(3), 597–603.

Tao, J., He, K., & Xu, J. (2021). The mediating effect of self-compassion on the relationship between childhood maltreatment and depression. Journal of Affective Disorders, 291, 288–293.

Timmins, F., McCausland, D., Brennan, D., Sheerin, F., Luus, R., McCallion, P., & McCarron, M. (2023). A national cohort study of spiritual and religious practices of older people with intellectual disability. Journal of Intellectual Disabilities, 28(2), 533–548.

Tolcher, K., Cauble, M., & Downs, A. (2024). Evaluating the effects of gratitude interventions on college student well-being. Journal of American College Health, 72(5), 1321–1325.

Valente, D., Theurel, A., & Gentaz, E. (2018). The role of visual experience in the production of emotional facial expressions by blind people: A review. Psychonomic Bulletin & Review, 25(2), 483–497.

van der Zee, Y. J., Kooiker, M. J., Talamante Ojeda, M., & Pel, J. J. (2019). Gestalt perception in children with visual impairments: Item-specific performance and looking behavior. Developmental Neuropsychology, 44(3), 296–309.

Vismaya, A., Gopi, A., Romate, J., & Rajkumar, E. (2024). Psychological interventions to promote self-forgiveness: A systematic review. BMC Psychology, 12(1), 258.

Vu, T. A., Fenwick, E. K., Gan, A. T., Man, R. E., Tan, B. K., Gupta, P., & Lamoureux, E. L. (2021). The bidirectional relationship between vision and cognition: A systematic review and meta-analysis. Ophthalmology, 128(7), 981–992.

Wang, T., Xiao, Q., Wang, H., Hu, Y., & Xiang, J. (2024). Self-compassion defuses the aggression triggered by social exclusion. PsyCh Journal, 13(6), 1014–1025.

Watermeyer, B., & Botha, M. (2025). Disability, trauma, and the place of affect in identity: Examining performativity in visual impairment rehabilitation. Feminism & Psychology, 35(2), 138–154.

Withagen, A., Kappers, A. M., Vervloed, M. P., Knoors, H., & Verhoeven, L. (2013). Short term memory and working memory in blind versus sighted children. Research in Developmental Disabilities, 34(7), 2161–2172.

World Health Organization. (2019). *World report on vision.* Geneva: World Health Organization. https://www.who.int/publications/i/item/9789241516570 [accessed 23 June 2026].

Yao, W., Cao, Y., Tian, Y., Liu, Y., Hua, X., & Chen, F. (2024). Were there any missing mediators between visual impairment and anxiety symptoms? Results from Chinese longitudinal healthy longevity survey. Frontiers in Public Health, 12, 1448638.

Zapata, M. A., & Pearlstein, J. G. (2022). Disability self-worth relates to lower anxiety and depression in people with visual impairment. Journal of Clinical Psychology, 78(7), 1491–1499.

Zhao, X., Liu, W., Lu, B., Zhu, X., Zhou, M., & Sun, X. (2022). Visual impairment and depression in China: A 7-year follow-up study from national longitudinal surveys. BMJ Open, 12(4), e055563.

Zheng, L., Luo, Y., & Chen, X. (2020). Different effects of attachment anxiety and attachment avoidance on depressive symptoms: A meta-analysis. Journal of Social and Personal Relationships, 37(12), 3028–3050.

Zou, X., & Zhou, Y. (2023). Spatial cognition of the visually impaired: A case study in a familiar environment. International Journal of Environmental Research and Public Health, 20(3), 1753.

14 Development of the Bladder Failure Self-Management Monitor (BFSMM)

A Patient-Centred Tool for Self-Care

Paul M. W. Hackett

INTRODUCTION

Bladder failure is a medical condition that encompasses neurogenic bladder dysfunction, detrusor underactivity and a series of other related conditions. Bladder failure is a condition that affects millions of individuals worldwide, which requires lifelong self-management so as to prevent serious complications and to enable quality of life to be maintained. The present chapter is concerned with a tool for self-managing bladder failure. In Chapter 17 in this book, I provide details about my bladder failure and its management. In order to effectively self-manage bladder failure, an individual with this condition must engage in a complex daily routine that includes clean intermittent self-catheterisation location and equipment acquisition and maintenance, infection prevention and psychological adaptation to chronic illness. However, it is often the case that clinical practice relies upon episodic healthcare check-ups along with very limited ongoing input and support for the continuous self-management behaviours essential for positive maintenance. Shortly after diagnosis the healthcare professionals passes over bladder care to the patient who must learn to self-manage their condition. Successfully developing and employing self-management competencies is important in order to avoid complications arising from the distended bladder and infections associated with its treatment and improvements in quality-of-life outcomes. Conversely, inadequate self-management skills associated with bladder failure contribute to increased infection rates, emergency medical visits, feeling ill and psychological distress. However, few tools exist to support patients in developing and maintaining self-management practices that are necessary for bladder failure care.

Support for individuals with bladder failure and who are employing self-management of this condition usually consist of a one-time educational session when first diagnosed with a demonstration of how to self-catheterise followed by a six-month and then regular meeting with a urologist. This level and type of education and on-going support fail to address the changing nature of bladder failure self-management and patient needs. This is true as the condition is constantly fluctuating and requires ongoing self-monitoring, problem-solving as symptoms change and behavioural adjustment. Chronic disease management models place an emphasis upon the importance of patient-centred tools that promote self-efficacy through providing regular feedback which supports continuous improvement in self-care behaviours. Furthermore, the development of patient-centred self-management tools for bladder failure is in accord with broader healthcare moves towards more personalised medicine and shared decision-making between the patient and professionals. Self-management tools need to be designed to balance clinical thoroughness with practical usability and must provide actionable insights for

DOI: 10.1201/9781003599074-16

the patient. For bladder failure, effective self-management tools must address the multifaceted nature of the condition and the skills the patient needs, including technical care skills, skills that support problem prevention (PP), psychological adaptation skills and practices that support social integration.

A review of the literature revealed a gap in bladder failure self-management support, which included the lack of brief instruments that patients can use independently for ongoing self-assessment and goal-setting. The quality-of-life measures that do exist for use in clinical assessment are typically lengthy. They also usually require professional interpretation of their scores and results and they focus on the measurement of outcomes rather than attempting to bring about behaviour change. For example, patient-reported outcome measures in bladder dysfunction have historically emphasised symptom severity and functional impact rather than self-management skill development.

In the foregoing paragraphs, I have considered my reasons for developing a tool to measure patient self-management of chronic bladder failure. Instruments exist that act as measures of bladder and bladder-related conditions; however, none of these instruments has been designed to be used with bladder failure or the treatment of this with clean intermittent self-catheterisation. In the sections that follow, I will provide details of how I developed such a tool.

BFSMM DEVELOPMENT

Having considered both anecdotal experience and the evidence from the literature, it was apparent that there is a need for an instrument to assess an individual with bladder failure's reactions to being diagnosed as needing to perform intermittent self-catheterisation, as well as for ongoing monitoring. I therefore designed an initial draft for such a tool, the BFSMM, which is reported below.

Initial Screening Requirements

It is important that a comprehensive screening tool for newly diagnosed bladder failure patients should assess the multiple domains or categories of patient experience of this condition, for instance: psychological adjustment to their diagnosis, perceived self-efficacy for bladder management, social support networks, coping mechanisms, and risk factors that may be associated with difficulties with the procedure or non-compliance. A tool designed around these categories of experience should, it was believed, enable healthcare professionals to identify individuals requiring immediate psychological input, or other forms of intervention, and should enable professionals to tailor support services according to responses given on the tool.

CONTENT OF BFSMM

The Bladder Failure Self-Management Monitor (BFSMM) is a weekly assessment tool that Has been designed to assess and improve self-management for an individual with bladder failure. The BFSMM attempts to achieve this through detailed self-monitoring resulting in action planning.

Introduction and Instructions

The BFSMM instrument commences with an introduction and instructions on how to complete the questions using their appropriate rating scales. Information is also provided about when and how to complete the tool and how to interpret the scores along with some insights on how to maintain the habit of completing the scales. It also stresses the importance of honest self-assessment.

The first and main section of the monitor is concerned with self-management over the past week. There are three sections to this part of the monitor which are: Care Routine Management

(CRM); PP; Confidence and Coping (CC). Each section comprised five questions each answered along a 5 point scale (from 1 = poor/never to excellent/always), followed by a rating of how confidence they felt to manage their condition over the last week answered along the same scale. The scale responses are additive to provide an index to management over the last seven days.

Care Routine Management (CRM) Section

In slightly more detail, the Care Routine Management (CRM) section takes the same format as the other two rating sections. The CRM **is** a 25-point assessment evaluates five forms of self-care behaviour. Users provide a numerical rating of their performance and, if they wish, annotate this in terms of their: adhering to catheterisation schedules; maintaining proper hygiene standards; keeping their equipment clean and well-organised, monitoring urine changes and maintaining appropriate levels of hydration.

Problem Prevention (PP) Section

The Problem Prevention (PP) section is also scored out of 25 points with five points for each of the five items. This section focuses on patients' proactive management strategies. The five areas that patients are asked to rate are: recognised early warning signs; took action when needed; kept supplies well-stocked; avoided risky situations; and followed prevention strategies.

Confidence and Coping (CC) Section

In the Confidence and Coping (CC) Section, the psychological adaptation was measured in terms of emotional and social management across five questions of a similar response format. Users were asked to assess how: Confident they felt in different locations; how well they handled unexpected situations; how well they maintained positive outlook; how they Managed stress effectively and the extent they stayed socially connected. This section recognised the importance of psychological adjustment in the management of a chronic health condition.

Quick Action Planning

The next part of the instrument is called Quick Action Planning. In this section, users are asked to supply textual responses to a series of open-ended questions about their successes over the past seven days. They were also asked about the problems they encountered. They were then asked about things they needed help with, and they then identified three goals and how they would achieve each and by what date. Next, users identified an overall rating for the severity of problems they had had that week, they listed the problems, what helped or didn't help them to address these problems and any action that was still needed. Overall, this section encouraged the weekly recognition of success and the identification of areas that still needed to be worked on. The identification of problems is achieved by focusing on lowest-scoring areas and seeing these as priority targets. Two priority problems were highlighted for specific attempts at improvement.

Support and Goal-Setting Components

In this section, attempts were made to assess an individual's support and needs. This was broken down into five categories: informational/educational needs; equipment or supply requirements; emotional support needs; healthcare provider contact requirements and family/friend support needs. Goal-setting allows for 1–3 specific objectives, each with open-ended strategies for achievement and completion timelines.

Problem and Progress Tracking

This problem monitor asks respondents to tick boxes to indicate their problems and to provide descriptive text responses. Users were asked to state what helped and did not help and to identify any action that was needed.

Monthly Review and Reference Materials

This is the end of the ratings and next those completing the tool are now asked to complete a monthly review, (this is completed every four weeks) in order to provide a profile of scores for the CRM, PP, and CC scales over the last month. This profile of scores is to enable self-management progress or difficulties to be monitored. Respondents were asked which were their biggest successes this month, their main problems and challenges, what they will focus on next month and, on a five-point scale, how confident they felt about managing their condition. The instrument closed with a list of emergency contact details, completed by the users of the monitor, for health professionals and medical supply companies along with a request to write a motivational statement of why they felt good self-management matters to them and their main goal for managing their condition.

DISCUSSION

The development of the Bladder Failure Self-Management Monitor (BFSMM) has been undertaken in an attempt to address the gap in patient-centred tools for the management of bladder failure. At the core of the BFSMM is a 15-item instrument that has been designed to be a comprehensive, practical instrument to assist with self-assessment that is absent in current clinical practice. It is hoped that the BFSMM will address the usual situation where patients typically receive only minimal ongoing support after their initial diagnosis and training. The BFSMM has a three-component internal structure that is made up of CRM, PP, and CC. This tripartite form is in accord with frameworks for chronic disease management, which emphasise the multifaceted nature of self-care. In the BFSMM I have incorporating both behavioural and attitudinal/emotional components in an attempt to acknowledges that in order to successfully self-manage bladder failure the patient must master technical catheterisation skills along with adapting emotionally to the condition, changing their social lives and solving problems. Adopting an integrated approach is particularly important due to the complex daily routines that those with bladder failure must engage in to facilitate effective bladder failure management and to avoid what are potentially significant quality of life impacts.

The weekly assessment frequency was adopted so as to balance between providing frequent enough feedback in order to allow for continuous improvement, whilst avoiding boredom or fatigue from completing more often. Action planning and goal setting were also incorporated into the monitor to enable the monitor to promote active intervention that promotes feelings of self-efficacy and concrete changes in behaviour. This feature is particularly appropriate due to the chronic, and fluctuating nature of bladder failure. Other features of the BFSMM are its brevity and self-administered format. Both of these characteristics are incorporated in order to facilitate practical implementation in clinical settings whilst promoting patient autonomy. As healthcare moves toward more personalised, patient-centred and co-design approaches, tools like the BFSMM that are able to span the gap between sporadic clinical appointments and a patient's daily self-management routines, offer a represent potentially valuable contributions to chronic disease management.

FUTURE RESEARCH

It is should be stress at this point that the BFSMM is still in the development stage and that there are several limitations to the instrument. For instance, the development of the tool has to date relied upon clinical experience and literature reviews rather than input from patients and medical staff. In this chapter, I have reflected upon how the instrument has come into existence, and also how, at the time of writing this chapter, the monitor had not been used in any health care settings and has not yielded any empirical data. It is therefore obvious that before the instrument can be used in a clinical setting it needs to be used on sample of respondents who have bladder failure. The monitor needs to be validated in order to assess the extent to which the monitor makes sense to those completing it (language, layout, etc.). Furthermore, the monitor also needs to have its clinical, diagnostic and management usefulness assessed. Finally, it would be useful to assess the psychometric properties of the monitor. All of the validation work for the monitor should focus on determining and improving the utility of the scale in terms of patient outcome.

Bladder Failure Self-Management Monitor (BFSMM)

A Short Self-Assessment and Action Planning Tool

Name: ______________________ **Date:** ______________

Weekly Use

- Complete every Sunday evening or Monday morning.
- Be honest in your answers – this is for YOU, and is not judging you!
- Focus on patterns and not on perfect scores.
- Celebrate any improvements you make, even small ones.

When Scores Are Low

- **1-2 = Red Zone:** Area of need, consider seeking professional help.
- **3 = Yellow Zone:** Room for improvement, good area to set as a goal.
- **4-5 = Green Zone:** Keep up the good work.

Making it a Habit

- Set a weekly reminder to complete the monitor and set an alarm on your phone.
- Keep this monitor somewhere visible.[1]
- Share your results and progress with someone who supports you.
- Review monthly patterns with your healthcare team and significant others.

Remember

- Progress isn't always along a straight line.
- Some weeks will be harder than others.
- The goal is overall improvement over time.
- By using this monitor, you're learning valuable self-management skills.

IMPORTANT

This health monitor is designed to complement, not replace, professional medical care. Always consult your healthcare provider about your medical concerns or anything that concerns you about your use of this monitor.

INSTRUCTIONS

This monitor helps you monitor the management of your bladder failure and to plan improvements.

Please complete the monitor once each week to stay on top of your self-management.

Rate each area from 1–5 and then focus on your lowest scores for action planning.

How to Score

- 1 = Never
- 2 = Rarely
- 3 = Sometimes
- 4 = Often
- 5 = Always

This Week's Self-Management Check List

Care Routine Management (CRM)

How well did you manage your bladder failure routine this week?

Area	Score (1–5)	Notes
I followed catheterisation schedule	_____	____________
I maintained proper hygiene	_____	____________
I kept equipment clean and organised	_____	____________
I monitored urine changes	_____	____________
I stayed hydrated appropriately	_____	____________

Care Routine Management (CRM) Score Total: _____/25

Problem Prevention (PP)

How well did you prevent problems with your bladder failure this week?

Area	Score (1–5)	Notes
I recognised early warning signs	_____	____________
I took action when needed	_____	____________
I kept supplies well-stocked	_____	____________
I avoided risky situations	_____	____________
I followed prevention strategies	_____	____________

Problem Prevention (PP) Score Total: _____/25

Confidence and Coping (CC)

How confident and positive did you feel about managing your bladder failure this week?

Area	Score (1–5)	Notes
I felt confident in different locations	_____	____________
I handled unexpected situations well	_____	____________
I maintained a positive outlook	_____	____________
I managed stress effectively	_____	____________
I stayed socially connected	_____	____________

Confidence and Coping (CC) Score Total: _____/25

Quick Action Planning

This Week's Successes

In terms of your bladder failure, what went really well this week? – List your successences.

- ______________________________
- ______________________________
- ______________________________

Problem Areas/Areas for Improvement

In terms of your bladder failure, what problems or difficulties did you have this week – which scores were lowest? (These are the areas you need to focus on).

Priority 1 (Lowest Score): ______________________________

What will you do differently next week? ______________________________

Priority 2: ______________________________

What will you do differently next week? ______________________________

Other difficulties: ______________________________

Support Needed

Do you need help with any of the following? ☐

Information/education about: ______________________________

Equipment or supplies: ______________________________

Emotional support: ______________________________

Healthcare provider contact: ______________________________

Family/friend support: ______________________________

Weekly Goals (Choose 1-3)

Goal 1: ______________________________

How will you achieve this? ______________________________

By when? ______________________________

Goal 2: ______________________________

How will you achieve this? ______________________________

By when? ______________________________

Goal 3: ______________________________

How will you achieve this? ______________________________

By when? ______________________________

Problem Monitor

Have You Had Any Problems or Difficulties This Week?

☐ No problems (great week)
☐ Minor issues (easily managed)
☐ Moderate problems (needed extra attention)
☐ Significant problems (considering professional help)

If you had problems, what were they?

___

___

What helped or did not help with your problems?

___

___

What action did you take:

- ☐ I handled my problems independently
- ☐ I contacted healthcare provider for help with my problems
- ☐ I got additional support with my problems
- ☐ I adjusted my routine/approach because of my problems

Notes:

___

___

Monthly Review (Complete every four weeks)

Your Overall Progress This Month

Week	Routine Score	Prevention Score	Confidence Score	What are Your Overall Feelings
	(CRM)	(PP)	(CC)	
Week 1	___/25	___/25	___/25	___
Week 2	___/25	___/25	___/25	___
Week 3	___/25	___/25	___/25	___
Week 4	___/25	___/25	___/25	___

Monthly Reflection

What were your biggest successes this month?

___

___

What were your main problems and challenges this month?

___

___

What will you focus on next month?

___

___

At this moment, how confident do you feel about managing your bladder failure?

Tick one

1 – Extremely Unsure ________

2 – Fairly Unsure ________

3 – Neither Confident nor Unsure ________

4 – Fairly Confident ________

5 – Extremely Confident ________

Emergency Contact Quick Reference

Healthcare Provider/Doctor: ______________________________

After-hours number: ______________________________

Chemist/**Pharmacy:** ______________________________

Medical supply company: ______________________________

Emergency contact person: ______________________________

Personal Motivation Statements

Why is good self-management important to you:

____

____

What is your main goal when managing your condition:

____

____

____

NOTE

1

15 Steering My Own Wheelchair
The Rehabilitation Journey from Dependency to Interdependency

Shane Clifton

INTRODUCTION

When invited to contribute to this volume on self-management in rehabilitation, I initially had only an intuitive grasp of the topic. My understanding was that readers would be keen on an insider's perspective: what it's truly like to take control of one's rehabilitation journey and ultimately thrive with a long-term injury. My intuition proved largely correct, as significant research now highlights how rehabilitation programs can empower individuals to effectively manage their conditions, often by enhancing self-efficacy—the belief in one's capacity to navigate daily challenges and shape a positive future (Jones and Riazi, 2011, Lorig and Holman, 2003).

While others in this volume will delve into the clinical literature and practice, I offer a personal account of my spinal cord injury rehabilitation since 2010. Fifteen years on, this chapter provides both an "insider's" and "outsider's" view. Rehabilitation was a profoundly challenging process, shaping me not just physically and emotionally, but also epistemically. Transformative experiences like spinal cord injury fundamentally alter one's way of knowing and understanding the world (Paul, 2014). My present self, armed with new values and insights, interprets those past events differently, weaving in later reflections to better understand both the accomplishments and setbacks.

The field of self-management in rehabilitation has developed a shared set of concepts and language that underpin its programs. However, that language is not mine, and reframing my experiences using its terminology would risk distorting my story. Before my injury, I was a theologian and ethicist, and I turned to the philosophical tradition of virtue ethics to make sense of my situation and build a new life. Virtue ethics, rooted in Greek philosophy, particularly the works of Aristotle and the Stoics, provided a valuable framework for understanding my experience. In Nicomachean Ethics (2012), Aristotle poses the question: What is the good or happy life? He answers that the good life (*eudaimonia*) is not one of mere pleasure—an unstable and fleeting pursuit—but one of purpose and meaning. He argues that the good life is achieved through the exercise of virtue: habits of character that promote success and balance, avoiding the vices of excess and deficiency that undermine flourishing. For example, courage lies between the vices of cowardice and recklessness. Only the courageous person is willing to fight effectively and judiciously in battle. Furthermore, Aristotle emphasises that virtue carries its own intrinsic reward; the inner satisfaction of knowing you have done your best to navigate a challenge (for a deeper discussion on the virtue tradition and its application to life with spinal cord injury and disability, see Clifton, 2018).

Virtue ethics became central to my adjustment, directly addressing how to find happiness (*eudaimonia*) amid immense loss and pain. Its answer was clear: pursue purpose and meaning and cultivate virtues. During my rehabilitation, virtues such as perseverance, courage, and patience were crucial, helping me push through recovery and move from dependency to maximising my independence.

Interestingly, virtue ethics aligns closely with the self-management literature. Both emphasise the pursuit of meaning and purpose, and the concept of self-efficacy shares much with virtue. I hope readers unfamiliar with virtue ethics will find its insights relevant and enriching, offering a deeper understanding of the principles underpinning self-management programs.

DOI: 10.1201/9781003599074-17

Finally, a note on my process: My academic writing skills proved invaluable in processing and adjusting to my injury. My 2015 memoir, Husband Should Not Break, co-authored with my wife Elly, was a vital resource for recalling those early experiences, and I draw extensively from it throughout this chapter.

And now, let me share my journey with you.

THE ACCIDENT

On October 7, 2010, just two weeks shy of my 40th birthday, my life irrevocably changed. While holidaying with my wife, Elly, and three children (then aged 10, 13, and 15) in the picturesque Shoalhaven region of New South Wales, Australia, I suffered a spinal cord injury that left me with C4/5 incomplete quadriplegia.

That morning, I'd enjoyed an idyllic early surf session, perfect waves, an offshore breeze, and dolphins swimming nearby. I was an active, healthy man: a runner, surfer, and golfer with a secure academic career teaching theology and ethics. I was at the height of my so-called "independence", living a fortunate life.

In the afternoon, we visited a church-based youth facility that featured a jump designed for skateboards and BMX bikes, complete with a foam pit for safe landing. Modelled after acrobatic pits in gymnasiums, it *looked* safe. But unknown to me, it was poorly constructed, with inferior foam and insufficient depth. As a playful parent who loved joining my kids' activities, I followed them onto the jump on a BMX. I landed upside down.

I knew instantly I was in trouble—trapped, head buried in the foam, unable to move. I shouted to Elly, "I've broken my neck". She laughed, disbelieving, but it soon became clear that I was not joking. I was struggling to breathe, feeling an "alien force… pinning me down, denying me movement, smothering me" (p. 19). That foam pit marked the abrupt ending of my independence and the beginning of my dependency. Paramedics carefully extracted me, and I was flown by helicopter to Prince of Wales Hospital in Randwick, Sydney, where I remained for the next seven months.

INDIGNITY AND DEPENDENCY

The initial days and weeks following my injury were a brutal and horrifying ordeal. Confined to the ICU, I was entirely dependent on nurses for nearly every bodily function, unable to even "scratch my bloody nose" (p. 18). Encased rigidly in a neck brace, I needed a ventilator for breathing support and a nasogastric tube to eat. I was trapped in bed, staring at the ceiling, pushed from pillar to post with X-rays, CAT scans, MRIs, procedures and surgery. With phlegm regularly clogging my airway, I relied on physiotherapists to assist me in coughing. Life was scary, out of control, and I was utterly dependent.

Basic bodily functions, once needing little thought, now demanded intimate assistance. Bladder and bowel care became a messy process of catheters and spilled urine, enemas, a manual per rectum (a finger up the bum), "shitting in bed", and the realisation that nurses or carers would ever after flush and clean my private parts. A month or so later, when I could sit on a commode, I would be taken to the toilet. I wasn't independent, and it took one to two hours to get ready in the morning. But I no longer "pooed" in bed. Small moves toward dignity make a big difference.

Seven years later, persistent complications with my bowel care, including chronic diarrhoea, bowel accidents, haemorrhoids, and autonomic dysreflexia, prompted me to pursue colostomy surgery. A peer worker had strongly recommended it, describing it as "life-changing", and I urged my doctor to arrange the procedure. The colostomy dramatically improved my life and independence. With only minimal assistance, I could change the bag myself. I reclaimed the hours previously lost to morning routines, and embarrassing bowel accidents became far less frequent. I became a "stoma evangelist", passionately advocating for its benefits.

Marcy Epstein (2010), who has an incomplete spinal cord injury, powerfully illustrates the profound shift in perspective that can accompany reliance on others. In her chapter "On Humility", she recounts an incident of soiling herself and being deeply moved by the humility and solicitude of the hospital volunteer who cleaned her:

> I cannot begin to describe to you the deliberation with which she cleaned my body, nor the relief, comfort, and sanctification I felt as I was being cleansed. Because she was gracious and helped me to collect myself, I learned that the taking of urine and feces from another person can be a holy act.
>
> **(Epstein, 2010: 132)**

Epstein notes that rehabilitating with spinal cord injury involves a series of humiliating indignities, but that the giving and receiving of care can transform humiliation into genuine humility.

In philosophical and theological tradition, humility is the virtue of being realistic and truthful about one's limitations and capacities. Humility is in the balance between thinking too highly of oneself (improper pride) and too lowly (false humility). Epstein emphasises the necessity of learning humility to adjust to her injury. My own theological background led me to reflect deeply on humility, which helped me assess and accept the new limits on my capacity (see my extended reflection on humility in Crippled Grace (2018)).

The disability rights movement is understandably suspicious of humility, often associating it with shame. Historically, humility has been weaponised by people in power to sustain the status quo and keep marginalised people in their place, including disabled people (Clifton, 2018: ch. 9, Dadlez and Woolvine, 2021). Shame and stigma in disability are manifestations of ableism; attitudes and behaviours that dehumanise people by categorising them as "other", abnormal, less than, and a burden (Campbell, 2009a, Clifton, 2020).

Ableism can be internalised, especially by people with spinal cord injury who bring pre-existing attitudes about disability to judgements about themselves and their new situation. My memoir, for example, describes my embarrassment and shame about my body, with its "ungainly neck", "shrunken" shoulders, "disappeared" chest, and "massive beer belly" [the "quad belly" comes from dysfunctional stomach muscles (Bailey et al, 2016)]. I wrote, "It is much harder to look in the mirror" (p.22).

Nearly 15 years later, I still don't love my quad body, but I've come to appreciate it as the price of being human and surviving in this dangerous world. Beyond negative self-perceptions, internalised ableism can become the tyranny within (Campbell, 2009b). In adjusting to spinal cord injury, this tyranny can either cause people to lose confidence, become passive, and fall into depression, or spur long-term efforts to "overcome disability" (Clifton and Bourke, 2026). The latter is preferable, but not without its negative effects.

ROLL WITH THE PUNCHES

The transition from complete dependence to a small but vital degree of self-control began with the move into a wheelchair. After weeks confined to bed, staring at ceilings, simply sitting upright was a surprising challenge; light-headedness and pain demanded a gradual approach. The process unfolded in bite-sized pieces; first sitting up in bed, then cautiously transferring to the wheelchair for a few minutes, extending for a few hours, and eventually, spending the entire day in the chair.

While outsiders, often viewing us with pity, might describe us as "wheelchair-bound", the wheelchair is, in fact, our liberation. When we eventually learn to drive it independently, whether by arm power, chin control, or a joystick (as in my case), we can at last escape the bedroom and chart our own course ... albeit within limits.

In the hospital, your autonomy is significantly curtailed by the environment and its routines. Clinicians issue proscriptions that dictate much of your day. Though self-management could involve choosing to skip a session for a smoke or, in my case, a coffee, I largely opted to do as I was told. Being away from home in a rehabilitation setting chips away at your spirit. My peers and I shared a common goal: to work diligently, maximise our function, and break free from Prince of Wales Hospital (our "POW"—prisoner of war confinement) to return home as soon as possible, and as strong as possible.

Much of the time was spent with physiotherapists and occupational therapists, who were critical to my journey and adjustment. My therapists were very special people. They guided me through work that was often tedious and painful, and progress was measured in millimetres; yet, small gains could make a profound difference. For example, to learn a tenodesis grasp, if your injury allows, as mine did, is to transition from having someone feed you to a messy but more independent meal. As my injury was incomplete, I eventually regained some finger movement in my right hand. Working with therapists to harness this improvement further increased my independence.

Quadriplegic bodies are frustrating and hilarious. You can either cry or laugh at another fall, another spilled meal, another failed exercise, and with my friends and therapists, I did both. By crying and laughing and shouting and swearing, you gradually improve and come to learn what your body is going to allow you to do.

VIRTUE

While much of the rehabilitation journey is guided by therapists—their training and experience truly make them the experts—my role was crucial. I had skin in the game, and my priorities, values, motivations, and passions profoundly impacted the outcomes. My rehabilitation team understood this, working with me to set goals and priorities, and shaping their program accordingly.

Rehabilitation, then, is fundamentally a partnership between clinicians and clients. Yet, ultimately, it was my own agency, my daily struggles, and my mood that truly determined what I gained from therapy as the days and months progressed.

Earlier, I identified the significance of virtue ethics for my rehabilitation. To adjust to my injury and manage the rehabilitation journey successfully, I needed to cultivate virtues that I sometimes lacked before the injury, particularly those that related to dependency and the slower pace of life. I needed to be:

- patient to cope with the endless waiting for doctors, tests, and the slow rate of progress – and, ultimately, a slower pace of life
- grateful for the help I received throughout the day, saying thank you even when the injury made me want to scream
- courageous, to face the day with an unwieldy and painful body, and the risks of bladder, bowel, and other complications
- resilient, to persevere against the relentless challenge of spinal cord injury and disability
- hopeful, to believe that better days were ahead and it was worth persevering

I've explored virtue through philosophical and theological traditions, but its contribution to wellbeing and resilience is also increasingly recognised by positive psychology. While delving into the connection between these two fields is beyond the scope of this paper (see Clifton, 2018). There's now substantial empirical evidence supporting the role of virtue—sometimes labelled as strengths—in successful rehabilitation (Clifton et al, 2018, Martz and Livneh, 2016, Wade et al, 2023).

THE POSITIVITY MYTH

There are dangers in overemphasising the significance of individual virtue and positivity for successful rehabilitation. First, no one, least of all me, can live up to these ideals. I regularly gave way to fear and panic, anger and frustration, ungratefulness, and hopelessness. It was not always easy to be my nurse, therapist, or family. In one instance, I shouted at the nursing unit manager who was attempting to move me from a private room to a shared four-bed room (p. 70). I told another patient to "f**k off" (p.69). So surprised and concerned was my doctor that he booked a cranial MRI to investigate the possibility that my accident had caused a brain injury. The MRI found no abnormality.

Like most people on the ward, I tried to exercise virtue for my own sake and the sake of others. But I also needed to be kind to myself when, time and again, I failed, because adjusting to quadriplegia is bloody hard and I have never been a saint.

Second, emphasising individual virtue, or its modern equivalent, "positivity", risks trapping people rehabilitating from an injury in the positivity myth. As a colleague and I explained:

> The positivity myth suggests that positive thinking can help the newly injured person overcome the limitations of disability, insisting that a positive attitude and hard work is the key determinant affecting the level of an individual's recovery. In religious contexts, faith is treated as the equivalent of positive thinking, so that recovery relies on belief in the divine capacity to heal; the faithful person will recover. While positive and faithful attitudes can play a role in resilience and recovery, the extent of an individual's biological injury presents a hard limit on what they can achieve. Positive thinking will not enable a person with a complete spinal cord injury to walk, and the dark side of the positivity myth is the psychological burden that inevitably follows the failure to satisfy social expectations and reach impossible goals.
>
> **(Clifton and Bourke, 2026)**

For the most part, I managed to avoid the positivity myth. The longer you live, the harder it is to believe in the positivity hype. I have experienced enough of life's sharp edges to be realistic about the future.

While in the hospital and for some years later, I was a Christian theologian, and the positivity of faith was harder to avoid. "Be strong in faith"; "Believe God has the power to heal"; "Can I pray for you? Lord Jesus, heal Shane, let him walk again". These were the well-meaning encouragements and prayers of many in the Christian community. They were deeply felt expressions of faith and hope, arising out of love and care for my well-being, so I tried to receive them with the generosity they were intended to convey. But prayer became tiring, a hindrance rather than a help to my adjustment. Unrealised prayer for healing and the pressure to exercise faith can wear you down.

The third and related danger of overemphasising virtue is the potential to blame the individual for failing to flourish when sociocultural factors shape a person's capacity to take control of their rehabilitation journey. I had the benefit of a loving family and friends, a stable job I could return to, and the financial resources to set up a home. Many individuals with spinal cord injury have no such luck. It's incredibly difficult to effectively self-manage rehabilitation when you don't own a home, accessible rentals are scarce, and the looming prospect of an aged care nursing home is your likely future (Smith and Caddick, 2015). Motivation can be harder to find when you're battling loneliness, or an injury shatters a beloved outdoor career.

While the grit displayed by many disadvantaged people who push through these immense challenges is a testament to their strength, we must never forget that disability is fundamentally a social challenge, not just an individual one. We, as a society, have a collective responsibility to create an environment where everyone can realistically exercise virtue and actively shape their lives with a disability. This responsibility is the driving force of the social model of disability.

DISABILITY IDENTITY AND PRIDE

My understanding of disability profoundly shifted after leaving rehabilitation and engaging with the social model of disability and the disability community. Works like Paul Longmore's *Why I Burned My Book and Other Essays on Disability* (2003) and Tom Shakespeare's *Disability*

Rights and Wrongs: Revisited (2014) revolutionised my self-understanding and reshaped my approach to the often-inaccessible society I inhabit. This newfound perspective highlighted key truths:

- Disability is not a tragedy.
- Disability is both a social and medical issue.
- The barrier isn't my inability to walk up steps, but buildings designed without ramps.
- My disability doesn't make me a burden.
- Disability doesn't equate to weakness; it reveals resilience and strength.
- My disability is nothing to be ashamed of.
- "Disability" is not a dirty word; it carries a proud history and identity.
- The disability community is a powerful force for collective action and advocacy.

While some of these ideas were implicit in the rehabilitation I received during rehabilitation, the social model and its powerful concepts were not a formal part of the program. For most of us who acquire disability, the medical model of disability is ingrained, and we begin our journey with disability shaped by ableism that we internalise (Campbell, 2009b). When we leave rehabilitation settings, many of us want very little to do with peers with spinal cord injury or the broader disabled community.

Of course, embracing a disabled identity and engaging with the disabled community is a personal choice. Yet, rehabilitation settings should actively challenge internalised ableism and introduce people to frameworks that have proven incredibly empowering for many disabled people.

In "Are standing and walking overrated? Ableism in spinal cord injury rehabilitation" (2025), Johnny Burke and I argued that rehabilitation settings can fall short in promoting and embodying these crucial disability concepts. Beyond critiquing the overemphasis on standing and walking, we raise the importance of peer support within the disabled community.

PEER SUPPORT

In the rehab unit, peer support begins with the shared learning from other injured residents. The in-ward camaraderie provides a raw and unfiltered space for shared realities, humour, and coping mechanisms. To regain control of life, you need to accept that spilled urine and faeces are no big deal, that a messy meal or a spasm that tips over a coffee is more funny than frustrating, that being carried upstairs need not be humiliating. These lessons are best learned with others. While the spinal ward brings together people from diverse backgrounds who might not ordinarily interact, shared experiences of both frustration and silliness generate unique connections that help one to come to recognise and accept "the absurdity of spinal cord injury" (p. 75).

My recovery journey was also significantly impacted by peer support workers, particularly Sheree Hurley, from Spinal Cord Injuries Australia. A few months into my stay at the rehab unit, Sheree, who was my age and had sustained a similar injury 13 years prior, visited with her beautiful support dog, Jade. Her unshakeable contentedness and generous sharing of her life offered invaluable insight into the potential for people with spinal cord injury. Her visits were a "godsend" (p.102). Sheree was a tangible example of flourishing and embodied practical independence by living independently and working full-time in a career she enjoyed. Her visits provided profound emotional validation and vital practical inspiration, directly challenging any notion I had that quadriplegia meant life was over. On the contrary, she showed it was possible to thrive.

In the months and years that followed, I had the privilege of meeting many other individuals who had lived well with their injuries. Each one became a vital source of practical advice, encouragement, and immense hope (Clifton et al., 2020, 2018). In my opinion, lived experience is often undervalued in rehabilitation. As mentioned, Sheree was employed by Spinal Cord Injuries Australia, which is a charity. There were no lived experience workers employed in the spinal unit at the hospital. Lived experience peer support workers provide an expertise that complements and transcends that of clinicians and other professionals, one that is essential to independence and self-management over the long term (Clifton and Bourke, 2025, Clifton et al, 2025a, 2025b).

HOME AT LAST

I left the hospital on May 11, 2011, seven months after arriving. Beyond the challenge of adjusting to my injury, lengthy hospital rehabilitation stays were emotionally fraught. I was desperate to escape the rigid hospital routines (especially the horribly bland and repetitive food) and return to "normal" family life. Yet, until I got home, it was hard to imagine what "normal" might even look like.

I returned to a house I had not seen before. Only 4% of all housing in Australia is properly accessible (Purple Orange, 2022) and our previous house was not one of them. We also needed to move closer to a train station to allow me greater independence, particularly for commuting to work. Thus, while I was in hospital rehabilitating, Elly had to shoulder the enormous task of buying and selling a house almost entirely on her own, all while supporting me through my recovery and managing family life.

I arrived home to balloons, a welcome banner, and a group hug. In the excitement, my middle son, Jacob, accidentally leaned against my wheelchair joystick, which sent us careening "like a rugby scrum" into the kitchen table. The table then smashed through the rear window, scattering glass everywhere (p. 102). While we laughed at the chaos of the moment, it also served as a symbolic reminder of the challenges that lay ahead. It wasn't until I was home that the full magnitude of the losses caused by spinal cord injury truly hit me.

CLINICAL AND SOCIAL SUPPORT SYSTEMS

It was surprisingly nerve-racking to find myself suddenly without the direct clinical support that was available during the months of rehabilitation. While I had come to be frustrated with the hospital routine, even sometimes resentful of the clinical control over my life, it was always comforting to know that help was nearby for the many bodily complications that flowed from the injury.

However, the staff in the rehabilitation unit had prepared me well, and I adjusted to the daily ritual of my body's needs relatively smoothly. Australia's public health system funds good quality in-house and outpatient support, including allocating patients to a spinal outreach service that provides ready contact for 18 months post-discharge (see https://royalrehab-ryde.com.au/public-rehab-services/spinal-outreach/). Six-monthly outpatient clinical consultations are also provided, services that I have continued to use to this day.

In Australia, the government also funds disability support, facilitated through the National Disability Insurance Scheme (NDIS). Access to the scheme is not dependent on private insurance but is available to all citizens and permanent residents. The scheme provides reasonable and necessary support and equipment to people with qualifying disabilities, enabling them to achieve goals that promote and maximise independence (see https://www.ndis.gov.au/). For people with spinal cord injury, this can include:

- assistive technology and equipment, such as wheelchairs, commodes, and voice recognition software
- personal support for daily living, like hoisting in and out of bed, toileting, dressing, domestic duties, and social and community support
- therapy needed for maintaining physical health and preventing secondary complications,
- capacity-building supports, such as skill development for people who need to retrain
- home modifications, such as ramps and accessible bathrooms
- transport assistance, such as the cost of accessible taxis

As I noted earlier, self-management cannot be an individual responsibility but depends on a social environment that empowers people to maximise their independence.

FAMILY AND RESILIENCE: REBUILDING TOGETHER

Even with this social support in place, adjusting to life at home with the injury was immensely challenging. For many years, I grieved my losses (Clifton, 2014). The most obvious were the physical changes, as the injury stole my ability to run, surf, play golf, and participate in other sports. Weekends, once filled with activity, became a void. I often found myself bored, questioning my identity. Since play was a huge part of my parenting style—indeed, it was the cause of my injury—I also struggled to know how to be a good dad. Above all, my marriage suffered for a time. Healthy relationships thrive on mutual giving and receiving, and sometimes, ours seemed unbalanced. The impact of the injury on intimacy and sexuality was particularly devastating and complex.

Yet, amid the profound challenges, connection and commitment forged a path forward. I've not yet highlighted the central role of my family during my in-house rehabilitation, but I could not have done it without them. Elly was a constant, unwavering bulwark of support from beginning to end, navigating every difficult stage while simultaneously managing our family life. Our children, too, demonstrated their love through countless hospital visits and by simply getting on with their lives and contributing at home. Our parents and siblings provided love and outstanding assistance, offering an extra set of hands around the house, moving in for a time to support Elly. My work colleagues and other friends visited relentlessly. In my seven months of rehabilitation, I never once felt forgotten or alone.

Once at home, my children and I found new ways to relate. They did some of my personal care work, especially at night. This gave me some flexibility at bedtime, allowed me to spend time with them rather than relying on external support workers, and provided them with valuable life skills. My wife and I, too, found ways to rebuild our relationship. Accepting our new reality, we reimagined domestic responsibilities, approached physical intimacy with creativity, and, above all, provided one another with the emotional support we both needed. Together, we began to reconstruct our lives, piece by piece.

THE JOY OF WORK

My return to work was a significant milestone. Fortunately, I was able to return to my preinjury vocation. At work, I felt less disabled. I was a theologian and ethicist first, with quadriplegia in the background. The simple act of commuting to work by train greatly renewed my sense of independence, making me "feel like an adult" (p. 96), free for a time from the hovering support of others. Surprisingly, quadriplegia provided me a unique advantage as a teacher, enabling me to speak to students from a deep well of experience of vulnerability, suffering, resilience, strength, and loving support. The Christian gospel and the ethical life are, in essence, about navigating the good life amid its vicissitudes and vulnerabilities (Clifton, 2018). I found classroom discussion to be wonderfully stimulating. For the first time since the accident, I felt like I was contributing to others and was not just a recipient of care.

Work was not without its challenges, and I still relied on the kind support of others. I regularly had to ask colleagues to unblock a catheter (a task involving some intimacy), and they were always willing and generous. I had some horrifying and messy bowel accidents, once in front of a classroom. In such instances, I was again reminded of the solicitude of work colleagues and care workers who willingly helped clean me up. I dealt with pain and tiredness and worked part-time for many years, and my workplace flexed with my needs.

Even so, work was immensely gratifying. It gave me financial independence and opportunities to teach and model what I was learning about disability values and inclusion. I redirected my research, taking the opportunity to explore the intersection between theology, virtue ethics, and disability. This proved a form of therapy—grappling in writing with the grief and loss of SCI, spinal cord injury, and pressing for a conception of happiness that I could bring to bear in my own life.

NARRATIVE RECONSTRUCTION OF PURPOSE AND MEANING

Reflecting on grief after the loss of a loved one, Robert Niemeyer (2001) emphasises the importance of narrative reconstruction. He notes that significant loss challenges one's sense of identity and narrative cohesion, "like a novel that loses a central character in the middle chapters, the life story disrupted by loss must be reorganised, rewritten, to find a new strand of continuity... searching for ways of assimilating the multiple meanings of loss into the overarching story of their lives" (Neimeyer, 2001: 264). Adjusting to spinal cord injury also entails processing the grief of lost function and identity—of the person you were before—and thus requires narrative reconstruction (Clifton, 2014).

In the years after returning home, I wrote several books and articles to process the grief and challenge of adjusting to a spinal cord injury, including the memoir cited throughout this chapter. I also searched for and interviewed people who had lived with the injury for a long time and had flourished. Writing about my journey alongside theirs helped me discover new meaning and envision a new future. Since the impact of the injury was a brutal loss of independence, narrative reconstruction was central to self-management and regaining some control of my life.

While this academic approach to narrative reconstruction may not suit everyone, spinal cord injury memoirs are relatively common, for example, Hanif Kureishi's brilliant novel, *Shattered* (2024). Many people adjusting to spinal cord injury use social media to explore their challenges and hopes. Others talk to psychologists and counsellors. Most people rewrite their story in conversation with family and friends.

In recent work with colleagues, we developed an intervention program aimed at helping individuals find meaning and purpose after a spinal cord injury. This program specifically targeted those who had left rehabilitation units and were struggling to adjust to their injury (Clifton et al, 2024, Dong et al, 2024). The intervention was rooted in the concept of post-traumatic growth, defined as "positive psychological change experienced as a result of the struggle with highly challenging life circumstances" (Tedeschi and Calhoun, 2004). Post-traumatic growth is characterised by five key components (Byra, 2016, Crawford et al, 2014, Jones et al, 2018, Kennedy et al, 2013, Wang et al, 2017):

- A greater sense of personal strength and the discovery of inner resources.
- A heightened appreciation of life and shifts in perspective, goals, and priorities.
- Stronger connections with others or a higher power.
- The identification of new possibilities or opportunities.
- A deeper sense of meaning and purpose in life.

The concept of post-traumatic growth aligns with the virtue ethics framework that has guided my journey, as described in this chapter. My recovery involved cultivating virtues or personal strengths, shifting perspectives and priorities, strengthening connections with others, embracing new opportunities, and reconstructing meaning through narrative. Post-traumatic growth involves maximising independence, but relies on interdependence. Our personal strength and inner resources emerge through stronger connections with others. Meaning is thoroughly relational. Our deepest meanings emerge from the deep giving and receiving between those we love and the larger communities we are a part of.

Meaning itself can be understood in two ways: global meaning and situational meaning. Global meaning encompasses our broader beliefs, values, identity, relationships, and long-term goals. Situational meaning, on the other hand, refers to the significance we find in specific daily events and activities. These two are interconnected; our global meaning can guide our daily actions, and the meaning we derive from those actions can, in turn, reshape our overarching beliefs and goals (Littooij et al, 2016, Park, 2010).

Reframing meaning is a lifelong task. From the earliest days in hospital, global meaning was on my mind. I had spent my life in church, and my injury raised complex questions about my faith and work. I had the privilege of spending many hours with close friends in the hospital exploring theological questions, many of which I subsequently wrote about (Clifton, 2018, 2015). Over time, my faith changed, and I drifted away from the church. The reasons for this are complex and beyond the scope of this paper. However, it is certainly true that spinal cord injury raised existential questions for me that I took many years to work through.

Today, my focus has shifted from contemplating global meaning to the more immediate question, "What do I get up for in the morning?"—a colloquial summation of situational meaning drawn from the Japanese term "ikigai" (Buettner and Skemp, 2016).

CONCLUSION

Life with quadriplegia remains challenging, bringing substantial limitations and pain. Despite this, it's mostly a good life. What gets me up in the morning is the joy of spending time with my wife and adult children (when they're around). My kids and I are close, and I'm incredibly proud of them. I must have done something right with my reconstructed parenting style.

I also cherish time with friends, especially the many wonderful people with disability who have broadened my horizons and enriched my life. I find immense purpose in my work as a faculty member at the University of Sydney, where I teach disability studies and ethics and conduct research on disability policy.

Weekends can still bring bouts of boredom, but whenever support is available, I combat this by riding my seated electric bike or rolling my wheelchair along the foreshore near my home. I'm now rarely jealous of the surfers. Instead, I find enjoyment watching them carve through the waves. I often take photos of the sunset, appreciating the beauty I had previously overlooked in my faster-paced pre-injury life. Reading consumes a good portion of my time, and I've started a science fiction book club with some friends.

You could say I've developed the skills and attitudes necessary to effectively manage my injury on my own. But the truth is that self-management is a myth. Living and thriving with spinal cord injury requires a community. Independence, as we often idealise it, is not truly achievable for anyone. Instead, interdependence forms the foundation of human life and flourishing.

For those of us living with permanent disability, robust networks of support are essential. These networks include medicos, therapists, support workers, family, and friends, together embedded within broader local and national social support systems. These systems provide vital resources and foster inclusive communities that enable people with disability to learn, play, work, and live fulfilling lives. In turn, they allow those of us with disability to contribute our unique strengths and perspectives, enriching the well-being of the entire community.

REFERENCES

Aristotle. (2012) *Nicomachean ethics*, Chicago: University of Chicago Press.

Bailey, K. A., Gammage, K. L., Van Ingen, C. and Ditor, D. S. (2016) 'Managing the stigma: Exploring body image experiences and self-presentation among people with spinal cord injury', *Health Psychology Open*, 3(1): 205510291665009.

Buettner, D. and Skemp, S. (2016) 'Blue zones: Lessons from the World's longest lived', *American Journal of Lifestyle Medicine*, 10(5): 318–21.

Byra, S. (2016) 'Posttraumatic growth in people with traumatic long-term spinal cord injury: Predictive role of basic hope and coping', *Spinal Cord*, 54(6): 478–82.

Campbell, F. K. (2009a) *Contours of ableism: The production of disability and abledness*, Springer.

Campbell, F. K. (2009b) *Internalised ableism: The tyranny within*, Basingstoke: Palgrave Macmillan UK, pp. 16–29.

Clifton, S. (2014) 'Grieving my broken body: An autoethnographic account of spinal cord injury as an experience of grief', *Disability and Rehabilitation*, 36(21): 1823–29.

Clifton, S. (2015) 'Theodicy, disability, and fragility: An attempt to find meaning in the aftermath of quadriplegia', *Theological Studies*, 76(4): 765–84.

Clifton, S. (2018) *Crippled grace: Disability, virtue ethics, and the good life*, Waco: Baylor University Press.

Clifton, S. (2020) *Hierarchies of power: Disability theories and models and their implications for violence against, and abuse, neglect, and exploitation of, people with disability*, Disability Royal Commission.

Clifton, S., & Bourke, J. (2026). Are standing and walking overrated? Ableism in spinal cord injury rehabilitation. *Disability and Rehabilitation*, *48*(4), 1141–1151. https://doi.org/10.1080/09638288.2025.2546070

Clifton, S., Bray, E., Dong, S., McCabe, R. and Siddall, P. (2024) 'Co-design of an intervention exploring meaning and purpose after spinal cord injury', *Disability and Rehabilitation*, 1–10. https://doi.org/10.1080/09638288.2023.2300655

Clifton, S., Cooper, E., Bourke, J., Connor, S., Denton, S., Dominish, B., Gibellini, C., Gilroy, J., Hallahan, L., Jessep, S., Katterl, S., Mellifont, D., Farrant, F. Q., O'Brien, B., Watharow, A., & Wynn, R. (2025). Disability lived experience and expertise: Recognising the expert contributions of people with disability. *Evidence & Policy*, *21*(4), 578–595. https://doi.org/10.1332/17442648Y2025D000000060

Clifton, S., Cooper, E., Bourke, J., Connor, S., Denton, S., Dominish, B., Drinkwater, A., Gibellini, C., Gilroy, J., Hallahan, L., Jessep, S., Katterl, S., Mellifont, D., O'Brien, B., Farrant, F. Q., Watharow, A., & Wynn, R. (2025). A framework for disability lived expertise. *Evidence & Policy*, *21*(4), 596–616. https://doi.org/10.1332/17442648Y2025D000000069

Clifton, S., Llewellyn, G. and Shakespeare, T. (2018) 'Quadriplegia, virtue theory, and flourishing: A qualitative study drawing on self-narratives', *Disability & Society*, 33(1): 20–38. https://doi.org/10.1080/09687599.2017.1379951

Clifton, S., Llewellyn, G. and Shakespeare, T. (2020) 'Faith, spirituality, and living the good life with quadriplegia', *Psychology of Religion and Spirituality*, 12(3): 356–65. https://doi.org/10.1037/rel0000215

Crawford, J. J., Gayman, A. M. and Tracey, J. (2014) 'An examination of post-traumatic growth in Canadian and American ParaSport athletes with acquired spinal cord injury', *Psychology of Sport and Exercise*, 15(4): 399–406.

Dadlez, E. M. and Woolvine, S. (2021) 'Ashamed of our selves: Disabling shame and humility', in M. Alfano, M. P. Lynch and A. Tanesini (eds): *The Routledge handbook of philosophy of humility*, Abingdon, Oxon; Routledge, pp. 117–26.

Dong, S., Bray, E., Clifton, S., McCabe, R. and Siddall, P. (2024) 'A qualitative exploration of the experiences of individuals with spinal cord injury participating in a community-based online intervention to support posttraumatic growth', *Disability and Rehabilitation*, 1–9. https://doi.org/10.1080/09638288.2024.2392035

Epstein, M. J. (2010) 'On humility', in T. Pettway and M. J. Epstein (eds): *Deep: Real life with spinal cord injury*, Ann Arbor, MI: University of Michigan Press.

Jones, F. and Riazi, A. (2011) 'Self-efficacy and self-management after stroke: A systematic review', *Disability and Rehabilitation*, 33(10): 797–810.

Jones, K. F., Dorsett, P., Simpson, G. and Briggs, L. (2018) 'Moving forward on the journey: Spirituality and family resilience after spinal cord injury', *Rehabilitation Psychology*, 63(4): 521–31.

Kennedy, P., Lude, P., Elfström, M. and Cox, A. (2013) 'Perceptions of gain following spinal cord injury: A qualitative analysis', *Topics in Spinal Cord Injury Rehabilitation*, 19(3): 202–10.

Kureishi, H. (2024) *Shattered: A memoir*, London: Penguin.

Littooij, E., Leget, C. J. W., Stolwijk-Swüste, J. M., Doodeman, S., Widdershoven, G. A. M. and Dekker, J. (2016) 'The importance of 'global meaning' for people rehabilitating from spinal cord injury', *Spinal Cord*, 54(11): 1047–52.

Longmore, P. K. (2003) *Why I burned my book and other essays on disability*, Philadelphia: Temple University Press.

Lorig, K. R. and Holman, H. R. (2003) 'Self-management education: History, definition, outcomes, and mechanisms', *Annals of Behavioral Medicine*, 26(1): 1–7.

Martz, E. and Livneh, H. (2016) 'Psychosocial adaptation to disability within the context of positive psychology: Findings from the literature', *Journal of Occupational Rehabilitation*, 26(1): 4–12.

Neimeyer, R. A. (2001) *Meaning reconstruction & the experience of loss*, Washington, DC: American Psychological Association.

Park, C. L. (2010) 'making sense of the meaning literature: An integrative review of meaning making and its effects on adjustment to stressful life events', *Psychological Bulletin*, 136(2): 257–301.

Paul, L. A. (2014) *Transformative experience*, Oxford University Press.

Purple Orange. (2022) *Urgent investment needed in accessible and affordable social housing*: https://purpleorange.org.au/news-resources/federal-election-2022/accessible-housing

Shakespeare, T. (2014) *Disability rights and wrongs revisited*, New York: Routledge. https://doi.org/10.4324/9781315887456

Smith, B. and Caddick, N. (2015) 'The impact of living in a care home on the health and wellbeing of spinal cord injured people', *International Journal of Environmental Research and Public Health*, 12(4): 4185–202.

Tedeschi, R. G. and Calhoun, L. G. (2004). 'Posttraumatic growth: conceptual foundations and empirical evidence', *Psychological Inquiry*, 15(1), 1–18.

Wade, L., Elliott, T. R., Schlegel, R. J., Williamson, M. L., Yoon, M. and Spooner, M. (2023) 'Resilience and well-being among persons with spinal cord injury/disorders', *Rehabilitation Psychology*, 68(3): 324.

Wang, Y., Wang, H., Wang, Z., Xie, H., Shi, J. and Zhao, X. (2017) 'The process of posttraumatic growth in individuals with traumatic spinal cord injury in mainland China: An interpretative phenomenological analysis', *Journal of Health Psychology*, 22(5): 637–49.

16 Our Liver Transplant Journey

Christopher Bushby and Cecilia (Nowak) Bushby

I spent a total of 140 days in hospitals, attending 34 separate appointments for investigations.

Personal hospital records, NHS UK, Google search

INTRODUCTION: ABOUT US

I was born at Colchester Hospital and was adopted, spending most of my early years on a farm in central Suffolk. Before attending agricultural college and university, I served three years in the Coldstream Guards. After completing my studies, I worked for the Suffolk Agricultural Association, a charity, for ten years as Showground Manager and 20 years as their Chief Executive. I then became Chief Executive of Big C Cancer Charity, a role I held for nine years until August 2024.

As a person, I am described as purposeful, resilient, determined, polite, and kind. Physically, I have an athletic build, standing 6 feet 2 inches (188 cm) tall; my weight at the time of surgery was 72 kg (11 st 4 lbs). Now, a year later, I weigh 103 kg (16 st 3 lbs).

My wife, Cecilia, has worked across the media, education, and health sectors. I would describe her as forthright and a defender, as she continuously advocates for me. Her inner strength during my illness was genuinely admirable.

SIGNS OF WHAT WAS TO COME

In late 2022, I started feeling exhausted and experienced irregular episodes of vomiting. This gradually worsened in the New Year, and I mistakenly believed I had a persistent stomach bug. It reached a point while travelling for work where I carried a bucket in the car, which was unfortunately needed several times.

On 26 April 2023, I was travelling to the Big C offices at Centrum in Norwich for a meeting with the Chairman and the Senior Leadership Team in preparation for the Board Trustees' Meeting the following day. During the meeting, I had to excuse myself several times to vomit, and I noticed blood in the vomit. After the meeting, the Company Secretary remarked that I looked very unwell and, along with others at the table, insisted that I go to the hospital, which is thankfully on the other side of the Research Park. They refused to let me travel alone.

I presented myself at Norfolk and Norwich University Hospital, A&E and was immediately taken through and a cannula was inserted (a cannula is a thin, hollow tube that can be inserted into the body, either to deliver fluids or medications, or to withdraw fluids or samples), a blood sample was taken, and I was attached infusion pump intravenously to administer saline drip (sodium chloride). After seeing a doctor, I was moved to the High Dependency Unit, where they began to treat me with 4 litres of plasma, vitamin K, and a spectrum of antibiotics. I was then taken for a CT scan. During this time, I was going in and out of consciousness and was eventually moved to the Gastroenterology Ward, into a private room.

I woke up in the morning after a difficult night to find myself surrounded by a team of medical practitioners. The lead Consultant (Gastroenterologist/Hepatologist) confirmed I had a serious liver condition, as shown by the CT scan and blood tests. This meant I had to stay in hospital for further investigations, including an endoscopy, ultrasound, and Fibroscan (to assess liver stiffness related to cirrhosis).

DOI: 10.1201/9781003599074-18

The endoscopy revealed several oesophageal varices, which required banding treatments over the coming year. For those who have not undergone an upper endoscopy, also known as gastroscopy, esophagogastroduodenoscopy (EGD), or upper GI, it is quite an experience. It did not matter how much sedation was administered; my body would fight the tube every time, and on one occasion, I managed to clamp down with my molars on the camera tube and would not let go without noticeable encouragement from the consultant. The speed at which they perform banding to the varices is incredible, along with taking biopsies.

The Fibroscan showed I had severe liver cirrhosis, stage 4. My score was 69 out of a possible 75. A healthy liver scores under 7; a compensated liver scores 35 and below; a decompensated liver scores 35 and above. These results indicated that I had a decompensated liver, and the chances of it reverting to a compensated state were unlikely. At this point, we both wondered how much time I might have left to live.

Surprisingly, I was discharged after just four days, with an appointment scheduled at the clinic for a month later, on 8 June 2023. I was prescribed several medications.

FIRST CLINIC APPOINTMENT

During a clinic appointment at the Norfolk and Norwich University Hospital, the Hepatologist confirmed that my liver had decompensated to stage 4 due to alcohol-related liver disease, which was caused by my love of wine. Only after the transplant and further investigations did I discover I had Hepatitis C and E, along with a genetic sensitivity affecting my organs' resilience. At best, I was given a year to live, making a liver transplant my only chance of survival. However, before I could be referred to the Addenbrooke's Hospital Liver Transplant Unit, I had to meet specific medical and lifestyle criteria. Medically, this involved examinations of my heart, lungs, kidneys, pancreas, gallbladder, and spleen to ensure I could withstand the operation if a transplant were performed. In terms of lifestyle, I had to abstain from alcohol for six months. We realised we needed to learn medical terminology to ask informed questions. The best source was the NHS England (National Health Service) website, and Cecilia also checked the chat rooms of the British Liver Trust and Addenbrooke's Liver Transplant Association. Cecilia kept detailed notes on her mobile phone, tablet, and notepad. We rehearsed questions beforehand for our appointments with medical practitioners.

> The liver performs over 500 vital functions, including filtering toxins from the blood, producing bile for digestion, metabolising nutrients, and storing vitamins and minerals. It also plays a key role in blood clotting, regulating blood sugar, and fighting infection.
>
> *NHS England (National Health Service)*

After this clinic, my wife and I travelled to Wiltshire to stay overnight on our way to Cornwall, as guests of the Royal Cornwall Show. Since we did not fully understand the implications of this diagnosis, our car journey was a mixture of mild despair and hope. I was unsure what my wife was thinking at the time, but I was already contemplating whether I had my affairs in order. We found that there were gaps which needed addressing.

Attending the Royal Cornwall Show was a boost for us both, especially being in an environment we are familiar with and among friends. During this time, Cecilia and I had in-depth conversations, beginning to realise the seriousness of my situation and the urgent need to understand the implications of my condition, as well as to explore the facts, treatments, and survival statistics related to the disease. Amid my medical investigations and treatments, I physically worsened, which resulted in 50 days in hospital at Ipswich and Norfolk and Norwich University Hospital on seven separate admissions – four in Ipswich and three in Norwich.

During my time in hospital, I was diagnosed with Hepatic encephalopathy, Clostridioides difficile (C. diff), colitis, ascites, peripheral neuropathy, and muscle atrophy (wastage). Symptom-wise, the high bilirubin levels not only caused jaundice but also led to severe irritation, causing me to scratch my legs until they bled. It was relentless, and combined with sleep deprivation, it was the most debilitating part of the illness and mentally exhausting. Cecilia now tells me I resembled a wounded animal whilst I was curled up in my bed, whether at home or in hospital. The loss of muscle mass prevented me from standing for long periods and limited my mobility, making it uncomfortable to sit down. It was a struggle to climb the stairs at home.

THE ASSESSMENT

In the New Year 2024, once I had met the criteria for a liver transplant assessment, Norfolk and Norwich University Hospital referred me to Addenbrooke's Hospital. I attended my pre-assessment appointments on 9 April 2024 and 23 April 2024, where I met with a transplant surgeon, anaesthetist, hepatologist, mental health and transplant nurses, and a registrar. During these assessments, I gained an understanding of the liver transplant procedure, associated risks, recovery process, and the lifestyle changes required after the operation. The multidisciplinary team met at the end of the week to review my case, and it was unanimously agreed that, for my survival, I needed a liver transplant.

Following their administrative procedures, I was now active on the National Liver Transplant Database on 2 May 2024.

It is not easy to comprehend the thoughts I had when I was told I was being referred to Addenbrooke's for assessment. Perversely, in my mind, I wanted my condition to be severe enough so that the only option would be a transplant to survive. I did not want to continue deteriorating and feeling the way I did. I am unsure what might have happened or what actions I would have taken if I hadn't been selected for transplant. My only caveat is my resilient nature and the belief that, throughout my life, things tend to work out right in the end, perhaps naively.

Cecilia was my solid support, keeping me grounded and hopeful; her kindness and compassion were visible not only to me but also to those around us. I now realise she was very anxious about me dying, especially after I was chosen for a transplant, as my condition deteriorated. Sometimes, Cecilia doubted I would make it to the operating table.

Without Cecilia, I would have struggled to adhere to the medication schedule, especially with lactulose, which was there to help with the Encephalopathy, along with a strong antibiotic, Rifaximin, taken twice daily. In addition to the protein drinks, which I came to hate, regardless of the flavour and had to consume three times a day, I also had to eat six meals/snacks a day, the last at 11 pm. She would march up the stairs and because of the nature of lactulose, would often find me sitting on the loo, and it became a joke when it came to finding me!

THE TRANSPLANT

I now continue with my admittance to hospital on the 19th May. We arrived at ward G5 on the 5th floor to meet the medical team again, and this time we were taken to a bed in the High Dependency Unit. Speaking with the consultant, he confirmed that the algorithm, which determines which patient receives a donated liver, prioritised me. If I did not receive the donated liver that day, he was confident that by the end of the week, I would be a recipient of a donor liver.

> The UK liver transplant algorithm, introduced in 2018, uses a computer algorithm to prioritise patients on the waiting list, aiming to maximise the benefit from each donated liver. This algorithm, known as the Transplant Benefit Score (TBS), considers various factors related to both the donor and the potential recipient to predict which patient would gain the most life-years from a transplant.
>
> *NHS England (National Health Service)*

As we waited, the team conducted several medical tests and performed various procedures. The registrar kept appearing to confirm that, hopefully, I would be taken to surgery at 6 pm. This was all dependent on the work currently being undertaken on the donated liver, with the aid of a liver perfusion machine. This pioneering technology keeps a donor liver alive outside the body by circulating oxygenated blood and nutrients, mimicking the natural process. At 5 pm, he confirmed that I would soon be collected by one of his colleagues. At that moment, Cecilia and I held hands as she sat on the bed with me. I telephoned Big C's Company Secretary to initiate communication with interested parties, which had been arranged in advance. Cecilia was ready to contact family and friends following the surgery.

As we travelled down on a trolley bed to the underground theatre, we remained silent in anticipation of what was to come. Cecilia gave me a lingering hug and kiss as I passed through the doors and down a long corridor, which I couldn't help but notice on either side: costly, portable, high-tech medical machines. I was wheeled into the theatre; my surroundings felt cramped, given that the medical team consisted of four surgeons, ten nurses, and two anaesthetists. After some introductions, I was asked if I needed assistance transferring from the trolley to the theatre table, which I did not. I lay there, and a hood was placed over my head with gas to make me unconscious. I was in theatre for 15 hours and 20 minutes, then taken to intensive care and kept in an induced coma for two days. This was to enable the medical team to deliver the intensive care required after such a significant operation, and also to allow my body to begin recovering without my consciousness interfering.

Cecilia, after leaving me at the door for the onward journey to the theatre, suddenly felt lost. She returned to the high dependency unit to find out where the accommodation that had been promised on campus was. After being passed around the hospital, the accommodation was sorted. In Cecilia's mind, the surgeon had said the operation should take 6 to 8 hours, so she was expecting a call early in the morning. She told me it was an extremely long night, just waiting for the phone to ring. By 8 am, she was feeling naturally anxious and contacted the liver transplant department, which confirmed that I was still in theatre. Eventually, at 9.15 am, she received a call from the surgeon confirming that there had been no complications and that she could visit at 12 noon.

At 12 noon prompt, Cecilia entered the Intensive Care Unit feeling nervous and apprehensive, unsure of what to expect. She was quite shocked to see the amount of tubing protruding from all over my body. She felt emotional as I lay there, peacefully breathing through the ventilator. Cecilia spent seven hours by my bedside. She was surprised at how quickly the time passed, as there was a constant flurry of medical activity and practitioners to talk to. She joked with the medical team that it was great to talk to me without my usual sarcastic response. She retired to her room at 7 pm for a well-deserved rest, sleeping from 8 pm to 8 am, safe in the knowledge that I was in good hands, and all those she had spoken to had reassured her that I was progressing well (Figure 16.1).

As I started to come out of the induced coma, I could hear an Irish voice, which turned out to be one of the transplant consultants performing an ultrasound on my stomach, while teaching medical students. The nurses were surprised by my memory, considering the drugs used to keep me asleep. As I regained consciousness, I noticed a large tube connected to the ventilator down my throat, with tubes on the side of my neck, and my head was secured to the bed so I could not move. My mouth was dry. Cecilia was sitting there, waiting to greet me. There was a flurry of nursing activity, with the ventilator tube being taken out and my head being released.

I was unaware of any pain, only that my body ached as if I hadn't been to the gym for ages and then overexerted myself. All my movements felt like they were in slow motion. I had a pain pump with a button that intravenously delivered a measured dose of a synthetic opioid, Fentanyl, which is a hundred times stronger than morphine. You could not overdose, but the drug does produce a high and makes patients susceptible to hallucinations. I am pleased to say that my hallucinations were pleasant, about family and, ironically, about work.

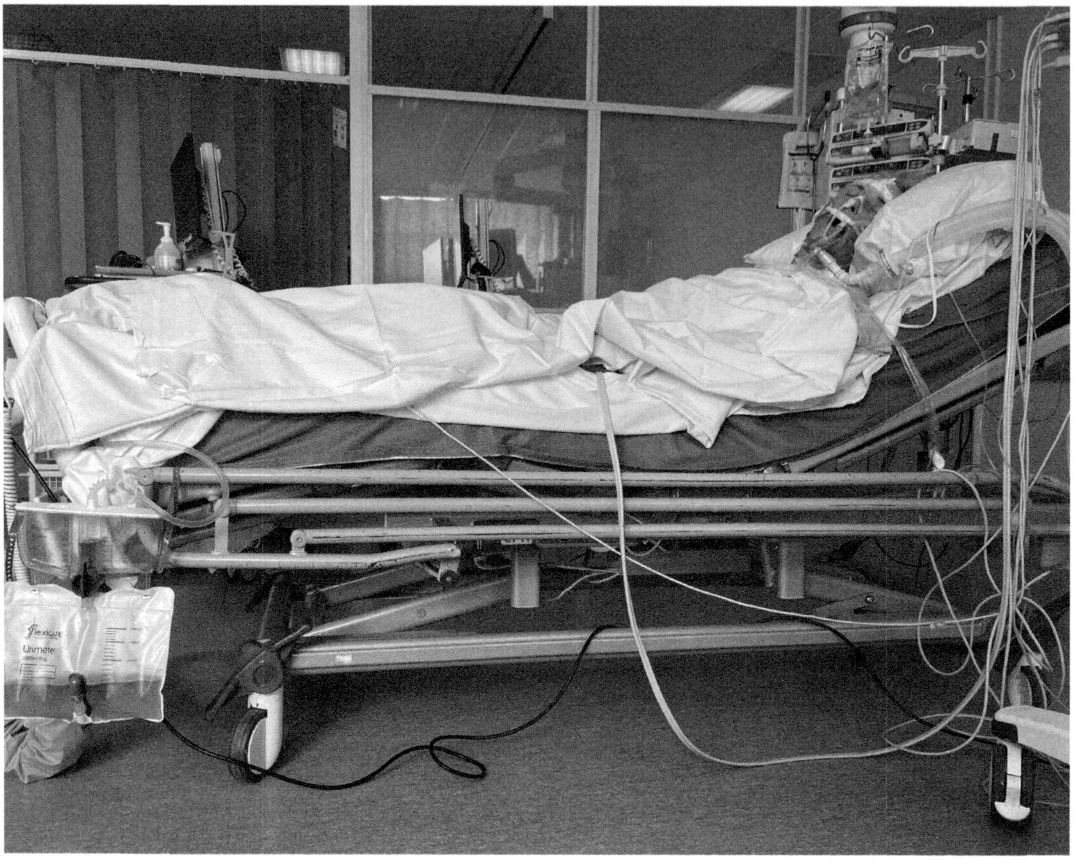

FIGURE 16.1 Waking up: Photo taken at Addenbrooke's Hospital Intensive Care Unit, 21 May 2024. (Photo courtesy of Mrs. C (Nowak) Bushby)

It is difficult to recall how many tubes were inserted into my body. There were two pipes in my stomach. I was fitted with a catheter, and besides the tubes in my neck, there was one running from my nose to my stomach, which was an irritation and became a point of contention in the days that followed.

I kept slipping in and out of consciousness, and on Tuesday afternoon, the 21 May· a team of physiotherapists and nurses gathered, eager to get me out of bed. However, it was not straightforward, given the attachments to my body and how weak and dizzy I felt. I was receiving instructions from all sides, which became overwhelming and confusing, so I had to ask them all to be quiet in a firm voice. One remarked that there are "too many chefs in the kitchen." I eventually managed to stand with the help of a support tool and take a few steps, then went straight back to bed. I could see Cecilia was concerned for me and felt they were rushing things.

During this period, I was consistently receiving medical treatment and medication, and I was being fed liquid protein directly into my stomach. I had significant difficulty swallowing my tablets because of the feeding tube. Some tablets are so large that they are often described as big enough for a horse. I developed a chest infection that, ironically, had no noticeable symptoms and did not cause any breathing difficulties. It was treated with antibiotics.

Cecilia, exhausted, went home, and the following day, my Scottish friend Ian visited me. His take on life kept me amused, even though I often found myself drifting off to sleep. Later that day, I was moved back to the high dependency unit for two days, then returned to the ward, which accommodated five patients.

RECLAIMING CONTROL

It became clear to me that I needed to start reclaiming control and adopting a more positive attitude in my interactions with the medical teams, especially the consultants and registrars. A point of contention was the feeding tube, which prevented me from eating solid foods. Dietitians wanted to continue feeding me this way because of my ongoing weight loss; however, I argued with the consultants, who questioned why I was not eating solid food. Sarcastically, I said that if they removed the tube, I could start eating normally again. This was actioned and another aspect of everyday life was realised. A treat for me at the end of the week was a Whopper burger from Burger King located in the hospital.

Each day, I set myself tasks to achieve specific important goals: having the catheter removed, using the toilet unassisted, discontinuing the use of bedpans, and taking a shower. I also aimed to shave and dress in regular clothing. This was complicated at first, due to the tube attachments and the need to protect the operation incision, which was 41cm (16 inches) long, running from the bottom of my rib cage down to my belly button and across the right side of my body to my waist. The incision was held together by 54 staples, which serve as a souvenir at home (Figure 16.2).

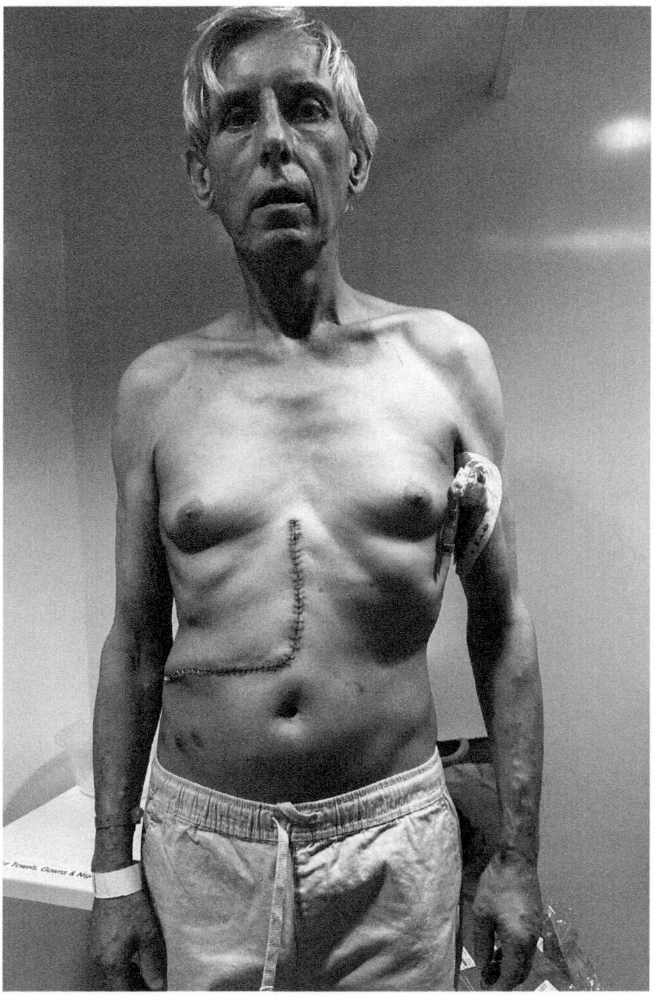

FIGURE 16.2 Photo taken at Addenbrooke's Hospital, 7 June 2024. (Photo courtesy of Mrs. C (Nowak) Bushby)

Cecilia established a pattern of visiting on two consecutive days, staying overnight at a local hotel or on campus. She would then stay at home for two days. I was particularly keen that she kept up with the garden maintenance and ensured the tomato plants given by my work colleague, the Director of Corporate Services, were planted and nurtured. She would send me photos, and I would check up on FaceTime calls. During her visits, we would go for a walk around the hospital or outside on the campus. I found this exertion quite tiring and had to rest many times along the journey. She would also read to me the news headlines, which I would often fall asleep to. She found this amusing and a chance to sneak away and grab a coffee.

My daily routine started with a blood test around 5:30 am. Medication was administered approximately every four hours, either intravenously or orally, as needed. Vital signs, including blood pressure, temperature, and oxygen levels, were checked every four hours. These measurements often did not align with the medication times. Breakfast at 8:30, lunch at 12:30, supper at 5:30, accompanied by plenty of coffee or tea and biscuits. The menu varied daily, and the food was consistently of high quality. I developed my favourites, especially the lasagna and broccoli. This was topped up with protein drinks and protein shots. My daily calorie intake was just over 4000 calories, and by the time I left the hospital, I weighed 78 kg (12st 8lb). From time to time, the dietitians checked in on me, and I was weighed every day. The physiotherapist also made regular visits to ensure the exercises I had been given showed signs of progress. At this time, I was experiencing severe tremors due to the immune suppression medication. This did affect my writing, making it more illegible than normal. This did settle down over time as my medication was finely adjusted to my medical needs.

INFORMATION SUPPORT

When you become a patient at Addenbrooke's, you are invited to join MyChart, which allows you to *view messages*, access your test results, manage your appointments, and complete questionnaires. It encourages proactive engagement with your healthcare team and enables you to ask relevant questions, especially in my case, regarding my blood results. Typically, I would receive my blood results by 10:30 am before the consultant or registrar's rounds. This system remains a valuable asset to me.

DISCHARGED TO HOME, SO I THOUGHT

Following a liver transplant, you are expected to stay in hospital for around two to three weeks. I was approaching the end of my fourth week when it was confirmed I could go home. However, I was moved to a different part of the hospital for two days, where I was placed in a single room as part of the preparation. Unfortunately due to my blood test results, it was found that I had hyperkalaemia, acute kidney injury (AKI), and a rare bacterial infection called Pseudomonas. This meant I was moved back to ward G5 for treatment and into the same bay with my fellow patients. There was great camaraderie between us, regardless of our conditions. During my time there, I was with seven different individuals, most of whom were kidney transplant patients. In total, I spent 50 days at Addenbrooke's.

During my stay, I asked friends and colleagues not to visit because of the risk of infection. However, I kept in touch through FaceTime, messaging, email, and Microsoft Teams. I even managed to hold a couple of work meetings via this platform, which was quite daring since I was not supposed to contact the office for three months to help aid my recovery.

All the staff I encountered, whether medical or administrative, were exceptional in their care and support. I will forever be indebted, along with the donor family, to the life they have provided, which I share with my wife, Cecilia, my daughters, my extended family, friends, colleagues, and society. It took several attempts to craft a letter to the donor family for the hospital to pass on that truly expressed our eternal gratitude for the gift of future life that their selfless action enabled.

GOING HOME

The next part of our story begins on the day I returned home, 27 June 2024. After exchanging heartfelt thank you with my fellow patients and the medical team, we took the customary photo of me outside Addenbrooke's Hospital main entrance, with my suitcase and sunglasses. A relative joked that the photo looked like a mafia boss going on holiday.

I could argue that true recovery began now, when I was back home. The hospital had completed their part, ensuring I survived the operation and preparing me to return home. Once out of this cocoon, it was now down to me, supported mainly by my wife and others, to physically and mentally reintegrate into an everyday home life and society. It had been agreed with Big C Cancer Charity that I would step down from my role at the end of September 2024, after nine years of service, which had provided me with personal privilege and enrichment. From the Chairman down, the charity's conduct towards me was exemplary, demonstrating empathy and kindness, which was invaluable to me. This was a significant step in leaving, allowing me to focus entirely on my recovery without the pressures and challenges of being a Chief Executive.

There are several rules that liver transplant patients must follow, some of which are only relevant during the recovery period, while others are lifelong. During your recovery, you need to be very careful not to cause a hernia through lifting, given the location of the operation incision. It is recommended that you are sensible about exercising. In my case, I was very eager to undertake light gardening tasks. However, I find walking fairly uncomfortable because of the nerve damage (peripheral neuropathy) that is irreversible in my feet and lower legs. I initially discovered that walking upstairs or doing any exercise left me exhausted, out of breath, and often dizzy. This gradually improved, and it was not until the end of March 2025 that these conditions virtually disappeared.

LIFESTYLE CHANGES

Part of the lifestyle changes involves avoiding certain foods that affect medication absorption, especially those that interact with immunosuppressants. It is essential that you take your immunosuppressants daily and imperative that you do not switch to a different brand. Therefore, the following are off the menu: Seville oranges, grapefruit, pomegranate seeds, a rare steak, and some seafood. It is also advisable to avoid buffets, as you cannot be certain how long the food has been sitting out. It is strongly recommended that you do not consume alcohol, regardless of the cause of the liver disease, as it has several effects. It can be harmful to your donated liver because of the immunosuppressants; you are more susceptible to cancer, and it can also interfere with your ability to absorb medications.

COMPLICATIONS

One week after returning home, I attended the transplant follow-up clinic at Addenbrooke's with Cecilia. During this appointment, the consultant considered readmitting me to the hospital. However, for my mental health, he felt I should remain at home, and this would be reviewed the following week at clinic. Little did I know I was now about to spend 34 days back in hospital on four separate occasions, and this was not to do with the donor liver. At my next clinic visit, I was immediately informed that I was being readmitted, with reasons including hyperkalaemia, AKI, and the reappearance of C. diff. I was initially treated in A&E before being moved to a different part of the hospital to continue my treatment for eight days. I continued to attend the clinic weekly, where blood tests were performed. When I returned home on 8th August, I received a phone call from a registrar at Addenbrooke's, asking me to go to A&E at Ipswich Hospital immediately. I was admitted once again with hyperkalaemia and AKI, remaining in hospital for 16 days. Hyperkalaemia can stop the heart, whether diseased or fit. Treatment for hyperkalaemia involved administering 30 mL of 10% calcium gluconate to me over 30 minutes, twice, through an infusion pump via a large peripheral vein in my arm, with continuous cardiac monitoring. The viscosity of the fluid as it was injected into the vein caused pain, and I watched the clock countdown, wishing it to finish. Treatment for acute kidney injury (AKI) focuses on addressing the underlying cause and providing supportive care. This included fluid management, medications to manage blood pressure and electrolytes, and in severe cases, dialysis. My treatment was predominantly infusion of 1 litre of saline every 12 hours for most of my time in hospital. It is also supported with antibiotics. This meant you were always connected to some form of medication intravenously, whether in bed or moving around the hospital when permitted. During this time, I received multiple medications and investigations, always in consultation with Addenbrooke's. This incident occurred again on 12 September. This time I was only in for seven days. At this point, it was determined that the immunosuppressant medication was affecting my kidneys, leading to hyperkalaemia. Considerable debate took place about changing the immunosuppressant; however, it was agreed not to, but to reduce the dosage. As you can imagine, this is a delicate balance of adjustment given the risk of rejection. Currently, the kidney markers continue to show a decline, but this has been discounted and is being closely monitored.

My final hospital stay was from 4 October and lasted only three days. This was due to Paroxysmal Atrial Fibrillation, which I had no previous experience of. Since then, an ultrasound has confirmed that my heart is healthy and there are no concerns. It was not until this period of hospital stays ended that I began to make progress. Cecilia was quite relieved to have a break from daily hospital visits. As you can appreciate, hospital stays did not help my recovery, especially since I was in semi-isolation in a room on my own.

LIFE IS RETURNING TO NORMAL

Life eventually started to feel normal again, and it was wonderful to begin going out, meeting friends and family, and having family stay. I still had to attend the transplant clinic, now monthly, but it was held in a satellite clinic in Ipswich, where I live. Cecilia always had questions to ask the consultants, and one of the most important was when we could go on holiday and what advice they would give! They suggested we stay within Europe in case I needed access to specialist medical treatment.

At the end of March, we managed to spend a week in the Algarve, Portugal. One of the recommended conditions is that when outdoors, you always apply factor 50 sun cream. This is because, with a weakened immune system, you are more susceptible to skin cancer. It is also advisable that you avoid sunbathing. This was not an issue during our holiday as, unexpectedly, this part of Portugal experienced terrible weather with three severe weather warnings. Nevertheless, we still enjoyed ourselves immensely, and I particularly valued the whole experience, from being at the airport, the flight from Stansted and staying in a hotel, to experiencing life in another country. One question I have been asked is whether travel insurance is costly given my medical status. I am pleased to say it was not excessive, especially within Europe. The situation does vary outside of Europe.

In April 2025 during a conversation with my consultant, he felt that I could start going to the gym, which I had not attended for over two years. This significantly improved my wellbeing, stamina, physical strength, and posture. My first session lasted only 30 minutes, but now my workouts last over an hour. My routine involves two days at the gym and one day of rest. Starting from a low point, the weights I can now lift are quite respectable, and the changing shape of my body has meant I need to update much of my wardrobe, much to Cecilia's dismay! I now weigh 103 kg, just over 16 stone, with a very healthy appetite. There is a slogan on the wall in the gym that I think is incredibly poignant: *"Progress not Perfection."* I have begun applying for voluntary Trustee positions and am now actively seeking a new role, as I believe I still have much to offer. I have a particular fondness for the charity sector, especially in health.

REALITY

It is only now, as I write this chapter, that I have become aware of some of Cecilia's most private thoughts, which revealed her genuine emotions that she rarely displayed outwardly, especially before the transplant.

There were nights when she lay in bed, planning my funeral and contemplating how to inform family, friends, and colleagues. Her primary concern was which Coldplay tracks to include in the service. She wanted it to be perfect. Her emotions could shift from calm to fear. Other times, she would be planning our world tour!

She did not want to contemplate a life without me. She found comfort in the support she received from her family, friends (particularly our Scottish friend Ian), and work colleagues.

She found sanctuary in sitting on what she calls "her rock" in Felixstowe, gazing out to sea with a latte in hand. This always helped ground her thoughts.

SIGNING OFF

As I finish writing this chapter of our liver transplant journey, I reflect on how fortunate I have been to have the support of a loving wife and family, as well as wonderful colleagues and friends, all of whom have been supportive and never judgmental. I have been given a chance at a future life because of the selfless act of the donor, their family, and an incredible—though sometimes understated—medical team across all the hospitals I attended. We are incredibly fortunate to have the NHS and the unmatched expertise within its ranks.

What this journey has taught me personally is the importance—albeit a challenge—of accessing your inner strength and survival instinct. It has also increased my awareness that millions of people worldwide face similar situations, just under different circumstances. You certainly need a supportive family around you who can act as a filter or barrier, so you can concentrate on your own condition and recovery. We now look back and sometimes chuckle with each other about some of the experiences we encountered and how we handled them. A sense of humour was invaluable.

SELF-MANAGEMENT

My wife and I were invited to contribute to this text on self-management. We were asked to share our life experiences. What have we learned about self-management that may help and support others?

For us, resilience means discovering our inner strength and focus, which enables us to navigate and understand varied outcomes and their impact. From these scenarios, develop supportive and practical plans, such as your Will.

It is essential to regain control, as previously stated. This includes acquiring knowledge to fully understand the condition and communicate effectively with medical specialists, which then helps in setting small, achievable goals towards recovery, such as going to the toilet unaided. Ask well-informed questions to the medical teams, especially during ward rounds and clinics.

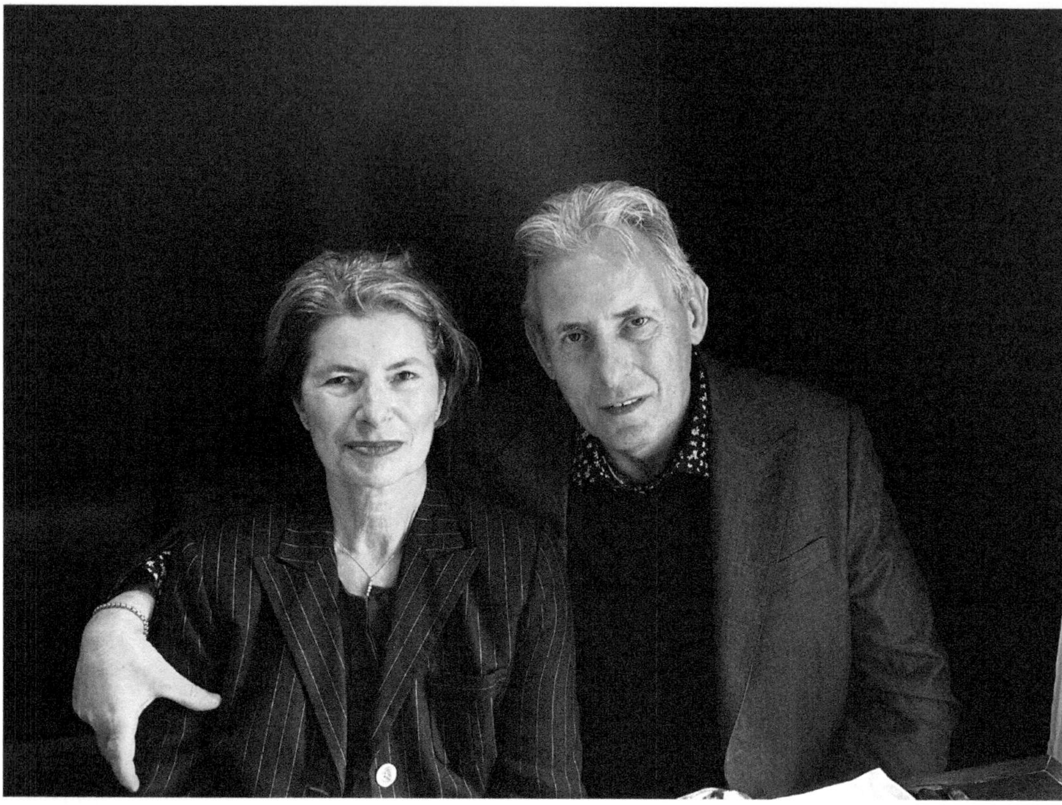

FIGURE 16.3 Photo Taken 3 August 2024. (Photo courtesy of Mrs C (Nowak) Bushby)

Having a wife, a supportive employer, and social support has been crucial, and to me, this has been invaluable. Without this network, the outcomes might have been very different (Figure 16.3).

Cecilia and I now sign off to continue enjoying our lives and, without doubt, the many adventures to come!

17 Living with and the Self-Management of Bladder Failure
A Transatlantic Autoethnography

Paul M. W. Hackett

POSITIONAL STATEMENT

In this chapter, I will present a personal account of having and self-managing a chronic medical condition. The condition has several names but may best be thought of as bladder failure (Kim, 2013). As bladder failure is not well-known, I will start this essay by providing a brief explanation of the condition. The opinions I express in this essay are inevitably coloured by many personal aspects of my life, both current and in the past. As this essay is a personal reflection on my own medical condition I do not, in any way expect, my comments to apply to others with a similar condition. Additionally, the comments I have made, both positive and negative, about the medical systems and professionals I have commented upon are purely my own very subjective perspectives. My perspective is particularly influenced by the fact that I am a British who lives in the United States and that I am a professor of health research. As I have already said: my opinions are entirely personal.

INTRODUCTION

Bladder Failure

Bladder failure (Kim, 2013; Kim and Kim, 2012; O'Leary, et al, undated) is not a commonly heard of medical condition, and it is often subsumed under names such as underactive bladder, non-neurogenic voiding disfunction, bladder outlet obstruction, distended bladder, and urinary retention. Several other common or medical terms have been used to describe this condition (D'Ancona, et al, 2019) including acontractile detrusor (Colaco, et al, 2018); atonic bladder (Michek, et al, 1992); bladder muscle sarcopenia (Fukushima, et al, 2018); chronic urinary retention (Barrisford and Steele, 2018); detrusor areflexia (Colaco, et al, 2018); detrusor failure (Osman, et al, 2014); detrusor underactivity (Osman, et al, 2014); flaccid bladder (Dorsher and McIntosh, 2012); hypotonic bladder (Weinberg, et al, 1974); impaired detrusor contractility (Griffiths, et al, 2002); lazy bladder (Stein, 2020); non-neurogenic bladder (Riccabona and Fotter, 2018); and overflow incontinence (Cleveland Clinic, 2024).

Because of lack of research into this condition, there is disagreement not only on the name for the condition but also on the definition of bladder failure. I include all of these terms to demonstrate how there is a lack of a universal definition of the condition and how this lack of condition unity has a significant negative effect upon self-managing the condition. Bladder failure is comprised of a group of urinary symptoms that result in an inability to empty the bladder. Individuals with bladder failure have difficulties emptying their bladder (micturition) or may not be able to empty or void their bladder at all. Voiding difficulty may lead to discomfort, infection, and leakage. It is apparent from the many names that are used to describe the condition, and also disagreement on standardised criteria to uphold a diagnosis, that research is needed to allow the appropriate application of treatments.

DOI: 10.1201/9781003599074-19

Bladder failure is a disorder that has no cure and those who have been diagnosed as having bladder failure have to learn to adapt their lives and to carry-on living as fully as possible. Bladder failure is one of the many illnesses or conditions that are associated with the function of the lower urinary tract (LUT) (Drake, et al, 2019). In my case, my bladder failure is due to my bladder being distended over many years, as a result of chronic urinary retention (Selius and Subedi, 2008). My bladder's distension has led to the bladder's detrusor muscles failing to function adequately enough to enable me to empty my bladder of urine. There is a lack of research into all aspects of detrusor underactivity (DU) (Chapple, et al, 2015; Osman, et al, 2014).[1] Furthermore, Chapple et al (2015) note how at the time they wrote their article, there were no effective treatments for detrusor underactivity[2] and this situation continues today. My bladder has become distended due probably to chronic enlargement of my prostate (benign prostatic hyperplasia (BPH)) (Bachman and de la Rosette, 2011) constituting an obstructive uropathy (Frøkiaer, 2020; Gallagher and Hughes, 2024) causing chronic urinary retention (NIDDKD, undated) causing me to retain a large volume of urine that I am unable to empty through normal micturition (Fowler, et al, 2008). Estimates vary of the normal urinary capacity of a healthy bladder: 300ml to 400 ml (Fitzgerald, et al, 2002; Latini, et al, 2004); 300ml to 600ml (Harrogate and District NHS Trust, 2016); 700ml in men (InformedHealth, 2022), whilst the bladder may be distended to a capacity of around 1.5 litres. As I noted earlier, when tested I managed to urinate 300ml with a residual 1.4 litres of urine in my bladder. This is the reason for my urologist saying, "you have an enormous bladder".

Having briefly described bladder failure as a condition, and more specifically my own condition, in the next section I will briefly describe my own experiences of being diagnosed with bladder failure before I then go on to describe how this diagnosis has changed many aspects of my day-to-day life. This personal account will take the form of an autoethnography, but before I present my account I will first briefly introduce the framework within which I will present my account: the declarative mapping sentence (DMS) (Hackett, 2018, 2020, 2021).

USING DECLARATIVE MAPPING SENTENCES TO EXPLORE PERSONAL EXPERIENCES OF URINARY RETENTION AND SELF-CATHETERISATION

The declarative mapping sentence is a methodological framework that is able to encompass and communicate the experience of multifaceted content domains and is therefore particularly well-suited to defining and exploring intricate personal health experiences such as bladder failure, urinary retention, bladder distension, and the necessity of self-catheterisation. The DMS has been developed as both a research methodology within qualitative social science and a way of thinking about such scholarship. Rather than being simply a research tool, the DMS comprises a hypothesised statement, or declaration, of a domain of interest that orients and communicates intricate health and well-being issues (Hackett, 2018, 2020). The DMS is a type of nomological network and a representation of the concepts associated with the experience of bladder failure, their observable manifestations, and the interrelationships between these components. The nomological validity of the DMS is a form of construct validity that assesses the consistency and rationality of the conceptual network model, confirming that the relationships between the facets in the DMS align with theoretical expectations.

A declarative mapping sentence can clearly express the different dimensions of an individual's experience of chronic urinary retention and the resultant need for self-catheterisation, from initial medical encounters and diagnostic processes to the ongoing realities of managing bladder dysfunction and adapting to self-catheterisation procedures. By mapping these interconnected elements, the DMS helps to communicate the full scope of patient experience in a coherent and structured manner. The DMS framework can help conceptualise the complexity of experiences faced by individuals using clean intermittent self-catheterisation (Logan, et al, 2008; Shaw, et al, 2008).

Using the DMS enables the understanding of the information gaps, emotional responses and adaptive strategies associated with patient experience and facilitating clearer communication of patient care needs.

A DMS for my experiences of being diagnosed and then managing bladder failure can be written as follows:

A DECLARATIVE MAPPING SENTENCE FOR BLADDER FAILURE DIAGNOSIS AND TREATMENT AUTOETHNOGRAPHY

This autoethnographic account explores my lived experience of bladder failure caused by detrusor underactivity through my:

Medical Diagnosis

(PSA investigation)
(unexpected diagnosis)
(bladder distension discovery)
(diagnostic procedures [ultrasound, urodynamics, cystoscopy])

with its associated:

Management Practices

(clean intermittent self-catheterisation frequency [six times daily])
(time investment [30–60 minutes daily])
(equipment sourcing [US and UK suppliers])
(environmental adaptations)
(life-style changes)

which has led me to experience:

Psychological Challenges

(anxiety about public catheterisation)
(adaptation to intimate medical procedures)
(coping with chronic invisible condition)

which have had impacts upon my:

Personal and Social Life

(misconceptions about temporary nature)
(conversational discomfort)
(taboo comparisons with dialysis)
(impact on daily social functioning)

which I have experienced within the two contexts of:

Healthcare Systems

(US diagnosis and management)
(UK care management and experiences)
(cross-national comparison of care approaches)

and where the condition has resulted in my experiencing and having to manage:

Complications Management

(frequent urinary tract infections)
(medication scheduling)
(ongoing distress)
(adaptive strategies)

which have resulted in my calling for mitigation and intervention in terms of:

Intervention

(self-management tool development)
(clinical understanding)
(research gap identification)
(condition visibility enhancement)

The above declarative mapping sentence defines my experience of having bladder failure and self-managing this condition within the context of limited research literature on detrusor underactivity and urinary retention. It also demonstrates how I also offer personal insights into chronic condition management across two different healthcare systems whilst I focus on experiential rather than comparative healthcare evaluation, after I have briefly described the autoethnographic methodology.

AUTOETHNOGRAPHY METHODOLOGY IN BLADDER AND LOWER URINARY TRACT DISORDERS RESEARCH

Autoethnography is a form of qualitative research methodology in which a researcher uses themself as a research tool in order to gather personal information through systematically exploring the researcher's own experiences as these exist within broader cultural and social contexts (Ellis and Adams, 2020; Ellis and Bochner, 2000). Autoethnography combines the two research methods of autobiography and ethnography, and through this amalgamation creates, "an approach to research and writing that seeks to describe and systematically analyze personal experience in order to understand cultural experience" (Ellis, et al, 2011, p. 1).

Within health research, the autoethnographic methodology has been used so as to shed-light upon the subjective experiences of those with illnesses and medical conditions and the interaction between patient and healthcare professionals and providers as these relate to the reality of living with a chronic health condition (see, for example, Belton and Sheridan, 2025; Greenhalgh, 2017; Nowakowski, 2016; Priddis, 2015; Wakelin, 2024) and closer to my condition (Toye and Barker's (2020)) metaethnography of incontinence. Within research into bladder and lower urinary tract disorders, autoethnography is especially valuable as it has the potential to provide a relatively clear view of what is the intimate, socially taboo and embarrassing nature of these conditions. Lower urinary tract symptoms (LUTS) (Gammack, 2010; Swavely, et al, 2019) include a range of disorders that include urinary incontinence, overactive and underactive bladder, and chronic pelvic pain, affect a significant proportion of people and are conditions that are frequently underreported and inadequately understood from the patient perspective (Milsom, et al, 2017). As these conditions have personal and social associations and consequences, they are particularly suited to investigation using an autoethnographic methodology based upon personal experiences, reflective journaling, institutional, and personal medical records, correspondence with healthcare providers and their own retrospective writing (Chang, 2008; Wikipedia, 2025).

In the context of bladder health research, an autoethnographer might examine entries they have made in their diary that document their experiences of symptoms, analyse and reflect upon their personal responses to treatment failures or successes and reflect critically and in-depth upon the encounters they had with healthcare professionals. The researcher must seek to establish an analytical distance from the information whilst also being emotionally engaged with this information. The researcher also attempts to connect their own subjective experiences to reports in the literature, etc., and to theoretical frameworks.

I used the autoethnographic approach in the research I report in this chapter as it allowed me to critically examine my personal experience of bladder dysfunction. Employing this approach also enabled me to make suggestion about such sequelae as feeling medically isolated and the psychosocial impacts of this urological condition. Autoethnography is a reflexive approach that is able to reveal how someone lives with a bladder disorder that more traditional research approaches (i.e., surveys, interviews) may fail to capture (Anderson, 2006). Using this method also allows for the development of how bladder failure relates to other aspects of the individual such as continence, sexuality, personal identity, gender, and aging. However, it is important to note that the autoethnographic approach in health research has been criticised due to it being extremely subjective. Furthermore, questions have been asked about the ability to generalise from results, the potential lack of stringency and rigour and the validity of the results produced through autoethnographic procedures (Reed-Danahay, 1997). These caveats warrant careful consideration when applying autoethnographic methods to bladder health research. However, if care is taken of these concerns, autoethnography can provide unique and valuable contributions to understanding how those with bladder and lower urinary tract disorders, live with their conditions, potentially offering insight into the self-management of bladder dysfunction. I end my description of methodology at this point and I now commence reporting of my experiences of bladder failure, commencing with my diagnosis.

DIAGNOSIS AND ASSESSMENT

It was that time of year when I had just had my annual health check, and my prostate specific antigen test (PSA) results had come in. I was not particularly concerned as I awaited the results as I had been diagnosed with an enlarged prostate over 15 years earlier. Urinating had however recently become a little more problematic, and I had discussed this with my primary health care practitioner in the US who had then given me a PSA test. I received the tests' results online and I noticed my PSA had risen significantly after years of little fluctuation. According to the information on the website of my US doctor's practice, my PSA was still in the normal or non-concerning range. However, my family doctor contacted me as she was concerned with the sudden jump in my PSA. "We'll wait for 3 months and get another PSA done" was her recommendation. She didn't feel overly concerned as my PSA was still low and she knew about my chronically enlarged prostate. So, I waited three, worrying, months.

My follow-up PSA was conducted and my doctor informed me that this was stable and had risen by just 0.1. However, this ruled out that my raised PSA had been a measurement artefact or due to some other specific event associated with the day I had the first test. "We'll get you to see a urologist just to be on the safe side" was her reaction. "Do you have any suggestions as to who I should see" I asked her? She did not so I told her that a person who was a slight friend of mine was a urologist and I suggested contacting him. After a few phone calls, I arranged a meeting with my acquaintance, the urologist, at his practice, which was an office, not too far from where I live. The office was in a large hospital with its familiarly comforting medical feel. I found his office and was received by a receptionist who asked me if I could provide a urine sample. I said I would try, and I managed to partially fill a plastic container. I was then asked if I could do some more if I tried. I said yes and I was again somewhat successful. I then lay on a couch and the nurse performed an ultrasound test (urodynamic test, Vignoli, 2016) to assess my ability to void my bladder of urine. This showed that whilst I had urinated around 300 ml of urine, that there was still about 1.4 litres of urine still remaining in my bladder. After she had told me these results, she left me. I sat and thought. I worried.

After waiting a quarter of an hour, my friend, the urologist came into the room in which I was sitting. "Well, your prostate is not our concern here" he said, "you have an enormously distended bladder, and you are retaining urine". This was a total shock to me as I had been preparing myself for a prostatic disease such as cancer of the prostate. I did not know whether to feel relieved or concerned. "If I were a benign dictator" he said, "you would leave here with a catheter. How do you feel about that?". I was in a state of shock. I had no idea what a distended bladder was, what its cause was, what my prognosis was, how this had to be treated…. "I don't really want to have a catheter" I said. My comment was totally founded in fear. I did not know what having a catheter really meant. Forty years before I had had a catheter when I was hospitalised after a car accident. However, I was unconscious at the time, and I had no memory of this save for being told that several times I had torn this out. So, the mention of a catheter simply aroused fear in me. My choice to not leave his office wearing a catheter was simply because I was ignorant and frightened. In hindsight, this was probably not a good decision even though it turned out that my lack of wearing a catheter on leaving the consultation did not have any negative consequences. "We need to do some more tests in my downtown office, make an appointment for as soon as I have an opening as you leave" I was told.

Within a week, I found myself driving to the hospital with my wife at 06.00 on a warm July morning. The traffic was bad, but we had left time to get into the city with time to spare. The hospital was pretty quiet, and my doctor's office had not yet opened. We waited and were greeted by the arriving nurses, who were all quite wonderful and who probably understood, or at least suspected, just how worried I was. A very professional and friendly nurse ushered me into a sterile room, and I undressed from the waist down. I was then seated with my legs open and raised. I have to admit that what happened over what felt like about 30 minutes is something of a blur. I believe that I remember having my bladder drained using a catheter and a rectal examination from my urologist. I was told by my urologist that I would have to self-catheterise six times a day.

The next thing I recall was standing in the same room with the nurse. She was truly kind and patient and inserted a catheter, describing what she was doing whilst I watched. It was my turn then. I was given a catheter, and I tried to insert this. I got it nearly all the way but found that it started to be painful. She changed the catheter to one with a coude tip and I tried again, and this time succeeded. "You have just bought yourself a life!" I was told by the nurse. "There are a lot of people who can't do that, and you can now live a normal life". I have to admit feeling elated that I could do this. I was told that I should drink eight glasses of water a day and no diuretics, such as coffee, tea, alcohol, and also things like green teas in case they included black tea. I have to admit this was quite shocking. I was also told that if I drank anything other than water, then I should drink three times the amount of water with this.

I was still in-shock and all I remember now was being given the details of a catheter supplier I could order catheters from and around a dozen catheters to give me enough before I received my order. I left the doctor's office and went to the bathroom. I was amazingly tender and I had to urinate. To my horror, I only produced a trickle of what looked more like blood than urine. Somewhat alarmed I went back to the doctor's reception and was told this was normal. My wife and I then went to a local café and sat and drank, water for my part. She was as shocked as I was, perhaps more. "How do you feel" she asked me?" "I'm relieved", I answered. "I expected to find out that I had cancer and that I had surgery coming up" I said happily, "I can live with this". She was amazed at my positive attitude, which I am usually still able to maintain.

The self-management of my condition commenced as departed from the office as I was left on my own to work out how I was going to cope with my new life situation. I contacted the catheter supplier and performed endless online searches trying to find out what catheters were available, how much these would cost me, whether my insurance would pay towards the cost for each manufacturer and how much of the cost they would cover. I found a couple of expensive academic medical research books and ordered these. I sent off for different catheters from different manufacturers, of different sizes, all with a coude tip. I started trying to insert the catheter alone which was painful and frightening. On the first day I could only manage to do this two or three times and not six. It hurt to do and I found the procedure more frightening than I had expected. Over the next couple of days, I was catheterising the requisite six times a day.

After another few days, we drove into the city and I returned to the hospital. I had been told that I would be having a cystoscopy, and I had looked this up on the internet. I discovered that I would be having a camera inserted into my urethra. The thought of this filled me with dread. I had looked up that there were two forms of cystoscopy: rigid and flexible. I had assumed I would be having a flexible cystoscopy as I read that a rigid form of the test required an anaesthetic and I had not been told to prepare for this. I was relieved to discover that my procedure would indeed use a flexible cystoscope, although I had also read that these were painful. I was shown into a room with procedure tables, cabinets, and other apparatuses. A nurse technician prepared me for the procedure and injected a numbing liquid into my urethra. My urologist then rolled up his sleeves (metaphorically) and inserted the cystoscope. The whole procedure was extremely unpleasant and at some points the pain took my breath away. "Breathe deeply, pant" I was told when I cried out in shock at the pain. During the procedure, I was able to see the monitor my doctor was continually looking at. All seemed grey and featureless, but he seemed to be able to distinguish important features. As I lay there, the thought occurred to me that I had seen the inside of my bladder, and what an eerie thought that was. Throughout the cystoscopy, the doctor seemed to be almost behaving like a sumo wrestler, positioning himself and wrestling with his opponent, who on this occasion was my urethra that was narrow and difficult to navigate due to my enlarged prostate. At the end of the procedure, he looked tired and I felt exhausted and extremely saw.

Following the procedure, I dressed and spoke with the doctor. He raised his eye-brows and in a resolute manner told me that it was as he had predicted, that I had an extremely distended bladder and that my prostate was moderately enlarged but did not show signs of cancer. Once again, and distressingly, following the cystoscopy I passed what looked like blood rather than urine. It also hurt to urinate. I was also told that they wanted to perform a prostate MRI to be sure that I did not have prostate cancer. A couple of days later I had to drive to another hospital location for my MRI. This was in a specialised wing that performed different forms of imaging. They were extremely professional and after undressing and donning a robe, I lay in the scanner and attempted to relax for around 40 minutes (it felt much longer, but I actually enjoyed the opportunity to unwind and rest). The diagnosis of non-malignancy was supported. Six months after my original diagnosis, I returned to my doctor's office for a check-up, which involved an ultrasound, a urine sample, questions, and thankfully little else. I was reassured that it appeared that I was doing everything correctly and I arranged for another check-up in six months' time. After the six months had passed, I had another follow-up meeting with my urologist which was very similar to the previous meeting and which ended in me receiving another appointment for six months later.

I have provided all of these details in regard to my diagnosis in order to emphasise how much of a shock this diagnosis was to me. I also include this information to enable the reader to understand just how confused and ill-informed I was for having to manage my distended bladder and its treatment. I also need to mention that throughout all of the diagnoses, I was accompanied by my wife. If I had not had her company and support, I am sure that these procedures would have been much more traumatic, and I am extremely grateful for her being with me. I am further grateful for her support over the following months; without her managing, my condition would have been much more of a problem and more distressing.

UK CONSULTANT

Approximately six weeks after I started to use catheters I travelled to the UK, where I stayed for a few weeks. Before coming to the UK, and given that we were frequent residents in the UK, I had discussed with my wife what I should do there in regard to managing my bladder failure. We decided that it was a good idea to have a urologist in the UK who I had met and who knew about my condition. This would also serve as a safety net if I needed any emergency input whilst in England. After searching online, I found a consultant urologist who worked locally to where I was located, and who sounded as if he might be a good fit for my condition. I contacted him and saw him privately. He confirmed much of my diagnosis, prognosis, and treatment regimen. However, there were significant differences such as he suggested I may be a candidate for a transurethral resectioning of the prostate, a procedure that my US urologist assured me would very likely leave me incontinent. However, he also made other suggestions regarding my ongoing management that I felt reflected a much more caring and humane approach. I felt that he saw me as a person and I had more confidence being in contact with him. Whilst in the UK, my GP practice also put me in contact with a continence nurse.

UK CONTINENCE NURSE

In the UK, I was fortunate to be able to access the services offered by a continence nurse. There were extreme difficulties accessing the nurse's services and after being sent to the community services rather than the continence services, and following a ten-month delay, I did meet with the nurse and have since met with her again. I have to say that this was, I felt, the most useful of any of the medical appointments I had had about my bladder failure on either side of the Atlantic. She was both humane and practical and made care suggestions that my US team had left me to attempt to discover on my own or through internet searches. When I told her I had had eight UTIs in 12 months, she responded that one or two perhaps, but eight were unacceptable. She gave me hygiene and other practices that have seemed to help reduce the number of UTIs I have had since seeing her. My UK consultant and continence nurse have given me confidence in my ability to self-manage my condition.

SELF-MANAGEMENT

I have already mentioned about self-management of my condition several times, but I will now present some details in regard to how I manage my bladder failure. I have broken the chapter into a series of sub-sections that consider such aspects as: catheters and where I get these from and how I have learnt to use them; the environment, by which I mean the location where I catheterise; traveling with catheterisation and catheterising outside of my home; urinary tract infections, which have become the bane my post-catheterising life.

CATHETERS

When I was first diagnosed, I did not really know what a catheter was, but I was soon to learn and to become incredibly familiar with these devices. I discovered through reading the websites of catheter producers and suppliers that catheters come in many different forms. I have found that catheter suppliers are a very useful source of information as well as where I get my catheters from in both the US and UK. I have discovered that the people who work at catheter suppliers in both the UK and US are compassionate and caring in their interactions with me. They are also, in the main, well informed and able to help me with problems I have encountered using catheters. In the UK, the Bladder and Bowel Community (who supply my catheters) have a nurse who works for them and who has called me to help me with the problems I have experienced. Within the US, my catheter supplier is 180 Medical. They too have been a great help as I manage my condition, although I have had great difficulties suspending my order when I am not in the US and catheters in the US are very expensive and even with health insurance paying around 75% of the costs, I still pay almost $300 a month.

THE ENVIRONMENT

As well as having to learn about and how to use catheters, I also had to make significant changes in my lifestyle and to adapt the place where I performed catheterisation. In the US, I am fortunate to have my own bathroom attached to my office where I am able to set out my catheterising materials. In the UK, we have a single toilet and we have had this re-fitted with a new basin and units so that I have a draw and cupboard in the vanity within which I keep my materials.

TRAVELING IN THE WIDER WORLD

I took me some weeks, if not months, before I felt confident enough to consider performing self-catheterisation outside of my own home. I found it daunting to consider the idea of inserting a catheter in an environment I did not have total control over and in which I was sure I would not be disturbed. I eased my way into catheterising outside of the home by visiting a café, local to my US home. I found this very traumatic and the procedure was even painful, due I suppose to me being tense. I then went to a local restaurant and then a nature centre. Gradually, I learnt a procedure for catheterising outside of the home. I have found that public toilets, and especially disabled toilets, are often hard to find and offer practically no privacy: handicapped toilets often being simply a wider access stall to allow wheelchairs to enter. Basins and other facilities are often dirty and unkept, and there is nowhere to lay out my materials or to catheterise in private. I have found this distressing and this has been restrictive. One extremely useful aspect of my condition management in the UK has been a "need to go" card and disability toilet key. Having this card and key, along with the websites that map where disabled and accessibility toilets are located, has enabled me to visit unknown places and to be able to find toilets every three hours. These websites even contain photographs of the insides of disabled toilets which has increased my confidence.

In order to help whilst I am outside the house, I have developed and taken to wearing a utility belt which I always wear away from home. In this I care a day's supply of catheters hand wipes, dry wipes, an incontinence pad, and disposal bags.

URINARY TRACT INFECTIONS (UTIs)

Easily the most distressing ongoing aspect of my failed bladder has been the series of urinary tract infections (Cooper, et al, 2021; Drekonja, 2024; Rane and Dasgupta, 2013; Royce, 2024; Sobel and Brown, 2020) that I have contracted subsequent to having to catheterise. Clean intermittent self-catheterisation (CISC) is a challenging process and one that took me some time to learn how to undertake. Initially, performing CISC involved me inserting a lubricated catheter into the urethra until it reaches the bladder and urine starts to flow. The catheter remains in position until the bladder is drained (usually this takes a minute or two). The catheter is them removed. I empty my bladder in this way first thing upon waking, and then six times during the day (approximately every three hours – using the timed alarm on my smart phone has proved priceless in keeping me to this schedule). Before each time I perform CISC, I void unaided, and I may urinate unaided an additional couple of times during the day. However, it is unusual for me to want to urinate, and my bladder never feels neither full nor empty. However, after developing UTIs, I was advised to take medication for this and to be pedantic in my cleanliness routine. I now wash my hands and then my penis with unscented soap and water, before using a cleansing wipe to clean. My penis. I then insert the catheter and drain the urine. After this stops, I move the catheter in and out very slowly a couple of time to drain as much urine as possible. After slowly removing the catheter, I wash my penis again. I then clean the area. However, I do occasionally have to urinate unexpectedly and then I am sometimes unable to stop leakage. I therefore will carry and use incontinence pads if I am attending a performance or I am in other situations in which my immediate access to a toilet may be problematic.

SELF-MANAGEMENT QUESTIONS FOR MEDICAL PROFESSIONS

Over the past 14 months, I have had many questions that have arisen about my management of my bladder failure. I have found answers to a good number of these online, in the literature and during my meetings with health professionals. However, there are still a few questions that remain unanswered. I provide examples of these below.

- The procedure is called clean intermittent self-catheterisation and not sterile intermittent self-catheterisation; I believe that this is to emphasise the need for cleanliness rather than sterileness. However, I would like to know how clean I should be aiming for? What are the exact steps I need to go through to achieve this?
- Sometimes I insert a catheter as far as possible, but no urine comes out. I withdraw and re-insert and urine does come out. What is happening and what does this mean?
- The skin on the glans of my penis peels due to excessive washing with soap and water or disinfecting hand wipes. This is not at all painful or sore. Is this to be expected? Does this need to be addressed?
- Should I be careful how far I insert the catheter and is it possible to insert this too far and to damage my bladder or the urethra?
- I was recently told that as I have developed eight UTIs in the first year of using catheters, I should attempt to drain all the urine from my bladder each time I use a catheter by moving the catheter slowly backwards and forwards until there is no stream or drips of urine coming out. Does this practice have any possible negative effects due to friction?

DISCUSSION

When I was first diagnosed with bladder failure, shown a catheter and told by the nurse that she was going to insert this 40cm piece of plastic into my urethra, my reaction was something along the lines of, "you're going to insert that, where! You must be joking". Similarly, when I started to use catheters, my initial thoughts about doing this myself were filled with horror. However, after successfully doing this, the first time I knew I could master the procedure. This has proven to be the case although the path to being able to effectively self-catheterise has not been a simple one. Being a very personal activity, self-catheterisation has many negative associations. Initially, I was awkward, and it hurt to insert a catheter. I also made mistakes and touched the tip of the catheter and had to discard it and use a new one. I did not feel embarrassed about self-catheterising and found it easy to talk about my condition to people I knew. However, as the procedure is associated with genitourinary aspects of the body, those to whom I was speaking often gave the impression they did not want to hear this type of information. I came to feel that I was rather like someone who had kidney failure and had to undergo dialysis, that is they had to regularly perform an intervention that kept them healthy. However, I sometimes feel that my intervention is like an unmentionable form of dialysis, and this made me feel isolated and, in some ways, unclean. I kept my catheters and other equipment in cupboards so they would not be seen. The process of clean intermittent self-catheterisation is something that you cannot talk about in everyday conversation.

CONCLUSIONS

In the preceding pages, I have provided details of my bladder failure and the ways in which I have learnt to adapt my life in order to manage this condition. It is appropriate that my account appears in a handbook that is concerned with patients' self-management of their health as throughout the time since I first diagnosed until the present time, I have had to rely largely upon my own initiative to devise ways to live healthily with this condition. This statement is not meant to minimise the excellent diagnostic procedures that were performed upon me and the peerless advice I have received from health professionals on both sides of the Atlantic. However, living day-to-day with a non-functioning bladder is inevitably something that I have to be aware of and to look after myself.

When I tell someone that I have recently experienced bladder failure, even if I do not use this exact phrase to describe my condition, the vast majority of people respond by wishing me well and saying that they hope that, or that they are sure that, I will get better very soon. If I tell them that this is not a curable condition, they usually become quiet. I get the feeling that a lot of people cannot imagine a condition that they have never heard of is incurable. According to the National Institute for Health and Care Excellence (NICE, 2024), over 50,000 individuals use intermittent catheters each year and with a mean catheter use of 4 per day this equals some 75 million intermittent urethral catheters are used in the NHS in England each year, whilst I do not know the number of people who experience having a failed bladder. However, perhaps because the condition is intimately associated with urine, toilets and genitals, it is something that we do not hear about. Even with millions of catheters being used each year, most people will never have seen one and they will not know how these are used. I have found that it can be a challenge to speak about my bladder failure as most people seem to not want to know the gory details. Friends may shudder if I talk about having to catheterise and say things such as: "I feel sick just thinking about doing that". "I don't know how you can do that", and "I couldn't do that".

A TOOL FOR SELF-MANAGEMENT OF BLADDER FAILURE

One thing that became apparent to me was that there is a need for a tool that individuals with bladder failure are given on diagnosis to help them to understand and manage their condition. It is beyond the scope of this essay to go into the nature of this tool. However, in a separate chapter (chapter XX), I provide details of such a monitor.

NOTES

1 Due to my personal medical history, it is interesting to note, though beyond the scope of this essay, that urinary retention and decreased bladder sensation have been associated with lesion in the midbrain PAG (Sakakibara, et al, 1998; Yaguchi, et al, 2004; Yamamoto, et al, 2005).
2 I believe that at the present time, this is still the case.

REFERENCES

Anderson, L. (2006). Analytic autoethnography. *Journal of Contemporary Ethnography*, 35(4), 373–395.

Bachman, A., and de la Rosette, J. (2011). *Benign Prostatic Hyperplasia and Lower Urinary Tract Symptoms in Men (Oxford Urology Library)*. Oxford University Press.

Barrisford, G.W., and Steele, G.S. (2018). Acute urinary retention. In T. Post (Ed.), *UpToDate*. UpToDate.

Belton, S., and Sheridan, K. (2025). 'The second arrow': A collaborative autoethnographic exploration of what can be learned from one long COVID journey. *Health Expect*, 28(3), e70227. https://doi.org/10.1111/hex.70227

Chang, H. (2008). *Autoethnography as Method*. Left Coast Press.

Chapple, C.R., Osman, N.I., Birder, L., van Koeveringe, G.A., Oelke, M., Nitti, V.W., Drake, M.J., Yamaguchi, O., Abrams, P., and Smith, P.P. (2015). The underactive bladder: A new clinical concept? *European Urology*, 68(3), 351–353. https://doi.org/10.1016/j.eururo.2015.02.030

Cleveland Clinic. (2024). Overflow incontinence. Retrieved from https://my.clevelandclinic.org/health/diseases/22162-overflow-incontinence

Colaco, M., Osman, N.I., Karakeçi, A., Artibani, W., Andersson, K.E., and Badlani, G.H. (2018). Current concepts of the acontractile bladder. *BJU International*, 122(2), 195–202. https://doi.org/10.1111/bju.14236

Cooper, K.L., Badalato, G.M., and Rutman, M.P. (2021). Chap 55. Infections of the urinary tract. In A.W. Partin, R.R. Dmochowski, L.R. Kavoussi, and C.A. Peters (Eds.), *Campbell-Walsh-Wein Urology* (12th ed., pp. 187–195). Elsevier.

D'Ancona, C.D., Haylen, B.T., Oelke, M., Herschorn, S., Abranches-Monteiro, L., Arnold, E.P., Goldman, H.B., Hamid, R., Homma, Y., Marcelissen, T., Rademakers, K., Schizas, A., Singla, A., Soto, I., Tse, V., and de Wachter, S. (2019). An international continence society (ICS) report on the terminology for adult male lower urinary tract and pelvic floor symptoms and dysfunction. *Neurology Urodynamics*, 38, 433–477. https://doi.org/10.1002/nau.23897

Dorsher, P.T., and McIntosh, P.M. (2012). Neurogenic bladder. *Advances in Urology*, 2012, 816274. https://doi.org/10.1155/2012/816274

Drake, M., Cocci, A., and Silva, P. (Eds.) (2019). *Lower Urinary Tract Symptoms in Adults: A Clinical Approach*. Springer.

Drekonja, D. (2024). Chapter 263, Approach to the patient with urinary tract infection. In L. Goldman, & K.A. Cooney (Eds.), *Goldman-Cecil Medicine* (27th ed.). Elsevier.

Ellis, C., Adams, T.E., and Bochner, A.P. (2011). Autoethnography: An overview. *Forum Qualitative Sozialforschung/Forum: Qualitative Social Research*, 12(1), 10.

Ellis, C., and Bochner, A.P. (2000). Autoethnography, personal narrative, reflexivity: Researcher as subject. In N.K. Denzin & Y.S. Lincoln (Eds.), *Handbook of Qualitative Research* (2nd ed., pp. 733–768). Sage Publications.

Ellis, C., and Adams, T.E. (2020). Practicing autoethnography and living the autoethnographic life. In P. Leavy (Ed.), *The Oxford Handbook of Qualitative Research* (2nd ed.). Oxford Handbooks.

Fitzgerald, M.P., Stablein, U., and Brubaker, L. (2002). Urinary habits among asymptomatic women. *American Journal of Obstetrics and Gynecology*, 187, 1384–1388. https://doi.org/10.1067/mob.2002.126865

Fowler, C.J., Griffiths, D., and de Groat, W.C. (2008). The neural control of micturition. *National Review of Neuroscience*, 9(6), 453–466. https://doi.org/10.1038/nrn2401

Frøkiaer, J. (2020). Chap 37, Urinary tract obstruction. In A.S.L. Yu, G.M. Chertow, V.A. Luyckx, P.A. Marsden, K. Skorecki, and M.W. Taal (Eds.), *Brenner and Rector's The Kidney* (11th ed.). Elsevier.

Fukushima, H., Takemura, K., Suzuki, H., and Koga, F. (2018). Impact of sarcopenia as a prognostic biomarker of bladder cancer. *International Journal of Molecular Sciences*, 19(10), 2999. https://doi.org/10.3390/ijms19102999

Gallagher, K.M., and Hughes, J. (2024). Chap 61, Urinary tract obstruction. In R.J. Johnson, J. Floege, and M. Tonelli (Eds.), *Comprehensive Clinical Nephrology* (7th ed.). Elsevier.

Gammack, J.K. (2010). Lower urinary tract symptoms. *Clinics in Geriatric Medicine*, 26(2), 249–260. https://doi.org/10.1016/j.cger.2010.02.006

Greenhalgh, T. (2017). Adjuvant chemotherapy: An autoethnography. *Subjectivity*, 10, 340–357. https://doi.org/10.1057/s41286-017-0033-y

Griffiths, D.J., McCracken, P.N., Harrison, G.M., Gormley, E.A., and Moore, K.N. (2002). Urge incontinence and impaired detrusor contractility in the elderly. *Neurourology and Urodynamics*, 21(2), 126–131. https://doi.org/10.1002/nau.10042

Hackett, P.M.W. (2018). Declarative mapping sentences as a co-ordinating framework for qualitative health and wellbeing research. *ResearchGate*. Retrieved from https://www.researchgate.net/publication/327775291_Declarative_Mapping_Sentences_as_a_Co-ordinating_Framework_for_Qualitative_Health_and_Wellbeing_Research

Hackett, P.M.W. (2020). *Declarative Mapping Sentences in Qualitative Research: Theoretical, Linguistic, and Applied Usages*. Routledge.

Hackett, P.M.W. (2021). A reflexive and adaptable framework for ethnographic and qualitative research: The declarative mapping sentences approach. *Academia.edu*. Retrieved from https://www.academia.edu/49086376/A_Reflexive_and_Adaptable_Framework_for_Ethnographic_and_Qualitative_Research_the_Declarative_Mapping_Sentences_Approach

Harrogate and District NHS Trust. (2016). *Patient and Carer Information The Overactive Bladder and Bladder Re-training*. Harrogate and District NHS Trust.

InformedHealth.org [Internet]. (2022). *In Brief: How Does the Urinary System Work?* Institute for Quality and Efficiency in Health Care (IQWiG). [Updated 2022 Mar 29]. Available from: https://www.ncbi.nlm.nih.gov/books/NBK279384/

Kim, J.H. (2013). Bladder failure: Still a Frontier; Commentary on "Bladder". *International Neurourology Journal*, 17(1), 41. https://doi.org/10.5213/inj.2013.17.1.41

Kim, K.H., and Kim, Y.H. (2012). Bladder failure? *International Neurourology Journal*, 16(4), 209–210. https://doi.org/10.5213/inj.2012.16.4.209

Latini, J.M., Mueller, E., Lux, M.M., et al (2004). Voiding frequency in a sample of asymptomatic American men. *The Journal of Urology*, 172, 980–984. https://doi.org/10.1097/01.ju.0000135890.08541.02

Logan, K., Shaw, C., Webber, I., Samuel, S., and Broome, L. (2008). Patients' experiences of learning clean intermittent self-catheterization: A qualitative study. *Journal of Advanced Nursing*, 62(1), 32–40. https://doi.org/10.1111/j.1365-2648.2007.04536.x

Michek, J., Sutory, M., and Zerhau, P. (1992). Surgical treatment of the atonic bladder. *Urological Research*, 20(3), 241–245.

Milsom, I., Altman, D., Cartwright, R., Lapitan, M.C., Nelson, R., Sillén, U., Tikkinen, K., et al (2017). Epidemiology of urinary incontinence (UI) and other lower urinary tract symptoms (LUTS), pelvic organ prolapse (POP) and anal incontinence (AI). In P. Abrams (Ed.), *Incontinence: 6th International Consultation on Incontinence* (pp. 1–141). ICUD-EAU.

National Institute for Health and Care Excellence (NICE). (2024). Late-stage assessment final scope: intermittent urethral catheters for long-term urinary management in adults. Retrieved from https://www.nice.org.uk/guidance/hte28/documents/final-scope#:~:text=In%20the%20UK%2C%20more%20than,NHS%20in%20England%20each%20year

National Institute of Diabetes and Digestive Kidney Diseases (NIDDKD). (undated). Urinary retention. Retrieved from https://www.niddk.nih.gov/health-information/urologic-diseases/urinary-retention (Accessed 27th July, 2025).

Nowakowski, A.C.H. (2016). Using paired depth interviews to collect qualitative data. *The Qualitative Report*, 21(9), 1615–1635.

O'Leary, M., Okonski, J., and Chancellor, M.B. (undated). *A Patient's Guide to Underactive Bladder.* Underactive Bladder Foundation. https://underactivebladder.org/index.php/a-patients-guide-to-underactive-bladder-syndrome/

Osman, N.I., Chapple, C.R., Abrams, P., Dmochowski, R., Haab, F., Nitti, V., Koelbl, H., van Kerrebroeck, P., and Wein, A.J. (2014). Detrusor underactivity and the underactive bladder: A new clinical entity? A review of current terminology, definitions, epidemiology, aetiology, and diagnosis. *European Urology*, 65(2), 389–398. https://doi.org/10.1016/j.eururo.2013.10.015

Priddis, H.S. (2015). Autoethnography and severe perineal trauma—an unexpected journey from disembodiment to embodiment. *BMC Women's Health*, 15, 88. https://doi.org/10.1186/s12905-015-0249-3

Rane, A., and Dasgupta, R., (Eds.) (2013). *Urinary Tract Infection: Clinical Perspectives on Urinary Tract Infection*. Springer.

Reed-Danahay, D.E. (1997). *Auto/ethnography: Rewriting the Self and the Social.* Berg Publishers.

Riccabona, M., and Fotter, R. (2018). Non-neurogenic bladder-sphincter dysfunction ("voiding dysfunction"). In M. Riccabona (Eds.), *Pediatric Urogenital Radiology. Medical Radiology.* Springer. https://doi.org/10.1007/978-3-319-39202-8_23

Royce, H. (2024). *The UTI Handbook: Your Guide to Urinary Tract Infection Symptoms and Solutions.* Independently published.

Sakakibara, R., Hattori, T., Fukutake, T., Mori, M., Yamanishi, T., and Yasuda, K. (1998). Micturitional disturbance in herpetic brainstem encephalitis; Contribution of the pontine micturition centre. *Journal of Neurology, Neurosurgery and Psychiatry*, 64, 269–272. https://doi.org/10.1136/jnnp.64.2.269

Selius, B.A., and Subedi, R. (2008). Urinary retention in adults: Diagnosis and initial management. *American Family Physician*, 77(5), 643–650.

Shaw, C., Logan, K., Webber, I., Broome, L., and Samuel, S. (2008). Effect of clean intermittent self-catheterization on quality of life: A qualitative study. *Journal of Advanced Nursing*, 61(6), 641–650. https://doi.org/10.1111/j.1365-2648.2007.04556.x

Sobel, J.D., and Brown, P. (2020). Chapter 72, Urinary tract infections. In J.E. Bennett, R. Dolin, and M.J. Blaser (Eds.), *Mandell, Douglas, and Bennett's Principles and Practice of Infectious Diseases* (9th ed.). Elsevier.

Swavely, N.R., Speich, J.E., Stothers, L., and Klausner, A.P. (2019). New diagnostics for male lower urinary tract symptoms. *Current Bladder Dysfunction Reports*, 14, 90–97. https://doi.org/10.1007/s11884-019-00511-0

Toye, F., and Barker, K.L. (2020). A meta-ethnography to understand the experience of living with urinary incontinence: 'is it just part and parcel of life?". *BMC Urology*, 20, 1. https://doi.org/10.1186/s12894-019-0555-4

Vignoli, G. (2016). *Urodynamics: A Quick Pocket Guide*. Springer.

Wakelin, K. (2024). Pain, shame, and power: An autoethnographic exploration of chronic pain. *Qualitative Health Research*. https://doi.org/10.1177/10497323241289805

Wikipedia. (2025, January 16). Autoethnography. *Wikipedia*. Retrieved from https://en.wikipedia.org/wiki/Autoethnography (Accessed 20 July, 2025).

Yaguchi, H., Soma, H., Miyazaki, Y., Tashiro, J., Yabe, I., Kikuchi, S., et al (2004). A case of acute urinary retention caused by periaqueductal grey lesion. *Journal of Neurology, Neurosurgery and Psychiatry*, 75, 1202–1203. https://doi.org/10.1136/jnnp.2003.027516

Yamamoto, T., Sakakibara, R., Uchiyama, T., Liu, Z., Ito, T., Yamanishi, T., et al (2005). Lower urinary tract function in patients with pituitary adenoma compressing hypothalamus. *Journal of Neurology, Neurosurgery and Psychiatry*, 76, 390–394. https://doi.org/10.1136/jnnp.2004.044644

18 Here's My Number
The Lived Experience of a Breast Cancer Survivor

Jessica B. Schwarzenbach

MY STORY

We had exited the hospital in shock and stood in the hot sun waiting for the street light to change. My husband Paul had been conclusively diagnosed with non-neurogenic bladder failure after several weeks of tests and three consultations with an urologist (see Chapters 14 and 17). I looked at Paul, his face was immobile, stunned; an expression of surprise perhaps. His eyes were shadowed by the brim of his hat. "How do you feel," I asked? "Actually, I feel relieved," he said. "I dreaded a diagnosis of prostate cancer. They didn't find any signs of cancer. I can deal with bladder failure and having to self-catheterize six times a day." "For the rest of your life?" I queried. "I was so afraid of having cancer," he replied simply.

We crossed the street and found an outdoor café to sit in while the enormity of the new life-changes loomed into reality. Paul is only 64 years old. "What comes next?" I asked. Paul shrugged, "That's it, until my next checkup in November, three months from now."

"What?" I felt my rage building. No follow-up, no support? I looked at Paul who was trying to process all of this overwhelming information and appeared to be doing amazingly well. Then I was crushed by his unvoiced vulnerability. I remembered how 30 years before I had been diagnosed with breast cancer at a hospital very much like the one in which he was now being treated. I too had been frozen with fear. Most of my peer group who had been diagnosed with cancer were dead. I had come to Boston from my home in New Mexico to attend a Master's program in art education. Four months into the course I found a lump in my right breast and went to my university's medical group where it was confirmed that I had breast cancer. I had had a mammogram in New Mexico only five months previously which had been determined negative for cancer!

When I returned to my apartment that evening so many years ago, I had called a friend to tell her my bad news. After some discussion, she put me in touch with Meg, a woman she knew, who had been successfully treated for breast cancer in the Boston area. I called Meg as soon as I could and still remember her clear and focused answers, her calm intelligence. She advised getting a second opinion, as well as seeking out a senior member of staff within an oncology department. She recommended her oncologist, Henry Sanger, whom she greatly respected. She also explained some of the protocols of cancer treatment. If the positive diagnosis was confirmed, I would most likely need surgery, probably chemotherapy, and even radiation treatment. After we hung-up, I decided the first step was to find a surgeon.

As part of my graduate program, I was working as a part-time art teacher at the Museum of Fine Arts. After sharing my health issues with colleagues, I was soon contacted by a woman in administration whom I had never met before. She knew of a well-respected surgeon through her family and friends and gave me the name of Dr. Clayton Ehrenman. A few days later I walked into Dr Ehrenman's office. While filling out the paperwork for my appointment, I saw a tall and elderly white-haired man looking through some medical records behind the receptionist's desk. "That must be him," I thought, "I don't want an old surgeon. I want someone who is on the cutting edge of technology, doing research, and has a strong steady hand." A few minutes later, I sat

 DOI: 10.1201/9781003599074-20

anxiously in the examination room, trying to think of ways to politely refuse Dr Ehrenman's services.

While my overtaxed brain was still struggling with ways to avoid making any commitment to his practice, Dr Ehrenman walked in. Blinking behind his eye glasses, he greeted me warmly and carried out a straightforward examination but with insight, as well as humor. We spoke of education, cancer, families, and how I had come to be in Boston. He even had me laughing (in this dire situation?). He knew I was asking for a second opinion. He looked at the X-rays and agreed with the initial assessment. "The tumor looks and feels like cancer," he concluded. "You will need treatment. Don't wait too long." He wished me good luck and went back to his office. After I dressed, I walked out to the receptionist, Teresa, to sign out. I was about to say good-bye when I suddenly hesitated. I trusted this man. I timidly asked her, "Would Dr. Ehrenman be able to do my surgery?" Behind Teresa, I saw his head lift in surprise. He and Teresa exchanged looks. She turned to me and said, "Yes, we will have to properly book you in for a pre-surgery appointment. Let's see what is available." This moment was the beginning of my almost six and a half years of treatment for breast cancer.

Dr. Ehrenman became my link to navigating the Boston medical system. He connected me to the hematologist/oncologist, Dr Henry Sanger (recommended by Meg), and the radiation oncologist, Dr Jim Mason (recommended by Dr. Sanger). They became my team: the persons with the knowledge, expertise, and understanding to be able to discuss my case stage by stage amongst themselves and with me.

In addition to my team of doctors, I was offered a support group at the hospital headed by Harriet Hilton, who was an oncology social worker as well as a breast cancer survivor. I was asked by her staff whether I would like to speak to another patient with a diagnosis similar to my own and one who had successfully passed through the same chemotherapy as prescribed for me. It was to establish a sort of "buddy" system to help new patients deal with their fears of the unknown, dispel rumors, and learn to accept the known at this dreaded time.

Harriet also presided over group meetings where women in different stages of breast cancer met and discussed their feelings and the difficulties encountered while trying to manage their lives. I found the group meetings too stressful. The terror was palpable. One woman was trembling while she told us she was waiting for her surgeon to return from holiday. "How long has he been gone?" I asked. "Oh, he is due to return in about 3 more weeks," she said. "I am not really sure." I wanted to beg her to take my surgeon, but I don't remember if I did. We were all so fragile. I felt as Harriet was presiding, she would not let someone be too reckless with their decisions about survival.

On the other hand, I did look forward to the calls and visits with Lynn, my former-cancer-patient volunteer. I now had someone with whom to compare notes and who was happy to answer my questions from a patient's perspective. Lynn's treatment notes were helpful but perhaps more importantly she normalized, or helped me accept some of the upsetting responses I had from family and friends. Lynn shared that people in general, even parents and close friends may have adverse reactions to my cancer diagnosis.

I had already experienced some of these situations. When I told a man with whom I was nearing the edge of a romantic relationship about my diagnosis, he responded positively. "You will need all the support you can get. I will be there for you," he said with affection. However, later on that same afternoon he called back and said, "I am so sorry. I was wrong. I cannot be there for you. I have too many things going on in my life right now, but I will keep in touch. Good luck." After he hung up, I was left staring at the wall not knowing what to think or feel. Another layer of expectation was stripped away when my friend, Mark, responded to my news with, "Well, yeah, call me when it's over?" Incredulous I answered, "What do you mean? Shall I have someone call you when I am dead?" He hysterically shouted, "You know I don't like death!" A former roommate from college came to stay with me for a few days during my treatment and the word cancer was never broached during the entire visit.

One of Lynn's stories that I remember was about her mother. Lynn's parents lived nearby and she went to stay with them one weekend during treatment. Her mother drew her aside, before the large family dinner party that night and gave Lynn a meaningful look. She whispered, "Not one word about your cancer, please." Recognizing how much fear of illness, pain, and death exists in our culture, I think I was able to better adjust to the hurtful abandonment I experienced. I believe I developed a greater understanding that many people would not respond the way I wanted them to, and denying a cancer patient attention and support is actually quite common.

Like Lynn, I also had a mother who was unable to sympathize with my situation even though she too was a cancer survivor of 25 years. In 1969, her treatment had been limited to a mastectomy and she had lived cancer free ever since. My lumpectomy surgery was scheduled for the day before the US holiday of Thanksgiving. My mother had recently remarried and had made plans with her husband, Earl, to attend his extensive family celebration in New York the day after my surgery. She was being pressured by my sister, Ann, to come up to Boston to visit me instead. She was invited to stay with my brother who had declined her invitation to join Earl's family. My brother, Max, had also invited me to spend Thanksgiving with him and his family on the North Shore about 40 minutes from my apartment.

When my mother called a few days before my surgery, I told her that I knew attending Earl's family Thanksgiving was important to her, and that she should go. I really didn't want more emotional complications as I was very concerned about what the biopsy would reveal. I did not have the energy to negotiate family dynamics at this time. Then, my mother suggested to me, "Perhaps the hospital could keep you overnight after surgery on Wednesday night. That way, you wouldn't be alone for the Thanksgiving holiday." I held my breath. She added, "It would be a shame to ruin Earl's family celebration if Max and his family do not attend." I was so shocked, I didn't know what to say. I blurted out, "I think Hospitals don't do that, Mom…. They are not hotels." After we hung up, I had to talk to someone about what she had said to me. I went down to the apartment below me and vented with some new friends, Linda and Mathew

At this time, no one knew how dangerous my cancer was. It would take days after surgery before I learned the results. It was one of those shakedown crazy unfathomable days. Eventually, my two siblings, Ann and Max, took care of the familial conflicts. I prepared myself for surgery. Dr Ehrenman, gowned and gloved, with hands in the air greeted me with a silly joke as I was being wheeled into the operating room. I was chuckling when the anesthesia mask was placed over my face. In the end, my mother did come up to Boston for the weekend, as did my sister (who stayed with me) and we all had a nice time at my brother's house over the holiday.

Not all of my interactions with friends and family were so precarious. I also experienced great acts of compassion in which people demonstrated unusual thoughtfulness and kindness. Sometime after Thanksgiving I ran into Mathew in the hall of our building. He hesitated a moment and then told me confidentially that after his wife Linda had heard the story about my mother, she told him she would not go with him to Connecticut if I was to be left alone. Linda and Mathew with their three-year-old son had planned to spend the holiday at her mother's house. If my family did not come through for me, Linda told Michael, she intended to stay home to make sure that when I was released from hospital, I was not going to return to an empty house. Thankfully, Linda, pregnant with her second child, was able to spend the weekend with her own family.

A few weeks after surgery, I encountered another person of remarkable compassion and committed responsibility. I had just received my schedule to start chemo and was crossing the street in front of my apartment building when a woman who lived opposite stopped me and asked how I was adjusting to my life as a grad-student. I gave a weak response and then said, "Actually, not very well. I have been diagnosed with breast cancer and start chemo at the end of this week." I had only spoken with this woman once previously when I had moved into my apartment several months ago. Her name was PJ. PJ looked at me with concern and took out her date book. "You are going to have to eat well," she said, "How about Wednesdays? Do you have classes or commitments on Wednesday evenings?" I didn't know what she was implying. PJ clarified, "I am a good cook and I am inviting you for dinner every Wednesday night that you are in treatment. It is important that you eat well." I was incredulous at this stranger's benevolence. In fact, I was speechless.

PJ kept her word. For the whole course of CMF chemotherapy (cyclophosphamide, methotrexate, and fluorouracil) which ended in August, including a six week "sandwich" period of radiation in the middle, PJ had me for dinner every Wednesday night. If she had other commitments, she would set up an alternative arrangement with me. Often, she also invited one or two of her friends to dine with us. When I told Dr Sanger about this amazing woman who had been previously unknown to me, his jaw dropped. He stood up and walked around his office. "Do you know how many awful, horrible stories I hear from patients about how family, friends, and co-workers treat them? This revives my belief in the human species." He looked at me with a questioning look. "May I share your story?" "Yes, of course," I smiled.

There were other acts of support from my family (Ann, Max) and friends (Hannah and Porter). My brother came with me to an early appointment and was an anchor during my initiation to chemotherapy. Porter spent the night at my apartment throughout the dreaded first night after chemo. My sister drove the 200+ miles to stay with me for the first two days of most of the six cycles of therapy. Hannah was a college friend who could actually talk about cancer. However, I think the greatest impact upon me of the power of empathy came from within the medical system, itself. During an early office visit with Dr Ehrenman, he said to me, "You live alone and you are in an unfamiliar city. The most difficult time for a cancer patient is often at 4 am in the morning." He wrote something on a scrap of paper and pushed it across his desk, "Here is my home phone number. Call me at any time if you need me." "Any time," he repeated, looking directly at me. I was so astonished that I took the torn page and religiously stuck it into my pocket, overwhelmed by his consideration and his trust that I would not abuse his kindness. I kept his number as a sort of talisman in the drawer of my night table for the next year and a half. I never called Dr Ehrenman at his home, yet during many an anxious night I was comforted to know that I had a rare choice which I was proud to honor.

My treatment was designed, organized, and carried out within an experimental oncology department, which relied on current research and the power of compassion to enhance the success of their patient's treatments. It was exactly what I had been looking for and I, in my arrogance, had almost thrown away the privilege to participate. With this new sense of community, I gained the courage to step into and through the cancer care world. It was Dr Ehrenman who helped me deal with the initial onslaught of the cancer reality. He managed the surgical stage but also kept involved after his medical role was complete.

Dr Ehrenman and Dr Sanger (whom I soon called Henry since all medical staff and patients did so) were my web of day-to-day support. In the hospital culture they were known for their compassion, intelligence and humor. For me, Dr Mason, the radiologist, was merely a kind presence during the shorter period of radiography. The radiation oncology nurses were the ones who offered information and self-care techniques to help me survive the effects of radiation exposure. Dr Ehrenman was a legend among staff, and beloved by all (He was always referred to as Dr Ehrenman). Henry was more difficult to work with, blunter, yet as we came to know each other better, he became an important presence in my life.

Although, Dr Ehrenman and Dr Sanger, continued to work together on my case, they did not always agree. During the first office visit after surgery, I sat with Henry as he was outlining my situation with the post-lumpectomy pathology report in hand. My eyes were starting to glaze over with the amount of disclosed information and the terror it produced. Henry estimated my risk of recurrence somewhere between 30% and 40%. I think I made a quick decision to explore this information only if I survived. My cancer stage classification was noted as T2-N0-M0 (T2 describes a tumor greater than 2cm, but less than 5cm; NO- signifies there was no cancer found in nearby lymph nodes; MO indicates there was no evidence that the cancer had metastasized to distant parts of the body). That was absorbable. However, one of the other tumor descriptions was LVI positive (or lymphovascular invasion positive) which indicated that cancer cells were found in the small blood or lymph vessels within the tumor. This could signify a more aggressive cancer and higher risk of the cancer spreading to the rest of the body. I was worried. These definitions of what I had and didn't have were not really clear to me at the time. I was slowly blanking out when Henry suddenly muttered, "I don't like this" and reached for the desk phone. He soon had Dr Ehrenman on speaker and asked why I had a dirty margin on the chest wall. I froze at the mention of cancer still living in my body and was unable to follow the conversation. I do not remember exactly what Ehrenman said but it had to do with making choices about breast conservation and my EIC-negative tumor which has lower rates of local recurrence and is generally successfully treated by CMF chemo and radiation therapy. I do remember, however, that Henry was satisfied with his answers. I asked him later, if he too was confident that the chemo and radiation would take care of the dirty margin. He said yes. I always wondered why, a doctor would ask these questions in front of a patient? However, after I escaped from the hospital into that wintry afternoon, I felt a strange but greater trust in my team. They were not hiding anything from me. I was a sharer in the decision-making process that was shaping my health. "Odd," I thought, "I feel more empowered?"

Henry became my prime contact during the chemotherapy stage. He too, asked questions, showed interest in my life, and provided emotional support. I was most afraid of chemo because I dread nausea. Henry took this very seriously and suggested I take my treatment intravenously. He could have the intravenous anti-nausea medication, a mixture of Zofran, Decadron, and Compazine administered prior to and adjusted during the chemo treatment. The administration of oral chemotherapy was not as easily controlled as it was usually taken in pill form by the patient at home. He said the infusion unit would make sure I did not get to the point where I would want to vomit. Henry explained that if I associated vomiting with chemo, I might start to feel ill as I walked into the hospital, even start to gag getting off the elevator before I entered the infusion area, etc., etc. On that first day of chemo, I tried very hard to monitor my fearful response as the needle was placed into my arm. Just the day before I had heard on the news of a fatal overdose of chemo given in error at a local hospital. I insisted on examining all the labels on the bags hanging on my IV pole. My oncology nurse, Lucy, was very accommodating. She helped me match the printed information on the bags to the treatment orders. I watched, as first the Zofran, and then the chemo, flowed into my body. At one point Henry came in and poked his head around the corner of my infusion chair. He looked at me with an intense stare which startled me but then he said, "You are doing well!" I felt relieved and suddenly hopeful. I was going to do it! In fact, we did seem to outwit my brain with this strategy and although I remember about two weeks of feeling crummy after each chemotherapy treatment, I had about a week of improved appetite and energy again before my next chemo administration. I never did vomit.

My turbulent life as a cancer patient had high moments filled with gratitude and aspirations for the future with many low points that were continually fraught with panic, fear, and a sense of defeat. An evening soon after my first chemo infusion, I received a call from an oncologist who was a friend of my new stepfather, Earl. The doctor was from out of state and had heard from Earl that I was in chemo for breast cancer. He asked me a series of questions, one of which was, what course of treatment I was on. After some more discussion he told me I was on the wrong drugs. I was flabbergasted that a doctor I did not know, nor who had spoken to my oncologist, would make such a diagnosis. He continued to tell me that because Earl was such a good friend, he would be glad to take me on as a patient. I should come down to New York and immediately start treatment under his guidance. I thanked him for his concern and told him I did not think I would do that as I was set up here in Boston. After I hung up, the impropriety of this doctor infuriated me. He should have spoken with Henry not to me. However, as the night progressed, a slow terror built up and pressured my chest. Perhaps he was right?! I should check with someone. In May, I had received a clean bill of health based on the mammogram taken in New Mexico. Within six months, a 1.5-inch tumor was discovered in my right breast. Could this be a very aggressive type of cancer?

First thing in the morning I called Dr Ehrenman's office and left a message. He soon returned my call and I was able to tell him what had happened with the oncologist from St Vincent's Hospital in N.Y.C. He responded thoughtfully and asked me what I was going to do. "I don't really want to do anything," I said. He told me that I was obviously very upset by this call and that I should talk to Henry. He was quite sure Henry would be able to alleviate my fears. I finally did call Henry's office and left a message. Late that night I received a very angry response from the usually composed Henry. "Who is this doctor who questions my treatment. How can he tell what is the appropriate chemotherapy without seeing the lab work, the biopsy results?! Where is he from? Oh, St. Vincent's, not exactly a research hospital, is it. I have patients coming in from all over the world. I am stretched beyond belief and some doctor tells my patient that she is on the wrong chemotherapy drugs? I don't have time for this. You are not on the wrong treatment. I have to go now." And that was the end of that.

And yet 30 years later here I stood on the hot pavement in Boston with Paul who had just received a devastating diagnosis; one that would limit the rest of his waking life to three-hour segments. He had no medical team to support him, no other patients to give him some kind of guideline to what the future holds. He had to learn to self-catheterize six-times a day or he was told he would die. There was nobody who had experienced this diagnosis of whom he could ask questions, share his doubts, his fears, trade stories… How have other patients' family and friends responded to their loved ones' newly obtained limitations? He did not have access to his doctors on fearful nights when he was sweating or having the shakes with another UTI. He was told to communicate through email with his doctor's PA with a 36 hour wait time for a response.

By the time Paul and I arrived home on the day of his diagnosis in August, 2024, I was determined to find out what support his hospital provided. I called the urology department and asked if there were any support groups available for persons diagnosed with bladder failure. I queried whether there were men who had been self-catheterizing for years who could talk to Paul: Does it get better? Is there a hotline to speak to someone when fearing the presence of the dreaded urinary tract infection and no quick access to antibiotics? What is the most effective manner of purchasing catheters? Are there recommended methods to confront the depression that this life change creates? Do patients farther along in the process adapt to the structured days, to the discouragement, the hopelessness, the shock? The woman who answered my call was apologetic. She told me, "No, we do not have any support groups here except for those who are undergoing a bladder transplant." I tried to tell her about the dynamic survivor culture offered at my former hospital, one in which I had been buoyed during my breast cancer treatment. She started to become defensive and answered, "We do not have anything like that here."

So, I could only try to boost up Paul and leave behind my perceived callousness of his urology doctor and the hospital staff. I tried to persuade him to seek out a second opinion which he refused to do at first. Paul said he didn't want contradicting opinions to confuse his perspective. However, two months later when we were in the UK, he did make arrangements to meet with a well-respected British urologist who basically agreed with his other doctor's evaluation. This gave Paul a greater sense of confidence in his American doctor, but also a resentment that he was not being treated in a more respectful way. The UK doctor made himself more accessible, and communicated personally with Paul by phone and email and showed a personal interest in the difficulties Paul was facing. As weeks passed, I watched Paul begin to negotiate his new lifestyle limits with resolution. However, Paul does not have a complex treatment aimed at a cure with a team of specialists to comfort him. He has to perform a procedure that may extend his life to that of an average life span for a male of his age but at this time there is no cure for his illness and no clear road map for the problems he might face in the future. Worries of kidney infection, prostate cancer and bladder cancer encircle him. Every day is an effort to maintain his focus on living a worthy life and creating good work: He is a writer and after a long dry spell is now once again producing publications of value.

On the other hand, when I was a cancer patient, I had had a cocoon of compassionate support at a time when breast cancer research was beginning to claim the public eye. Before my diagnosis, I had never heard anyone speak of "cure" in regard to breast cancer. Dr Ehrenman was the first person I knew to use the word. He told me with pride, "We are now using the word cure for many forms of breast cancer." I hoped I was on that road. At first, I did not accept the belief that there was a "cure" for me, but as time and treatment progressed, I too began cautiously to look forward to a future. I waited for over two years after my chemo therapy concluded (the recurrence window for my type of cancer) before I could smile and reply to queries from family and friends when they carefully phrased, "Are you in remission now?" "No," I brightly responded, "I am not. I am considered cured."

Paul does not have this possible route; there is no cure. Bladder failure is not a sexy topic. Much of the conversation is held undercover; a topic not discussed at dinner tables or elegant brunches. I had experienced the diminishing of the breast cancer taboo in the wake of Dr Susan Love's efforts to popularize the plight of women and cancer which began in the 1980s. She was a prominent surgeon and breast cancer awareness advocate who brought the disease into mainstream culture by appearing on talk shows and developing multiple avenues for media presentations. With the growth of the women's movement, funding became more available and research increased. Lives were saved.

When Paul asked his urologist about improving the support for bladder patients at his hospital, his doctor said that he had tried to solicit funding to make his department more patient friendly. However, the hospital had denied his requests. Bladder failure is not that common and, apparently, donors were not interested in providing money to humanize care for what is considered an old man's disease. I queried, "No money even for emotional support? Not economically feasible? How much could it cost a world-famous hospital to organize a few long-term patients with bladder failure to speak about their experiences with newly diagnosed people?"

Times have changed. The role of compassion is belittled. Medicine has become big business. "Everything is about money, now," Paul's urologist told him. Even while I was still consulting with Henry, he was complaining that he was now being told to cut his patient appointments down to 15 minutes! "I won't do that," he said. "How do I find out who my patient is, if I am confined by such a time limit?" As I muse now, I wonder if perhaps that is part of the key to better health and survival in medicine. Someone wants to know you.

As I was finishing up my last course of chemo, I had an appointment with Henry to discuss what I was going to do and what I needed to know about navigating the world post- cancer therapy. I was quite exultant. After almost a year I would finally be free of the hospital routines, appointment after appointment, labs, worries about platelets, white cell counts, etc., etc. I would now be free to travel further than an hour from a major hospital. I was fully enrolled in my graduate program again, and I was making plans to visit my sister in upstate New York before classes started. I didn't feel my life was on hold anymore. I was ready to really live again. Henry was pleased with how my last tests came back. We sat in his office as I prattled on about how I was so glad to be finishing up. "Not quite," he said. "I would like you to go on Tamoxifen for five years. As you know you had hormone receptor-positive breast cancer. Taking tamoxifen will greatly reduce the risk of the cancer returning or new cancer developing."

Tamoxifen is an antiestrogen drug. It blocks estrogen activity which helps stop the growth of breast tumors that need estrogen to multiply. I knew my cancer was ER positive but I thought we had opted for chemo over hormone treatment. "Five more years? No way!" I exclaimed. Henry calmly explained the benefits, primarily increasing protection (up to 50%) against cancer recurrence, also bone strengthening effects, and acting as a false estrogen in my body. I obviously looked as if I wasn't convinced, so he continued, "Since you are already entering menopause from the effects of the chemo, you will start having physiological changes. For example, you will start to grow facial hair…." "What!?" I responded in shock. I had to think a moment, "Are you appealing to my vanity?" A small grin appeared on his face. I looked at him in disbelief. I knew I was being unreasonable. So, I could only shrug my shoulders and say in defeat, "Okay."

Months or perhaps even years later, I sat in an examining room again with Henry for my annual oncology checkup and he was going over my case notes. He casually looked up and said, "How did you feel when I told you your diagnosis gave you a sixty percent chance of survival? "I was angry," I said trying to keep my tone even. "I was angry. Angry that my life was being assessed, defined by a universal standard made up of numbers. How dare the medical world treat me as a statistic.

Numbers don't show who I am…." Then, I thought for a moment and sheepishly added, "Of course, I was very frightened," Henry wrote down some notes and we talked on about other matters.

Lucy, my chemo nurse advised me that although it was wonderful to be completing my regimen, I should be aware that people often became depressed when finishing treatment. "Oh," I laughed, "Not me. I will have more energy, a normal appetite. I am going to feel better!" However, a few weeks after I finished all my hospital appointments, I was walking in a wooded park. I stopped to look at a solitary and graceful tree standing in the sunlight. For no apparent reason, I started to cry. And cry. And cry. I thought to myself, "Lucy was right. It is all so very sad." I don't know if I was crying because I felt so sorry for myself, or if it was looking at a future without the safety of the structured support to which I was accustomed, or perhaps it was the realization that I would never again be the person I was before cancer.

19 Self-Management
Reflections of a 44-Year Pediatric Survivor

Brason Lee

INTRODUCTION

It happened on January 20, 1981, at 4:30 p.m. I fell off a three-wheel motorcycle. My friends called for help. An ambulance came. I was taken to a local hospital and admitted under an emergency situation as a minor with a severe cerebral contusion—one of the most serious forms of traumatic brain injury. I was barely 18 years old and not expected to live. The nurses and doctors at the hospital didn't know how to reach my family. My panicked mom and sisters finally found me the next day. They were told, if I lived, I wasn't expected to ever walk again by myself. And I was a junior karate champion!

After a week in a coma and a month in the hospital, the neurosurgeon and his medical team placed me on a waiting list for inpatient rehabilitation care, and I was sent home with my older sisters. The kids from the neighborhood lined up to welcome me back. A few guys about my age were on the sidewalk in front of my house, but I recognized no one. I never thought about asking myself why. I was too busy concentrating on stepping out of the car and walking to the sidewalk leading to my house.

Therapy did not start for about another 35 days.

Fast-forward nearly half a century to August 8, 2025. I am now a 63-year-old retiree married to a wonderful woman and a proud father of a daughter in college. I completed a bachelor's degree and two graduate degrees within ten years. I started a 30-year career as a lobbyist for the National Association of Social Workers and a research consultant for AARP Public Policy Institute in Washington, D.C. I finished my career as a maternal and child health research scientist for the California Department of Public Health. I worked full time during my entire career except for four to five months between 1992 and 1993.

What can I say about self-management for survivors of traumatic brain injury? Self-management is a popular term in the health education field that emphasizes patient responsibility for his or her day-to-day care. Five core skills underline the principles of self-management: problem solving, decision making, resource utilization, patient-provider partnership, and action taking (Lorig and Holman, 2003). Yet, self-management is a vision that has eluded me for stretches of time during my lifetime as a survivor.

With five decades of lived experience, I can now offer the opinion that I wasn't always a good candidate for self-management. My view on this matter might be considered exploratory in nature. One reason is that the literature in self-management for persons with traumatic brain injury is still early in its development (Sander et al., 2024). This is further complicated by the limited research focusing on the successful lives of adults who sustained a traumatic brain injury in their youth.

Let's dive into this topic by exploring my varied thoughts and experiences by each decade post-trauma.

DECADE ONE: 1981 TO 1990

The first decade of life post-trauma was perhaps the most consequential period of time and would lay the foundation to my lifelong recovery as a survivor. Everything about my life post-trauma can be routed back to my experiences within this decade—the first three years, the middle years, and the last three years.

 DOI: 10.1201/9781003599074-21

During the first three years, I was cognitively, emotionally, and physically unprepared to take on the tasks required to self-manage. At the beginning, I was not able to make any informed decision on my own. I needed guidance in every aspect of life, even with directions on how to find my way between my therapy appointments.

This came across after one particularly exhausting session sometime in April of 1981—about a month after the start of my therapy at Sharp Rehabilitation Center, located in San Diego, California. My physical therapist, Pat, led me into a corridor with handrails. It was the largest hallway that I'd ever been in. There were tables with white-covered sheets against the wall. On top of these tables were rows of red-colored fruit drinks and chocolate chip cookies. Everything looked wonderfully delicious.

She poured a drink and handed it to me.

The next day, after my session, I returned to the same hall by myself, beaming expectantly for another treat of snacks, but they were no longer in sight. It puzzled me. I walked up and down the hall. My eyes inspected the area more intensely. When I reached one end, I saw another hallway with handrails connecting to the one I was in.

Maybe the snacks were there?

I walked halfway down the second corridor, but something felt wrong. This hallway was also empty, with no trace of fruit drinks. I paused, trying to decide what to do. I turned around to head back, but I had forgotten my way. Everything looked the same: the plain white walls, the mahogany-colored rails, the shiny waxed floors. I was terrified.

I turned a few more corners before reaching a walkway near the midpoint. My eyes locked onto the opening as I stepped closer. Then, a blast of cool air came rushing from the opening. Pat was in the distance, working with another patient. She must have sensed my presence because her head perked up and she greeted me with a smile. I had found my way back!

Pat pointed to the door across the dining area to the occupational therapy room. I headed for my next session, still not knowing that the halls connected to form a square.

My problem-solving and decision-making skills remained limited during the initial years. My speech pathologist, Bridget, taught me how to ask myself what I knew and didn't know as one way to analyze and solve problems. This was a difficult task. I needed lots of hints in order to come up with the right answer. My ability to accurately interpret, organize, and think about information was assessed to be equivalent to a seven-year-old child. My ability to understand words and identify similarities between two related ideas was assessed to be equal to a 12-year-old. I needed tutors to help me complete school assignments and other everyday tasks that I took for granted before my accident.

During the middle years of the first decade, from about 1984 to 1987, I began to regain or develop skills needed for self-management. However, they were limited, mostly to my ability to function within the academic environment as an undergraduate college student—going to class without a map of the school, reading assigned chapters of textbooks, recording class lectures, and studying for upcoming exams. This was my routine for almost every day of the week, since I had enrolled in a community college as a part of my therapy in 1981. By now, I did not require the help of tutors as much as before, in part because I was beginning to know how to prepare for class. I was beginning to learn how to plan the semester on my own.

I utilized resources only to the extent that I knew how to use the library and how to contact my school counselors whenever I needed help with editing my term papers and other major written assignments. It was not until 1985 that I began to take a full-load of four classes—the most that I had ever taken in one semester since my accident, four years post-trauma. I wanted to be prepared for the upper-division classes, which sounded frightening because I had barely survived my class on the fundamental of chemistry—a general education course that I passed only with extra home instructions from my sister, Rose, a chemist at the Salk Institute for Biological Studies.

In time, I discovered that I could receive free sessions of speech therapy by enrolling in a university clinic where graduate speech pathology students were able to practice what they learned.

Obtaining this help was significant because I had never reached out for help without the assistance of a therapist or social worker at the rehabilitation center to initiate the service.

Being a college student consumed almost all of my time. I didn't know how to function outside of the university, except for ordering food at local cafés or paying the bill with a credit card. My older sister, Anna, a 26-year-old microbiologist who always watched out for her younger siblings, balanced my checkbook every couple of months. Anna was also the person I sought out for help communicating with medical doctors. She handled all medical-related questions and concerns because my dad was too busy working and my mom did not speak English fluently.

My responsibilities were mostly geared to showing up for office visits. I made sure of this by arriving to appointments and anywhere else I needed be about an hour early, just so I wouldn't feel rushed. I showed up to nearly all appointments far in advance because I wanted to feel okay with myself. I didn't recognize then that this was my way of handling the stress and anxiety that had developed after my injury.

The last three years of the first decade was a period of growth as a person because, at about 26 years of age, I moved out of my parents' house in San Diego to pursue my graduate studies at the University of Southern California, located about 130 miles away in Los Angeles. I wasn't completely alone, however, because my brother, Coke, was an undergraduate student at another university in Los Angeles. We lived about five miles apart in separate apartments with our own group of roommates. But he was always there to help whenever I was in trouble, like when my car battery died in the parking lot of a shopping center.

I drove home on most weekends and always bought back a box of cooked Chinese food that my mother prepared for my brother and me.

During the last three years of the first decade, I continued to develop skills needed for self-management. I knew how to plan my studies and, if needed, how to adjust my study habits midway through the school semester. I knew the steps that needed to be taken to succeed in the classroom. For example, during my first year as a graduate student, I received a failing "F" grade on my first exam in a class on the psychology of aging. After some intense studying, I received an "A" grade by my second exam. Dr. Knight, my psychology professor at the school of gerontology at the University of Southern California, commented, "This is the strongest comeback that I have ever seen", as he returned the exam to me with a smile.

Outside of the academic environment, I knew how to take care of myself by going to the grocery store, doing my own laundry, and eating out. I must have eaten out at least once every day. I didn't know how to cook anything except for chicken soup, baked chicken, and turkey sandwiches. In a way, I did not recognize that I continued to have problems, partly because I had few interactions with groups of people and I was working mostly by myself in the silence of my bedroom.

Without knowing it, from about 1987 to 1990, I was building a marketable skill in the job market for my future work in policy-oriented research. Beyond my developing ability to research information and write papers, I really did not have too much confidence in my own actions. My belief in myself was fragile and too easily shaken by any uncomfortable looks from my fellow students. I often questioned my own decisions and asked for reassurance from others—my professors, my classmates, and almost anyone else who came into contact with me. I often depended on a few classmates whom I felt closest to for a sense of peace.

DECADES TWO AND THREE: 1991 TO 2010

I was probably a good candidate for self-management during the second and third decades of life post-trauma. With my professional training, I knew how to define a problem, arrive at a solution, and implement an action plan. I knew—or, at least, I thought I knew—how to manage my problems with memory. The only glitch was that, in the initial years after completing my education, I had nearly forgotten about my history of traumatic brain injury.

This may be hard to explain. I never denied my history with people who knew about my past. I just never said anything about it to people I recently met. I never considered the consequences of my brain injury as a possible reason for my continuing troubles. I was lost within the image that I created as an entrepreneurial student who found ways to write solid term papers and connect with people to complete projects, such as bringing together organizations with competing interests to support my research into the implications of a federal nursing home reform law on nursing homes in Los Angeles.

By 1995, I began to reconnect the notion of my continuing difficulties with speech, attention, and memory with my medical history of brain injury. I sought help from a team of neurologists, neuropsychologists, and speech pathologists at the University of California Los Angeles Health. The only problem was that, after their evaluations and recommendations for care, I refused to follow up on them. One speech therapist wrote in her medical notes that I appeared to have problems with severe dysnomia—a language disorder characterized by difficulty in recalling words, names, and objects. The speech pathologist wrote about me:

> Patient had a number of concerns regarding a group therapy program; one of which seemed to be a bit inappropriate. For example, his perception is that educated people like himself are very competitive with respect to what school they attended and he expressed concern that this competitive school spirit would interfere with group dynamics.

Did I sabotage my own care out of a misguided notion? I think so, which I believe illustrates the limits of my ability to utilize resources and form partnerships with healthcare providers to fully engage in the practice of self-management, even after 14 years post-trauma. All of this directly impacted my ability to act on the advice—to work with my treatment team to address what I knew deep inside was a problem.

Outside of the work environment, I continued to experience problems with managing money and balancing my checkbook. Sometimes, my sister helped reconcile my bank account. Other times, I simply closed an account and reopened another account, which I thought was more efficient. I created monthly spreadsheets to record every dollar spent by expense category so that I wouldn't spend more money than I earned. Here again, this worked until I would accidentally miss a month or two and forget about recording my spending. I lost control of my spending two or three times during these two decades. I accumulated a debt of a few thousands, which my mother helped bail me out, once she learned about my troubles.

My ability to manage my funds somewhat improved after my marriage to my wife, Ling, in 2003, and the birth of my daughter, Amanda, in 2004. I only lost control of my spending once.

DECADE FOUR: 2011 TO 2020

I was probably at my strongest overall point during the first half of my fourth decade post-trauma, from about 2011 to 2015. I continued to define problems, arrive at solutions, and implement plans to address those problems. I did this in both my personal life and my professional life. I continued to develop a reputation of writing good reports, which helped me overcompensate for my continued problems with speech and memory. It seemed that most people were able to overlook my difficulties in favor for my strengths in writing.

In terms of my medical and psychiatric needs, I had established a solid doctor-patient relationship with my primary care physician, who directed all my care, and my psychiatrist, who monitored my medication treatment for attention deficit disorder and other mental health concerns.

DECADE FIVE: 2021 TO PRESENT

The fifth decade is turning into a period a peace and comfort in terms of the path I have taken in my life so far. Some problems that I had in the initial months or years after my injury have returned to some degree, such as misplacing my wallet and, now, my cell phone. I lost a few jackets along the way by forgetting to pick them up after a stop at the bookstore. I have, at times, temporarily lost track of the direction of my driving. That is, do I turn right or left at the street to arrive at my doctor's office or my hairstylist's salon?

In 2021, after two decades with continuous health insurance with the same doctor, my primary care physician made a referral for a neuropsychological re-evaluation to assess my cognitive, physical, and behavioral functioning and to examine my cognitive status since my last neuropsychological assessment in 1995. In 2023, she ordered another neuropsychological re-evaluation. Taken together, a picture emerged with a decline in attention, working memory and processing speed over time.

My team of doctors advised me to restrict my driving to daytime hours and familiar places. The doctors diagnosed me with mild cognitive impairment, describing it to me as somewhere between what might be expected as normal aging and a degenerative brain disease. The good news for me was learning that my abilities to think at an abstract level and to solve problems under non-timed conditions continued to be intact and as strong as any person my age.

With that, I came up with a clever idea of buying a new sporty car to drive. I wanted to have fun driving in my final years, just in case my doctors might decide to restrict my driving by the next neuropsychological exam. Instead, my wife became the official manager of my funds, which was okay with me.

CONCLUSION

Self-care—and even the perception of self-care—is important. This is one reason why self-management may be a useful intervention for survivors of traumatic brain injury that will need to be further studied and examined. One recent study suggested that, among adults 65 years and older with traumatic brain injury, cognitive functioning had limited predictive ability to engage in self-management activities with the aid of additional support, such as extending the time spent on specific tasks (Kemp et al., 2025). This finding should be followed with the qualification that most (73.7%) of the survivors in this study sustained a mild traumatic brain injury and more than half (57.8%) were 4 to 15 years post-trauma.

My reflections on self-management are based on personal experience over 44 years post-trauma.

It is possible that self-management may be more easily applied to survivors of a mild traumatic brain injury than to survivors of a severe traumatic brain injury. One reasoning is based on the finding that most patients with mild traumatic brain injury tend to recover within a few months with only a subgroup experiencing more persistent symptoms (Rabinowitz et al., 2025).

I suspect that survivors of severe traumatic brain injury, like mine, may be able to engage in self-management activities at varying levels based on the time since injury and the context and situation. Over time, my ability to solve problems and make day-to-day decisions post-trauma was episodic in nature and complicated by varying levels of self-awareness of my own limitations. I may have been least able to engage in self-management activities during my first five years post-trauma, with improving abilities up to my 34th year before I began to decline by my 42nd year post-trauma. As the state of literature on self-management advances in the field of traumatic brain injury rehabilitation, it will be interesting to see if the practice of self-management might be partitioned by severity of the injury and individualized based on each survivor's strengths and limitations.

REFERENCES

Kemp AM, Love K, O-Brien KH. Exploring demographic and cognitive predictors of self-management in quasi-randomized fall prevention intervention for older adults with and without traumatic brain injury. Journal of Head Trauma Rehabilitation. 2025;40(3):E216–E225.

Lorig, KR, Holman HR. Self-management education: history, definition, outcomes, and mechanisms. Annals of Behavioral Medicine. 2003;26(1):1–7.

Rabinowitz AR, Li Xiaoqi, McCauley SR, Wilde EA, Barnes A, Hanten G, et al. Prevalence and predictors of poor recovery from mild traumatic brain injury. Journal of Neurotrauma. 2025;32(19):1488–1496.

Sander AM, Pappadis MR, Bushnik T, Chiaravalloti ND, et al. An umbrella review of self-management interventions for health conditions with symptom overlap with traumatic brain injury. Journal of Head Trauma Rehabilitation. 2024;28(2):140–151.

Section III

Perspectives of Self-Management

20 Self-Management for Neurorehabilitation in Low- and Middle-Income Countries

Eugene Nizeyimana

INTRODUCTION

The global burden of neurological disorders continues to escalate, with an estimated 3.4 billion people affected worldwide, representing a 59% increase since 1990 (Vos et al., 2020). This burden falls disproportionately on low- and middle-income countries, where 85% of the world's population resides but where access to specialized neurological care and rehabilitation services remains critically limited (Owolabi et al., 2022). The World Health Organization estimates that over 2.4 billion people globally require rehabilitation services, yet in many low- and middle-income countries, more than 50% of people who need rehabilitation do not get it (World Health Organization, 2021). Barriers to rehabilitation access in low- and middle-income countries include inadequate infrastructure and resources, workforce shortages and training gaps, policy deficiencies and governance issues, geographic isolation and high costs, limited community-based programs, and insufficient awareness shaped by cultural factors and social support systems (Ohnmar et al., 2024).

Integrating self-management strategies within rehabilitation programs offers a promising pathway to overcome many of these systemic barriers. Self-management approaches can reduce dependency on specialized healthcare infrastructure by empowering patients and caregivers with skills and knowledge to manage conditions independently, while community-based self-management programs can overcome geographic barriers and reduce costs associated with frequent clinical visits (Parke et al., 2015). Furthermore, culturally adapted self-management interventions show promise for enhancing engagement and addressing barriers to care within local contexts in low- and middle-income countries. When these interventions are tailored to address specific community needs such as language barriers, cultural beliefs about health, and structural constraints, they can improve intervention acceptability and feasibility (Naderbagi et al., 2024). This approach supports the development of contextually appropriate, scalable solutions that work within the resource constraints of low- and middle-income countries.

This chapter examines self-management approaches for neurorehabilitation, exploring the conceptual foundations of self-management, evidence-based interventions for major neurological conditions, multi-level barriers to implementation in low- and middle-income countries, and the potential of digital technologies to enhance accessibility and patient engagement in resource-constrained settings.

CONCEPTUAL FOUNDATIONS OF SELF-MANAGEMENT

The concept of self-management has emerged as a potentially transformative approach to address healthcare disparities. Self-management in health is defined as 'an individual's ability to manage the symptoms, treatment, physical and psychological consequences, and lifestyle changes

DOI: 10.1201/9781003599074-23

inherent in living with a chronic condition' (Barlow et al., 2002). Self-management in neurorehabilitation encompasses the knowledge, skills, and confidence that individuals with neurological conditions require to effectively manage their condition and maintain optimal functioning in daily life (Barlow et al., 2002; Taylor et al., 2014). This definition extends beyond simple adherence to prescribed treatments to include active problem-solving, goal setting, resource utilization, and partnership with healthcare providers in decision-making processes (Lorig & Holman, 2003).

Rather than viewing patients as passive recipients of care, self-management paradigms recognize individuals and their caregivers as active partners in the rehabilitation process, capable of making informed decisions about their health and implementing evidence-based interventions with appropriate support (Lorig & Holman, 2003). This approach is particularly relevant in neurorehabilitation, where the chronic nature of many conditions necessitates long-term adaptation and ongoing skill development that extends far beyond the acute care setting.

The conceptual framework of self-management in neurorehabilitation is built upon three core principles: patient empowerment, self-efficacy, and active participation in care. Patient empowerment involves enabling individuals to take control of their health by providing them with the necessary knowledge, skills, and confidence to make informed decisions about their care (Anderson & Funnell, 2010). Self-efficacy, as defined by Bandura (1978), refers to an individual's belief in their capacity to execute behaviors necessary to produce specific performance attainments. In the context of neurorehabilitation, this translates to patients' confidence in their ability to manage their condition and perform rehabilitation activities independently.

Active participation in care represents a fundamental shift from traditional medical models where patients are passive recipients of treatment. Instead, it emphasizes collaborative partnerships between patients, caregivers, and healthcare providers, where individuals are recognized as experts in their own lived experience of their condition (Hibbard & Greene, 2013).

The burden of neurological rehabilitation needs in low- and middle-income countries is particularly acute, with 70% of strokes occurring in these settings and subsequent disease burden being greater than in high-income countries (Prvu Bettger et al., 2019). On average, low- and middle-income countries have just ten total skilled rehabilitation experts for every one million population. In contrast, high-income countries average over 400 occupational therapists, 900 physical therapists, 400 speech therapists and 20 physical medicine and rehabilitation physicians per one million population (Kayola et al., 2023). This critical shortage necessitates innovative approaches to service delivery, making self-management interventions particularly relevant for conditions such as stroke, spinal cord injury, traumatic brain injury, and Parkinson's disease.

THEORETICAL FRAMEWORKS SUPPORTING SELF-MANAGEMENT

Several behavioral and psychological theories provide a theoretical foundation for self-management interventions in neurorehabilitation. The Health Belief Model (Alyafei & Easton-Carr, 2024) suggests that health behaviors are influenced by individuals' perceptions of susceptibility to health problems, the severity of consequences, the benefits of preventive action, and barriers to action. In neurorehabilitation contexts, this model helps explain why patients may or may not engage in self-management activities and provides a framework for addressing potential barriers.

Social Cognitive Theory (Bandura, 1986) offers another crucial theoretical foundation, emphasizing the reciprocal interaction between personal factors, environmental influences, and behaviors. This theory's emphasis on self-efficacy, observational learning, and self-regulation processes is particularly relevant to neurorehabilitation, where patients must develop new skills and adapt to functional limitations while navigating environmental challenges.

The Chronic Care Model (Wagner et al., 2001) provides a systems-level framework that emphasizes the importance of prepared, proactive practice teams working with informed, activated patients to achieve optimal outcomes. This model's focus on community resources, health system organization, and decision support aligns well with the multi-faceted nature of neurological conditions and the need for comprehensive, long-term management strategies.

COMPONENTS OF EFFECTIVE SELF-MANAGEMENT IN NEUROREHABILITATION

Effective self-management programs in neurorehabilitation represent a comprehensive approach that empowers patients to become active participants in their recovery journey. These programs incorporate multiple interconnected components that address the cognitive, emotional, behavioral, and practical aspects of living with neurological conditions. The following components form the foundation of evidence-based self-management interventions.

Foundational Knowledge and Skills Development

Education and skill development form the cornerstone of effective self-management, providing patients and caregivers with essential knowledge about their condition, treatment options, and practical skills for daily management (Lorig & Holman, 2003). This foundation enables informed decision-making and builds confidence in managing the complexities of neurological conditions. Health literacy, encompassing functional, communicative, and critical dimensions, plays a crucial role in self-management by enabling individuals to access, understand, and apply health information effectively (Nutbeam, 2000).

Goal Setting and Self-Monitoring Systems

Goal setting and action planning help individuals identify specific, achievable objectives and develop concrete steps to achieve them, promoting a sense of ownership and progress in their rehabilitation journey. Meaningful goal setting that incorporates personal values and life aspirations significantly enhances motivation and rehabilitation outcomes (Dekker et al., 2020). Closely integrated with goal setting is self-monitoring, which involves the systematic observation and recording of one's own behavior, providing essential feedback for behavior change and self-regulation (Korotitsch & Nelson-Gray, 1999). Self-monitoring enables patients to track practice and exercise activities, providing data-driven feedback that supports adherence to rehabilitation programs (Dobkin & Dorsch, 2011).

Problem-Solving and Adaptive Thinking Skills

Problem-solving skills training enables patients to identify challenges, generate potential solutions, and evaluate outcomes, building confidence in their ability to manage unexpected situations or setbacks (D'zurilla & Goldfried, 1971). This component is particularly crucial in neurorehabilitation, where patients must frequently adapt to changing abilities and circumstances. Self-awareness, defined as the ability to understand one's own thoughts, feelings and behaviors, serves as a fundamental prerequisite for effective problem-solving and adaptation (Master ABA, 2024).

Behavioral Self-Regulation and Motivation Enhancement

Behavioral self-management strategies require education, ongoing contact, tailored information, goal setting, monitoring, feedback, and motivational enhancement (Dobkin & Dorsch, 2011). Self-determination theory provides a framework for understanding motivation in neurorehabilitation, emphasizing the importance of autonomy, competence, and relatedness in sustaining therapeutic engagement (Kusec et al., 2019). Motivation in rehabilitation is influenced by multiple factors including patients' goals, experiences of success and failure, physical condition, resilience, and social relationships (Yoshida et al., 2021).

Technology Integration and Digital Literacy Skills

Digital technology skills have become increasingly important in neurorehabilitation, enabling patients to access eHealth applications for self-monitoring, symptom tracking, and remote therapeutic engagement (Banakou et al., 2018). Technology allows for guided self-management through hybrid treatment programs that incorporate both therapist-led and self-guided interventions (Cetinkaya et al., 2024). Digital literacy encompasses not only technological skills but also cognitive abilities for critical thinking about information and social skills for communication and collaboration (Ng, 2012).

Health Advocacy and Communication Skills

Patient self-advocacy, defined as the willingness to challenge providers and actively participate in decision-making, is significantly associated with health literacy skills, particularly speaking and listening abilities (Martin et al., 2011). Communication and partnership skills help patients develop confidence and the ability to communicate effectively with healthcare providers, advocate for their needs, and participate meaningfully in treatment decisions. Self-advocacy involves taking an active role in health management, learning about conditions and treatment options, and working in partnership with healthcare teams (Canberra Health Literacy, 2024).

Resource Utilization and Support Network Development

Resource utilization involves helping patients identify and access available community resources, support services, and technological tools that can support their self-management efforts. Supported self-management interventions, including peer support, self-management education, and health coaching, significantly increase knowledge, skills, and confidence in managing health conditions (NHS England, 2024). Social support serves as a critical factor that enhances self-efficacy and self-management behaviors in chronic conditions (Xu et al., 2018).

Emotional Regulation and Psychological Coping

Emotional coping and stress management components address the psychological aspects of living with a neurological condition, including strategies for managing anxiety, depression, and adjustment challenges that commonly accompany these conditions (Dobson & Kendall, 1993). Self-monitoring of emotional states, thoughts, and behaviors provides crucial awareness that supports cognitive-behavioral interventions and emotional regulation (Psychology Tools, 2024). Anhedonia and reduced motivation to engage in rehabilitation programs can significantly impact recovery, requiring specific interventions to address these psychological barriers (Segura et al., 2024).

Self-Efficacy and Confidence Building

Self-efficacy, defined as confidence in one's capabilities to develop and meet planned goals, increases as self-management proceeds successfully and is enhanced through positive mastery experiences, vicarious learning, verbal persuasion, and physiological feedback (Bandura, 1997; Dobkin & Dorsch, 2011). The relationship between health literacy and self-efficacy is particularly strong in the communicative and critical domains, suggesting that interventions should focus on enhancing communication skills and critical thinking abilities (Xu et al., 2018).

These interconnected components of self-management in neurorehabilitation work synergistically to promote patient autonomy, engagement, and optimal outcomes. The integration of traditional skills training with modern technological approaches, combined with attention to psychological and social factors, creates a comprehensive framework for supporting individuals with neurological conditions in their journey toward independence and improved quality of life.

EVIDENCE OF SELF-MANAGEMENT INTERVENTIONS IN LOW- AND MIDDLE-INCOME COUNTRIES

Despite demonstrated cost-effectiveness, self-management interventions remain underutilized in low- and middle-income countries, indicating incomplete integration into healthcare systems despite empirical support (Akhal et al., 2025).

STROKE SELF-MANAGEMENT INTERVENTIONS

The strongest evidence emerges from stroke rehabilitation research. In Iran, Amiri et al. conducted a randomized controlled trial of 72 stroke patients examining a 5A-based self-management program (Assess, Advise, Agree, Assist, Arrange). The intervention group (n=36) received a comprehensive six-week program including needs assessment, goal setting, symptom management education, psychological coping strategies, medication management, and problem-solving skills training. Results demonstrated significantly greater self-efficacy improvements compared to controls both immediately (p=0.047) and at three months (p=0.009) post-intervention (Amiri et al., 2022).

Similarly promising results were observed in West Africa, where Natta et al. evaluated a self-management program for chronic stroke patients with upper-limb impairment in Benin. Twenty-eight participants performed supervised home-based exercises for eight weeks, demonstrating 20% improvement in manual ability, enhanced grip force, and improved quality of life, with effects sustained eight weeks post-treatment (Natta et al., 2021).

In Bangladesh, Afrin et al. conducted a large-scale randomized controlled trial (n=432) evaluating comprehensive health education including face-to-face counseling, educational materials, self-monitoring tools, and monthly follow-ups over 12 months. The intervention significantly reduced mortality and enhanced medication adherence, providing robust epidemiological evidence for healthcare system integration (Afrin et al., 2025).

A feasibility study in Uganda examined F@ce™, a mobile phone-supported family-centered intervention. Despite technical challenges, including mobile connectivity issues, the eight-week program involving goal setting, daily self-management reminders, and twice-weekly occupational therapist calls demonstrated significant improvements in performance scores and self-efficacy among 28 participants (Kamwesiga et al., 2018).

However, not all stroke interventions proved effective. The ATTEND Collaborative Group's large randomized controlled trial across 14 Indian hospitals (n=1,250) found no significant benefits from family caregiver-led rehabilitation training. At six months, 47% of both intervention and control groups were dead or dependent, with no improvements in quality of life, caregiver burden, or functional measures (Lindley et al., 2017).

SPINAL CORD INJURY SELF-MANAGEMENT INTERVENTIONS

Evidence for spinal cord injury self-management in low- and middle-income countries remains limited. Hossain et al. conducted a randomized controlled trial in Bangladesh with 410 wheelchair-dependent participants, implementing comprehensive community-based care including 36 phone calls and three home visits over two years. Results showed no significant differences in mortality rates (7.4% intervention vs 7.8% control) or secondary outcomes including complications, depression, participation, quality of life, and independence (Hossain et al., 2017). Evidence from disaster-affected low-resource settings also highlights persistent shortcomings in spinal cord injury management and rehabilitation (Rathore et al., 2008).

Qualitative research provides valuable insights into existing self-management strategies. Baniya et al. found that 84.3% of 115 community-dwelling people with spinal cord injury in Nepal experienced depressive mood, with 60.8% reporting moderate to severe symptoms. Participants primarily employed non-pharmacological approaches including internet/social media use (50.5%), family support (31.9%), religious practices (31.9%), and substance abuse (15.5%), often due to limited rural healthcare access (Baniya et al., 2022).

Begum et al. identified nine self-management strategy groups across four components through photoelicitation focus groups in Bangladesh. Beyond traditional medical, emotional, and role management components, they identified "management of social complexities" as a fourth component particularly relevant to low- and middle-income countries, encompassing environmental relocation, assertive behavior, and advocacy for social change (Begum et al., 2022).

Traumatic Brain Injury and Parkinson's Disease Self-Management Interventions

Despite traumatic brain injury prevalence rates being three times higher in low- and middle-income countries than high-income countries (Allen et al., 2023; Dulf et al., 2021) and Parkinson's disease prevalence of 49 per 100,000 in sub-Saharan Africa (Pereira et al., 2024), no specific self-management intervention studies were identified for these conditions in low- and middle-income countries. This research gap exists alongside severely limited rehabilitation access, where unprepared families manage survivors independently (Soule et al., 2024). While emerging evidence demonstrates potential benefits of culturally adapted self-management interventions in low- and middle-income countries, significant research gaps persist.

IMPLEMENTATION STRATEGIES OF SELF-MANAGEMENT IN LOW- AND MIDDLE-INCOME COUNTRIES

Implementing effective self-management programs in low- and middle-income countries requires innovative, culturally adapted approaches that address resource constraints, healthcare system limitations, and diverse population needs. Successful strategies must leverage available infrastructure, community resources, and technology while ensuring sustainability and scalability within existing healthcare frameworks and economic realities of these settings.

Cultural Adaptation

Successful implementation of self-management in low- and middle-income country settings necessitates systematic cultural adaptation that extends beyond translation to encompass deep structural modifications addressing local beliefs, practices, and healthcare contexts. Cultural adaptation must link culture with contextual factors including economic conditions and social systems to ensure intervention accessibility and sustainability (Naderbagi et al., 2024).

Contemporary frameworks emphasize both surface-level modifications (language, visual elements, delivery methods) and deep structural changes addressing cultural values, health beliefs, family structures, and traditional healing practices. Spanhel et al. identified 17 components of cultural adaptation across 55 studies of internet- and mobile-based interventions, comprising ten content components (characters, activities, environments, values, language translation, text tailoring, visualization, mental health concepts, treatment aims, and methods), four methodological components (structure, functionality, design aesthetics, and guidance format), and three procedural components (information gathering methods, stakeholder involvement, and theoretical frameworks) (Spanhel et al., 2021).

In neurorehabilitation contexts, cultural adaptation must particularly address disability beliefs, traditional recovery concepts, family caregiving roles, and indigenous healing practice integration.

Bautista-Gomez et al. distinguish between cultural adaptation (modifying delivery to reflect community values) and structural adaptation (modifying interventions to encourage attendance and completion) (Bautista-Gomez et al., 2024).

Patient and Caregiver Training

Effective implementation requires comprehensive, health literacy-informed training programs addressing both patients and caregivers while accommodating diverse educational backgrounds and cultural preferences prevalent in low- and middle-income country settings.

Patient Education and Self-Management Training

Patient education interventions demonstrate significant effectiveness across multiple chronic conditions in low- and middle-income countries. Heine et al.'s systematic review and meta-analysis of health education interventions for adults with non-communicable diseases in low- and middle-income countries provided compelling evidence that health literacy interventions effectively promote disease knowledge and behavior change, particularly for diabetes patients across 53 studies spanning cancer, cardiovascular disease, chronic respiratory disease, and diabetes (Heine et al., 2021).

Meherali et al. (2020) found that all 23 health literacy intervention studies reviewed significantly improved knowledge and awareness, employing four main strategies: traditional health literacy approaches, art-based interventions, active learning strategies, and technology-based interventions across diverse populations (Meherali et al., 2020). According to Zou et al. (2024), health literacy significantly affects disease management self-efficacy, with social support mediating and illness perception moderating these relationships.

Caregiver Health Literacy and Training

Caregiver training represents a critical component given family caregivers' central role in low- and middle-income countries healthcare contexts. O'Conor et al. (2023) found that caregivers with marginal or low health literacy demonstrate poorer performance on everyday health tasks. Dorsey et al. (2023) demonstrated that poor caregiver health literacy significantly associates with healthcare communication and navigation difficulties, with low health literacy caregivers being 2.52 times more likely to experience high difficulty levels. Moore et al. (2024) found that 7% of cancer caregivers had inadequate health literacy, scoring lowest on social support, information seeking, and care recipient preference understanding domains.

Integration with Healthcare Systems through Task-Shifting

The evidence suggests that task sharing/shifting transforms self-management from a specialist-dependent activity to a community-supported, accessible process that builds local capacity and provides culturally relevant, ongoing support for individuals with neurological conditions.

Capacity Building and Skill Transfer

Task sharing enables the training of non-physician healthcare workers to deliver lifestyle counselling, self-management skill adoption, and protocol-led treatment that can be effectively implemented by community health workers, nurses, and other non-specialists (Anand et al., 2019). This approach significantly expands the workforce capable of teaching and supporting self-management techniques. Task-sharing models improve accessibility of services for patients and caregivers, bringing neurological care closer to communities where specialist services are scarce. In low- and middle-income countries, where skilled rehabilitation practitioners' number fewer, task sharing allows community-based delivery of self-management support (Bernhardt et al., 2020).

Peer Support and Community Integration

Non-specialist providers often serve as trusted community figures who can deliver culturally appropriate self-management support. Studies show that community health workers apply intervention skills, such as problem-solving techniques, to their own lives, creating authentic peer models for self-management (Sangraula et al., 2024).

Family and Caregiver Engagement

Family members and caregivers serve as valuable "therapy extenders," assisting patients with mobility, wheelchair activities, balance, self-care, and speech and language activities. Task sharing formalizes this natural support system through structured training, enabling continuous reinforcement of therapeutic exercises and self-care techniques between formal sessions. This approach transforms family members from passive observers into skilled participants who can provide daily motivation, early problem detection, and culturally appropriate support, creating a sustainable self-management system (Bernhardt et al., 2020).

BARRIERS TO SELF-MANAGEMENT ADOPTION IN LOW- AND MIDDLE-INCOME COUNTRIES

Systemic Barriers

The adoption of self-management approaches in low- and middle-income country settings faces numerous systemic barriers that operate at policy, organizational, and funding levels. Healthcare policies in many low- and middle-income countries continue to emphasize acute care and hospital-based treatment models, with limited recognition or support for self-management approaches (Atun et al., 2013). This policy environment can create regulatory barriers, funding challenges, and professional resistance to implementing self-management programs.

Funding constraints represent perhaps the most significant systemic barrier to implementing self-management interventions in low- and middle-income countries, directly limiting the development and sustainability of programs that empower patients to manage their own health conditions. High out-of-pocket expenses are among the most commonly reported barriers to accessing rehabilitation services globally, with over 50% of people with disabilities in low- and middle-income countries lacking access to rehabilitation due to insufficient pooled funding mechanisms (World Health Organization, 2023). This financial constraint forces healthcare systems to prioritize acute care over preventive self-management programs.

Systematic reviews consistently identify lack of financing for rehabilitation services by government and organizations, alongside high out-of-pocket costs, as significant financial barriers that prevent the establishment of comprehensive self-management support systems (Ohnmar et al., 2024). Current reimbursement mechanisms, frequently based on global budgets and salary structures, while helpful for cost control, represent important barriers to expanding supply and quality of self-management services (Bachani et al., 2024).

Healthcare system infrastructure limitations compound these financial challenges, creating additional systemic barriers that undermine the delivery and effectiveness of self-management interventions. The three most prevalent infrastructure-related barriers in developing countries are lack of basic infrastructure (14%), inadequate equipment (12%), and technology gaps (12%), all of which are essential for supporting patient self-monitoring and program delivery (Kruse et al., 2019). Without proper information systems to support self-management programs, healthcare staff struggle to track the large volume of patients seen daily, resulting in poor quality reports and compromised ability to provide ongoing support and monitoring essential for successful self-management (Fraser & Blaya, 2010). Technological and infrastructural hurdles, including limited internet and phone coverage, system malfunctions, and lack of software interoperability, prevent the implementation of digital self-management tools and compromise patient tracking, follow-up support, and outcome monitoring that are fundamental to effective self-management interventions (Qureshi et al., 2013).

Provider-Related Barriers

Healthcare providers in low- and middle-income country settings face numerous barriers that can impede the adoption of self-management approaches. Training gaps represent a primary concern, as many healthcare providers lack specific training in self-management principles, behavior change techniques, and patient education strategies (Bloom et al., 2020). The training that does exist is frequently brief with limited subsequent support. Health professionals may need to develop specific skills to provide effective self-management support for patients with progressive neurological conditions, as these conditions are associated with problems such as fatigue and cognitive impairment which may make self-management more challenging (Davies et al., 2017).

Workload and time constraints present additional barriers, as implementing self-management approaches often requires significant time investment for patient education, skill training, and ongoing support. In resource-constrained settings where healthcare providers are already managing heavy patient loads, the additional time requirements for self-management implementation may be perceived as burdensome.

Patient-Related Barriers

Patients and caregivers in low- and middle-income country settings face numerous barriers that can impede their participation in self-management programs. Health literacy represents a fundamental challenge, as many individuals may lack the basic knowledge and skills necessary to understand their condition, interpret health information, and make informed decisions about their care (Berkman et al., 2011). Socioeconomic barriers significantly impact the ability of patients and families to participate in self-management programs. People experiencing socioeconomic deprivation face competing priorities between immediate economic survival needs and long-term health management activities, often forcing difficult choices between basic necessities and health-related expenses (Woodward et al., 2023). Additionally, patients from lower socioeconomic backgrounds may lack the educational resources, health literacy, and stable living environments necessary to effectively implement complex self-management routines and what impact do chronic disease self-management support interventions have on health inequity gaps related to socioeconomic status (Hardman et al., 2020), while time availability becomes compromised when individuals must prioritize immediate economic needs over time-intensive self-management activities (Woodward et al., 2023).

Digital Technologies and Self-Management

The rapid expansion of mobile technology in low- and middle-income countries has created unprecedented opportunities for supporting self-management in neurorehabilitation. Mobile health (mHealth) applications offer several advantages for self-management support, including portability, accessibility, interactive features, and the ability to provide real-time feedback and support (Stephani et al., 2016). Innovative mHealth applications show significant promise for neurorehabilitation self-management in low- and middle-income countries. The 9zest Stroke App®, implemented in Ghana, delivered individualized, goal-targeted exercise programs remotely supervised by tele-therapists for 12 weeks. The feasibility study demonstrated excellent user satisfaction and motor deficit improvements, proving tele-rehabilitation is feasible in resource-limited settings. This highlights how digital infrastructure enhances self-management by providing accessible, personalized interventions that overcome geographical barriers (Sarfo et al., 2018).

CONCLUSION

This review reveals both the transformative potential and critical limitations of self-management interventions in neurorehabilitation within low- and middle-income countries. While the theoretical foundations and conceptual frameworks strongly support self-management approaches as viable solutions to address the overwhelming rehabilitation burden in low- and middle-income countries, the empirical evidence base remains concerningly narrow and geographically concentrated.

The most significant finding is the stark evidence gap for traumatic brain injury and Parkinson's disease conditions with disproportionately high prevalence in low- and middle-income countries yet completely absent from the self-management intervention literature in these settings. The available evidence derives predominantly from stroke interventions, creating a misleading impression of comprehensive coverage while leaving vast populations with neurological conditions without evidence-based self-management guidance. Furthermore, many studies cited were conducted in high- and upper-middle-income countries, raising questions about the applicability and generalizability of findings to resource-constrained low- and middle-income countries contexts.

The successful interventions identified primarily from Iran, Bangladesh, Benin, and Uganda demonstrate that culturally adapted, family-centered approaches incorporating technology can achieve meaningful improvements in self-efficacy, functional outcomes, and quality of life. However, these isolated successes cannot mask the fundamental research inequity that mirrors the broader healthcare disparities affecting low- and middle-income countries.

Moving forward, urgent priorities include conducting rigorous self-management intervention research specifically for traumatic brain injury and Parkinson's disease in low- and middle-income country settings, expanding geographical representation beyond the current limited scope, and developing implementation frameworks that address the unique systemic, provider, and patient-level barriers identified. Without addressing these critical evidence gaps, the promise of self-management in reducing neurological rehabilitation disparities will remain unrealized for millions of individuals in low- and middle-income countries who need these interventions most. The field requires a fundamental shift toward equity-focused research that prioritizes the most underserved populations and conditions.

REFERENCES

Afrin, M., Huq, K.E., Khan, S.U., Das, S.C., Chowdhury, M.S.J.H., Fukuoka, Y., Fukushima, Y. and Moriyama, M. (2025) 'Effectiveness of a health education program to reduce recurrence of stroke by controlling modifiable risk factors in a specialized hospital in Bangladesh: Randomized controlled trial', JMIR Public Health and Surveillance, 11(1), p. e72233.

Akhal, T., Gabra, M., Adesokan, M. and Babatunde, O.O. (2025) 'Self-management interventions for common long-term conditions in low-and middle-income countries: A synthesis of current evidence', Journal of Global Health, 15, p. 04148.

Allen, B.C., Cummer, E. and Sarma, A.K. (2023) 'Traumatic brain injury in select low-and middle-income countries: A narrative review of the literature', Journal of Neurotrauma, 40(7–8), pp. 602–619.

Alyafei, A. and Easton-Carr, R. (2024) The health belief model of behavior change. Treasure Island, FL: Stat Pearls Publishing.

Amiri, F.S., Abolhassani, S., Alimohammadi, N. and Roghani, T. (2022) 'Investigating the effect of self-management program on stroke's patients' self-efficacy', BMC Neurology, 22(1), p. 360.

Anand, T.N., Joseph, L.M., Geetha, A.V., Prabhakaran, D. and Jeemon, P. (2019) 'Task sharing with non-physician health-care workers for management of blood pressure in low-income and middle-income countries: A systematic review and meta-analysis', The Lancet Global Health, 7(6), pp. e761–e771.

Anderson, R.M. and Funnell, M.M. (2010) 'Patient empowerment: Myths and misconceptions', Patient Education and Counseling, 79(3), pp. 277–282.

Atun, R., Jaffar, S., Nishtar, S., Knaul, F.M., Barreto, M.L., Nyirenda, M., Banatvala, N. and Piot, P. (2013) 'Improving responsiveness of health systems to non-communicable diseases', The Lancet, 381(9867), pp. 690–697.

Bachani, A.M., Bentley, J.A., Kautsar, H., Neill, R. and Trujillo, A.J. (2024) 'Suggesting global insights to local challenges: Expanding financing of rehabilitation services in low and middle-income countries', Frontiers in Rehabilitation Sciences, 5, p. 1305033.

Banakou, D., Kishore, S. and Slater, M. (2018) 'Virtually being Einstein results in an improvement in cognitive task performance and a decrease in age bias', Frontiers in Psychology, 9, p. 368309.

Bandura, A. (1978) 'Self-efficacy: Toward a unifying theory of behavioral change', Advances in Behavior Research and Therapy, 1(4), pp. 139–161.

Bandura, A. (1986) Social foundations of thought and action. Englewood Cliffs: Prentice-Hall.

Bandura, A. (1997) Self-efficacy: The exercise of control. New York: W.H. Freeman and Company.

Baniya, M., Kitrungrote, L. and Damkliang, J. (2022) 'Prevalence, severity, and self-management of depressive mood among community-dwelling people with spinal cord injury in Nepal', Belitung Nursing Journal, 8(2), pp. 101–107.

Barlow, J., Wright, C., Sheasby, J., Turner, A. and Hainsworth, J. (2002) 'Self-management approaches for people with chronic conditions: A review', Patient Education and Counseling, 48(2), pp. 177–187.

Bautista-Gomez, M.M., Zuluaga, L.S. and Medina-Tabares, M.F. (2024) 'Cultural adaptation of health interventions for ethnic communities in vulnerable settings: A qualitative data synthesis', New Trends in Qualitative Research, 20(3), p. e920.

Begum, S., Alve, Y.A. and Bontje, P. (2022) 'Self-Management embedded in daily activities: A photoelicitation focus group study among persons with spinal cord injury and their primary caregivers in Bangladesh', Occupational Therapy International, 2022(1), p. 2705104.

Berkman, N.D., Sheridan, S.L., Donahue, K.E., Halpern, D.J. and Crotty, K. (2011) 'Low health literacy and health outcomes: An updated systematic review', Annals of Internal Medicine, 155(2), pp. 97–107.

Bernhardt, J., Urimubenshi, G., Gandhi, D.B. and Eng, J.J. (2020) 'Stroke rehabilitation in low-income and middle-income countries: A call to action', The Lancet, 396(10260), pp. 1452–1462.

Bloom, D.E., Chen, S., Kuhn, M., McGovern, M.E., Oxley, L. and Prettner, K. (2020) 'The economic burden of chronic diseases: Estimates and projections for China, Japan, and South Korea', The Journal of the Economics of Ageing, 17, p. 100163.

Canberra Health Literacy. (2024) Self-advocacy. Available at: https://cbrhl.org.au/consumers-carers/communicating-with-a-provider/self-advocacy/ (Accessed: 15 September 2025).

Cetinkaya, B., Twomey, K.E. and Conroy, P. (2024) 'Initial evaluation of the TALES (technology and literacy engagement after stroke) programme targeting functional literacy and social engagement in people with aphasia after stroke', Aphasiology, 38(10), pp. 1589–1607.

D'zurilla, T.J. and Goldfried, M.R. (1971) 'Problem solving and behaviour modification', Journal of Abnormal Psychology, 78(1), pp. 107–126.

Davies, F., Wood, F., Bullock, A., Wallace, C. and Edwards, A. (2017) 'Interventions to improve the self-management support health professionals provide for people with progressive neurological conditions: Protocol for a realist synthesis', BMJ Open, 7(3), p. e014575.

Dekker, J., De Groot, V., Ter Steeg, A.M., Vloothuis, J., Holla, J., Collette, E., Satink, T., Post, L., Doodeman, S. and Littooij, E. (2020) 'Setting meaningful goals in rehabilitation: Rationale and practical tool', Clinical Rehabilitation, 34(1), pp. 3–12.

Dobkin, B.H. and Dorsch, A. (2011) 'The promise of mHealth: daily activity monitoring and outcome assessments by wearable sensors', Neurorehabilitation and Neural Repair, 25(9), pp. 788–798.

Dobson, K.S. and Kendall, P.C. (1993) Psychopathology and cognition. San Diego: Academic Press.

Dorsey, B.F., Cook, L.J., Katz, A.D., Sapiro, H.K., Kadish, H.A. and Holsti, M. (2023) 'Health care provider bias in estimating the health literacy of caregivers in a pediatric emergency department', Pediatric Emergency Care, 39(12), pp. e80–e85.

Dulf, D., Coman, M.A., Tadevosyan, A., Chikhladze, N., Cebanu, S. and Peek-Asa, C. (2021) 'A 3-country assessment of traumatic brain injury practices and capacity', World Neurosurgery, 146, pp. e517–e526.

Fraser, H.S. and Blaya, J. (2010) 'Implementing medical information systems in developing countries, what works and what doesn't', AMIA Annual Symposium Proceedings, 2010, p. 232.

Hardman, R., Begg, S. and Spelten, E. (2020) 'What impact do chronic disease self-management support interventions have on health inequity gaps related to socioeconomic status: A systematic review', BMC Health Services Research, 20(1), p. 150.

Heine, M., Lategan, F., Erasmus, M., Lombaard, C.M., Mc Carthy, N., Olivier, J., van Niekerk, M. and Hanekom, S. (2021) 'Health education interventions to promote health literacy in adults with selected non-communicable diseases living in low-to-middle income countries: A systematic review and meta-analysis', Journal of Evaluation in Clinical Practice, 27(6), pp. 1417–1428.

Hibbard, J.H. and Greene, J. (2013) 'What the evidence shows about patient activation: Better health outcomes and care experiences; Fewer data on costs', Health Affairs, 32(2), pp. 207–214.

Hossain, M.S., Harvey, L.A., Rahman, M.A., Bowden, J.L., Islam, M.S., Taylor, V., Muldoon, S. and Herbert, R.D. (2017) 'A pilot randomised trial of community-based care following discharge from hospital with a recent spinal cord injury in Bangladesh', Clinical Rehabilitation, 31(6), pp. 781–789.

Kamwesiga, J.T., Eriksson, G.M., Tham, K., Fors, U., Ndiwalana, A., von Koch, L. and Guidetti, S. (2018) 'A feasibility study of a mobile phone supported family-centred ADL intervention, F@ce™, after stroke in Uganda', Globalization and Health, 14(1), p. 82.

Kayola, G., Mataa, M.M., Asukile, M., Chishimba, L., Chomba, M., Mortel, D., Nutakki, A., Zimba, S. and Saylor, D. (2023) 'Stroke rehabilitation in low-and middle-income countries: Challenges and opportunities', American Journal of Physical Medicine & Rehabilitation, 102(2S), pp. S24–S32.

Korotitsch, W.J. and Nelson-Gray, R.O. (1999) 'An overview of self-monitoring research in assessment and treatment', Psychological Assessment, 11(4), pp. 415–430.

Kruse, C., Betancourt, J., Ortiz, S., Luna, S.M.V., Bamrah, I.K. and Segovia, N. (2019) 'Barriers to the use of mobile health in improving health outcomes in developing countries: Systematic review', Journal of Medical Internet Research, 21(10), p. e13263.

Kusec, A., Velikonja, D., DeMatteo, C. and Harris, J.E. (2019) 'Motivation in rehabilitation and acquired brain injury: Can theory help us understand it?, Disability and Rehabilitation, 41(19), pp. 2343–2349.

Lindley, R.I., Anderson, C.S., Billot, L., Forster, A., Hackett, M.L., Harvey, L.A., Jan, S., Li, Q., Liu, H., Langhorne, P. and Maulik, P.K. (2017) 'Family-led rehabilitation after stroke in India (ATTEND): A randomised controlled trial', The Lancet, 390(10094), pp. 588–599.

Lorig, K.R. and Holman, H.R. (2003) 'Self-management education: history, definition, outcomes, and mechanisms', Annals of Behavioral Medicine, 26(1), pp. 1–7.

Martin, L.T., Schonlau, M., Haas, A., Derose, K.P., Rosenfeld, L., Buka, S.L. and Rudd, R. (2011) 'Patient activation and advocacy: Which literacy skills matter most?, Journal of Health Communication, 16(sup3), pp. 177–190.

Master ABA. (2024) Developing effective self-management skills in ABA programs: Strategies and techniques. Available at: https://masteraba.com/developing-effective-self-management-skills-in-aba-programs-strategies-and-techniques/ (Accessed: 15 September 2025).

Meherali, S., Punjani, N.S. and Mevawala, A. (2020) 'Health literacy interventions to improve health outcomes in low-and middle-income countries', HLRP: Health Literacy Research and Practice, 4(4), pp. e251–e266.

Moore, C., Gallagher, P. and Dunne, S. (2024) 'Health literacy, eHealth literacy and their association with burden, distress, and self-efficacy among cancer caregivers', Frontiers in Psychology, 15, p. 1283227.

Naderbagi, A., Loblay, V., Zahed, I.U.M., Ekambareshwar, M., Poulsen, A., Song, Y.J., Ospina-Pinillos, L., Krausz, M., Mamdouh Kamel, M., Hickie, I.B. and LaMonica, H.M. (2024) 'Cultural and contextual adaptation of digital health interventions: Narrative review', Journal of Medical Internet Research, 26, p. e55130.

Natta, D.D.N., Lejeune, T., Detrembleur, C., Yarou, B., Sogbossi, E.S., Alagnide, E., Kpadonou, T., Selves, C. and Stoquart, G. (2021) 'Effectiveness of a self-rehabilitation program to improve upper-extremity function after stroke in developing countries: A randomized controlled trial', Annals of Physical and Rehabilitation Medicine, 64(1), p. 101413.

Ng, W. (2012) 'Can we teach digital natives digital literacy?', Computers & Education, 59(3), pp. 1065–1078.

NHS England. (2024) Supported self-management. Available at: https://www.england.nhs.uk/personalised-care/supported-self-management/ (Accessed: 15 September 2025).

Nutbeam, D. (2000) 'Health literacy as a public health goal: A challenge for contemporary health education and communication strategies into the 21st century', Health Promotion International, 15(3), pp. 259–267.

O'Conor, R., Bonham, M., Magnuson, G., Opsasnick, L., Hurtado, J., Benavente, J.Y., Curtis, L.M. and Wolf, M.S. (2023) 'Caregiver health literacy and health task performance: Findings from the LitCog caregiver cohort study', PEC Innovation, 3, p. 100240.

Ohnmar, H.T.W.E., Yuliawiratman, B.S., Tannor, A.Y., Asikin, M.Z.N., Elaine, S.O.H., De Groote, W., Naicker, M.S. and Naicker, A.S. (2024) 'Barriers and facilitators for increased accessibility to quality rehabilitation services in low-and middle-income countries: A systematic review', European Journal of Physical and Rehabilitation Medicine, 60(3), p. 514.

Owolabi, M.O., Thrift, A.G., Mahal, A., Ishida, M., Martins, S., Johnson, W.D., Pandian, J., Abd-Allah, F., Yaria, J., Phan, H.T. and Roth, G. (2022) 'Primary stroke prevention worldwide: Translating evidence into action', The Lancet Public Health, 7(1), pp. e74–e85.

Parke, H.L., Epiphaniou, E., Pearce, G., Taylor, S.J., Sheikh, A., Griffiths, C.J., Greenhalgh, T. and Pinnock, H. (2015) 'Self-management support interventions for stroke survivors: A systematic meta-review', PloS One, 10(7), p. e0131448.

Pereira, G.M., Teixeira-dos-Santos, D., Soares, N.M., Marconi, G.A., Friedrich, D.C., Saffie Awad, P., Santos-Lobato, B.L., Brandão, P.R.P., Noyce, A.J., Marras, C. and Mata, I.F. (2024) 'A systematic review and meta-analysis of the prevalence of Parkinson's disease in lower to upper-middle-income countries', NPJ Parkinson's Disease, 10(1), p. 181.

Prvu Bettger, J., Liu, C., Gandhi, D.B., Sylaja, P.N., Jayaram, N. and Pandian, J.D. (2019) 'Emerging areas of stroke rehabilitation research in low-and middle-income countries: A scoping review', Stroke, 50(11), pp. 3307–3313.

Psychology Tools. (2024) Self-monitoring. Available at: https://www.psychologytools.com/professional/techniques/self-monitoring (Accessed: 15 September 2025).

Qureshi, Q.A., Shah, B., Kundi, G.M., Nawaz, A., Miankhel, A.K., Chishti, K.A. and Qureshi, N.A. (2013) 'Infrastructural barriers to e-health implementation in developing countries', European Journal of Sustainable Development, 2(1), pp. 163–170.

Rathore, F.A., Farooq, F., Muzammil, S., New, P.W., Ahmad, N. and Haig, A.J. (2008) 'Spinal cord injury management and rehabilitation: Highlights and shortcomings from the 2005 earthquake in Pakistan', Archives of Physical Medicine and Rehabilitation, 89(3), pp. 579–585.

Sangraula, M., Chauhan, J., Best, C., McEneaney, C., Shah, C., Brown, A.D. and Kohrt, B.A. (2024) 'The impact of task-sharing scalable mental health interventions on non-specialist providers: A scoping review', Cambridge Prisms: Global Mental Health, 11, p. e134.

Sarfo, F.S., Adusei, N., Ampofo, M., Kpeme, F.K. and Ovbiagele, B. (2018) 'Pilot trial of A tele-rehab intervention to improve outcomes after stroke in Ghana: A feasibility and user satisfaction study', Journal of the Neurological Sciences, 387, pp. 94–97.

Segura, E., Vilà-Balló, A., Mallorquí, A., Porto, M.F., Duarte, E., Grau-Sánchez, J. and Rodríguez-Fornells, A. (2024) 'The presence of Anhedonia in individuals with subacute and chronic stroke: An exploratory cohort study', Frontiers in Aging Neuroscience, 16, p. 1253028.

Soule, A.C., Fish, T.J., Winegardner, J. and Schrieff-Brown, L. (2024) 'Implementing neuropsychological rehabilitation following severe traumatic brain injury in a low-to-middle income country: A case report', Frontiers in Rehabilitation Sciences, 5, p. 1393302.

Spanhel, K., Balci, S., Feldhahn, F., Bengel, J., Baumeister, H. and Sander, L.B. (2021) 'Cultural adaptation of internet-and mobile-based interventions for mental disorders: A systematic review', NPJ Digital Medicine, 4(1), p. 128.

Stephani, V., Opoku, D. and Quentin, W. (2016) 'A systematic review of randomized controlled trials of mHealth interventions against non-communicable diseases in developing countries', BMC Public Health, 16(1), p. 572.

Taylor, S.J., Taylor, S., Pinnock, H., Epiphaniou, E., Pearce, G., Parke, H.L., Parke, H., Schwappach, A., Purushotham, N., Jacob, S. and Griffiths, C.J. (2014) 'A rapid synthesis of the evidence on interventions supporting self-management for people with long-term conditions (PRIMS practical systematic review of self-management support for long-term conditions)', Health and Social Care Delivery Research, 2(53), pp. 1–580.

Vos, T., Lim, S.S., Abbafati, C., Abbas, K.M., Abbasi, M., Abbasifard, M., Abbasi-Kangevari, M., Abbastabar, H., Abd-Allah, F., Abdelalim, A. and Abdollahi, M. (2020) 'Global burden of 369 diseases and injuries in 204 countries and territories, 1990–2019: A systematic analysis for the Global Burden of Disease Study 2019', The Lancet, 396(10258), pp. 1204–1222.

Wagner, E.H., Austin, B.T., Davis, C., Hindmarsh, M., Schaefer, J. and Bonomi, A. (2001) 'Improving chronic illness care: Translating evidence into action', Health Affairs, 20(6), pp. 64–78.

Woodward, A., Davies, N., Walters, K., Nimmons, D., Stevenson, F., Protheroe, J., Chew-Graham, C.A. and Armstrong, M. (2023) 'Self-management of multiple long-term conditions: A systematic review of the barriers and facilitators amongst people experiencing socioeconomic deprivation', PLoS One, 18(2), p. e0282036.

World Health Organization. (2021) Rehabilitation. Geneva: World Health Organization. Available at: https://www.who.int/news-room/fact-sheets/detail/rehabilitation (Accessed: 15 September 2025).

World Health Organization. (2023) Rehabilitation in health financing: Opportunities on the way to universal health coverage. Geneva: World Health Organization. ISBN 978-92-4-008182-6. Available at: https://iris.who.int/bitstream/handle/10665/375712/9789240081826-eng.pdf

Xu, X.Y., Leung, A.Y.M. and Chau, P.H. (2018) 'Health literacy, self-efficacy, and associated factors among patients with diabetes', HLRP: Health Literacy Research and Practice, 2(2), pp. e67–e77.

Yoshida, T., Otaka, Y., Osu, R., Kumagai, M., Kitamura, S. and Yaeda, J. (2021) 'Motivation for rehabilitation in patients with subacute stroke: A qualitative study', Frontiers in Rehabilitation Sciences, 2, p. 664758.

Zou, H., Liu, J., Jiang, D., Hou, L., Wang, W. and Zhang, L. (2024) 'The effect of health literacy on disease management self-efficacy in chronic disease patients: The mediating effects of social support and the moderating effects of illness perception', Patient Preference and Adherence, 18, pp. 657–666.

21 Participatory Approaches to Developing Self-Management Interventions

Ebuka Miracle Anieto, Ijeoma Blessing Anieto, and Israel Ikechukwu Adandom

INTRODUCTION

Self-management has emerged as a cornerstone of contemporary rehabilitation practice, reflecting a shift from paternalistic models of healthcare towards approaches that empower individuals to take an active role in managing their health and wellbeing. Defined as the tasks that individuals must undertake to live well with their conditions, self-management is especially important in long-term conditions where ongoing adaptation and behaviour change are critical (Velde *et al.*, 2019). Evidence from a systematic review demonstrates that effective self-management interventions can improve clinical outcomes, enhance quality of life, and reduce healthcare utilization across a wide range of conditions such as diabetes, cardiovascular disease, respiratory, and mental health issues (Panagioti *et al.*, 2014).

Despite these benefits, the impact of many self-management interventions is limited by poor adherence and uptake, or lack of sustainability when implemented in real-world contexts (Roberts *et al.*, 2012; Subedi *et al.*, 2020). One key explanation is that interventions are often designed using top-down approaches that inadequately reflect the lived experiences, values, and contexts of the people they are intended to support (Greenhalgh *et al.*, 2016). Hence, there is an increasing awareness that interventions must not only be evidence-based, but also experience-based, developed in genuine partnership with patients, carers, clinicians, and other stakeholders (Greenhalgh *et al.*, 2016; Slattery, Saeri and Bragge, 2020).

Participatory approaches, including community-based participatory research, participatory action research, co-design, co-production, and co-creation, have therefore gained prominence in health research and rehabilitation. These methodologies (especially co-creation) seek to democratize the research process, ensuring that stakeholders are actively engaged across all stages of intervention development, from identifying priorities to designing, testing, and implementing solutions (Pearce *et al.*, 2020). By fostering collaboration, ownership, and contextual relevance, participatory approaches hold promise in addressing longstanding challenges in self-management research and practice (Jagosh *et al.*, 2012). This chapter explores these approaches, with a particular focus on co-creation as a strategy for developing effective, acceptable, and sustainable self-management interventions in rehabilitation.

THE CONCEPT OF PARTICIPATION IN HEALTH INTERVENTION DEVELOPMENT

Participation in the design and implementation of health interventions has become a fundamental element of contemporary rehabilitation science, embodying both a philosophical commitment to patient-centred care and a practical strategy for enhancing intervention effectiveness (Greenhalgh *et al.*, 2016). Evidence demonstrates that the meaningful involvement of patients and stakeholders

DOI: 10.1201/9781003599074-24

increases contextual relevance and facilitates uptake across healthcare and community settings, thereby accelerating translation into practice (Esmail, Moore and Rein, 2015; Gröne, 2022). Nevertheless, the terminology surrounding participation remains contested. Terms such as *involvement, engagement,* and *empowerment* are often employed interchangeably, obscuring important conceptual distinctions (Hickmann, Richter and Schlieter, 2022). Recent analyses suggest these terms are not isolated or unrelated concepts, but are rather stages of a progression: *involvement* is generally restricted to information exchange, *engagement* entails active contribution to decision-making, and *empowerment* signifies shared authority whereby patients and stakeholders directly shape priorities, processes, and outcomes (Bergerum *et al.*, 2019; Ocloo and Matthews, 2016). Conceptualizing participation in this way highlights the need to progress beyond tokenistic consultation toward authentic co-creation in healthcare innovation.

Some frameworks have been developed to classify and operationalize varying degrees of stakeholder engagement. Arnstein's *Ladder of Citizen Participation* offered an early hierarchical model, ranging from non-participation to citizen control, which continues to inform assessments of patient and public involvement (PPI) (Arnstein, 1969). Expanding this perspective, the International Association for Public Participation (IAP2) introduced the *Spectrum of Public Participation,* comprising five progressive levels: informing, consulting, involving, collaborating, and empowering (International Association for Public Participation, 2018). By situating stakeholders along this spectrum, healthcare professionals and researchers can adopt structured, context-sensitive approaches to engagement, ensuring that participation transcends symbolic gestures and meaningfully contributes to decision-making, service design, and knowledge co-creation (Ocloo and Matthews, 2016).

The rationale for participation is further reinforced by its philosophical underpinnings, which reveal why it has gained prominence within rehabilitation science. Three traditions are particularly influential. First, **constructivism** asserts that knowledge is socially constructed through lived experience, positioning participatory methods such as action research as vital for incorporating patient perspectives into knowledge generation (Thomas *et al.*, 2024; Vaughn and Jacquez, 2020). Second, **user-centred design (UCD)**, originating in engineering and human-computer interaction, emphasizes iterative collaboration to ensure rehabilitation technologies and practices align with users' routines, accessibility needs, and cultural expectations (Hardy *et al.*, 2018; Ortiz-Escobar *et al.*, 2023). Finally, the **democratization of healthcare** situates participation within broader policy movements toward shared decision-making, reflecting a normative commitment that healthcare interventions should be developed *with*, not merely *for*, those they are intended to serve (Maleševic´ and Čartolovni, 2025; Singh, 2022).

Together, these conceptual, practical, and philosophical perspectives underscore the profound implications of participation for rehabilitation science. Active patient involvement, particularly in collaborative goal-setting, has been shown to enhance functional outcomes and improve goal attainment (Sagen *et al.*, 2024). Similarly, co-design and co-production strategies foster engagement and generate interventions that are more relevant, acceptable, and sustainable (Brotherdale *et al.*, 2024). Beyond improving effectiveness, participatory approaches cultivate ownership and empowerment, aligning rehabilitation practices more closely with patients' lived realities. Consequently, embedding participatory methodologies within rehabilitation science is not only a methodological advancement but also an ethical imperative, ensuring that the field remains responsive, inclusive, and patient-centred as it continues to evolve.

RATIONALE FOR PARTICIPATORY APPROACHES IN SELF-MANAGEMENT

Traditional rehabilitation models often follow a top-down approach, where clinical experts define problems, design solutions, and deliver them to patients. While scientifically rigorous, these models frequently fail to support long-term behaviour change or real-world adoption. For instance,

Wen *et al.* (2025) found that although digital health tools for stroke rehabilitation achieved positive trial results, long-term engagement declined due to poor alignment with patients' daily contexts. Participatory approaches offer an alternative by embedding patient voices into the design process. Lynch *et al.* (2024) used Experience-Based Co-Design with stroke survivors and clinicians to develop implementation strategies, finding the process both feasible and empowering. Similarly, Wittink *et al.* (2024) co-designed a walking intervention for stroke survivors that integrated patient context and embedded behaviour change techniques, supporting more sustained use.

Involving users throughout intervention development yields multiple benefits including relevance, acceptability, adherence, equity and empowerment, and sustainability of interventions (Chao *et al.*, 2023; Domecq *et al.*, 2014; Federman *et al.*, 2024; Murray *et al.*, 2015; Ocloo and Matthews, 2016). In chronic disease management, participatory methods have demonstrated consistent benefits. Studies have reported that co-created interventions lead to improvement in health outcomes in multiple patient populations including patients with diabetes, COPD, peripheral arterial disease, stroke, and mental health conditions (Anieto *et al.*, 2025a; Wiesmüller *et al.*, 2025).

Despite their strengths, participatory methods face challenges. In high-acuity or highly technical settings, such as acute neurorehabilitation, intensive participation may be less feasible. Additional barriers include resource demands, representational bias, and institutional resistance (Davies, Arana-Catania and Procter, 2022; Gilfoyle, 2025). Scaling participatory approaches also require careful planning and ongoing reflexivity to ensure inclusivity (Zahlsen, Parmiggiani and Dahl, 2023). Nonetheless, participatory approaches offer a vital pathway to more equitable, effective, and sustainable interventions, particularly for self-managed chronic conditions where patient agency and lived experience are central.

METHODOLOGIES FOR PARTICIPATORY INTERVENTION DEVELOPMENT

Among the array of participatory methods available there are several 'co-' approaches such as co-design, co-production, and co-creation, which have been historically used for intervention development. These terms are often erroneously used interchangeably in literature; however, each offers varying degrees of stakeholder involvement, timing, and purpose. Furthermore, many 'co-' approaches fail to reflect the values of equal participation and practical benefit that define genuine co-research, leading to a confusing mix of terms and methods starting with 'co-', which Williams *et al.* (2020) described as 'cobiquities'. Recent studies have provided clarifications on the conceptual distinctions between the terms co-design, co-production, and co-creation (Grindell *et al.*, 2022; Vargas *et al.*, 2022).

Co-design involves working closely with various stakeholders to develop solutions for a pre-identified issue (Vargas *et al.*, 2022). It encourages public involvement in addressing or enhancing particular challenges, such as improving services or products, strengthening prevention efforts, increasing available resources, enhancing staff training in health promotion, and creating initiatives based on evidence (Guía, Cazorla and de-Miguel-Molina, 2017). Co-design approaches prioritize end-user input in shaping specific components, often resulting in user-friendly, tailored tools or services (Guía, Cazorla and de-Miguel-Molina, 2017). However, its application is mainly at the design, implementation and evaluation phase, with limited involvement of stakeholders in the earlier framing of the problem (Vargas *et al.*, 2022).

Co-production, on the other hand, centres on collaborative delivery problems (Vargas *et al.*, 2022). It focuses on sharing responsibility and resources in implementing pre-designed solutions but does not typically involve stakeholders in the ideation, development or refinement stages (Etgar, 2008; Guía, Cazorla and de-Miguel-Molina, 2017). Co-production is distinct from co-design and co-creation in that its aim is to enhance an existing service/intervention that can be refined (Vargas *et al.*, 2022).

Co-creation distinguishes itself through its holistic, end-to-end collaboration with stakeholders (Voorberg, Bekkers and Tummers, 2015). Unlike co-design or co-production, which focus on discrete stages, co-creation involves community members, practitioners, researchers, and policymakers throughout the entire process, from identifying the problem to developing, implementing, and evaluating solutions (Vargas *et al.*, 2022). The key critical difference between co-creation, co-design, and co-production lies in how much and when stakeholders are involved in the process (Vargas *et al.*, 2022). The extensive collaborative nature of co-creation helps to build trust, mutual learning, and a sense of ownership among stakeholders. This is crucial not only for the intervention's relevance but also for its sustainability. Co-creation facilitates iterative learning, real-time adaptation, and collective decision-making, critical features for any intervention hoping to operate effectively in dynamic, real-world conditions (Vargas *et al.*, 2022). It ensures that interventions are not imposed on communities but developed with them, increasing both feasibility and legitimacy. This makes co-creation especially well-suited to self-management interventions in rehabilitation, where both patient engagement and theoretical robustness are essential.

Co-creation is not without challenges. It requires considerable facilitation skills, resources, and institutional support to maintain genuine participation, and risks superficial engagement if stakeholders are not empowered as equal partners. Yet, when implemented systematically and transparently, co-creation offers a comprehensive approach that balances scientific rigour with experiential insight, ultimately increasing intervention acceptability, adherence, and sustainability (Agnello *et al.*, 2025).

FRAMEWORKS FOR IMPLEMENTING PARTICIPATORY APPROACHES

While participatory methodologies provide philosophical and methodological guidance, frameworks are required to structure and operationalize these approaches in the context of complex health intervention development. Frameworks help ensure transparency, replicability, and theoretical alignment, while supporting meaningful stakeholder involvement. Among the most prominent frameworks relevant to participatory intervention development are the Medical Research Council (MRC) framework for complex interventions, the Behaviour Change Wheel (BCW) Framework for intervention development, and the more recently proposed Problem, Objective, Design, User, Co-creators, Evaluation, and Scalability (PRODUCES) framework.

The MRC framework is widely recognized as the gold standard for developing and evaluating complex interventions in health (Skivington *et al.*, 2021, 2024). It provides a four phased structure to guide intervention development process comprising: development (identifying evidence and theory), feasibility/piloting, evaluation, and implementation (Skivington *et al.*, 2021). The revised framework emphasizes iterative processes, systems perspectives, and stakeholder involvement (Skivington *et al.*, 2024). Its strength lies in promoting theoretical rigour and systematic evaluation. However, while it acknowledges the importance of patient and public involvement (PPI), it does not prescribe specific strategies for embedding participatory practices. As such, researchers may struggle to integrate stakeholder input consistently across phases, resulting in varying depth of engagement.

The BCW framework for intervention development provides a systematic, theory-driven approach to developing behaviour change interventions, consisting of three stages and eight steps (Michie, Atkins and West, 2014).

- **Stage 1 (Understanding the Behaviour):** involves defining the problem (Step 1), selecting the target behaviour (Step 2), specifying the behaviour (Step 3), and understanding what needs to change (Step 4).

- **Stage 2 (Identifying Intervention Options):** involves identifying intervention functions (Step 5) and identifying relevant policy categories (Step 6).
- **Stage 3 (Identifying Content and Implementation Options):** involves selecting behaviour change techniques (BCTs) that can address the problem (Step 7) and determining mode of intervention delivery (Step 8).

This staged process ensures interventions are not only theoretically sound but also practically targeted to the barriers and facilitators of a target behaviour (Michie, Atkins and West, 2014). The BCW framework has been widely applied across health domains, including physical activity, smoking cessation, and diet change, and is increasingly combined with participatory approaches where stakeholders contribute to defining target behaviours and identifying feasible intervention techniques (Michie, Atkins and West, 2014). Critically, while the BCW provides strong guidance for behaviourally informed intervention content, it is less explicit about how to manage stakeholder involvement and co-creation processes. As such, it is often combined with participatory frameworks (such as PRODUCES) to balance scientific rigour with inclusive design.

The PRODUCES framework addresses the gap between participatory principles and practical guidance for developing complex health interventions (Leask *et al.*, 2019). Unlike the MRC and BCW frameworks, PRODUCES explicitly integrates participatory processes with structured intervention development. It ensures that stakeholder engagement is not tokenistic but embedded throughout, from defining the problem to planning for long-term sustainability. Moreover, PRODUCES complements behaviour change frameworks like BCW by providing a participatory scaffold within which behavioural diagnosis and intervention specification can be collaboratively achieved (Leask *et al.*, 2019). See Table 21.1 for a description of the components of the Framework.

The three frameworks each offer unique strengths. The MRC framework ensures methodological credibility and is widely accepted by funders and policymakers, but is less explicit on participatory processes. The BCW framework is invaluable for translating theory into specific intervention content, but without an emphasis on participatory approach risks producing interventions misaligned with user contexts. The PRODUCES framework directly addresses this gap by explicitly structuring co-creation, ensuring that interventions are problem-focused, user-centred, and sustainable. Its limitation is that it is relatively new, with fewer empirical applications compared to MRC or BCW. However, when combined, PRODUCES and BCW offer a powerful synergy: PRODUCES provides the participatory 'how', while BCW provides the behavioural 'what', all within the evaluative rigour of the MRC framework.

TABLE 21.1
Components of the PRODUCES Framework[a]

PR	**Pr**oblem	What is the rationale for the process?
O	**O**bjective	What is the aim of the process?
D	**D**esign	What specific participatory methodology is used for co-creation?
U	(End-) **U**ser	Who will use the co-created intervention?
C	**C**o-creators	Who is engaging in the process?
E	**E**valuation	How is success measured?
S	**S**calability	How can the solution be scaled to a population level?

[a] Table adapted from (Leask *et al.*, 2019).

ENSURING RIGOUR AND TRUSTWORTHINESS IN PARTICIPATORY RESEARCH

Participatory approaches in intervention development are adaptive, iterative, and embedded in community realities, which strengthens contextual relevance but complicates conventional markers of rigour. To preserve scientific integrity without erasing community voice, four pillars are essential: credibility, dependability, confirmability, and transferability (Belone *et al.*, 2016; Lincoln and Guba, 1985).

Credibility

Credibility improves when stakeholders shape the study from agenda setting to dissemination. Member checking, peer debriefing, and triangulation ensure that interpretations align with lived experience rather than researcher expectations (Israel *et al.*, 2001). Mixed-method triangulation, pairing qualitative accounts with clinical or behavioural outcomes, bolsters evidential weight. Co-creation projects in physiotherapy education in the United Kingdom (UK) have demonstrated that inclusivity in curriculum designs builds credibility and relevance (Dairo *et al.*, 2025). Youth participatory action research (YPAR) shows that credibility is also social: sustained engagement cultivates agency and leadership among participants, and projects that channel youth priorities tend to yield actions that communities recognize as valid (Anyon *et al.*, 2018).

Dependability

Dependability requires transparent documentation of decision points as partnerships evolve. Audit trails, meeting logs, and reflexive journals allow others to trace how evidence prompted adaptations. Doctoral-led participatory projects reveal the strain of balancing institutional milestones with authentic partnership rhythms, making systematic documentation indispensable for accountability (Lambley, 2025). In work with children and adolescents, sustained participation often wanes during analysis or dissemination, signalling the need to plan role continuity and training in advance (Freire *et al.*, 2022).

Confirmability

Confirmability emphasizes that findings are grounded in participant perspectives, not researcher bias. Reflexive positionality statements, collaborative analysis sessions, and explicit attention to power are core practices. Community-based participatory research (CBPR) with sexual and gender minority communities shows that reflexivity is vital for navigating divergent priorities while protecting cultural relevance (Ricks *et al.*, 2022). Trust is both mechanism and outcome; its conceptualization and measurement should be specified a priori and revisited during the project lifecycle (Gilfoyle, MacFarlane and Salsberg, 2022; Jagosh *et al.*, 2015)

Transferability

Thick description of context and process enables others to judge applicability across settings. In low- and middle-income countries, participatory programs such as Health Workers for Change demonstrate how locally led problem-solving produces context-fit improvements with portable principles (Olude *et al.*, 2023). In professional education, co-creation of racial-inclusivity resources shows how participatory methods can surface situated inequities while generating models that inform wider practice (Dairo *et al.*, 2025).

Quality Appraisal Tool for Participatory Research

While there is no widely recognized quality appraisal tool for assessing the rigour of participatory research process, the Adapted Checklist for Reporting Intervention Co-creation (A-CRIC) tool offer a starting point for quality appraisal (Anieto *et al.*, 2023). The tool was designed for assessing the reporting quality of intervention co-creation studies. It is intended to evaluate how well studies conduct and describe co-creation processes, rather than focusing on outcomes alone (Anieto *et al.*, 2023). The checklist is divided into three main domains: Planning of the intervention co-creation project, Conducting of the intervention co-creation project, and Evaluation of the co-creation project. The tool contains a total of 22 specific items spread across the three domains. Examples include whether the study clearly describes its sampling procedure, setting, characteristics of co-creators, facilitators; whether the iterative nature of co-creation is detailed; whether prototyping is described; whether co-creators' experiences are evaluated; and whether plans for testing scalability or effectiveness are presented (Anieto *et al.*, 2023).

Studies assessed using the A-CRIC tool are given a score out of 22. Based on the score, reporting quality is categorized as: Low (< 7 items satisfied), Moderate (7–14), High (15–22) (Anieto *et al.*, 2023). The tool helps in evaluating process transparency, which is important for understanding which components of co-creation contribute to effectiveness, replicability, and scalability. It also supports systematic reviews and researchers to compare and synthesize co-creation studies more fairly, considering not only outcomes but how well the development process has been described. Furthermore, it encourages better reporting in future co-creation studies, which in turn enhances trustworthiness, replicability, and usefulness of the interventions developed (Anieto *et al.*, 2023).

BARRIERS AND CHALLENGES IN PARTICIPATORY APPROACHES

Tokenism and Power Asymmetries

Superficial involvement remains common: participants are consulted but excluded from agenda control or analysis. Reviews of participatory projects with children/adolescents document invitation fatigue, proceduralism, and limited downstream influence (Freire *et al.*, 2022). Doctoral researchers report structural pressures (timelines, authorship conventions) that re-centralize academic authority (Lambley, 2025).

Resource Intensity and Sustainability

Co-creation workshops, iterative testing, and stakeholder training demand time and financing that are frequently underestimated (Olude *et al.*, 2023). Misalignment between funding cycles and community rhythms lead to premature closure or diluted outputs (Minkler *et al.*, 2003).

Conflicting Priorities and Outcome Definitions

Patients, clinicians, and policymakers often value different outcomes (e.g., quality-of-life vs. throughput). Evidence from a systematic review of co-created lifestyle interventions highlights the need for negotiated outcome sets and staged decision rules (Anieto *et al.*, 2025a). Without such scaffolding, consensus defaults to the most powerful actors (Volkmann, Dresel and Jochems, 2023).

Ethical Complexities

Participatory work intensifies obligations around ongoing consent, data stewardship, and recognition. Inadequate remuneration and lack of authorship pathways reproduce extractive dynamics (Ricks *et al.*, 2022). Where histories of medical mistrust exist, failure to address structural harm jeopardizes engagement (Gilfoyle, MacFarlane and Salsberg, 2022).

Structural Constraints in Clinical Practice

European health systems are facing acute workforce shortages, with more than 20 EU countries reporting deficits of doctors and nurses in 2022–2023, alongside an estimated shortfall of 1.2 million health professionals across the region (Gholipour *et al.*, 2023; OECD, 2024). These constraints are driven by an ageing workforce, high retirement rates, and declining interest among younger people in health careers. Such shortages restrict the scope for participatory practice by limiting the time and specialist capacity needed for co-creation with patients. Similar constraints have been documented in Nigeria, where fracture rehabilitation settings face scarce specialists, reliance on subjective judgements, and financial obstacles that limit referrals (Adandom *et al.*, 2020). Together, these contexts illustrate how workforce and resource pressures shape the practical realities of participatory health research and practice.

Cultural and Literacy Challenges

Efforts to broaden participation in the UK and Europe frequently contend with cultural diversity and varying levels of health literacy, particularly among migrant and older populations (Gogoi *et al.*, 2025). Approaches such as plain-language communication, culturally adapted materials, and community partnerships are used to support inclusion. Comparable challenges appear in Nigeria, where physical literacy among older adults is shaped by beliefs, communication norms, and access barriers (Adandom *et al.*, 2025a). Additionally, personality traits and health behaviours linked to fall risk highlight the need for contextually sensitive participatory designs (Adandom *et al.*, 2025b).

FACILITATORS OF SUCCESSFUL PARTICIPATORY INTERVENTION DEVELOPMENT

Trust and Relationship Infrastructure

Trust underpins recruitment, disclosure, and adherence. Scoping evidence recommends making trust an explicit construct with indicators for transparency, reciprocity, and reliability, monitored across the project lifecycle (Gilfoyle, MacFarlane and Salsberg, 2022).

Clear, Accessible Communication

Visual storyboards, journey maps, and plain-language summaries widen participation and enhance shared understanding (Freire *et al.*, 2022). In clinical teams, iterative two-level communication (provider-provider; provider-patient/family) supported timely identification and management of psychosocial and cognitive (PSC) issues (Adandom *et al.*, 2020).

Institutional Backing and Policy Alignment

Endorsement by health systems, universities, and funders legitimizes participatory work, stabilizes resourcing, and embeds dissemination pathways to practice (Olude *et al.*, 2023).

Capacity Building for All Partners

Training community members in inquiry methods and researchers in facilitation and cultural humility reduces power asymmetries. For instance, rehabilitation exemplar suggests targeted upskilling to administer and interpret brief cognitive screens within routine workflows (Adandom *et al.*, 2020). In education settings, co-creation around racial inclusivity required facilitation competencies and safe-space protocols (Dairo *et al.*, 2025).

Iterative Feedback Loops and Visible Influence

Showing when and how stakeholder input changes designs fosters ownership, adherence, and sustained participation. Meta-analytic evidence indicates that co-created lifestyle interventions can improve health behaviours and mental health among adults with non-communicable diseases, particularly when participants can see their fingerprints on intervention content (Anieto *et al.*, 2025a).

Context-Attuned Design Logics

Integrating physical literacy considerations (language, cultural meanings, access to safe spaces) into co-design improves fit for older adults' immigrants (Gogoi *et al.*, 2025). Personality-informed tailoring (e.g., aligning messaging with conscientiousness or neuroticism profiles) may enhance adoption of fall-prevention behaviours (Adandom *et al.*, 2025).

CASE EXAMPLES OF PARTICIPATORY APPROACHES IN SELF-MANAGEMENT

Participatory approaches to self-management intervention development have been applied across a range of long-term conditions, yielding valuable lessons about the benefits and challenges of co-creation. The following case examples drawn from diabetes, stroke, and peripheral arterial disease (PAD) with claudication, illustrate both the diversity of contexts and the consistent value of stakeholder engagement.

Diabetes

In diabetes care, participatory design has been used to build digital self-management tools that leverage patients' social networks and lived experience. For example, the Diabetes Networking Tool (DNT) was developed using participatory design with low-income, minority communities to ensure the app addressed local support needs and usability barriers (Zachary *et al.*, 2017). More recently, co-design work has produced digital dietary interventions for adults at risk of type 2 diabetes where users shaped content, language and functionality; these studies report improved perceived usability and stronger alignment with users' daily routines compared with top-down designs (Tay *et al.*, 2021; Zachary *et al.*, 2017).

Stroke

Stroke rehabilitation presents unique challenges for self-management, particularly with motor recovery and long-term adherence to exercise. Stroke research has applied participatory approaches to develop self-management interventions for people with communication impairment and during inpatient rehabilitation. Wray *et al.* (2021) combined co-production with behaviour-change theory to create a supported self-management intervention for stroke survivors with aphasia; the process produced accessible prototypes and clear links between user-identified needs and intervention components. Likewise, inpatient co-creation work identified concrete, implementable solutions (peer support, early family meetings, environmental adaptations) to start self-management support during hospital stays (Dobe *et al.*, 2023). These studies illustrate how participatory approaches can surface system-level changes as well as individual materials.

Peripheral Arterial Disease and Claudication

The project that led to the development of the 'Living Well with PAD' intervention prototype exemplifies co-creation applied to a traditionally underserved group (Anieto, 2025b). Through iterative workshops, patients with claudication and healthcare professionals jointly identified barriers to physical activity in individuals with claudication. Through co-creation, an intervention prototype comprising a digital hub and printable resources providing tailored physical activity guidance, motivational support, and peer interaction was developed (Anieto., 2025b). Patients valued the sense of ownership and clinicians reported that the process deepened their understanding of patient priorities. A key lesson from this case example is that co-creation can bridge the gap between guideline recommendations and patient realities, producing interventions that are both evidence-informed and acceptable (Anieto, 2025b).

Across conditions, the common takeaways are that participatory methods increase acceptability and context fit, expose system barriers early, and produce prototypes that stakeholders are more likely to adopt, but they also require explicit theory linkage and formal evaluation to move from prototypes to sustained, scalable programmes.

EVALUATING PARTICIPATORY SELF-MANAGEMENT INTERVENTION DEVELOPMENT

Evaluation is a critical stage in participatory intervention development, ensuring that interventions are not only co-created but also effective, acceptable, and sustainable in real-world rehabilitation contexts. Unlike traditional top-down programmes, participatory interventions require evaluation approaches that capture both outcomes and processes, recognizing that the 'how' of development is as important as the 'what' of delivery (Skivington *et al.*, 2024). The recently designed PROcesS Evaluation framework for CO-creation (PROSECO) framework offers practical guidance on how to conduct process and outcome evaluation of co-creation process (Longworth *et al.*, 2025).

Process Evaluation

Process evaluation is essential to understand fidelity, reach, dose, and the quality of implementation. For participatory interventions, process measures should capture the depth and quality of stakeholder involvement. During the design of the 'Living Well with PAD' intervention, for example, process evaluation involved documenting workshop participation, monitoring adaptations made in response to feedback, and assessing whether co-creators perceived their contributions as meaningfully integrated (Anieto, 2025b). Tools such as participation logs, reflexive field notes, and post-workshop surveys can provide rich insights into how interventions evolve during co-creation (Moore *et al.*, 2015).

Outcome Evaluation

Outcome evaluation remains central to demonstrating effectiveness. For self-management interventions, outcomes may include clinical measures (e.g., walking distance in PAD, HbA1c in diabetes), behavioural indicators (e.g., adherence to walking or exercise plans), and patient-reported outcomes such as quality of life, self-efficacy, and empowerment. However, because participatory interventions are often context-specific, outcome measures should be co-selected with stakeholders to ensure they reflect patient priorities as well as clinical relevance (Longworth *et al.*, 2025). During the design of the 'Living Well with PAD' intervention, for example, co-creators highlighted functional mobility and psychological wellbeing as outcomes of equal importance to traditional walking performance metrics (Anieto, 2025b).

Sustainability and Scalability Evaluation

Sustainability is a frequent weakness in self-management interventions. Participatory approaches can mitigate this by embedding scalability considerations into evaluation. The PRODUCES framework explicitly includes scalability as a stage, prompting early discussion of how interventions can be adapted across settings (Leask *et al.*, 2019). Evaluation strategies may therefore examine not just whether an intervention works, but how it can be delivered within existing service structures, with acceptable resource requirements, and in a way that addresses health inequities (Leask *et al.*, 2019).

CONCLUSION

Participatory approaches have transformed how self-management interventions are developed in rehabilitation, moving from top-down models to inclusive, collaborative designs that embed the perspectives of patients, carers, clinicians, and researchers. Across diverse conditions including diabetes, stroke, and peripheral arterial disease, it has been consistently demonstrated that the use of participatory approaches may produce interventions that are more acceptable, relevant, and sustainable. It has been established that participatory approaches (especially co-creation) foster ownership, enhance adherence, and increase the likelihood of real-world impact (Anieto *et al.*, 2025a).

Frameworks provide the structure to embed these methods rigorously. The MRC framework ensures methodological legitimacy, while the Behaviour Change Wheel offers precision in specifying behavioural targets and techniques. The PRODUCES framework adds a unique layer by explicitly structuring stakeholder involvement at every stage, from defining the problem to planning for scalability. Together, these frameworks ensure that co-created interventions are both theoretically sound and contextually grounded.

Ultimately, this chapter underscores that self-management interventions cannot succeed without addressing the lived realities of the people they serve. Co-creation offers a practical and evidence-based pathway to develop interventions that are not only effective in controlled trials but also sustainable in everyday rehabilitation practice.

REFERENCES

Adandom, I. *et al.* (2025a) “Physical literacy among older adults: How feasible is this in the Nigerian context? A qualitative exploration of the concept among physiotherapists,” *Physical Education and Sport Pedagogy*, pp. 1–20. Available at: https://doi.org/10.1080/17408989.2025.2536692.

Adandom, H.C. *et al.* (2025b) “Personality traits and health behaviors as predictors of fall among community-dwelling older adults: Findings from the Canadian longitudinal study on aging,” *Journal of Applied Gerontology*, p. 07334648251328427. Available at: https://doi.org/10.1177/07334648251328427.

Adandom, I.I. *et al.* (2020) “Managing psycho-social-cognitive factors during Hip/knee fracture rehabilitation for older adults: Clinicians’ experiences,” *Nigerian Hospital Practice*, 26(1–2), pp. 23–32.

Agnello, D.M., Anand-Kumar, V., An, Q., de Boer, J., Delfmann, L.R., Longworth, G.R., Loisel, Q., McCaffrey, L., Steiner, A. and Chastin, S., 2025. Co-creation methods for public health research—characteristics, benefits, and challenges: a Health CASCADE scoping review. *BMC Medical Research Methodology*, *25*(1), p.60.

Anieto, E.M. (2025b). Co-*creation of an intervention to increase physical activity in individuals with peripheral arterial disease and intermittent claudication* [Doctor of Philosophy (PhD) thesis]. Glasgow Caledonian University. Available at: https://doi.org/10.59019/WJYQ8412.

Anieto, E.M. *et al.* (2023) “Cocreators’ experiences and effectiveness of cocreated interventions in improving health behaviours of adults with non-communicable diseases: A systematic review protocol,” *BMJ Open*, 13(10), p. e073153. Available at: https://doi.org/10.1136/bmjopen-2023-073153.

Anieto, E.M., Dall, P.M., *et al.* (2025a) “The effectiveness of co-created lifestyle interventions in improving health behaviour, physical and mental health in adults with non-communicable diseases: A systematic review with meta-analysis,” *Public Health*, 248, p. 105929. Available at: https://doi.org/10.1016/j.puhe.2025.105929.

Anyon, Y. *et al.* (2018) “A systematic review of youth participatory action research (YPAR) in the United States: Methodologies, youth outcomes, and future directions,” *Health Education & Behavior*, 45(6), pp. 865–878. Available at: https://doi.org/10.1177/1090198118769357.

Arnstein, S.R. (1969) “A ladder of citizen participation,” *Journal of the American Institute of Planners*, 35(4), pp. 216–224. Available at: https://doi.org/10.1080/01944366908977225.

Belone, L. *et al.* (2016) "Community-based participatory research conceptual model: Community partner consultation and face validity," *Qualitative Health Research*, 26(1), pp. 117–135. Available at: https://doi.org/10.1177/1049732314557084.

Bergerum, C. *et al.* (2019) "How might patient involvement in healthcare quality improvement efforts work – A realist literature review," *Health Expectations: An International Journal of Public Participation in Health Care and Health Policy*, 22(5), pp. 952–964. Available at: https://doi.org/10.1111/hex.12900.

Brotherdale, R. *et al.* (2024) "Co-producing digital mental health interventions: A systematic review," *Digital Health*, 10, p. 20552076241239172. Available at: https://doi.org/10.1177/20552076241239172.

Chao, E.C. *et al.* (2023) "Collaboratively designing an app for a more personalized, community-endorsed continuous glucose monitoring onboarding experience: An early study," *Journal of Diabetes Science and Technology*, 18(1), pp. 14–21. Available at: https://doi.org/10.1177/19322968231213654.

Dairo, Y. *et al.* (2025) "Co-creation methodology for developing a racial inclusivity training resource in physiotherapy education," *Health Expectations*, 28(4), p. e70363. Available at: https://doi.org/10.1111/hex.70363.

Davies, J., Arana-Catania, M. and Procter, R. (2022) *Embedding Digital Participatory Budgeting Within Local Government: Motivations, Strategies and Barriers Faced*, in Proceedings of the 15th International Conference on Theory and Practice of Electronic Governance (ICEGOV '22). New York, NY, USA: Association for Computing Machinery (ACM), p. 104. Available at: https://doi.org/10.1145/3560107.3560124.

Dobe, J. *et al.* (2023) "Co-creation of self-management support during inpatient stroke rehabilitation," *PEC Innovation*, 3, p. 100191. Available at: https://doi.org/10.1016/j.pecinn.2023.100191.

Domecq, J.P. *et al.* (2014) "Patient engagement in research: A systematic review," *BMC Health Services Research*, 14(1), p. 89. Available at: https://doi.org/10.1186/1472-6963-14-89.

Esmail, L., Moore, E. and Rein, A. (2015) "Evaluating patient and stakeholder engagement in research: Moving from theory to practice," *Journal of Comparative Effectiveness Research*, 4(2), pp. 133–145. Available at: https://doi.org/10.2217/cer.14.79.

Etgar, M. (2008) "A descriptive model of the consumer co-production process," *Journal of the Academy of Marketing Science*, 36(1), pp. 97–108. Available at: https://doi.org/10.1007/s11747-007-0061-1.

Federman, A.D. *et al.* (2024) "Feasibility trial of a comprehensive, highly patient-centered COPD self-management support program," *Chronic Obstructive Pulmonary Diseases (Miami, Fla.)*, 11(1), pp. 13–25. Available at: https://doi.org/10.15326/jcopdf.2023.0419.

Freire, K. *et al.* (2022) "Engaging with children and adolescents: A systematic review of participatory methods and approaches in research informing the development of health resources and interventions," *Adolescent Research Review*, 7(3), pp. 335–354. Available at: https://doi.org/10.1007/s40894-022-00181-w.

Gholipour, K. *et al.* (2023) "Barriers to community participation in primary health care of district health: A qualitative study," *BMC Primary Care*, 24(1), p. 117. Available at: https://doi.org/10.1186/s12875-023-02062-0.

Gilfoyle, M. (2025) "A square peg in a round hole: Reflecting on using a participatory health research approach during my PhD," *Educational Action Research*, 33(1), pp. 172–182. Available at: https://doi.org/10.1080/09650792.2024.2325058.

Gilfoyle, M., MacFarlane, A. and Salsberg, J. (2022) "Conceptualising, operationalising, and measuring trust in participatory health research networks: A scoping review," *Systematic Reviews*, 11(1), p. 40. Available at: https://doi.org/10.1186/s13643-022-01910-x.

Gogoi, M. *et al.* (2025) "Migrants living in the United Kingdom and their perceptions of participation in health research: A mixed-methods study," *Health Expectations : An International Journal of Public Participation in Health Care and Health Policy*, 28(4), p. e70337. Available at: https://doi.org/10.1111/hex.70337.

Greenhalgh, T. *et al.* (2016) "Achieving research impact through co-creation in community-based health services: Literature review and case study," *The Milbank Quarterly*, 94(2), pp. 392–429. Available at: https://doi.org/10.1111/1468-0009.12197.

Grindell, C. *et al.* (2022) "The use of co-production, co-design and co-creation to mobilise knowledge in the management of health conditions: A systematic review," *BMC Health Services Research*, 22(1), p. 877. Available at: https://doi.org/10.1186/s12913-022-08079-y.

Gröne, O. (2022) "Patient Involvement in Health Care: Conceptualisation, Measurement, Uptake and Future Improvement," in B. Schmitz-Luhn and C. Woopen (eds.) *Justice Over the Course of Life*. Cham: Springer International Publishing, pp. 107–127. Available at: https://doi.org/10.1007/978-3-030-86449-1_10.

Guía, L.S., Cazorla, M.P. and de-Miguel-Molina, B. (2017) "Terms and meanings of 'participation' in product design: From 'user involvement' to 'co-design,'" *The Design Journal* [Preprint]. Available at: https://www.tandfonline.com/doi/abs/10.1080/14606925.2017.1352951 (Accessed: August 7, 2025).

Hardy, A. *et al.* (2018) "How inclusive, user-centered design research can improve psychological therapies for psychosis: Development of SlowMo," *JMIR Mental Health*, 5(4), p. e11222. Available at: https://doi.org/10.2196/11222.

Hickmann, E., Richter, P. and Schlieter, H. (2022) "All together now – Patient engagement, Patient empowerment, and associated terms in personal healthcare," *BMC Health Services Research*, 22(1), p. 1116. Available at: https://doi.org/10.1186/s12913-022-08501-5.

Hickey, G., Brearley, S., Coldham, T., Denegri, S., Green, G., Staniszewska, S., Tembo, D., Torok, K., and Turner, K. (2018). *Guidance on co-producing a research project.* Southampton: INVOLVE. Updated as: https://www.learningforinvolvement.org.uk/wp-content/uploads/2021/04/NIHR-Guidance-on-co-producing-a-research-project-April-2021.pdf

International Association for Public Participation. (2018) "IAP2 Spectrum of Public Participation." Available at: https://iap2.org.au/wp-content/uploads/2020/01/2018_IAP2_Spectrum.pdf (Accessed: September 13, 2025).

Israel, B.A. *et al.* (2001) "Community-based participatory research: Policy recommendations for promoting a partnership approach in health research," *Education for Health (Abingdon, England)*, 14(2), pp. 182–197. Available at: https://doi.org/10.1080/13576280110051055.

Jagosh, J. *et al.* (2012) "Uncovering the benefits of participatory research: Implications of a realist review for health research and practice," *The Milbank Quarterly*, 90(2), pp. 311–346. Available at: https://doi.org/10.1111/j.1468-0009.2012.00665.x.

Jagosh, J. *et al.* (2015) "A realist evaluation of community-based participatory research: Partnership synergy, trust building and related ripple effects," *BMC Public Health*, 15(1), p. 725. Available at: https://doi.org/10.1186/s12889-015-1949-1.

Lambley, R. (2025) "The challenges of navigating participatory research: The perspective of a doctoral student who co-ordinates a team of researchers with lived experience of mental health challenges," *Educational Action Research*, 33(1), pp. 143–152. Available at: https://doi.org/10.1080/09650792.2024.2429444.

Leask, C.F. *et al.* (2019) "Framework, principles and recommendations for utilising participatory methodologies in the co-creation and evaluation of public health interventions," *Research Involvement and Engagement*, 5, p. 2. Available at: https://doi.org/10.1186/s40900-018-0136-9.

Lincoln, Y.S. and Guba, E.G. (1985) *Naturalistic Inquiry.* Newbury Park: Sage Publications.

Longworth, G.R. *et al.* (2025) "Evaluating the co-creation process in public health interventions: The PROSECO framework," *Public Health*, 245, p. 105783. Available at: https://doi.org/10.1016/j.puhe.2025.105783.

Lynch, E.A. *et al.* (2024) "Codesigning implementation strategies to improve evidence-based stroke rehabilitation: A feasibility study," *Health Expectations: An International Journal of Public Participation in Health Care and Health Policy*, 27(1), p. e13904. Available at: https://doi.org/10.1111/hex.13904.

Maleševic´, A. and Čartolovni, A. (2025) "Healthcare 5.0 Paradigm Shift: Empowered Patients and Democratisation of Healthcare," in M. Bertolaso, M.L. Ilardo, and J. Ribera (eds.) *Healthcare in the Digital Age: Perspectives for Sustainable Innovation and Assessment.* Singapore: Springer Nature, pp. 139–162. Available at: https://doi.org/10.1007/978-981-96-1437-0_7.

Michie, S., Atkins, L. and West, R. (2014) *The Behaviour Change Wheel: A Guide to Designing Interventions.* Sutton, Surrey: Silverback.

Minkler, M. *et al.* (2003) "Community-based participatory research: Implications for public health funding," *American Journal of Public Health*, 93(8), pp. 1210–1213. Available at: https://doi.org/10.2105/ajph.93.8.1210.

Moore, G.F. *et al.* (2015) "Process evaluation of complex interventions: Medical research council guidance," *BMJ*, 350, p. h1258. Available at: https://doi.org/10.1136/bmj.h1258.

Murray, E. *et al.* (2015) "HeLP-diabetes: Randomised controlled trial protocol," *BMC Health Services Research*, 15(1), p. 578. Available at: https://doi.org/10.1186/s12913-015-1246-9.

Ocloo, J. and Matthews, R. (2016) "From tokenism to empowerment: Progressing patient and public involvement in healthcare improvement," *BMJ Quality & Safety*, 25(8), pp. 626–632. Available at: https://doi.org/10.1136/bmjqs-2015-004839.

OECD. (2024) *Health at a Glance: Europe 2024: State of Health in the EU Cycle.* Paris: Organisation for Economic Co-operation and Development. Available at: https://www.oecd.org/en/publications/health-at-a-glance-europe-2024_b3704e14-en.html.

Olude, O. *et al.* (2023) "A systematic review of participatory approaches to empower health workers in low- and middle-income countries, highlighting health workers for change," *International Health*, 15(4), pp. 462–473. Available at: https://doi.org/10.1093/inthealth/ihac070.

Ortiz-Escobar, L.M. *et al.* (2023) "Assessing the implementation of user-centred design standards on assistive technology for persons with visual impairments: A systematic review," *Frontiers in Rehabilitation Sciences*, 4, p. 1238158. Available at: https://doi.org/10.3389/fresc.2023.1238158.

Panagioti, M. *et al.* (2014) "Self-management support interventions to reduce health care utilisation without compromising outcomes: A systematic review and meta-analysis," *BMC Health Services Research*, 14(1), p. 356. Available at: https://doi.org/10.1186/1472-6963-14-356.

Pearce, T. *et al.* (2020) "What is the co-creation of new knowledge? A content analysis and proposed definition for health interventions," *International Journal of Environmental Research and Public Health*, 17(7), p. 2229. Available at: https://doi.org/10.3390/ijerph17072229.

Ricks, J.M. *et al.* (2022) "A systematic literature review of community-based participatory health research with sexual and gender minority communities," *Health Equity*, 6(1), pp. 640–657. Available at: https://doi.org/10.1089/heq.2022.0039.

Roberts, N. *et al.* (2012) "Barriers to the implementation of self management support in long term lung conditions," *London Journal of Primary Care*, 5(1), pp. 35–47. Available at: https://doi.org/10.1080/17571472.2013.11493370.

Sagen, J.S. *et al.* (2024) "Patient involvement in the rehabilitation process is associated with improvement in function and goal attainment: Results from an explorative longitudinal study," *Journal of Clinical Medicine*, 13(2), p. 320. Available at: https://doi.org/10.3390/jcm13020320.

Singh, A. (2022) "The democratisation of healthcare is an integral part of public health principles - Some examples from a medical college affiliated hospital, Chandigarh," *Bharati Vidyapeeth Medical Journal*, 2(1), p. 1. Available at: https://doi.org/10.56136/BVMJ/2022_00025.

Skivington, K. *et al.* (2021) "A new framework for developing and evaluating complex interventions: Update of medical research council guidance," *BMJ*, 374, p. n2061. Available at: https://doi.org/10.1136/bmj.n2061.

Skivington, K. *et al.* (2024) "A new framework for developing and evaluating complex interventions: Update of medical research council guidance," *International Journal of Nursing Studies*, 154, p. 104705. Available at: https://doi.org/10.1016/j.ijnurstu.2024.104705.

Slattery, P., Saeri, A.K. and Bragge, P. (2020) "Research co-design in health: A rapid overview of reviews," *Health Research Policy and Systems*, 18(1), p. 17. Available at: https://doi.org/10.1186/s12961-020-0528-9.

Subedi, N. *et al.* (2020) "Implementation of telerehabilitation interventions for the self-management of cardiovascular disease: Systematic review," *JMIR mHealth and uHealth*, 8(11), p. e17957. Available at: https://doi.org/10.2196/17957.

Tay, B.S.J. *et al.* (2021) "Co-design of a digital dietary intervention for adults at risk of type 2 diabetes," *BMC Public Health*, 21(1), p. 2071. Available at: https://doi.org/10.1186/s12889-021-12102-y.

Thomas, E. *et al.* (2024) "Participatory action research among people with serious mental illness: A scoping review," *Qualitative Health Research*, 34(1–2), pp. 3–19. Available at: https://doi.org/10.1177/10497323231208111.

Vargas, C. *et al.* (2022) "Co-creation, co-design, co-production for public health – A perspective on definition and distinctions," *Public Health Research & Practice*, 32(2), p. 3222211. Available at: https://doi.org/10.17061/phrp3222211.

Vaughn, L.M. and Jacquez, F. (2020) "Participatory research methods – Choice points in the research process," *Journal of Participatory Research Methods*, 1(1), p. 13244. Available at: https://doi.org/10.35844/001c.13244.

Velde, D.V. de *et al.* (2019) "Delineating the concept of self-management in chronic conditions: A concept analysis," *BMJ Open*, 9(7), e027775. Available at: https://doi.org/10.1136/bmjopen-2018-027775.

Volkmann, T., Dresel, M. and Jochems, N. (2023) "Balancing Power Relations in Participatory Design: The Importance of Initiative and External Factors," in *Extended Abstracts of the 2023 CHI Conference on Human Factors in Computing Systems*. New York: Association for Computing Machinery (CHI EA '23), pp. 1–6. Available at: https://doi.org/10.1145/3544549.3585864.

Voorberg, W.H., Bekkers, V.J.J.M. and Tummers, L.G. (2015) "A systematic review of co-creation and co-production: Embarking on the social innovation journey," *Public Management Review*, 17(9), pp. 1333–1357. Available at: https://doi.org/10.1080/14719037.2014.930505.

Wen, X. *et al.* (2025) "Enhancing long-term adherence in elderly stroke rehabilitation through a digital health approach based on multimodal feedback and personalized intervention," *Scientific Reports*, 15(1), p. 14190. Available at: https://doi.org/10.1038/s41598-025-95726-z.

Wiesmüller, F. *et al.* (2025) "Support of home-based structured walking training and prediction of the 6-minute walk test distance in patients with peripheral arterial disease based on telehealth data: Prospective cohort study," *JMIR Formative Research*, 9, p. e65721. Available at: https://doi.org/10.2196/65721.

Williams, O. *et al.* (2020) "Lost in the shadows: Reflections on the dark side of co-production," *Health Research Policy and Systems*, 18(1), p. 43. Available at: https://doi.org/10.1186/s12961-020-00558-0.

Wittink, H. *et al.* (2024) "Co-design of a walking activity intervention for stroke survivors," *Frontiers in Rehabilitation Sciences*, 5, p. 1369559. Available at: https://doi.org/10.3389/fresc.2024.1369559.

Wray, F. *et al.* (2021) "Development of a self-management intervention for stroke survivors with aphasia using co-production and behaviour change theory: An outline of methods and processes," *PLOS ONE*, 16(11), p. e0259103. Available at: https://doi.org/10.1371/journal.pone.0259103.

Zachary, W.W. *et al.* (2017) "Participatory design of a social networking app to support type II diabetes self-management in low-income minority communities," *Proceedings of the International Symposium of Human Factors and Ergonomics in Healthcare. International Symposium of Human Factors and Ergonomics in Healthcare*, 6(1), pp. 37–43. Available at: https://doi.org/10.1177/2327857917061010.

Zahlsen, ØK., Parmiggiani, E. and Dahl, Y. (2023) "Challenges of Scaling Participatory Design: A Systematic Literature Review," in *Proceedings of the 34th Australian Conference on Human-Computer Interaction*. New York: Association for Computing Machinery (OzCHI '22), pp. 143–159. Available at: https://doi.org/10.1145/3572921.3572924.

22 Beyond Compliance

Science Capital, Funds of Knowledge, and Self-Management in Rehabilitation

Jerome Atutornu

INTRODUCTION

Self-management has become a central tenet of modern rehabilitation. Across clinical disciplines and care settings, patients are increasingly expected to take responsibility for monitoring symptoms, adhering to treatment, and making informed decisions about their care (Freilich et al., 2020; Riegel et al., 2021; Whittaker et al., 2024). Patients are increasingly being empowered to take a more active role in their care through approaches such as education, goal setting, health coaching, and peer support (Benzo, 2024). This model aligns with wider healthcare goals of patient-centredness, efficiency, and empowerment (Dineen-Griffin et al., 2019). However, it often presumes a uniform set of knowledge, values, and behaviours that patients are expected to adopt, frequently without adequate regard for their social, cultural, and epistemological contexts along with the inherent power dynamics (Fletcher et al., 2019).

While structured interventions to support self-management can yield positive outcomes (Fønhus et al., 2019; Kidd et al., 2022), they also risk reinforcing assumptions about who is capable of managing and on what terms. When individuals appear to disengage, are labelled non-compliant, or fail to meet clinical expectations, the dominant response often frames this as a deficit, one of literacy, motivation, or cultural alignment (Reincke et al., 2020). This framing obscures the everyday realities and structural barriers that shape people's capacities and decisions, particularly for those from minoritised or historically marginalised communities.

This chapter offers an alternative framing of self-management by drawing on two conceptual frameworks: **science capital** and **funds of knowledge**. These concepts shift the focus from individual deficits to the assets and cultural resources that people use to make sense of health and science. In doing so, they invite us to consider what forms of knowledge are recognised in clinical settings, how people engage with health-related information on their own terms, and what supports more equitable participation in health systems.

The analysis is grounded in findings from a mixed-methods study exploring the attitudes of Ghanaian publics (both in Ghana and the UK) towards genomics and the sharing of health data. While situated within genomic medicine, the study offers wider insights into how people from culturally diverse backgrounds engage with unfamiliar or specialised forms of biomedical knowledge. Participants drew upon a range of knowledge systems, including cultural narratives, familial roles, language practices, lived experiences, and spiritual worldviews. Rather than being "outside" science, these knowledge systems represent legitimate ways of knowing that, when acknowledged and appropriately legitimised, can enrich rehabilitation and support more meaningful engagement.

In this chapter, I argue that self-management in rehabilitation should be reframed not only as a behavioural practice but also as an epistemic process—one that involves how people understand, interpret, and respond to health-related information in light of their own values and experiences. Acknowledging and integrating these systems of knowledge is central to achieving equitable,

DOI: 10.1201/9781003599074-25

culturally responsive care. From a social justice point of view, I argue that doing this enables epistemic justice, the elevation of marginalised voices and hopefully the decolonisation of rehabilitation knowledge and practice (Pratt & De Vries, 2023; Rosen, 2021). Epistemic injustice (portraying the knowledge systems of others as deficient) renders people powerless to self-describe or define (Fanon, 1961; Said, 1995).

The chapter proceeds as follows. Section 2 outlines the conceptual foundations of science capital and funds of knowledge and discusses their relevance to rehabilitation. Section 3 applies these frameworks to empirical findings from the study, illustrating how participants navigated biomedical concepts through sociocultural and linguistic tools. Section 4 draws implications for rehabilitation practice, arguing for engagement strategies that centre justice, inclusion, and the co-production of knowledge. Section 5 concludes by offering a vision of self-management that is not imposed but collaboratively constructed; rooted in mutual recognition and shared understanding.

Ultimately, this chapter contends that for self-management to fulfil its promise, it must attend to whose knowledge counts, whose capacities are recognised, and whose realities are centred in rehabilitation policy and practice.

THEORETICAL FRAMEWORK: SCIENCE CAPITAL AND FUNDS OF KNOWLEDGE

To reimagine self-management in rehabilitation through a more inclusive and equitable lens, it is vital to understand how people relate to scientific and medical knowledge in ways that go beyond institutional expectations. This section introduces two theoretical lenses (**science capital** and **funds of knowledge**) that provide a framework for recognising the assets individuals and communities already possess, and how these may be leveraged or excluded within rehabilitation contexts.

Science Capital: Beyond Scientific Literacy

Science capital, a concept developed by Archer et al. (2015), extends the idea of scientific literacy by focusing on the broader cultural, social, and symbolic resources that shape individuals' engagement with science. Drawing on Bourdieu's concept of social reproduction, science capital critiques deficit models of science communication that blame underrepresented groups for non-engagement, instead arguing that social positioning, familiarity with science, and embodied dispositions (habitus) shape access to science participation and in this context, meaningful engagement with rehabilitation regimes (Archer et al., 2015).

Social advantage/disadvantage is created and reproduced by an interplay between the environment in which one finds themselves (their field), the resources available to them to navigate the environment (their capital) and their predispositions (habitus) (Bourdieu, 1998; Dawson, 2019). This in essence is what Bourdieu calls cultural capital which is the familiarity one needs to be competent in a field (Bourdieu et al., 1991).

Consequently, science capital encompasses not only what people know about science but also:

- Whether they see science as "for people like them"
- Their exposure to scientific ideas at home, school, or work
- The networks and relationships they have with people in science
- Their confidence in talking about and applying scientific knowledge

Crucially, these attributes of Science Capital (familiarity, exposure, networks) are mediated by the legitimacy that are attributed to them. What counts as legitimate knowledge, legitimate exposure or legitimate network is largely arbitrary and dependent on the values of dominant groups in society. Dominant group values/knowledges are normalised as "usual" while those of minoritised groups become peripheral and "exotic", oriental (Said, 1995). Therefore, knowledge emanating from one social background could be classed as deficient while another could be legitimised: creating hierarchies of value.

In the context of rehabilitation, the notion of science capital challenges assumptions that patients who do not readily adopt clinical recommendations are unmotivated or uninformed. Instead, it prompts a more nuanced inquiry into how people's social backgrounds, cultural histories, and lived experiences shape their confidence and capacity to engage with biomedical frameworks. It allows us to consider, for example, how historical exclusion from healthcare systems or negative clinical encounters might reduce someone's perceived legitimacy or comfort in healthcare spaces, regardless of their actual interest or intelligence.

Importantly, science capital is not fixed. It can be accumulated, transformed, or constrained depending on context (Archer et al., 2015, 2015; Bourdieu et al., 1990; King & Nomikou, 2018). Rehabilitation professionals can play a role in either reinforcing or disrupting the structural inequalities that shape science capital. When clinical environments rely on rigid, biomedical models that fail to accommodate and legitimise diverse knowledges and ways of understanding health, they inadvertently reproduce existing hierarchies of value.

Funds of Knowledge: Valuing Everyday Expertise

The concept of funds of knowledge, originally developed in educational research by Moll et al. (1992), refers to the historically accumulated and culturally developed bodies of knowledge that households use to sustain their well-being. These include skills, know-how, language practices, belief systems, and informal modes of problem-solving that are embedded in daily life.

From its early use in personal and family finances (Wolf, 1966), this concept has evolved to a broader range of uses, such as well-being (Oughton, 2018), popular culture (Moje et al., 2004), 'knowledges, experiences, histories, identities, and images of themselves, attitudes, dispositions, desires, values, beliefs and social relationships' (Oughton, 2010, p. 67). Far from being marginal, these knowledges are central to how people navigate complex systems, including health systems.

When applied to rehabilitation, funds of knowledge help reframe how we understand patient behaviours and decisions. For example, someone managing a chronic condition may draw on intergenerational practices of herbal medicine, religious beliefs about healing, or collective decision-making processes within the family. These practices are often invisible in clinical settings, not because they are irrelevant, but because they are not institutionally recognised or legitimised.

Recognising funds of knowledge does not mean romanticising all forms of non-biomedical practice or abandoning clinical standards. Rather, it means acknowledging that people come to rehabilitation with existing frameworks for understanding the body, pain, care, and healing. This is similar to Kelly's (Kelly, 1963) description of how people make sense of their world through personal constructs that are usually borne out of their life experiences (Taber, 2020). If clinicians fail to recognise these frameworks, they risk creating friction or disengagement. By contrast, when practitioners engage with these knowledges in a spirit of respect and curiosity, they create space for mutual understanding and shared decision-making.

This is based on the notion that people draw on a variety of sources (such as those from their sociocultural experiences and formal science) to make sense of the world (Moje et al., 2004).

Intersection and Complementarity

Together, science capital and funds of knowledge offer complementary perspectives. Science capital focuses on the *institutionalised* dimensions of knowledge (how people navigate the field, i.e., formal structures and gatekeeping mechanisms of science). Funds of knowledge, by contrast, centres the *experiential* and *cultural* knowledge embedded in everyday life and attempts to posit it as legitimate knowledge worthy of science capital.

In rehabilitation, this intersection is particularly valuable. For example, a person recovering from a stroke may need to learn new biomedical information about neuroplasticity or medication regimes (science capital), while simultaneously drawing on culturally meaningful routines, family support structures, or spiritual practices to sustain motivation and emotional wellbeing (funds of knowledge). Acknowledging both as valid and necessary, means the rehabilitation process becomes not simply a transfer of medical knowledge, but a collaborative negotiation of how different knowledges can work together to support recovery. Crucially, I argue that these funds of knowledge should legitimately contribute to one's science capital; the knowledges and attributes required to be competent in this field.

Furthermore, both concepts underscore that the problem is not an individual's failure to conform to a clinical script, but the healthcare system's failure to recognise and incorporate alternative ways of knowing. This reframing enables a shift from deficit thinking (i.e., what patients lack) to an asset-based approach (i.e., what patients bring). In practical terms, this might involve using metaphors drawn from a patient's linguistic and cultural context, engaging family or community members as knowledge brokers, or inviting patients to co-design aspects of their care based on their lived realities.

Creating spaces (such as a responsive rehabilitation environment), where formal 'scientific' knowledges and those borne out of people's socio-cultural circumstances are acknowledged, enables recovery, not only physically but gives the added value of justice in terms of recognition (Fraser, 2020).

Fraser and Honneth (2003) conceptualise justice in terms redistribution and recognition. While redistributive justice seeks equitable access to resources, recognition seeks an environment friendly to difference and of equal respect for all. They assert that the core principle against which justice should be measured is that of *parity of participation* where members of a society can interact with each other as peers. For justice in terms of recognition, to be present, there needs to be intersubjective participatory parity. This means that there needs to be equal value and respect for all such that they can attain social esteem (Fraser & Honneth, 2003). For redistributive justice to be present, there need to be objective parity. This means social systems are structured equally to allow an equal voice on how resources are distributed. Acknowledging people's knowledge assets drawn from their lived experiences feeds into creating parity of participation.

APPLYING THE FRAMEWORK – INSIGHTS FROM PUBLICS OF GHANAIAN ORIGIN AND GENOMICS

To make science capital and funds of knowledge meaningful in the context of rehabilitation, we need grounded, empirical examples of how these frameworks operate in real-world settings. This section draws on findings from my doctoral research, a mixed-methods study exploring the attitudes of Ghanaian publics (both in Ghana and in the UK diaspora) towards genomics and the sharing of genomic and health data. While the topic may appear distant from rehabilitation at first glance, the implications for self-management, trust, and engagement in healthcare are, I would argue, highly relevant.

Study Overview

The study included focus groups and a large-scale survey in Twi and Ewe; two of Ghana's widely spoken languages. It aimed to uncover how Ghanaians (in Ghana and in the UK diaspora) understood genomic science, what they thought about contributing their data to research, and what conditions would foster or impede their participation. A core finding was that the decision to engage with genomics was not based simply on access to information or biomedical literacy. Rather, it involved complex negotiations of trust, history, identity, and power, all of which are also present in rehabilitation encounters. The study showed that, participants did actually possess Science capital, and this was evident in the nuanced discussions they were able to make around the topic of genetics and genetic data. What remains is how these knowledges are legitimised and made mainstream in the research and clinical environment, such that people are empowered to utilise appropriate, contextualised knowledge in the appropriate circumstances.

Notably, participants demonstrated *low familiarity* with the formal language of genomics, consistent with previous studies (Ipsos Mori, 2018; Middleton et al., 2020). They however, expressed *rich, nuanced reflections* about inheritance, health, and health data. Their knowledge was mediated through everyday experiences, cultural metaphors, religion, historical memory, and family conversations. For instance, many used analogies involving "blood" to make sense of genetic inheritance—linking it to ancestral ties, spiritual significance, and physical health.

This suggests that while formal scientific terminology (as defined by dominant biomedical discourse) appeared limited, *alternative forms of knowledge* were abundant and meaningfully applied. These were drawn from participants' funds of knowledge; culturally rooted, shared, and often embodied understandings of health and self. The gap between biomedical assumptions and these lay knowledges is not a matter of ignorance, but of misrecognition. Misrecognition is seen by some theorists as going beyond the absence of respect to inflicting injury to an important human need which can lead eventually to a damaged self-identity (Honneth, 1992; Taylor & Gutmann, 1992).

Relevance to Rehabilitation

Although genomics and rehabilitation are different domains, they share a common challenge: how to engage publics (particularly those from marginalised or minoritised communities)in processes of care that require active participation, trust, and alignment with biomedical recommendations.

In rehabilitation, self-management strategies often rely on the assumption that patients will follow prescribed exercises, adhere to medication, monitor symptoms, and report progress (Dineen-Griffin et al., 2019; Riegel et al., 2021). Yet, similar to genomic data donation, compliance and engagement depend not only on information but on how individuals relate to the system, the messenger, and the meaning of the care being offered.

Drawing from the study, three insights can be applied to rehabilitation practice:

Knowledge Is Relational, Not Deficit-Based

Many participants did not trust genomic researchers, not due to superstition or resistance to science, but because of historical and contemporary experiences of exclusion and exploitation. Some referenced slavery, colonialism, and unethical medical practices in the past (Atutornu et al., 2022). Others expressed concerns about how their data might be misused or sold for profit without their consent. Referring to their genes and the idea of donating their data for research, one participant said…

> That is "me" in a code. That's me giving "me" up to a system that has not been trustworthy in the past. It's tricky.

In rehabilitation, similar dynamics may arise. Patients may not fully trust the system because of past neglect, perceived bias, or systemic barriers. If professionals interpret disengagement as disinterest or noncompliance, they risk missing the relational work needed to build safety, transparency, and shared purpose. Science capital, in this light, includes relational trust, cultivated, not assumed. The quote below also, underscores the need for demonstrating trustworthiness in such relationships.

> Naturally, someone can be in the lab and do that [create a virus to target specific people]. The only way we can all agree to what we are doing is that when something is being prepared in the kitchen, we Black people too need to be in the kitchen to see what is being prepared so that everyone can believe that nobody has put anything poisonous into the food

> As far as trust is concerned, it does not matter who the person is. It would be difficult to just trust somebody. We would have to sign legal agreements for such DNA data to be released. I think that would be better. Then, there would have to be an agreement that it would be held confidentially. But saying you would trust someone without signing an agreement? No, you cannot trust someone like that.

Language and Metaphor Matter

The study found that using local languages (Twi and Ewe) and culturally relevant metaphors (e.g., talking about "blood" rather than "DNA") significantly improved comprehension and comfort. Participants responded positively to audio-visual explanations and appreciated that the study had been translated and localised. While that may not in itself lead to decisions to participate in research or follow rehabilitation recommendations, they act as a source of communication accommodation and the creation of common ground which might serve as critical foundations for future desired goals (Kecskes, 2014; Zhang & Imamura, 2017).

Rehabilitation often involves abstract concepts (such as muscle strength, neuroplasticity, gait mechanics) that are challenging to understand, especially when English is not the first language. By adopting metaphors and examples from patients' cultural and linguistic worlds, practitioners can create a shared language of healing. This is not about simplification but about translation into meaningful, linguistically and culturally appropriate terms (Sharif et al., 2020).

In the quote below, a participant referred to colonialism and past history of unethical medical research and expressed his preference to donating his genetic data to a person who matches them in terms skin colour and language.

> There is no doubt in me that I will donate my DNA to a Black person like me. Someone who speaks the same language as me. I would trust such a person more than a White person who (in my opinion) is acting like he wants to help me. So, if the person is a Black person and speaks my language, Ewe, then I would trust them because as Ewes, our language unites us a lot. For us Ewes, the moment you hear a person speak your language, you connect to the person naturally, unlike other tribes such as Akan or Ga. The moment you hear a person speaking Ewe, it feels like the person is your brother or sister

A key and quite incidental finding in my study was the phenomenon of code switching. While the study was meant to be and largely conducted in Ewe/Twi, it was noticed that participants felt comfortable switching between the Ewe/Twi and English. This is a usual phenomenon in bilingual societies, especially those with a history of colonisation (Flamenbaum, 2013) where these are used in creating common ground and showing solidarity with people of common ancestry (Amuzu, 2012). As the above quote suggests that some people might only engage with scientists or clinicians due to trust issues, there might be the need to use staff who culturally and linguistically match the patients such that room is made for code switching.

Communities Are Resources, Not Obstacles

The Ghanaian publics (in the Ghana and the UK) consulted often spoke of decision-making as a collective process. Some participants said they would consult family or community leaders before agreeing to share genomic data. This notion is argued also as indigenous data sovereignty among indigenous communities across close knit communities in countries like the US, Australia, New Zealand and Canada (Kukutai, 2023). This is not a rejection of individual autonomy, but an alternative model of decision-making rooted in their relational identity.

In rehabilitation, this insight challenges the lone-patient model of self-management. For many people (especially in collectivist cultures)health is negotiated within networks of care (Cho et al., 2021; Moleiro et al., 2017; Naramore & Marquez, 2024). Family, religious groups, and community norms may influence adherence, interpretation of symptoms, and what is considered a "successful" recovery. Engaging these networks, rather than bypassing them, can enhance outcomes and sustainability.

> The Western individualistic approach means the person's DNA is his DNA, he doesn't care, he can give it out. He can make that decision without any cultural influences, any external influences, but my submission is that, in the African context, specifically in my Ewe context where I'm coming from, my DNA is not my individual matter for me to say 'take it, it's my information'. That is not our understanding; I mean we are a communal people, different from the individualistic approach of the Western world.

Implications for Culturally Responsive Rehabilitation

The findings point to several practical implications for making rehabilitation more inclusive and responsive to people's lived realities:

- **Designing materials and conversations that acknowledge multiple ways of knowing**: This includes using culturally resonant language, metaphors, accommodating code-switching, and being open to lay interpretations of health and illness. That is being able to use contextualised language in the appropriate circumstances.
- **Creating space for patient narratives that draw on their funds of knowledge**: This could be through structured narrative interviewing, group consultations, or patient-led goal-setting that incorporates spiritual, cultural, or familial dimensions of recovery.
- **Training clinicians in cultural sensitivity and science communication**: Professionals need tools to communicate complex ideas in ways that are both accurate and accessible. This includes listening skills, flexibility in explanation, and awareness of how their own authority may be perceived.
- **Building systems that enable shared decision-making across different cultural logics**: Consent processes, treatment planning, and follow-up mechanisms should allow for family involvement, community brokerage, and iterative dialogue, rather than one-off instructions.

In summary, the case study illuminates how people use their funds of knowledge and social capital to make sense of their world and complex health information. By recognising and working with these assets (rather than dismissing them) rehabilitation professionals can build more just, effective, and culturally grounded care pathways.

PRACTICAL IMPLICATIONS AND RECOMMENDATIONS

The preceding sections have made the case that culturally responsive rehabilitation must move beyond models that assume a universal pathway to self-management. Drawing from the Ghanaian publics' engagement with genomics and applying the lens of science capital and funds of knowledge, we see how engagement, trust, and knowledge are socially and culturally situated. This section outlines concrete recommendations for practitioners, educators, and policy makers to create more inclusive and effective rehabilitation systems.

Recognise the Value of Lay Expertise

Recommendation: Treat patients and their communities as knowledge-holders, not just knowledge-receivers.

In both genomics and rehabilitation, people bring knowledge rooted in everyday life: how bodies feel, how pain is interpreted, how priorities shift based on family, work, and belief systems. These knowledges are not inferior to biomedical ones, they are simply different. Making room for these perspectives, through narrative elicitation and co-designed care plans, fosters ownership and engagement. The idea of co-creation requires that the care of patients reflect their personal circumstances and priorities.

- **Example**: A rehabilitation practitioner could begin assessments with open-ended questions such as: "How do you understand what's going on in your body?" or "What does recovery mean to you and your family?".

Tailor Communication to Cultural Contexts

Recommendation: Use metaphors, languages, and formats that reflect the patient's lived reality.

Just as participants in the genomic study responded more positively to local language versions of the survey and culturally familiar metaphors (e.g., "blood" as a proxy for DNA), rehabilitation conversations could benefit from language that resonates. Communication is more than clarity, and it is cultural alignment.

- **Example**: Work with interpreters not just to translate words, but to co-create metaphors or analogies that suit a patient's background (e.g., comparing rehabilitation exercises to walking a child to school, or dancing—whatever fits the patient's context).
- **Practice Point**: Consider producing or using bilingual rehabilitation guides that incorporate visuals, storytelling, or recorded audio in multiple dialects. These might be QR codes that link to appropriate audio-visual content.

Embed Relational Approaches to Engagement

Recommendation: Support collective decision-making and community involvement where appropriate.

In my research, it was clear that decision-making was not always individualistic. Family, elders, faith leaders, and social networks played crucial roles in shaping how participants understood science and decided on data sharing. In rehabilitation, assuming the patient acts in isolation can miss key enablers (or barriers) to self-management. This is particularly relevant to collectivist communities.

- **Example**: Where culturally appropriate, invite trusted family members or caregivers into consultations and goal-setting processes. In some cases, "community health brokers" or peer navigators can act as bridges between clinical systems and patients' social worlds.

Expand the Concept of Science Capital in Training

Recommendation: Introduce the concept of science capital and funds of knowledge into the professional education of rehabilitation specialists.

Science capital training encourages future clinicians to see beyond "compliance" and instead ask: What knowledge resources does this person already hold? How can we link rehabilitation goals to those resources?

- **Training Module Suggestion:**
  - Explore case studies where patients' funds of knowledge supported or clashed with rehabilitation advice.
  - Reflect on the clinician's own science capital: how were they taught to value certain knowledges over others?
  - Practise reframing common rehabilitation language using patient-informed metaphors.

Design Systems that Enable Recognition and Redistribution

Recommendation: Build systems that both recognise diverse ways of knowing and address structural inequities.

Drawing on Fraser's theory of justice, we must go beyond individual-level adaptation and embed structural changes that allow for redistributive justice (e.g., equitable access to rehabilitation) and recognition justice (e.g., valuing non-dominant knowledge systems).

- **Policy Action:**
  - Allocate funding for co-designed materials that reflect multilingual, multicultural contexts.
  - Support the development of minoritised patient panels, advisory boards, or community-based participatory research in rehabilitation.
  - Evaluate existing programmes using justice-oriented metrics: Who is benefitting? Whose knowledge is reflected in the process?

Embrace a Post-Trust Paradigm in Engagement

Recommendation: Do not assume trust; build it through transparency, procedural fairness, and mutual accountability.

In my genomics research, participants were hesitant to share data not due to apathy, but due to historically grounded mistrust. I call this a post-trust paradigm which is marked by a departure from automatic trust in mere assurances to seeking legally binding agreements. Similarly, in rehabilitation, patients may not automatically trust clinicians or systems, especially if their communities have experienced neglect or exclusion. A post-trust model does not expect automatic deference but earns participation through honesty and care.

Best Practice:

- Be transparent about uncertainties, limits of rehabilitation, and shared risks.
- Honour patients' right to disagree, disengage, or reshape the terms of care.
- Document and act on patient feedback about feeling heard and respected.

CONCLUSION

Culturally responsive rehabilitation requires more than adding a translator or checking a cultural competence box. It requires structural sensitivity, creative communication, and a commitment to justice. The case of Ghanaian publics in Ghana and the diaspora navigating genomics demonstrates that people already have science capital, they already engage with complex biomedical ideas when the invitation is respectful, situated, and dialogic.

Similarly, patients in rehabilitation contexts can and do manage their care when systems recognise the assets they bring. This chapter has argued for a reframing, from deficit to dialogue, from compliance to co-creation, from universalism to situated justice.

REFERENCES

Amuzu, E. (2012). Socio-pragmatics of conversational codeswitching in Ghana. *Ghana Journal of Linguistics, 1*(2), 1–22. https://www.ajol.info/index.php/gjl/article/view/86782

Archer, L., Dawson, E., DeWitt, J., Seakins, A., & Wong, B. (2015). "Science capital": A conceptual, methodological, and empirical argument for extending Bourdieusian notions of capital beyond the arts. *Journal of Research in Science Teaching, 52*(7), 922–948. https://doi.org/10.1002/tea.21227

Archer, L., Dewitt, J., & Osborne, J. (2015). Is science for us? Black students' and parents' views of science and science careers. *Science Education, 99*(2), 199–237. https://doi.org/10.1002/sce.21146

Atutornu, J., Milne, R., Costa, A., Patch, C., & Middleton, A. (2022). Towards equitable and trustworthy genomics research. *EBioMedicine*, *76*, 103879. https://doi.org/10.1016/J.EBIOM.2022.103879

Benzo, R. P. (2024). Self-management programs and the pursuit of behavior change. *Respiratory Care*, *69*(6), 678. https://doi.org/10.4187/RESPCARE.11987

Bourdieu, P. (1998). Practical *r*eason: On the *t*heory of *a*ction. Stanford University Press. https://philpapers.org/rec/BOUPRO

Bourdieu, P., Darbel, A., & Schnapper, D. (1991). The love of art: European art museums and their public (p. 182). Polity Press. https://www.wiley.com/en-gb/The+Love+of+Art%3A+European+Art+Museums+and+Their+Public-p-9780745619149

Bourdieu, P., Passeron, J., & Claude (1990). *Reproduction in education, society and culture*. Sage. https://books.google.co.uk/books?id=vl0n9_wrrbUC&dq=Reproduction+in+education,+society+and+culture&hl=en&sa=X&ved=0ahUKEwjGiZf2nNriAhXPSxUIHWkiA5IQ6AEIKDAA

Cho, H., Guo, Y., & Torelli, C. (2021). Collectivism fosters preventive behaviors to contain the spread of COVID-19: Implications for social marketing in public health. *Psychology & Marketing*, *39*(4), 694. https://doi.org/10.1002/MAR.21613

Dawson, E. (2019). Equity, *e*xclusion and *e*veryday *s*cience *l*earning. Routledge. https://doi.org/10.4324/9781315266763

Dineen-Griffin, S., Garcia-Cardenas, V., Williams, K., & Benrimoj, S. I. (2019). Helping patients help themselves: A systematic review of self-management support strategies in primary health care practice. *PLoS ONE*, *14*(8), e0220116. https://doi.org/10.1371/JOURNAL.PONE.0220116

Fanon, F. (1961). The wretched of the earth/Frantz Fanon ; Preface by Jean-Paul Sartre ; tr. by Constance Farrington. *Penguin Classics*, 256. https://bookshop.thephotographersgallery.org.uk/products/frantz-fanon-the-wretched-of-the-earth

Flamenbaum, R. (2013). The pragmatics of codeswitching on Ghanaian talk radio. *International Journal of Bilingualism*, *18*(4), 346–362. https://doi.org/10.1177/1367006913481136

Fletcher, S., Kulnik, S. T., Demain, S., & Jones, F. (2019). The problem with self-management: Problematising self-management and power using a Foucauldian lens in the context of stroke care and rehabilitation. *PLOS ONE*, *14*(6), e0218517. https://doi.org/10.1371/JOURNAL.PONE.0218517

Fønhus, M. S., Dalsbø, T. K., Johansen, M., Fretheim, A., Skirbekk, H., & Flottorp, S. (2019). Patient-mediated interventions to improve professional practice: A summary of a cochrane systematic review. *Patient Education and Counseling*, *102*(3), 474–485. https://doi.org/10.1016/J.PEC.2018.10.022

Fraser, N. (2020). From redistribution to recognition? : Dilemmas of justice in a "postsocialist" age. In *The New Social Theory Reader* (pp.188–196). Routledge. https://doi.org/10.4324/9781003060963-30

Fraser, N., & Honneth, A. (2003). *Redistribution or Recognition? : A Political-Philosophical Exchange*. Verso.

Freilich, J., Nilsson, G. H., Ekstedt, M., & Flink, M. (2020). Standing on common ground" - A qualitative study of self-management support for patients with multimorbidity in primary health care. *BMC Family Practice*, *21*(1), 1–12. https://doi.org/10.1186/S12875-020-01290-Y/TABLES/2

Honneth, A. (1992). Integrity and disrespect: Principles of a conception of morality based on the theory of recognition. *Political Theory*, *20*(2), 187–201. https://www.jstor.org/stable/192001

Ipsos Mori. (2018). Genomics England polling. Ipsos MORI. http://www.ipsos-mori.com/terms.http://www.ipsos-mori.com/terms

Kecskes, I. (2014). Common ground. In *Intercultural pragmatics*. Oxford University Press. https://doi.org/10.1093/acprof:oso/9780199892655.001.0001

Kelly, G. (1963). *A theory of personality: The psychology of personal constructs*. W.W. Norton.

Kidd, L., Millar, J. D., Mason, H., Quinn, T., Gallacher, K. I., Jones, F., Fisher, R. J., Lebedis, T., Barber, M., Brennan, K., & Smith, M. (2022). Supported self-management in community stroke rehabilitation: What is it and how does it work? A protocol for a realist evaluation study. *BMJ Open*, *12*(1), e055491. https://doi.org/10.1136/BMJOPEN-2021-055491

King, H., & Nomikou, E. (2018). Fostering critical teacher agency: The impact of a science capital pedagogical approach. *Pedagogy, Culture and Society*, *26*(1), 87–103. https://doi.org/10.1080/14681366.2017.1353539

Kukutai, T. (2023). Indigenous data sovereignty—A new take on an old theme. *Science*, *382*(6674), eadl4664. https://doi.org/10.1126/SCIENCE.ADL4664

Middleton, A., Milne, R., Almarri, M. A., Anwer, S., Atutornu, J., Baranova, E. E., Bevan, P., Cerezo, M., Cong, Y., Critchley, C., Fernow, J., Goodhand, P., Hasan, Q., Hibino, A., Houeland, G., Howard, H. C., Hussain, S. Z., Malmgren, C. I., Izhevskaya, V. L., & Morley, K. I. (2020). Global public perceptions of genomic data sharing: What shapes the willingness to donate DNA and health data? *The American Journal of Human Genetics*, *107*(4), 743–752. https://doi.org/10.1016/J.AJHG.2020.08.023

Moje, E. B., Ciechanowski, K., Mci., Kramer, K., Ellis, L., Carrillo, R., & Collazo, T. (2004). Working toward third space in content area literacy: An examination of everyday funds of knowledge and discourse. *Reading Research Quarterly*, *39*(1), 38–70. https://doi.org/10.1598/RRQ.39.1.4

Moleiro, C., Ratinho, I., & Bernardes, S. (2017). Autonomy-connectedness in collectivistic cultures: An exploratory cross-cultural study among Portuguese natives, Cape-Verdean and Chinese people residing in Portugal. *Personality and Individual Differences*, *104*, 23–28. https://doi.org/10.1016/J.PAID.2016.07.031

Moll, L. C., Cathy, A., Neff, D., & Gonzale, N. (1992). Funds of knowledge for teaching: Using a qualitative approach to connect homes and classrooms. *Theory into Practice*, *31*(2), 132–141. https://doi.org/10.1080/00405849209543534/ASSET//CMS/ASSET/7A24816B-8754-444D-9DCA-DCCF92293C0B/00405849209543534.FP.PNG

Naramore, R., & Marquez, E. (2024). A choice not to choose: Respecting patient autonomy in collectivist cultures. *Journal of Pain and Symptom Management*, *67*(5), e636. https://doi.org/10.1016/J.JPAINSYMMAN.2024.02.074

Oughton, H. (2010). Funds of knowledge-a conceptual critique. *Studies in the Education of Adults*, *42*(1), 63–78. https://doi.org/10.1080/02660830.2010.11661589

Oughton, H. (2018). Disrupting dominant discourses: A (re)introduction to social practice theories of adult numeracy. *Numeracy*, *11*(1), Article 2. https://doi.org/10.5038/1936-4660.11.1.2

Pratt, B., & De Vries, J. (2023). Where is knowledge from the global South? An account of epistemic justice for a global bioethics. *Journal of Medical Ethics*, *49*(5), 325. https://doi.org/10.1136/JME-2022-108291

Reincke, C. M., Bredenoord, A. L., & van Mil, M. H.. (2020). From deficit to dialogue in science communication: The dialogue communication model requires additional roles from scientists. *EMBO Reports*, *21*(9), e51278. https://doi.org/10.15252/EMBR.202051278

Riegel, B., Dunbar, S. B., Fitzsimons, D., Freedland, K. E., Lee, C. S., Middleton, S., Stromberg, A., Vellone, E., Webber, D. E., & Jaarsma, T. (2021). Self-care research: Where are we now? Where are we going? *International Journal of Nursing Studies*, *116*, 103402. https://doi.org/10.1016/J.IJNURSTU.2019.103402

Rosen, L. T. (2021). Mapping out epistemic justice in the clinical space: Using narrative techniques to affirm patients as knowers. *Philosophy, Ethics, and Humanities in Medicine*, *16*(1), 1–6. https://doi.org/10.1186/S13010-021-00110-0/METRICS

Said, E. W. (1995). *Orientalism*. Penguin Books. https://books.google.co.uk/books?id=66sIHa2VTmoC&pg=PP1&source=kp_read_button&redir_esc=y#v=onepage&q&f=false

Sharif, S. M., Blyth, M., Ahmed, M., Sheridan, E., Saltus, R., Yu, J., Tonkin, E., & Kirk, M. (2020). Enhancing inclusion of diverse populations in genomics: A competence framework. *Journal of Genetic Counseling*, *29*(2), 282–292. https://doi.org/10.1002/jgc4.1263

Taber, K. (2020). Constructive alternativism: George Kelly's personal construct theory. In B. Akpan & T. Kennedy (Eds.), *Science education in theory and practice*. SPRINGER NATURE. https://www.researchgate.net/publication/340266621_Constructive_Alternativism_George_Kelly's_Personal_Construct_Theory

Taylor, C., & Gutmann, Amy. (1992). *Multiculturalism and "The politics of recognition" : An essay*. Princeton University Press.

Whittaker, S. L., Brusco, N. K., Hill, K. D., & Taylor, N. F. (2024). Self-management programs within rehabilitation yield positive health outcomes at a small increased cost compared with usual care: A systematic review and meta-analysis. *Archives of Physical Medicine and Rehabilitation*, *105*(10), 1946–1960. https://doi.org/10.1016/J.APMR.2024.05.007/ATTACHMENT/B0805A9A-A9B9-4A93-9766-5E2D260932A0/MMC1.DOCX

Wolf, E. (1966). *Peasants*. Prentice-Hall.

Zhang, Y. B., & Imamura, M. (2017). Communication accommodation theory and intergroup communication. In *Oxford research encyclopedia of communication*. Oxford University Press. https://doi.org/10.1093/ACREFORE/9780190228613.013.484

23 Integrating Dyadic Self-Management into Rehabilitation

Theoretical Perspectives, Practical Applications, and Considerations for Implementation

Olivia Crozier, Stephanie R. Cimino, Jacobi Elliott, Jeffrey D. Holmes, Janelle Unger, and Dalton L. Wolfe

HISTORY OF SELF-MANAGEMENT

The concept of self-management emerged in the mid-19th century, initially through interventions aimed at improving patient adherence to medications and treatments and promoting positive health behaviors (Creer, Renne and Christian, 1976). Early contributions include Thomas Creer's work in pediatric asthma, which emphasized how patient education and behavioral conditioning could be effective strategies to support disease management (Creer, Renne and Christian, 1976). Around the same time, Dr. Albert Bandura developed self-efficacy theory, highlighting the central role of an individual's perceived confidence in their ability to exert control over health-related behaviors, tasks, or disease management activities (Bandura, 1977; Creer, 1976).

Other early contributors to self-management include Corbin and Strauss (1985), who introduced a framework identifying three overarching tasks: medical, emotional, and role management, and five essential self-management skills: problem-solving, decision-making, resource utilization, forming partnerships with healthcare providers, and taking action (Corbin and Strauss, 1988). This framework has become a fundamental tool for designing interventions that promote patient autonomy, skill development, and goal setting across diverse health domains and patient populations. However, many health promotion and patient education programs have not been able to integrate all tasks and skills into this framework, prompting the evolution of new perspectives aimed at expanding and refining these traditional perspectives (Lorig and Holman, 2003). For instance, programs may emphasize disease-specific knowledge and symptom monitoring while neglecting relational skills such as communication, shared decision-making, or strategies to support care partner involvement.

One of these new perspectives came from Barlow and colleagues. In 2002, they provided an updated definition of self-management that integrated work done by previous investigators (Alderson *et al.*, 1999; Barlow, 2001; Clark *et al.*, 1991; D'Zurilla and Nezu, 1999; Nakagawa-Kogan *et al.*, 1988), which is now one of the most widely cited definitions of self-management in the chronic illness literature:

> …the individual's ability to manage the symptoms, treatment, physical and psychosocial consequences, and lifestyle changes inherent in living with a chronic condition. Efficacious self-management encompasses ability to monitor one's condition and the effect the cognitive, behavioural and emotional responses necessary to maintain a satisfactory quality of life.
>
> **(Barlow *et al.*, 2002)**

DOI: 10.1201/9781003599074-26

Lorig and collaborators at Stanford University, California, emerged as key pioneers in the development of self-management programming throughout the 1990s, independently advancing the field by embedding core behavioral principles into chronic disease interventions (Lorig *et al.*, 1999, 2001). Their work played a central role in shaping contemporary understandings of self-management, and in 2003, Lorig and Holman conceptualized self-management as an individual's ability to manage the symptoms, treatment, physical and psychosocial consequences, and the lifestyle changes inherent to living with a chronic condition (Lorig and Holman, 2003). In this work, they articulated a skill-based model that built upon and refined earlier conceptual foundations, most notably expanding Barlow's (2002) five core self-management skills with the additional principle of self-tailoring, influenced by the behavioral strategies of D'Zurilla and Nezu (1999). Self-tailoring refers to the ability of individuals to apply learned self-management knowledge in ways that are personally meaningful, contextually appropriate, and responsive to their evolving needs and circumstances (D'Zurilla and Nezu, 1999; Lorig and Holman, 2003). Together, these foundational perspectives established the underpinnings of self-management as it is understood today.

While traditional perspectives on self-management have contributed to improved clinical outcomes and reduced healthcare costs by empowering patients to manage their health and symptoms more effectively, they are often criticized for being overly focused on the individual (Dineen-Griffin *et al.*, 2019; Lorig and Holman, 2003). For example, by predominantly focusing on the individual's ability to manage symptoms, treatment, and lifestyle changes, this individualistic perspective aligns with neoliberal discourses of personal responsibility while underrepresenting the relational, and broader systemic, contextual factors that simultaneously shape the experiences of chronic disease management (Barlow *et al.*, 2002; Fletcher *et al.*, 2019; Newman, Steed and Mulligan, 2004). For example, some of these critical contextual factors that could impact an individual's capacity to engage in self-management include socioeconomic status, health literacy, geographic access to services, and cultural context (Fletcher *et al.*, 2019; Satink *et al.*, 2015).

While individual-focused models of self-management have been critiqued for neglecting relational and contextual influences, these limitations are particularly evident for individuals who require substantial daily support, such as older adults experiencing frailty or those living with neurological conditions. In such contexts, the active involvement of a care partner is often integral to effective management (Helgeson and Zajdel, 2017; Rosland, Heisler and Piette, 2012; Van Houtven, Voils and Weinberger, 2011). In this chapter, the term "care partner" refers to a family member or a friend who provides unpaid, informal support, rather than a paid caregiver or healthcare professional (Chai *et al.*, 2014). Support provided by care partners can include behavioral cueing (e.g., reminders to take medications, take smaller bites at mealtimes, or use bigger steps when walking), motivational support (e.g., positive words of encouragement), logistical coordination (e.g., scheduling, coordination and transportation to and from appointments), and physical assistance (e.g., helping in and out of the bathtub, bed, chair, or car). Despite the critical role care partners play in disease management, they are rarely acknowledged in mainstream definitions of self-management, leaving a critical dimension of self-management insufficiently addressed (Berger *et al.*, 2019; Clare *et al.*, 2018; Crozier *et al.*, 2025; Pigott *et al.*, 2022). Understandably, recognizing these limitations has prompted an evolution in self-management approaches, moving towards frameworks that take the interdependence between the patient and the care partner into consideration (Audulv *et al.*, 2021; Lorig and Holman, 2003; Lyons and Lee, 2018).

INTRODUCTION TO DYADIC SELF-MANAGEMENT PERSPECTIVES

The evolution towards dyadic self-management perspectives reflects the shift away from viewing the individual as the sole manager of their condition, towards conceptualizing disease management as a shared, relational, and co-constructed process. Early theoretical contributions that have guided this field include the coping congruence model by Revenson (1994); the relationship-focused model; Bodenmann's systemic-transactional model (1995); and the relational-cultural coping model by Kayser, Watson, and Andrade (2007). Among these perspectives, one particularly influential early theory was Interdependence Theory, first articulated by Thibaut and Kelley in 1959, but further developed in later decades (Van Lange and Balliet, 2015). Interdependence Theory states that individuals in close relationships can influence each other's outcomes through mutual responsiveness, shared goals, and coordinating behaviors (Thibaut and Kelley, 1959; Van Lange and Balliet, 2015). From this perspective, health-related decisions and actions are deeply embedded within relational contexts that influence motivation, meaning, and the capacity to act and make decisions (Thibaut and Kelley, 1959; Van Lange and Balliet, 2015). These theoretical perspectives paved the way for Bodenmann's Systemic-Transactional Model of Dyadic Coping (1997) which framed the management of stress and illness as a collaborative process in which two individuals jointly appraise challenges and engage in coordinated emotional behavioral strategies. Central to this model was the notion that relational attunement, mutual support, and joint problem-solving are not ancillary but essential when navigating the demands of chronic illness and disease (Bodenmann, 1995; Bodenmann *et al.*, 2008).

Looking forward to 2018, Lyons and Lee proposed the Theory of Dyadic Illness Management (TDIM) responding to more than a decade of empirical and theoretical research that primarily conceptualized illness management from the perspective of the patient alone or with incidental involvement from informal care partners. This theory reframes illness as a shared experience that requires coordinated appraisal, collaborative action, and mutual emotional adaptation between the patient and the care partner, otherwise known as the dyad (Lyons and Lee, 2018). The TDIM marks a shift from an individual focus on skills and capacities to an emphasis on the interactive and interdependent processes such as communication, goal alignment, empathy, and relational quality, as determinants of health for both partners. The central concepts within this model include dyadic appraisal, dyadic management, and dyadic health, which when taken together offer a structured framework for understanding and supporting joint illness management (Lyons and Lee, 2018).

Dyadic Appraisal

A central and novel principle of the TDIM is its shift from the individual appraisal of symptoms to the focus on the extent to which both members of the dyad share a common understanding of symptom severity and illness or disease impact (Lyons and Lee, 2018). This shared appraisal plays a pivotal role in shaping how dyads coordinate disease management activities and influences the overall health of both partners. For example, in Parkinson's disease, congruent symptom appraisals may foster greater collaboration and engagement in self-management behaviors, leading to improved outcomes for each member of the dyad. Dyadic appraisals are not static, and they vary according to contextual factors such as relationship dynamics, disease stage, and symptom experience (Lyons and Lee, 2018; Weitkamp *et al.*, 2021).

Importantly, dyadic appraisal is not just about agreeing on how severe symptoms are, it also applies to alignment in care values and preferences. For example, it may include discussions about what matters most to the person receiving care and how that individual wants that care delivered. In dementia care, a common problem is that the person living with dementia and their care partner do not always share the same understanding of these values due to forgotten, misinterpreted, or unknown care preferences (Lyons and Lee, 2018). The TDIM emphasizes that reducing incongruences early on and continuously re-evaluating throughout the disease process can ensure care decisions align with the patient's wishes while the care partner can proceed with confidence and legitimacy if they need to make decisions on the patient's behalf (Lyons and Lee, 2018).

While greater congruence can enhance dyadic management and, in some cases, directly improve dyadic health, adopting a dyadic perspective does not diminish the agency of either individual.

Instead, it broadens the analytic lens to reflect the inherently relational nature of disease management and the ways it is enacted collaboratively in daily life.

Dyadic Management

The next component of the TDIM emphasizes that patients and care partners engage in illness management along a continuum of collaboration, tailoring their approach to meet the needs of both individuals, a dimension rarely used in other theoretical models (Lyons and Lee, 2018). At one end of this spectrum, a single partner assumes primary responsibility for illness management behaviors and at the other, both members actively participate in actions aimed at promoting the health of the dyad as a whole.

Behaviors central to dyadic management can include shared decision-making, responding to changes in function or worsening symptoms, maintaining health-promoting behaviors, co-developing care plans, and implementing agreed-upon goals (Lyons and Lee, 2018). These activities can be placed along the continuum based on how responsibilities are distributed, and the degree of collaboration involved. This framing underscores that effective illness management is not solely about individual capacity, but about how both partners work together to sustain mutual health and well-being (Lyons and Lee, 2018).

Dyadic Health

The third central component is dyadic health, which emphasizes that the needs of both members of the dyad should be equally prioritized and effectively balanced (Lyons and Lee, 2018). Evidence indicates that the physical and emotional health of patients and care partners are inherently interconnected, often shifting in relation to one another (Bodenmann, 1995; Weitkamp *et al.*, 2021). Although numerous studies have examined dyadic self-management, many focus on individual patient or care partner outcomes to infer interpersonal dynamics. Such approaches do not constitute true dyadic research, as they fail to examine the dyad as an interdependent unit, limiting our understanding of how illness shapes shared health and functioning (Lyons and Lee, 2018). For example, an important consideration in this context is the language and terminology we often use to describe each member of the dyad. In many situations, particularly among older adults or individuals with neurological conditions, one member is designated as the "care partner" and the other is classified as the "patient." While this is common practice in clinical environments, this distinction can inadvertently minimize the health needs of the care partner and reinforce a hierarchy that positions one member's well-being as the priority (Lyons and Lee, 2018). Moreover, it is important to recognize that care partners themselves are often managing their own health challenges, and/or simultaneously providing care for multiple people, such as balancing responsibilities for an aging parent while also caring for a child, further underscoring the need for dyadic approaches that address the health and well-being of both partners (Applebaum, 2015; Choi *et al.*, 2019; Holliday, Quinlan and Schwartz, 2022; Vriendt *et al.*, 2012).

Contextual Factors

In addition to the three foundational concepts, and in contrast to traditional self-management definitions and models, the TDIM explicitly addresses the contextual factors that can either support or challenge dyadic appraisal and self-management behaviors. The influence of the contextual factors operates across micro-, meso-, and macro-levels, including individual (e.g., health literacy, coping style), dyadic (e.g., relationship quality, communication patterns), family/social (e.g., availability of family member and larger support networks), and cultural (e.g., norms, values, beliefs, and expectations) contexts. Recognizing and addressing these factors is essential for tailoring interventions that strengthen the capacity of both members to engage in effective, equitable illness management.

IMPACTS OF DYADIC SELF-MANAGEMENT APPROACHES

From a health system perspective, dyadic approaches such as the TDIM have the potential to improve healthcare efficiency and sustainability by empowering patients and care partners to manage symptoms, maintain therapy gains, and recognize early signs of decline which may reduce hospitalizations, emergency visits, and use of high-intensity services (e.g., goal-directed therapy or specialized treatment programs) (Lorig and Holman, 2003; Wensing, Grol and Grimshaw, 2020). Care partners often act as the navigator, ensuring continuity across care settings. By equipping both members of the dyad with shared knowledge and skills, these interventions can extend the benefits of rehabilitation well beyond the formal clinical encounter between patients and providers.

Emerging evidence suggests that dyadic self-management approaches can generate benefits across multiple levels. For patients, these interventions have been associated with improved adherence to rehabilitation programs, especially when care partners are involved in monitoring progress, cueing therapeutic activities, and reinforcing disease management behaviors (Lorig and Holman, 2003; Lyons and Lee, 2018). Structured joint sessions can help align patient and care partner's expectations and strategies, allowing patients to experience consistent reinforcement both in the clinic and at home. Programs that integrate communication and coping skills training can also help patients navigate frustration, uncertainty, and the emotional impact of functional change (Badr *et al.*, 2010). Over time, this approach could strengthen patients' self-efficacy in their ability to manage symptoms and trust in their support system (Chan, 2018).

Care partners have also benefitted from participating in dyadic interventions. Meaningful involvement in rehabilitation planning can clarify care partner roles, reduce uncertainty, and provide practical tools for supporting the patient's activities of daily living (Karlstedt *et al.*, 2017). When care partners feel prepared and supported, their own health and resilience improves, sustaining their ability to provide effective care over longer periods of time (Gutierrez-Baena, Gilart and Romero-Grimaldi, 2024; Uhm *et al.*, 2023). Training in stress management, communication, and adaptive coping can lessen the risk of burnout, anxiety, and depression which are common concerns among those caring for someone with a chronic or neurological condition (Anderson *et al.*, 2019; Chiu *et al.*, 2020).

Perhaps most distinctively, dyadic self-management has shown to strengthen the dyad as a relational unit (Lyons and Lee, 2018; Weitkamp *et al.*, 2021; Weitkamp and Bodenmann, 2022). By promoting joint problem-solving, shared decision-making, and emotional reciprocity, these approaches can improve relationship quality which is a factor linked to better rehabilitation engagement and long-term health outcomes for both partners (Lyons and Lee, 2018). This relational strengthening can help buffer against the strains of disease progression, supporting both members in adapting together rather than in parallel.

APPLICATIONS AND IMPLEMENTATION OF DYADIC SELF-MANAGEMENT IN REHABILITATION

The growing evidence base for dyadic self-management leads to questions about how these approaches can be systematically embedded into rehabilitation practice. Rehabilitation is broadly defined as a goal-oriented, person-centered process that enables individuals with health conditions or impairments to optimize functioning, independence, and quality of life through coordinated interventions delivered by interdisciplinary teams (World Health Organization, 2024). While early studies demonstrate promising outcomes for both patients and care partners, moving from theory to implementation requires attention to feasibility, staff training, contextual adaptations, and rigorous and continuous evaluation. Implementation science offers a variety of frameworks, theories, methods, and tools to guide this process, enabling interventions to be adapted, scaled, and sustained in real-world clinical settings (Bowen, 2009; Damschroder *et al.*, 2022; Roundtable on Translating Genomic-Based Research for Health *et al.*, 2016).

Rehabilitation environments are conducive to the relational and collaborative processes involved with dyadic self-management perspectives due to its participatory and function-oriented nature (Lyons and Lee, 2018). Rehabilitation programs aim not only to restore or optimize physical function but also to foster long-term self-management, enhance community participation, and address psychosocial needs; goals that often necessitate the active involvement of care partners or family members (Choo *et al.*, 2022; Cianci, 2007; Clare *et al.*, 2018; Noonan *et al.*, 2019; Quinn *et al.*, 2020). This is particularly critical in progressive and often unpredictable conditions such as Parkinson's disease, multiple sclerosis, and dementia, where care demands can extend over years and require ongoing adaptation to shifting needs (Clare *et al.*, 2018; Lutz *et al.*, 2016; Quinn *et al.*, 2016).

In such contexts, engaging both members of the dyad is essential for sustaining therapy participation, preventing secondary complications, and preserving quality of life for both patient and care partner (Bäckström and Sundin, 2009; Rosland, Heisler and Piette, 2012, 2012; Weitkamp and Bodenmann, 2022). Despite the clear relevance, care partner engagement remains underrepresented in many rehabilitation-based self-management programs, especially for neurological conditions. For example, Kessler and Liddy (2017) identified 18 self-management programs for Parkinson's disease, of which only three included family members. Similarly, Crozier *et al.* (2025) found only 34 self-management interventions involving care partners of individuals with neurodegenerative movement disorders, with just over half (n = 17) meaningfully involved both members of the dyad either through joint education or a mix of individual and blended learning strategies.

Barriers to Implementing Dyadic Approaches into Rehabilitation Practice

Although dyadic models of illness management have gained increasing attention over recent years, their translation into rehabilitation clinical practice remains inconsistent. The gap in dyadic-oriented programs and interventions highlights a critical implementation challenge, as despite well-documented evidence supporting their value, their translation into routine rehabilitation practice remains inconsistent due to a range of practical, relational, organizational, and systemic challenges (Karlstedt *et al.*, 2017; Lyons and Lee, 2018; Rosland, Heisler and Piette, 2012; Weitkamp and Bodenmann, 2022). The following section of this chapter examines the practical barriers that may impede the adoption of dyadic models in rehabilitation settings, followed by strategies grounded in implementation science to overcome these challenges.

Lack of Conceptual Clarity and Standardization

One of the most persistent barriers to integrating dyadic approaches into rehabilitation practice is the lack of conceptual clarity and consistent operationalization across research and clinical contexts. While the TDIM (Lyons and Lee, 2018) and related dyadic models offer structured frameworks, definitions of "dyadic self-management" and "dyadic health" vary widely, both in scope and in the behaviors they involve. This variability complicates the translation of theory into practice, as clinicians may be uncertain about the core components that must be addressed to constitute a true dyadic intervention. For example, some programs emphasize joint symptom appraisal and shared decision-making, whereas others focus on broader relational factors such as communication quality or emotional support (Badr *et al.*, 2010; Lyons and Lee, 2018; Weitkamp and Bodenmann, 2022).

The lack of standardized outcome measures further exacerbates the problem. Existing tools often capture individual health status or caregiver burden separately, without assessing the dyad as an interdependent unit (Weitkamp and Bodenmann, 2022). This gap limits the ability to evaluate intervention effectiveness and to compare findings across studies or settings. In rehabilitation, where time and resources are already constrained, the absence of a clear, consensus-driven model can result in fragmented adoption, where only select dyadic elements are incorporated rather than a comprehensive, integrated approach (Rosland, Heisler and Piette, 2012). The theoretical appeal of dyadic models may thus fail to translate into routine practice unless supported by operational guidelines and validated measures (Audulv *et al.*, 2021).

Interpersonal and Relational Complexities among the Dyad

Many dyadic models implicitly assume that patient-care partner relationships are cooperative, communicative, and mutually supportive, when in reality dyads may face substantial relational challenges that complicate the implementation of collaborative, dyadic approaches. These barriers may include pre-existing interpersonal conflict, differences in coping styles, imbalances in caregiving responsibilities, and emotional strain linked to the disease trajectory (Holmes *et al.*, 2025; Lyons and Lee, 2018). In progressive conditions involving cognitive decline, such as Parkinson's disease, dementia, stroke, multiple sclerosis, or Alzheimer's disease, communication breakdowns can further limit the feasibility of shared decision-making, with care partners taking on an increasingly directive role (Clare *et al.*, 2018; Rosland, Heisler and Piette, 2012).

Building on these challenges, the focus on shared processes within dyadic models can inadvertently obscure the distinct needs of care partners, who may experience fatigue, stress, or role overload. Some care partners also use the time their partner is engaged in rehabilitation sessions for their own self-care needs (e.g., going for a coffee or reading a book) and therefore feel little motivation to attend sessions as part of a dyad. The resulting increase in caregiver burden and competing demands may diminish the capacity of care partners to effectively participate in rehabilitation programs. This is particularly salient in high-intensity programs, where session frequency and complexity can place substantial demands on both members of the dyad. Without adequate support, care partners may disengage or resist participation, undermining the intended benefits of the intervention (Rosland, Heisler and Piette, 2012). Addressing these relational complexities requires interventions that are flexible, sensitive to interpersonal histories, and supported by services that support the mental health and resilience of both partners.

Logistical and Organizational Challenges

Rehabilitation programs and interventions are often time-limited (e.g., outpatient day programs commonly occurring for up to 12 weeks), which may not align with the ongoing, evolving nature of dyadic illness management. Thus, coordinating the participation of both patient and care partner in rehabilitation sessions poses significant logistical challenges. Scheduling difficulties are compounded in health systems with fragmented services, long wait times, or limited capacity of health care professionals to address the needs of both members of the dyad during a joint appointment. Even when attendance is feasible, differences in readiness to engage, whether due to emotional factors, competing priorities, or uncertainty about the relevance of the intervention, can limit the effectiveness of dyadic approaches (Karlstedt *et al.*, 2017). Many health systems also prioritize efficiency, leaving minimal room for the additional time required to assess both members of the dyad, facilitate shared goal setting, and adapt care plans accordingly (Dineen-Griffin *et al.*, 2019). Furthermore, funding models and performance metrics tend to focus on individual patient outcomes, creating systemic disincentives for the sustained involvement of care partners.

Clinicians themselves may face barriers related to workload, competing clinical priorities, and a lack of organizational support for dyadic practice. Rehabilitation professionals require advanced skills in relational facilitation and conflict resolution, skills not traditionally included in discipline-specific training, to navigate these dynamics and maintain therapeutic momentum (Bodenmann *et al.*, 2008; Lyons and Lee, 2018). Additional logistical barriers also arise from the constraints of working with care partners, who are not formally recognized as patients, creating uncertainty around scope of practice, liability, and institutional responsibility. Without clear protocols, integrated referral pathways, and administrative support, even motivated clinicians may struggle to embed dyadic approaches within existing workflows (Lyons and Lee, 2018).These challenges highlight the need for organizational commitment, including policy changes, staffing models that support dyadic care, and investment in interdisciplinary training to operationalize dyadic principles within rehabilitation settings.

Equity and Contextual Considerations

Access to rehabilitation and overall healthcare is shaped by a complex interplay of socioeconomic, cultural, and geographic factors. Much of the existing research on dyadic approaches to self-management has been conducted in high-resource, urban settings with relatively homogenous populations, raising questions about the transferability of findings to more diverse or underserved communities (Audulv *et al.*, 2021). In rural or remote areas, geographic distance, limited rehabilitation infrastructure, and inadequate access can restrict participation.

Cultural norms and expectations about caregiving roles may also influence the acceptability and uptake of dyadic approaches. For example, in some cultural contexts, family members may prioritize the patient's needs above their own to such an extent that care partner well-being is overlooked (Satink *et al.*, 2015). In other cases, illness management may be viewed as a collective responsibility shared among extended family networks (Satink *et al.*, 2015). Dyadic models that do not account for such variability risk imposing culturally incongruent expectations that undermine engagement.

Socioeconomic barriers, including lower health literacy, competing employment demands, and limited financial resources, can further constrain participation in dyadic rehabilitation. These factors may not only limit access to the intervention but also affect the sustainability of behavioral changes promoted by dyadic interventions. Addressing equity considerations requires tailored strategies that incorporate culturally competent practices, flexible delivery models, and support mechanisms that reduce logistical and financial burdens for both partners (Fletcher *et al.*, 2019; Pigott *et al.*, 2022).

Given the barriers described here, it is evident that the integration of the TDIM into rehabilitation practice is constrained, despite the compelling nature of this framework to conceptualize illness as a shared process and positioning the dyad as the unit of care. However, it may be possible to overcome these barriers using implementation science and capacity building. While the value of dyadic approaches is increasingly recognized in chronic disease and rehabilitation research, their integration into care remains inconsistent, often limited to small-scale programs or isolated pilot studies (Audulv *et al.*, 2021; Lyons and Lee, 2018).

Leveraging Implementation Science to Integrate Dyadic Approaches in Rehabilitation

The translation of dyadic illness management approaches into rehabilitation practice is a complex process that requires structured, evidence-informed strategies. This variability underscores the importance of implementation science, a discipline concerned with the systematic uptake of research evidence into healthcare policy and practice to improve quality and effectiveness (Damschroder *et al.*, 2022; ; Nilsen, 2015; Roundtable on Translating Genomic-Based Research for Health *et al.*, 2016).

Implementation science provides both conceptual and practical tools for understanding why promising interventions can succeed or fail in real-world settings and how they can be adapted for sustainability (Bowen *et al.*, 2009; Nilsen, 2015; Roundtable on Translating Genomic-Based Research for Health *et al.*, 2016). The Consolidated Framework for Implementation Research (CFIR) and Reach, Effectiveness, Adoption, Implementation, and Maintenance (RE-AIM) framework are two implementation science frameworks that are particularly well-suited to understand the influences impacting how dyadic approaches can be integrated into rehabilitation contexts and/or to systematically evaluate implementation (Damschroder *et al.*, 2022; Glasgow *et al.*, 2001, 2019).

The CFIR is a determinant framework that offers a theoretical structure that consolidates multiple implementation theories into a comprehensive taxonomy of 39 constructs across the following five domains (Table 23.1): (1) Intervention Characteristics; (2) Outer Setting; (3) Inner Setting; (4) Characteristics of Individuals; and (5) Process (Damschroder *et al.*, 2022). When applied to dyadic rehabilitation, the CFIR can identify both barriers and facilitators to implementation by highlighting context-specific dynamics. Potential barriers may include perceptions that dyadic care increases workflow complexity or evidence of limited organizational readiness, whereas facilitators

TABLE 23.1
The Consolidated Framework for Implementation Research (CFIR) Constructs

CFIR Domains	Domain Constructs
Intervention Characteristics	1. Intervention Source
	2. Evidence Strength & Quality
	3. Relative Advantage
	4. Adaptability
	5. Trialability
	6. Complexity
	7. Design Quality & Packaging
	8. Cost
Outer Setting	9. Patient Needs & Resources
	10. Cosmopolitanism
	11. Peer Pressure
	12. External Policy & Incentives
Inner Setting	13. Structural Characteristics
	14. Networks & Communications
	15. Culture
	16. Implementation Climate
	a. Tension for Change
	b. Compatibility
	c. Relative Priority
	d. Organizational Incentives & Rewards
	e. Goals & Feedback
	f. Learning Climate
	17. Readiness for Implementation
	a. Leadership Engagement
	b. Available Resources
	c. Access to Knowledge & Information
Characteristics of Individuals	18. Knowledge & Beliefs about the Intervention
	19. Self-efficacy
	20. Individual Stage of Change
	21. Individual Identification with Organization
	22. Other Personal Attributes
Process	23. Planning
	24. Engaging
	a. Opinion leaders
	b. Formally Appointed Internal Implementation Leaders
	c. Champions
	d. External Change Agents
	25. Executing
	26. Reflecting & Evaluating

may involve visible leadership engagement or recognition of the relative advantage of dyadic approaches compared with traditional individualized models. Within the domain of *Intervention Characteristics*, constructs such as adaptability (i.e., tailoring dyadic protocols to align with the practices of different rehabilitation disciplines) and trialability (i.e., piloting dyadic strategies on a small scale before broader integration) serve as key levers for adoption. Similarly, within the *Inner Setting* domain, examining organizational culture, communication networks, and established norms regarding care partner involvement in care can provide critical insight into the degree of readiness to embed dyadic approaches into routine rehabilitation practice. Importantly, care partners are not always family members; they may include friends, neighbors, or paid caregivers, which introduces additional layers of relational and role complexity for clinicians to navigate. Ultimately, by mapping these constructs onto local rehabilitation contexts or programs, the CFIR enables systematic identification of the specific barriers that must be addressed to support successful and sustainable implementation.

The RE-AIM, in contrast, is an evaluation framework that focuses on the pragmatic evaluation of health interventions across five dimensions (Table 23.2) (Glasgow *et al.*, 2001, 2019).

In practice, CFIR and RE-AIM often complement each other. The CFIR is most useful in the diagnostic stages to assist with identifying the barriers and facilitators to implementation, while the RE-AIM is focused on helping teams determine the reach and sustainability of interventions. Together, they encourage a cycle of continuous quality improvement in which barriers are identified, addressed, and monitored over time. For example, a rehabilitation program piloting a dyadic Parkinson's self-management program could use CFIR to assess readiness (e.g., staff perceptions of value, leadership engagement, resource availability) and RE-AIM to track participation rates, dyadic outcomes, and maintenance of practices. Importantly, implementation science emphasizes stakeholder engagement, including patients, care partners, clinicians, and administrators, throughout design, testing, and scaling, ensuring that dyadic programs are contextually relevant and feasible (Damschroder *et al.*, 2022; Nilsen, 2015).

In addition to these frameworks, there are many other implementation science theories, models and frameworks that can help researchers translate theory and concepts such as dyadic management into clinical practice. Process models can guide the step-by-step planning and execution of implementation strategies (i.e., Quality Implementation Framework, the Exploration, Adoption/Preparation, Implementation, Sustainment (EPIS) model); determinant frameworks can identify contextual barriers and enablers (i.e., the CFIR, Active Implementation Framework, Theoretical Domains Framework); classic theories can explain behavior change mechanisms (i.e., Behavioral theories, Organizational theories); implementation theories can offer detailed constructs to design tailored interventions (i.e., Organizational readiness for change, Implementation climate); and evaluation frameworks can support the assessment of implementation outcomes across different levels

TABLE 23.2
RE-AIM Framework Constructs

RE-AIM Construct	Description
Reach	The extent to which eligible dyads are engaged, accounting for equity considerations such as cultural and linguistic appropriateness.
Effectiveness	The degree to which the approach improves outcomes for *both* patient and care partner, including quality of life, emotional well-being, and functional independence.
Adoption	The proportion and representativeness of rehabilitation settings and clinicians that choose to implement dyadic care.
Implementation	The fidelity, consistency, and adaptations made during delivery.
Maintenance	The extent to which dyadic practices are sustained over time within clinical workflows.

of care (i.e., RE-AIM, Stages of Implementation Completion) (Damschroder *et al.*, 2022; Nilsen, 2015; Roundtable on Translating Genomic-Based Research for Health *et al.*, 2016).

The deliberate use of implementation models, frameworks, and theories in dyadic rehabilitation shifts the focus from isolated program innovation to system-wide integration. By embedding these methods, rehabilitation services can improve the likelihood that dyadic approaches move beyond experimental pilot studies to become a consistent approach to care.

Capacity Building and Workforce Training for Dyadic Rehabilitation

Dyadic approaches require clinicians to extend their focus from the patient as the sole unit of care to the patient-care partner dyad as an interdependent system. This reframing changes not only how assessments are conducted but also how interventions are designed, delivered, and evaluated. It involves engaging both members in goal setting, balancing competing needs, navigating interpersonal dynamics, and facilitating collaborative problem-solving (Northouse *et al.*, 2012). Without targeted training, many clinicians may feel ill-equipped to manage the emotional complexity or communication challenges that can arise, especially in the context of progressive illnesses, cognitive decline, or strained relationships (Holmes *et al.*, 2025).

A critical barrier to implementing dyadic illness management in rehabilitation is the lack of training and minimal capacity to deliver dyad focused interventions. While most rehabilitation professionals such as physiotherapists, occupational therapists, speech-language pathologists, nurses, and social workers are trained in discipline-specific therapeutic skills, very few receive formal education in dyadic engagement, relational facilitation, or family systems theory (Glasgow *et al.*, 2001, 2019). This gap not only limits clinician confidence but can also perpetuate a default to individual-focused models of care, even when the presence of a care partner is central to the success of rehabilitation.

Capacity building is also important because dyadic care often requires interdisciplinary coordination. For example, a physiotherapist working with a patient living with Parkinson's disease on falls prevention strategies might need to coordinate with a speech-language pathologist to ensure the care partner and patient understand the importance of caloric intake for muscle mass, or with a social worker to discuss safe transportation options. These connections are strengthened when all team members have a shared understanding of dyadic principles and their relevance to rehabilitation outcomes.

Advancing dyadic approaches in rehabilitation will require a deliberate focus on clinician training that equips the workforce to address the relational, emotional, and practical complexities of patient-care partner partnerships. Priority content areas for professional development include foundational knowledge of dyadic theories, such as the TDIM (Lyons and Lee, 2018) skill-building in relational facilitation (e.g., mediating differences in symptom appraisal, aligning goals, and negotiating roles), and competence in using and interpreting validated dyadic assessment tools to inform care planning (Badr *et al.*, 2010; Weitkamp and Bodenmann, 2022; Whitlatch *et al.*, 2006). Organizational support, in the form of protected time for training, structured care pathways that incorporate care partners, and access to evidence-based tools and resources, will be critical to sustain implementation and ensure these skills translate into improved outcomes for both members of the dyad (Fixsen, Barrett, and Shimonovich, 2022).

FUTURE CONSIDERATIONS FOR RESEARCHERS

While dyadic coping theories such as the TDIM have become more common, Lyons and Lee (2018) emphasize the need for targeted research to advance its application and validity across diverse clinical and community contexts. A priority area is the longitudinal study of dyadic appraisal, which includes exploring how congruence or incongruence in perceptions of illness severity, impact, and care values evolves over time, and how these shifts reciprocally influence dyadic management behaviors (Lyons and Lee, 2018; Weitkamp *et al.*, 2021). Understanding the temporal dynamics of appraisal could illuminate critical intervention points that optimize collaborative care (Lyons and Lee, 2018).

A second area involves the comprehensive examination of dyadic management behaviors. Existing research has often been limited to symptom monitoring and care tasks; however, a broader investigation into decision-making, role negotiation, shared daily health behaviors, and balancing the needs of both members is essential. Such studies should also account for contextual factors, including relationship quality and communication, health literacy, and cultural norms, which may influence the dyads' capacity for collaboration (Audulv *et al.*, 2021; Holmes *et al.*, 2025). The TDIM also calls for the development and evaluation of dyad-focused interventions or programs in which the dyad is both the target and the unit of change. Research should investigate not only the timing, mechanisms, and conditions under which such interventions are most effective, but also how their effectiveness may vary depending on illness type, stage of disease progression, and dyad configuration (e.g., spousal, adult child-parent, friend, or paid caregiver relationships) (Orsulic-Jeras *et al.*, 2019). In addition, future work is needed to determine which components of dyadic interventions (e.g., joint goal setting, communication training, stress management, shared problem-solving) are most impactful, and how these elements interact with contextual factors such as cultural expectations, health system structures, and resource availability. This level of inquiry will not only advance theory but also inform the design of flexible, scalable models of dyadic care that can be meaningfully integrated into rehabilitation.

CONCLUSION

The evolution of self-management from individual-focused models to dyadic approaches reflects a necessary shift in rehabilitation science. Early frameworks by Creer, Bandura, Corbin, and Strauss advanced autonomy and self-efficacy but often overlooked the relational and contextual realities of chronic illness management. The TDIM (Lyons and Lee, 2018) reframes illness and disease as a shared, interdependent process, emphasizing joint appraisal, collaborative management, and dyadic health. This perspective is particularly relevant in progressive and complex conditions, where patient and care partner outcomes are inherently linked.

Evidence demonstrates that dyadic approaches can enhance adherence, functional outcomes, relationship quality, and care partner well-being, while reducing healthcare utilization ((Badr *et al.*, 2010; Lyons and Lee, 2018). However, their implementation in rehabilitation remains inconsistent due to conceptual ambiguity, staff and healthcare capacity gaps, logistical constraints, and access inequities. Addressing these challenges requires targeted training in relational facilitation, conflict resolution, and dyadic assessment, supported by organizational infrastructure and policy incentives.

Implementation science frameworks such as CFIR and RE-AIM offer structured pathways for integrating dyadic care into routine practice, enabling context-sensitive adaptation, rigorous evaluation, and sustainability. Future research should prioritize the development of dyad-specific outcome measures, longitudinal studies on dyadic processes, and testing in diverse and underserved populations.

Embedding dyadic self-management as a standard in rehabilitation will require coordinated efforts across research, clinical practice, and policy. By positioning the dyad as the unit of care, rehabilitation can better reflect the lived realities of disease management, improve outcomes for both members, and advance health system sustainability.

REFERENCES

Alderson, M. *et al.* (1999) "The program for rheumatic independent self-management: A pilot evaluation," *Clinical Rheumatology*, 18(4), pp. 283–292. Available at: https://doi.org/10.1007/s100670050103.

Anderson, J.G. *et al.* (2019) "A fine line that we walk every day': Self-care approaches used by family caregivers of persons with dementia," *Issues in Mental Health Nursing*, 40(3), pp. 252–259. Available at: https://doi.org/10.1080/01612840.2018.1499156.

Applebaum, A. (2015) "Isolated, invisible, and in-need: There should be no 'I' in caregiver," *Palliative & Supportive Care*, 13(3), pp. 415–416. Available at: https://doi.org/10.1017/S1478951515000413.
Audulv, Å *et al.* (2021) "Managing everyday life: Self-management strategies people use to live well with neurological conditions," *Patient Education and Counseling*, 104(2), pp. 413–421. Available at: https://doi.org/10.1016/j.pec.2020.07.025.
Bäckström, B. and Sundin, K. (2009) "The experience of being a middle-aged close relative of a person who has suffered a stroke, 1 year after discharge from a rehabilitation clinic: A qualitative study," *International Journal of Nursing Studies*, 46(11), pp. 1475–1484. Available at: https://doi.org/10.1016/j.ijnurstu.2009.04.009.
Badr, H. *et al.* (2010) "Dyadic coping in metastatic breast cancer," *Health Psychology : Official Journal of the Division of Health Psychology, American Psychological Association*, 29(2), pp. 169–180. Available at: https://doi.org/10.1037/a0018165.
Bandura, A. (1977) "Self-efficacy: Toward a unifying theory of behavioral change," *Psychological Review*, 84(2), pp. 191–215. Available at: https://doi.org/10.1037//0033-295x.84.2.191.
Barlow, J. (2001) "How to use education as an intervention in osteoarthritis," *Best Practice & Research Clinical Rheumatology*, 15(4), pp. 545–558. Available at: https://doi.org/10.1053/berh.2001.0172.
Barlow, J. *et al.* (2002) "Self-management approaches for people with chronic conditions: A review," *Patient Education and Counseling*, 48(2), pp. 177–187. Available at: https://doi.org/10.1016/S0738-3991(02)00032-0.
Berger, S. *et al.* (2019) "The self-management balancing act of spousal care partners in the case of Parkinson's disease," *Disability and Rehabilitation*, 41(8), pp. 887–895. Available at: https://doi.org/10.1080/09638288.2017.1413427.
Bodenmann, G. (1995) "A systemic-transactional conceptualization of stress and coping in couples," *Swiss Journal of Psychology*, 54(1), pp. 34–49.
Bodenmann, G. *et al.* (2008) "Effects of coping-oriented couples therapy on depression: A randomized clinical trial," *Journal of Consulting and Clinical Psychology*, 76(6), pp. 944–954. Available at: https://doi.org/10.1037/a0013467.
Bowen, D.J. *et al.* (2009) "How we design feasibility studies," *American Journal of Preventive Medicine*, 36(5), pp. 452–457. Available at: https://doi.org/10.1016/j.amepre.2009.02.002.
Bowen, G. (2009) "Document analysis as a qualitative research method," *Qualitative Research Journal*, 9, pp. 27–40. Available at: https://doi.org/10.3316/QRJ0902027.
Chai, H. *et al.* (2014) "The magnitude, share and determinants of unpaid care costs for home-based palliative care service provision in Toronto, Canada," *Health & Social Care in the Community*, 22(1), pp. 30–39. Available at: https://doi.org/10.1111/hsc.12058.
Chan, B. (2018) "An evaluation of the influence of the care (compassion and respect at the end-of-life) program on registered nurses' knowledge and comfort about end-of-life care and care delivery for patients with life-limiting illnesses," *Dissertation Abstracts International: Section B: The Sciences and Engineering*, 79(8-B(E)), pp. 1–9.
Chiu, Y.-C. *et al.* (2020) "The mediating effects of leisure engagement on relationships between caregiving stress and subjective wellbeing among family caregivers of persons with cognitive impairment: A cross-sectional study," *Geriatric Nursing (New York, N.Y.)*, 41(2), pp. 124–131. Available at: https://doi.org/10.1016/j.gerinurse.2019.08.017.
Choi, S.-M. *et al.* (2019) "Analysis of characteristics affecting instrumental activities of daily living in Parkinson's disease patients without dementia," *Neurological Sciences: Official Journal of the Italian Neurological Society and of the Italian Society of Clinical Neurophysiology*, 40(7), pp. 1403–1408. Available at: https://doi.org/10.1007/s10072-019-03860-0.
Choo, W.T. *et al.* (2022) "Effectiveness of caregiver-mediated exercise interventions on activities of daily living, anxiety and depression post-stroke rehabilitation: A systematic review and meta-analysis," *Journal of Advanced Nursing*, 78(7), pp. 1870–1882. Available at: https://doi.org/10.1111/jan.15239.
Cianci, H.J. (2007) "Rehabilitation Interventions in Parkinson's Disease," in Comprehensive Nursing Care for Parkinson's Disease. New York: Springer Publishing Company, pp. 233–253. https://books.google.co.mz/books?id=ngMyzHmrjN4C&pg=PR3&hl=pt-PT&source=gbs_selected_pages&cad=1#v=onepage&q&f=false
Clare, L. *et al.* (2018) "Cognitive rehabilitation, self-management, psychotherapeutic and caregiver support interventions in progressive neurodegenerative conditions: A scoping review," *NeuroRehabilitation*, 43(4), pp. 443–471. Available at: https://doi.org/10.3233/NRE-172353.
Clark, N.M. *et al.* (1991) "Self-management of chronic disease by older adults: A review and questions for research," *Journal of Aging and Health*, 3(1), pp. 3–27. Available at: https://doi.org/10.1177/089826439100300101.

Corbin, J., and Strauss, A. (1985). "Managing chronic illness at home: Three lines of work," *Qualitative Sociology*, 8(3), pp. 224–247. Available at: https://doi.org/10.1007/BF00989485.

Corbin, J.M. and Strauss, A.L. (1988) *Unending Work and Care: Managing Chronic Illness at Home*. Minnesota: Jossey-Bass Publishers. https://books.google.ca/books?id=RLH8V527HqwC

Creer, T.L. (1976) *Chronically Ill and Handicapped Children: Their Management and Rehabilitation*. Champaign: Research Press.

Creer, T.L., Renne, C.M. and Christian, W.P. (1976) "Behavioral contributions to rehabilitation and childhood asthma," *Rehabilitation Literature*, 37(8), pp. 226–232, 247.

Crozier, O. *et al.* (2025) "Self-management interventions involving care partners of individuals with neurodegenerative movement disorders: A scoping review," *Disability and Rehabilitation*, pp. 1–20. Available at: https://doi.org/10.1080/09638288.2025.2496784.

D'Zurilla, T.J. and Nezu, A.M. (1999) *Problem-Solving Therapy: A Social Competence Approach to Clinical Intervention*. New York: Springer Pub.

Damschroder, L.J. *et al.* (2022) "The updated consolidated framework for implementation research based on user feedback," *Implementation Science*, 17(1), p. 75. Available at: https://doi.org/10.1186/s13012-022-01245-0.

Dineen-Griffin, S. *et al.* (2019) "Helping patients help themselves: A systematic review of self-management support strategies in primary health care practice," *PloS One*, 14(8), p. e0220116. Available at: https://doi.org/10.1371/journal.pone.0220116.

Fixsen, D. A., Barrett, D. S., and Shimonovich, M. (2022). "Supporting vulnerable populations during the pandemic: Stakeholders' experiences and perceptions of social prescribing in Scotland during Covid-19," *Qualitative Health Research*, *32*(4), pp. 670–682. Available at: https://doi.org/10.1177/10497323211064229.

Fletcher, S. *et al.* (2019) "The problem with self-management: Problematising self-management and power using a Foucauldian lens in the context of stroke care and rehabilitation," *PLoS ONE*, 14(6), p. e0218517. Available at: https://doi.org/10.1371/journal.pone.0218517.

Glasgow, R.E. *et al.* (2001) "The RE-AIM framework for evaluating interventions: What can it tell us about approaches to chronic illness management?," *Patient Education and Counseling*, 44(2), pp. 119–127. Available at: https://doi.org/10.1016/s0738-3991(00)00186-5.

Glasgow, R.E. *et al.* (2019) "RE-AIM planning and evaluation framework: Adapting to new science and practice with a 20-year review," *Frontiers in Public Health*, 7, p. 64. Available at: https://doi.org/10.3389/fpubh.2019.00064.

Gutierrez-Baena, B., Gilart, E. and Romero-Grimaldi, C. (2024) "Factors associated with and predictive model for resilience in family caregivers of care-dependent adults," *Nursing Reports*, 14(4), pp. 3476–3487. Available at: https://doi.org/10.3390/nursrep14040253.

Helgeson, V.S. and Zajdel, M. (2017) "Adjusting to chronic health conditions," *Annual Review of Psychology*, 68(1), pp. 545–571. Available at: https://doi.org/10.1146/annurev-psych-010416-044014.

Holliday, A.M., Quinlan, C.M. and Schwartz, A.W. (2022) "The hidden patient: The CARE framework to care for caregivers," *Journal of Family Medicine and Primary Care*, 11(1), pp. 5–9. Available at: https://doi.org/10.4103/jfmpc.jfmpc_719_21.

Holmes, J.D., Rempel, H.A. *et al.* (2025) "Voices of care: Navigating difficult conversations among caregivers and individuals with Parkinson's disease," *Disability and Rehabilitation*, 47(8), pp. 1–12. Available at: https://doi.org/10.1080/09638288.2025.2486456.

Karlstedt, M. *et al.* (2017) "Determinants of dyadic relationship and its psychosocial impact in patients with Parkinson's disease and their spouses," *Parkinson's Disease*, 2017, p. 4697052. Available at: https://doi.org/10.1155/2017/4697052.

Kayser, K., Watson, L. E., and Andrade, J. T. (2007). "Cancer as a "we-disease": Examining the process of coping from a relational perspective," *Families, Systems, & Health*, *25*(4), pp. 404–418. Available at: https://doi.org/10.1037/1091-7527.25.4.404.

Kessler, D., and Liddy, C. (2017). "Self-management support programs for persons with Parkinson's disease: An integrative review," *Patient Education and Counseling*, *100*(10), pp. 1787–1795. Available at: https://doi.org/10.1016/j.pec.2017.04.011.

Lorig, K.R. *et al.* (1999) "Evidence suggesting that a chronic disease self-management program can improve health status while reducing hospitalization: A randomized trial," *Medical Care*, 37(1), pp. 5–14. Available at: https://doi.org/10.1097/00005650-199901000-00003.

Lorig, K.R. *et al.* (2001) "Chronic disease self-management program: 2-year health status and health care utilization outcomes," *Medical Care*, 39(11), pp. 1217–1223. Available at: https://doi.org/10.1097/00005650-200111000-00008.

Lorig, K.R. and Holman, H. (2003) "Self-management education: History, definition, outcomes, and mechanisms," *Annals of Behavioral Medicine: A Publication of the Society of Behavioral Medicine*, 26(1), pp. 1–7. Available at: https://doi.org/10.1207/S15324796ABM2601_01.

Lutz, S.G. *et al.* (2016) "Clinical presentation of anxiety in Parkinson's disease: A scoping review," *OTJR: Occupation, Participation and Health*, 36(3), pp. 134–147. Available at: https://doi.org/10.1177/1539449216661714.

Lyons, K.S. and Lee, C.S. (2018) "The theory of dyadic illness management," *Journal of Family Nursing*, 24(1), pp. 8–28. Available at: https://doi.org/10.1177/1074840717745669.

Lyons, K. S. *et al.* (2021). "Benefits of a self-management program for the couple living with Parkinson's disease: A pilot study," *Journal of Applied Gerontology : The Official Journal of the Southern Gerontological Society*, 40(8), pp. 881–889. Available at: https://doi.org/10.1177/0733464820918136.

Nakagawa-Kogan, H. *et al.* (1988) "Self-management of hypertension: Predictors of success in diastolic blood pressure reduction," *Research in Nursing & Health*, 11(2), pp. 105–115. Available at: https://doi.org/10.1002/nur.4770110206.

Newman, S., Steed, L. and Mulligan, K. (2004) "Self-management interventions for chronic illness," *Lancet (London, England)*, 364(9444), pp. 1523–1537. Available at: https://doi.org/10.1016/S0140-6736(04)17277-2.

Nilsen, P. (2015) "Making sense of implementation theories, models and frameworks," *Implementation Science*, 10(1), p. 53. Available at: https://doi.org/10.1186/s13012-015-0242-0.

Noonan, M.C. *et al.* (2019) "Involving caregivers in self-management interventions for patients with heart failure and chronic obstructive pulmonary disease. A systematic review and meta-analysis," *Journal of Advanced Nursing*, 75(12), pp. 3331–3345. Available at: https://doi.org/10.1111/jan.14172.

Northouse, L. *et al.* (2012) "Psychosocial care for family caregivers of patients with cancer," *Journal of Clinical Oncology*, 30(11), pp. 1227–1234. Available at: https://doi.org/10.1200/JCO.2011.39.5798.

Orsulic-Jeras, S. *et al.* (2019) "The SHARE program for dementia: Implementation of an early-stage dyadic care-planning intervention," *Dementia (London, England)*, 18(1), pp. 360–379. Available at: https://doi.org/10.1177/1471301216673455.

Pearce, G. *et al.* (2016) "The PRISMS taxonomy of self-management support: Derivation of a novel taxonomy and initial testing of its utility," *Journal of Health Services Research & Policy*, 21(2), pp. 73–82. Available at: https://doi.org/10.1177/1355819615602725.

Pigott, J.S. *et al.* (2022) "Systematic review and meta-analysis of clinical effectiveness of self-management interventions in Parkinson's disease," *BMC Geriatrics*, 22(1), p. 45. Available at: https://doi.org/10.1186/s12877-021-02656-2.

Quinn, C. *et al.* (2016) "A pilot randomized controlled trial of a self-management group intervention for people with early-stage dementia (the SMART study)," *International Psychogeriatrics*, 28(5), pp. 787–800. Available at: https://doi.org/10.1017/S1041610215002094.

Quinn, L. *et al.* (2020) "Clinical recommendations to guide physical therapy practice for Huntington disease," *Neurology*, 94(5), pp. 217–228. Available at: https://doi.org/10.1212/WNL.0000000000008887.

Revenson, T. A. (1994). "Social support and marital coping with chronic illness," *Annals of Behavioral Medicine*, 16(2), 122–130.

Rosland, A.-M., Heisler, M. and Piette, J.D. (2012) "The impact of family behaviors and communication patterns on chronic illness outcomes: A systematic review," *Journal of Behavioral Medicine*, 35(2), pp. 221–239. Available at: https://doi.org/10.1007/s10865-011-9354-4.

Roundtable on Translating Genomic-Based Research for Health *et al.* (2016) "Implementation Science: Methods and Approaches," in *Applying an Implementation Science Approach to Genomic Medicine: Workshop Summary*. National Academies Press (US). Available at: https://www.ncbi.nlm.nih.gov/books/NBK373700/ (Accessed: August 13, 2025).

Satink, T. *et al.* (2015) "How is self-management perceived by community living people after a stroke? A focus group study," *Disability and Rehabilitation*, 37(3), pp. 223–230. Available at: https://doi.org/10.3109/09638288.2014.918187.

Thibaut, J. W., and Kelley, H. H. (1959). *The Social Psychology of Groups* (pp. xiii, 313). John Wiley.

Uhm, K.E. *et al.* (2023) "Influence of preparedness on caregiver burden, depression, and quality of life in caregivers of people with disabilities," *Frontiers in Public Health*, 11, p. 1153588. Available at: https://doi.org/10.3389/fpubh.2023.1153588.

Van Houtven, C.H., Voils, C.I. and Weinberger, M. (2011) "An organizing framework for informal caregiver interventions: Detailing caregiving activities and caregiver and care recipient outcomes to optimize evaluation efforts," *BMC Geriatrics*, 11(1), p. 77. Available at: https://doi.org/10.1186/1471-2318-11-77.

Van Lange, P.A.M. and Balliet, D. (2015) "Interdependence Theory," in *APA Handbook of Personality and Social Psychology, Volume 3: Interpersonal Relations*. Washington, DC: American Psychological Association, pp. 65–92. Available at: https://doi.org/10.1037/14344-003.

Vriendt, P.D. *et al.* (2012) "The process of decline in advanced activities of daily living: A qualitative explorative study in mild cognitive impairment," *International Psychogeriatrics*, 24(6), pp. 974–986. Available at: https://doi.org/10.1017/S1041610211002766

Weitkamp, K. *et al.* (2021) "Dyadic coping in couples facing chronic physical illness: A systematic review," *Frontiers in Psychology*, 12, p. 722740. Available at: https://doi.org/10.3389/fpsyg.2021.722740.

Weitkamp, K. and Bodenmann, G. (2022) "Couples coping together: A scoping review of the quantitative and qualitative evidence and conceptual work across three decades," *Frontiers in Psychology*, 13, p. 876455. Available at: https://doi.org/10.3389/fpsyg.2022.876455.

Wensing, M., Grol, R. and Grimshaw, J. (eds.) (2020) *Improving Patient Care: The Implementation of Change in Health Care*. Third edn. Hoboken: John Wiley & Sons. Available at: https://doi.org/10.1002/9781119488620.

Whitlatch, C.J. *et al.* (2006) "Dyadic intervention for family caregivers and care receivers in early-stage dementia," *Gerontologist*, 46(5), pp. 688–694. Available at: https://doi.org/10.1093/geront/46.5.688.

World Health Organization. (2024, April 22). *Rehabilitation*. Available at: https://www.who.int/news-room/fact-sheets/detail/rehabilitation.

24 Toward Responsive Rehabilitation Systems

Rethinking Self-Management as a Behavioral and Contextual Practice

Nicola Diviani and Enxhi Qama

INTRODUCTION

Self-management has become a cornerstone of contemporary rehabilitation discourse, widely promoted as a means of enhancing autonomy, improving health outcomes, and optimizing the use of healthcare resources for individuals living with chronic conditions (Barlow *et al.*, 2002; Grady & Gough, 2014). Across clinical settings and policy frameworks, self-management is commonly conceptualized as a set of behaviors—such as medication adherence, symptom monitoring, physical activity, or dietary regulation—supported through patient education, goal-setting, and behavioral interventions (Bodenheimer *et al.*, 2002). While this framing has helped to formalize and legitimize the role of individuals in managing their health, it often rests on implicit assumptions of linearity, stability, and individual agency.

This chapter argues that such assumptions risk obscuring the complex, situated, and negotiated nature of self-management as it is experienced in daily life. In reality, individuals must integrate self-management into broader personal routines, shifting identities, and social contexts (Audulv, 2013). As any other health-related behavior, self-management does not occur in isolation but is deeply entangled with other life domains—work, caregiving, relationships, emotional wellbeing—frequently involving trade-offs, re-prioritizations, and adaptations over time (Qama, Rubinelli & Diviani, 2022). Drawing on recent qualitative research in rehabilitation contexts, this chapter adopts a behavioral and contextual lens to better understand how self-management is enacted, sustained, or sometimes resisted by individuals in their everyday environments.

Crucially, this perspective also raises questions about the role of rehabilitation systems and professionals. If self-management is to be sustainable and meaningful, it must be supported by systems that are flexible, responsive, and attentive to the lived realities of individuals, not merely those captured in clinical assessments or standardized protocols (Nguyen & Kane, 2024). In line with consensus definitions from rehabilitation research, a responsive rehabilitation system is a collaborative and person-centered process that acknowledges variability across individual trajectories, listens to personal goals and constraints, and tailors interventions accordingly to optimize functioning and participation (Negrini *et al.*, 2022).

The aim of this chapter is threefold: (1) to critically examine prevailing assumptions about self-management in rehabilitation; (2) to present alternative conceptualizations grounded in lived experience and behavioral adaptation; and (3) to explore implications for rehabilitation professionals and service design. By shifting the lens from compliance to context, this chapter contributes to ongoing efforts to reimagine rehabilitation as a truly person-centered and relational process—capable of engaging with complexity, uncertainty, and the diversity of everyday life.

DOI: 10.1201/9781003599074-27

THE DOMINANT FRAMING OF SELF-MANAGEMENT IN REHABILITATION

Over the past 20 years, self-management has increasingly become a cornerstone in rehabilitation research and clinical practice, emerging as a powerful framework for supporting individuals' autonomy and long-term health outcomes (Audulv *et al.*, 2019). Influenced by broader paradigms of patient empowerment, chronic care models, and behavioral medicine, self-management is typically defined as an individual's ability to manage symptoms, treatment, physical and psychosocial consequences, and lifestyle changes associated with chronic illness (Barlow *et al.*, 2002; Lorig & Holman, 2003). Within rehabilitation, this has often translated into a structured set of behaviors that patients are encouraged to adopt, supported by educational interventions, coaching techniques, and behavior change frameworks such as the health belief model, social cognitive theory, or the COM-B model (Bandura, 1997; Champion & Skinner, 2008; Michie, van Stralen & West, 2011).

This framing has several advantages. It has enabled the development of replicable interventions, integration into clinical pathways, and alignment with performance metrics and health service efficiency goals. It has also allowed rehabilitation professionals to articulate their role in enabling patients to take responsibility for their health—a central tenet of person-centered care (Wagner, Austin & Von Korff, 1996). Yet, the widespread adoption of this framework has also led to conceptual narrowing. Self-management is often equated with compliance to medical advice, goal achievement, and behavior modification, with success defined by measurable outcomes such as increased physical activity, reduced hospital admissions, or improved biomedical markers (Brady *et al.*, 2013).

Such an approach, however, tends to decontextualize the lived experience of self-management. It assumes that once individuals are informed, motivated, and equipped with the right skills, they will be able to incorporate health-related behaviors into their routines in a rational and sustained manner. This risks underestimating the complex realities in which self-management must occur—realities shaped by social roles, emotional states, structural constraints, competing priorities, and changing life circumstances (Qama *et al.*, 2025a).

Furthermore, this framing of self-management is often overly linear and individualistic. It typically presents self-management as a progression from ignorance to awareness, from passivity to action, from dependence to autonomy (Bandura, 2001). This teleological model assumes that patients are on a predictable path toward becoming "good self-managers"—an ideal that may not reflect the values, goals, or capacities of many individuals navigating chronic conditions. Research in rehabilitation and chronic illness has increasingly shown that self-management is not simply a matter of acquiring skills or following routines but is embedded in relational, temporal, and existential dimensions of life (Riegel, Jaarsma & Strömberg, 2012).

Moreover, the dominant model often reflects a professional rather than patient-centered perspective. Interventions are usually designed by clinicians or researchers based on normative expectations of what patients *should* do, with limited attention to how people *actually* make sense of their condition, their health-related goals, and the feasibility of recommended actions (Pulvirenti, McMillan & Lawn, 2014; Sadler, Wolfe & McKevitt, 2014). One common practice illustrates this: evaluating self-management progress by tracking digital app usage or medication adherence rates. These indicators may be readily measurable, but they offer a narrow lens on engagement. This, in fact, ignores whether the behaviors in question are meaningful, sustainable, or aligned with individuals' broader life circumstances. A person may skip a logging task not due to apathy, but because completing it would interfere with caregiving duties or amplify distress. This gap is particularly evident in marginalized populations or those facing multiple social disadvantages, for whom access to resources, continuity of care, and trust in institutions may significantly shape self-management capacity (Boucher *et al.*, 2022).

While the dominant framing of self-management in rehabilitation has brought important gains, it is also constrained by several assumptions: that behaviors can be detached from their context;

that individuals are rational and self-directed actors; and that health management is universally prioritized. These assumptions risk producing interventions that are well-designed in theory but misaligned with the messy, dynamic, and negotiated nature of everyday life. The next section offers an alternative lens—one that treats self-management as a behavioral and contextual practice, deeply embedded in the lived realities of rehabilitation.

SELF-MANAGEMENT AS A CONTEXTUAL AND BEHAVIORAL PRACTICE

To move beyond the dominant framing of self-management as a set of predefined behaviors, this section proposes an alternative lens: self-management as a contextual and behavioral practice. This perspective acknowledges that while self-management does involve actions—monitoring symptoms, adjusting medication, performing exercises—these actions are not isolated events. They are interwoven with daily routines, social relationships, emotional experiences, environmental factors, and personal meaning-making processes. Self-management, in this sense, is not something added *onto* life, but something lived *through* it. Below, we illustrate this perspective with concrete evidence, which highlights how individuals negotiate, adapt, and sometimes resist self-management in the flow of everyday life.

A Contextual Practice

Individuals living with chronic conditions rarely experience health management as a standalone domain. Instead, they must integrate it with work schedules, family obligations, mobility constraints, economic pressures, and cultural norms (Hörnsten *et al.*, 2011). Contextual factors are shaped by systemic and structural conditions such as health system accessibility, workplace accommodations, social protection policies, and even urban infrastructure (Munce *et al.*, 2014; Siabani, Leeder & Davidson, 2013). These broader determinants often dictate which self-management options are realistically available and sustainable, highlighting the need for health systems to address barriers beyond the individual level.

Context also includes the temporal dimension of everyday life. People do not manage their health in a static or linear way; they respond to fluctuations in symptoms, unexpected life events, changes in social support, or shifts in priorities. Self-management practices may evolve or regress over time, with phases of experimentation, avoidance, adaptation, or reframing. In this sense, consistency is not always a realistic or even desirable goal; rather, adaptability and situational awareness may be more meaningful indicators of effective self-management (Audulv, 2013; Qama, Rubinelli & Diviani, 2022).

Qualitative research strongly supports this point. Narrative analyses (Franklin *et al.*, 2023; Qama *et al.*, 2025a) describe phases of hesitation, experimentation, and deliberation in the early stages of living with a chronic condition, underscoring how routines are woven into everyday life through trial and error. These adaptations are rarely linear; they are cyclical and fragile, shaped by shifting energy, priorities, and social context. A study by Sadeghi *et al.* (2024) further highlights that this work is not just physical or cognitive but also emotional and relational—what has been described as invisible labor.

Theories such as normalization process theory emphasize that embedding health practices into daily life requires continuous effort to maintain coherence, participation, and monitoring, a process that is always at risk of disruption (May & Finch, 2009). Moreover, excessive emphasis on rigid adherence can backfire, increasing feelings of burden and guilt (Liddy, Blazkho & Mill, 2014). Flexible strategies that respect personal rhythms and priorities may foster more sustainable engagement than prescriptive, one-size-fits-all approaches.

A Behavioral Practice

Much of the literature on self-management draws on behavioral science, employing models focused on decision-making, motivation, or compliance. However, these frameworks often do not capture the lived complexity of self-management among individuals with chronic conditions. In particular, behaviorist models tend to assume linear causality—that knowledge leads to motivation, which leads to action—overlooking how behavior is often emergent, situated, and constrained by systemic, relational, and temporal factors (Barlow *et al.*, 2002). This risks framing lapses as individual failure rather than as consequences of structural or contextual barriers. This chapter emphasizes a behavioral process that unfolds through adaptation, frequently improvised, relational, and deeply influenced by emotion and context (Allegrante, Wells & Peterson, 2019; Franklin *et al.*, 2023; Sadeghi *et al.*, 2024).

Recent research underscores that behavior is not merely a set of isolated actions, but an ongoing process of negotiating identity—who a person was before diagnosis, who they are now, and who they strive to become (Ould Brahim, 2019). Peters and Brown (2022), for instance, found that acceptance of illness as part of the self positively correlates with successful self-management, while rejection or identity engulfment is associated with reduced engagement and poorer outcomes. Importantly, this identity work is rarely performed in isolation. Partners, peers, and professionals often participate in shaping what "good" self-management looks like, sharing or delegating tasks and co-producing routines (Qama *et al.*, 2025b).

Qualitative research confirms that people draw on a wide repertoire of behavioral strategies. These range from strategic planning (e.g., developing structured routines or back-up plans) to reflexive adjustments (e.g., responding intuitively to bodily cues) and avoidant coping (e.g., disengaging from tasks to preserve emotional energy). Such adaptations are not always empowering or sustainable, but they make sense within the constraints of daily life. People experiment, form or break habits, and craft routines that best fit their circumstances—even when these diverge from clinical recommendations (Franklin *et al.*, 2023; Qama *et al.*, 2025a; Sadeghi *et al.*, 2024).

This spectrum of strategies mirrors what naturalistic decision-making research describes as "bounded rationality": individuals rely on heuristics and satisficing rather than optimization, especially under uncertainty, fatigue, or competing demands (Klein, 2008). Recognizing this helps shift expectations from perfect compliance to pragmatic, good-enough solutions that sustain engagement over time.

Motivation in this context is profoundly tied to meaning and identity. Self-management behaviors endure when they support valued roles, social participation, and personal autonomy (Franklin *et al.*, 2023). Conversely, when routines undermine these priorities, individuals may resist or reframe them. Trade-offs in this sense are not merely logistical but also moral: they express what and who people value, how they prioritize relationships, and what constitutes a meaningful life beyond disease control. Care ethics scholarship highlights that such decisions are often guided by responsibility to others as much as by self-interest (Tronto, 1998). For example, an individual might skip a physiotherapy session to attend a child's school event, framing this choice as meaningful and consistent with personal identity even when it contradicts medical advice (Moore-Bouchard *et al.*, 2024).

Emotions and relationships further shape self-management behavior. Anxiety, frustration, hope, guilt, and pride can drive or inhibit action. Family, peer, and professional support may facilitate adherence or create friction, depending on how well these supports align with the individual's goals and understanding of their condition. Invisible labor—planning, monitoring, and adjusting behind the scenes—also plays a critical role. People frequently adjust medication schedules around work, manage intimate care in inaccessible spaces, time conversations with caregivers, or mask challenges for social ease. These efforts are rarely captured in conventional metrics, yet they are foundational to autonomy and are particularly exhausting for those managing multiple conditions or navigating fragmented care systems (Allegrante, Wells & Peterson, 2019; Dwyer *et al.*, 2024; Sadeghi *et al.*, 2024).

Implications of a Contextual and Behavioral Lens

Reframing self-management in this way has significant implications. First, it shifts the evaluative focus from adherence to appropriateness—from asking "Is the patient following instructions?" to "Is this behavior meaningful and sustainable in this person's context?" Second, it highlights the agency and creativity of individuals, without romanticizing the substantial burden placed upon them. People are not passive recipients of care, nor are they always rational actors. Rather, they are engaged in continuous negotiation, shaped by values, environments, and relationships. Finally, this lens invites a critical reflection on system-level expectations. If the success of self-management depends on its integration into everyday life, then rehabilitation must move beyond linear goal-setting and behavior modification. It must consider how recommendations are translated, adapted, or resisted in context—and how systems can support flexibility, experimentation, and person-centered negotiation over time.

These contrasts are summarized in Table 24.1, which juxtaposes the dominant prescriptive framing of self-management with a contextual and behavioral perspective. The table makes visible how assumptions about patients as rational actors, linear progress, and biomedical indicators of success give way, in a contextual lens, to notions of negotiation, fluctuation, and subjective fit. Importantly, it also illustrates how the role of professionals and systems must evolve—from primarily educating and monitoring behavior to facilitating, co-navigating, and creating flexible environments that recognize the lived realities of individuals.

The differences outlined in Table 24.1 are not merely theoretical but become visible in the realities of everyday rehabilitation. The following example illustrates this point. A 45-year-old woman lives with multiple sclerosis. In a prescriptive model, her rehabilitation plan emphasizes strict adherence to a daily exercise routine and systematic fatigue monitoring, with success measured by whether she completes each task as instructed. Yet, her daily life is shaped by fluctuating energy levels, part-time employment, and caregiving responsibilities for her children. On some days she cannot perform the prescribed exercises, while on others she adapts creatively, for instance climbing stairs at work, stretching while helping with homework, or conserving energy to attend family

TABLE 24.1
Reframing Self-Management in Rehabilitation: From Prescriptive to Contextual Practice

Framing	Prescriptive	Contextual and Behavioral
Core assumption	Self-management is a set of behaviors to be learned and executed	Self-management is a dynamic process integrated into everyday life
Primary goal	Behavioral compliance with clinical advice	Sustainable integration into personal routines and priorities
Temporal view	Linear progression toward autonomy and stability	Fluctuating, non-linear, shaped by life changes and transitions
Context consideration	Often abstracted or treated as secondary	Central: includes physical, social, emotional, and structural factors
Role of identity	Stable "patient" identity expected	Identity is fluid and negotiated in relation to illness and life roles
Measurement of success	Biomedical indicators and adherence metrics	Meaningfulness, adaptability, and subjective fit with everyday life
View of the individual	Rational actor, passive recipient of expert knowledge	Active negotiator, navigating constraints and making trade-offs
Role of professionals	Educators and behavior change agents	Supporters, facilitators, co-navigators of lived self-management strategies
System responsibility	Provide standardized tools and education	Create responsive, flexible environments that adapt to individuals' realities

events. From a contextual and behavioral perspective, these choices are not failures but forms of negotiation, showing how she integrates health management into her routines and priorities. For professionals, the lesson is clear: support must focus on co-adaptation, flexibility, and shared definitions of meaningful progress.

IMPLICATIONS FOR REHABILITATION

Despite growing recognition of self-management as a cornerstone of rehabilitation, current clinical systems often struggle to support it in ways that are meaningful and sustainable for individuals. Much of this difficulty stems from a persistent gap between how self-management is conceptualized by professionals—typically as a list of desirable behaviors—and how it is experienced by individuals—messy, negotiated, emotionally charged, and deeply embedded in daily life. This challenge is not just interpersonal but structural. High caseloads, time constraints, rigid reimbursement models, and fragmented care pathways all limit professionals' ability to engage in person-centered dialogue (Esmaeili, Cheraghi & Salsali, 2014). Meaningful self-management support therefore requires not only individual clinician effort but also organizational commitment to allocate time, resources, and incentives for this work. To bridge this gap, rehabilitation practice must move beyond prescriptive protocols and embrace a more person-centered, responsive, and dialogical approach. The following sections outline two complementary levels of change: (1) practice-level adjustments in how professionals engage with individuals, and (2) system-level adaptations to make services more flexible, coordinated, and person-aligned.

PRACTICE-LEVEL RESPONSIVENESS

Asking Different Questions

Professionals often frame their interactions with individuals around task-oriented questions such as, "Are you doing your exercises?", "How often are you monitoring your symptoms?", or "Have you reached your goal?". While these questions may seem clinically relevant, they tend to reduce self-management to a checklist of behaviors and risk overlooking the complexity of lived experience (Hashim, 2017). A more responsive approach involves shifting the focus from compliance to integration, inviting conversations that acknowledge how health practices intersect with the rest of a person's life. Instead of asking whether exercises are being completed, professionals might explore how routines are fitting into someone's day, and whether they can be sustained alongside work, caregiving, or fluctuating energy levels. Rather than simply checking symptom monitoring, they might ask what is helping—or getting in the way—of doing what matters most to the individual, opening space to identify meaningful facilitators and barriers. And instead of assuming stability in goals, they could inquire whether priorities have changed since the last encounter, recognizing that values and motivations often shift over time. These kinds of questions shift the focus of the clinical encounter from compliance co-exploration, positioning the person not as a passive respondent but as an active partner in shaping what self-management can realistically and meaningfully look like in their daily life. Also, they open up space for individuals to share not only their behaviors but also the meaning behind them, as well as the constraints they are navigating. This aligns with approaches such as motivational interviewing and shared decision-making, which emphasize curiosity, collaborative agenda-setting, and eliciting the individual's own reasons for change rather than prescribing solutions (Carr, 2017; Mapes, DePergola & McGee, 2020).

Listening Differently

Listening, in this context, requires more than clinical empathy or polite attentiveness. It involves a deeper attunement to the messiness of people's lives—their moments of resistance and doubt, the fatigue that disrupts even the best intentions, the improvisations that make care feasible, and the setbacks or failures that are part of the process. Professionals must become comfortable with the reality that individuals' decisions will not always align neatly with clinical recommendations. Instead of framing such divergences as non-compliance, they can be interpreted as signals for adaptation—openings to revisit underlying assumptions, adjust strategies, and co-design alternatives that better fit the individual's circumstances (Qama et al., 2025b).

This form of listening also recognizes the narrative dimension of self-management. People do not experience their health as a series of isolated behaviors; they understand it through stories—stories of loss and recovery, of shifting identity, of striving for control in the face of uncertainty. These stories give meaning to routines, and meaning often determines whether a practice is sustained. Supporting self-management, therefore, also means supporting the stories through which individuals make sense of their experiences. Practically, this may involve narrative-based interventions, guided reflection, or structured storytelling tools that enable individuals to articulate what matters to them and to co-create meaning together with professionals (Petraglia, 2007). By listening for the story behind the behavior, rehabilitation professionals can move beyond surface-level adherence and engage with the values, struggles, and aspirations that shape how self-management unfolds in everyday life.

Co-Adapting Interventions

Finally, rehabilitation professionals must shift from implementing standardized interventions to co-adapting them in collaboration with individuals. This does not mean abandoning structure altogether, but rather allowing existing frameworks to bend and flex so they remain meaningful in practice. Co-adaptation may take many forms. For some, it could involve adjusting the scheduling or intensity of prescribed routines, recognizing that what is sustainable varies depending on a person's energy, responsibilities, and health fluctuations. For others, it might mean integrating care into existing roles and environments—embedding exercises into workplace routines, reframing them as family activities, or finding ways to carry out tasks within the flow of daily life rather than as additional burdens. Co-adaptation also requires rethinking what counts as progress. Instead of measuring success solely through biomedical markers or strict adherence, professionals can recognize milestones that align with what individuals themselves value—whether that is maintaining the ability to attend social gatherings, balancing self-care with caregiving, or sustaining a sense of autonomy. In this sense, co-adaptation represents a shift from rigid implementation to flexible partnership, where structure provides guidance but meaning and feasibility are defined together with the person living with a chronic condition.

Implementation frameworks such as Normalization Process Theory remind us that for interventions to 'stick,' they must fit into people's routines and make sense to them (coherence), be doable with available resources (capacity), and be continually evaluated and reconfigured (reflexive monitoring). Co-adaptation is therefore not a one-off adjustment but an ongoing process of embedding and renegotiation (Gallacher *et al.*, 2011). Such flexibility can only emerge through partnership. Co-adaptation depends on trust, shared decision-making, and a willingness to modify plans over time.

In sum, for self-management to succeed outside the clinic, it must first make sense inside the person's life. Rehabilitation professionals have a crucial role to play—not as instructors, but as facilitators of a process that is inherently behavioral, contextual, and deeply human.

SYSTEM-LEVEL RESPONSIVENESS

Adapting Structures and Pathways

Practice-level responsiveness cannot succeed in isolation; it must be supported by structural and organizational changes that create space for adaptation. System-level responsiveness entails rethinking how rehabilitation services are organized and delivered. Standardized pathways, though efficient in principle, often fail to accommodate variation in individual circumstances. Individuals with fluctuating conditions, limited resources, or low health literacy may fall through the cracks if services are rigid or overly protocol-driven (Khan *et al.*, 2021).

A more responsive system would embed flexibility at key points—allowing for timing adjustments, alternative modes of engagement (e.g., home visits, telehealth, community-based touchpoints), and iterative reassessments of needs. For example, follow-up after discharge might be tailored based on the person's evolving self-management strategies, rather than predetermined timelines (Saba *et al.*, 2014). Services could adopt modular models, offering varying levels of intensity or support modes that individuals can opt into or out of as life demands change.

Responsiveness also means improving continuity and coordination. Many individuals report fragmentation in care—receiving conflicting messages from different providers, or feeling abandoned once structured rehabilitation ends (Kern, Bynum & Pincus, 2024). Supporting self-management across the care continuum requires stronger integration of services, shared records, and coordinated handovers between acute, outpatient, and community settings. Moreover, involving peer navigators or community-based workers can help bridge gaps between formal services and lived environments.

Expanding Notions of Success

A truly responsive rehabilitation system requires rethinking how success is defined and measured. Traditional indicators—such as goal attainment, functional gains, or adherence rates—may not fully capture the complexities and personal value of self-management as experienced in daily life. Individuals may judge success not by whether they followed instructions precisely, but by whether they maintained social roles, managed stress, avoided exacerbation, or simply found workable routines that preserved their quality of life (Duprez *et al.*, 2020; Trappenburg *et al.*, 2013).

Evaluations should therefore include subjective, relational, and contextual indicators—what matters most to the person, and how well their routines fit within the fabric of their life. This might involve incorporating narrative outcome measures, routine assessment of person-defined goals, or the use of reflective tools that allow individuals to track their own progress in meaningful terms. Importantly, such tools should not be treated as static forms to be completed, but as opportunities for dialogue and shared understanding.

More broadly, rehabilitation institutions and funders should support models of care that prioritize adaptability and co-production, even if they require more time, negotiation, or iteration (Pielenz *et al.*, 2022). Responsiveness is not inefficiency—it is an investment in sustainable, person-aligned outcomes that are more likely to endure once formal services end.

Responsiveness as a System Ethic

Finally, responsiveness should not be understood as a series of small adjustments to existing practices, but as a core ethical orientation that shapes the very foundations of rehabilitation (Bradd et al., 2022). At its heart, responsiveness acknowledges that people's realities are dynamic and diverse, and that their ability to manage health is often shaped as much by conditions beyond their control—structural barriers, cultural expectations, social roles—as by personal motivation or skill. To respond meaningfully requires more than technical solutions; it calls for humility, openness, and a willingness to co-create care pathways in partnership with individuals.

A truly responsive rehabilitation system is one that learns continuously from the people it serves, embedding feedback loops and mechanisms that allow services to evolve in real time. It creates space for adaptation, recognizing that goals and strategies must be renegotiated as life circumstances shift. Crucially, it acknowledges that health is lived in context—not in isolation, and not according to standardized timelines. Within this model, both professionals and systems share responsibility for shaping environments that support rather than demand self-management, validating that there are multiple legitimate ways to live well with chronic conditions. Responsiveness, therefore, is not only a matter of efficiency or effectiveness, but of ethics: an affirmation that sustainable rehabilitation must honor diversity, uncertainty, and the lived realities of those at its center.

CONCLUSION

This chapter has challenged dominant models of self-management in rehabilitation that emphasize standardized behaviors and linear progressions. Drawing on qualitative insights and behavioral reasoning, we proposed an alternative framing: self-management as a contextual and behavioral practice embedded in the fabric of everyday life. From this perspective, individuals are not simply recipients of guidance but active agents navigating routines, constraints, relationships, and meanings in ways that often exceed—or diverge from—clinical expectations. We have shown how this rethinking calls for a shift in professional practice: from delivering protocols to co-adapting them with individuals; from focusing on adherence to supporting integration; and from evaluating outcomes by clinical metrics alone to recognizing success through person-defined goals and sustainable routines. But person-centered support requires more than a change in mindset. It also demands responsive systems—those capable of accommodating diversity in needs, trajectories, and life circumstances. Flexible service design, continuity of care, and community-based engagement are not luxuries but necessities if rehabilitation is to equitably support people living with chronic conditions. A shift toward responsive rehabilitation means accepting that complexity, fluctuation, and negotiation are not obstacles to care but inherent features of real-life self-management. The role of rehabilitation, then, is not to eliminate this complexity, but to accompany it—supporting individuals as they navigate uncertainty, redefine priorities, and develop strategies that make sense in their own lives. Such a shift is not easy, but it is urgent. By aligning rehabilitation with the realities of everyday living, we move closer to a model of care that is not only effective, but also ethical, sustainable, and meaningful.

REFERENCES

Allegrante, J.P., Wells, M.T. & Peterson, J.C., 2019. Interventions to support behavioral self-management of chronic diseases. Annual Review of Public Health, 40, pp. 127–146. doi:10.1146/annurev-publhealth-040218-044008.

Audulv, Å, 2013. The over time development of chronic illness self-management patterns: A longitudinal qualitative study. BMC Public Health, 13(1), p. 452. doi:10.1186/1471-2458-13-452.

Audulv, Å, Ghahari, S., Kephart, G., Warner, G. & Packer, T.L., 2019. The taxonomy of everyday self-management strategies (TEDSS): A framework derived from the literature and refined using empirical data. Patient Education and Counseling, 102(2), pp. 367–375. doi:10.1016/j.pec.2018.08.034.

Bandura, A., 1997. Self-efficacy: The exercise of control. New York: Macmillan.

Bandura, A., 2001. Social cognitive theory: An agentic perspective. Annual Review of Psychology, 52, pp. 1–26. doi:10.1146/annurev.psych.52.1.1.

Barlow, J., Wright, C., Sheasby, J., Turner, A. & Hainsworth, J., 2002. Self-management approaches for people with chronic conditions: A review. Patient Education and Counseling, 48(2), pp. 177–187. doi:10.1016/S0738-3991(02)00032-0.

Bodenheimer, T., Lorig, K., Holman, H. & Grumbach, K., 2002. Patient self-management of chronic disease in primary care. JAMA, 288(19), pp. 2469–2475. doi:10.1001/jama.288.19.2469.

Boucher, L.M., Shoemaker, E.S., Liddy, C.E., Leonard, L., MacPherson, P.A., Presseau, J., Martin, A., Pineau, D., Lalonde, C., Diliso, N., Lafleche, T., Fitzgerald, M. & Kendall, C.E., 2022. "They're all struggling as well": Social and economic barriers and facilitators to self-managing chronic illness among marginalized people who use drugs. International Journal of Qualitative Studies on Health and Well-Being, 17, p. 2082111. doi:10.1080/17482631.2022.2082111.

Bradd, P., Johnson, T., Marussinszky, N. & Williams, K., 2022. Responsive care and reflective practice: Learning from ethical issues faced during 2020 and 2021. Journal of Clinical Practice in Speech-Language Pathology, 24(1), pp. 51–53.

Brady, T.J., Murphy, L., O'Colmain, B.J., Beauchesne, D., Daniels, B., Greenberg, M., House, M. & Chervin, D., 2013. A meta-analysis of health status, health behaviors, and health care utilization outcomes of the chronic disease self-management program. Preventing Chronic Disease, 10, p. E07. doi:10.5888/pcd10.120112.

Carr, D.D., 2017. Motivational interviewing supports patient centered-care and communication. Journal of the New York State Nurses Association, 45(1), pp. 39–43.

Champion, V.L. & Skinner, C.S., 2008. The health belief model. In K. Glanz, B.K. Rimer & K. Viswanath (Eds.) Health behavior and health education: Theory, research, and practice. 4th ed. San Francisco: Jossey-Bass, pp. 45–65.

Duprez, V., Beeckman, D., Van Hecke, A. & Verhaeghe, S., 2020. Nurses' perceptions of success in self-management support: An exploratory qualitative study. Research in Nursing & Health, 43(3), pp. 274–283. doi:10.1002/nur.22032.

Dwyer, L., Barber, C., Dowding, D. & Kearney, R., 2024. Barriers and facilitators to self-management of chronic conditions reported by women: A systematic review of qualitative studies. BMJ Open, 14(9), p. e088568. doi:10.1136/bmjopen-2024-088568.

Esmaeili, M., Ali Cheraghi, M. & Salsali, M., 2014. Barriers to patient-centered care: A thematic analysis study. International Journal of Nursing Knowledge, 25(1), pp. 2–8. doi:10.1111/2047-3095.12007.

Franklin, M., Willis, K., Lewis, S. & Smith, L., 2023. Chronic condition self-management is a social practice. Journal of Sociology, 59(1), pp. 215–231. doi:10.1177/14407833211038059.

Gallacher, K., May, C.R., Montori, V.M. & Mair, F.S., 2011. Understanding patients' experiences of treatment burden in chronic heart failure using normalization process theory. The Annals of Family Medicine, 9(3), pp. 235–243. doi:10.1370/afm.1249.

Grady, P.A. & Gough, L.L., 2014. Self-management: A comprehensive approach to management of chronic conditions. American Journal of Public Health, 104(8), pp. e25–e31. doi:10.2105/AJPH.2014.302041.

Hashim, M.J., 2017. Patient-centered communication: Basic skills. American Family Physician, 95(1), pp. 29–34.

Hörnsten, Å, Jutterström, L., Audulv, Å & Lundman, B., 2011. A model of integration of illness and self-management in type 2 diabetes. Journal of Nursing and Healthcare of Chronic Illness, 3(1), pp. 41–51. doi:10.1111/j.1752-9824.2010.01078.x.

Kern, L.M., Bynum, J.P. & Pincus, H.A., 2024. Care fragmentation, care continuity, and care coordination—how they differ and why it matters. JAMA Internal Medicine, 184(3), pp. 236–237. doi:10.1001/jamainternmed.2023.6309.

Khan, G., Kagwanja, N., Whyle, E., Gilson, L., Molyneux, S., Schaay, N., et al. 2021. Health system responsiveness: A systematic evidence mapping review of the global literature. International Journal for Equity in Health, 20(112), pp. 1–20. doi:10.1186/s12939-021-01440-y.

Klein, G., 2008. Naturalistic decision making. Human Factors, 50(3), pp. 456–460. doi:10.1518/001872008X288385.

Liddy, C., Blazkho, V. & Mill, K., 2014. Challenges of self-management when living with multiple chronic conditions: Systematic review of the qualitative literature. Canadian Family Physician, 60(12), pp. 1123–1133.

Lorig, K.R. & Holman, H.R., 2003. Self-management education: History, definition, outcomes, and mechanisms. Annals of Behavioral Medicine, 26(1), pp. 1–7. doi:10.1207/S15324796ABM2601_01.

Mapes, M.V., DePergola, P.A. & McGee, W.T., 2020. Patient-centered care and autonomy: Shared decision-making in practice and a suggestion for practical application in the critically ill. Journal of Intensive Care Medicine, 35(11), pp. 1352–1355. doi:10.1177/0885066620927625.

May, C. & Finch, T., 2009. Implementing, embedding, and integrating practices: An outline of normalization process theory. Sociology, 43(3), pp. 535–554. doi:10.1177/0038038509103208.

Michie, S., van Stralen, M.M. & West, R., 2011. The behaviour change wheel: A new method for characterising and designing behaviour change interventions. Implementation Science, 6, p. 42. doi:10.1186/1748-5908-6-42.

Moore-Bouchard, C., Martel, M.-E., Develay, E., Côté, J., Durand, M. & Pagé, M.G., 2024. Prioritizing chronic pain self-management amid coexisting chronic illnesses: An exploratory qualitative study. International Journal of Nursing Studies Advances, 6, p. 100175. doi:10.1016/j.ijnsa.2024.100175.

Munce, S.E., et al. 2014. Perceived facilitators and barriers to self-management in individuals with traumatic spinal cord injury: A qualitative descriptive study. BMC Neurology, 14, p. 48. doi:10.1186/1471-2377-14-48.

Negrini, S., Selb, M., Kiekens, C., Todhunter-Brown, A., Arienti, C., Stucki, G. & Meyer, T., 2022. Rehabilitation definition for research purposes. American Journal of Physical Medicine & Rehabilitation, 101(12), pp. e100–e107. doi:10.1097/PHM.0000000000002031.

Nguyen, T.V. & Kane, S., 2024. Towards an agenda of action and research for making health systems responsive to the needs of people with disabilities. The Lancet Regional Health – Western Pacific, 52, p. 101225. doi:10.1016/j.lanwpc.2024.101225.

Ould Brahim, L., 2019. Reconsidering the 'self' in self-management of chronic illness: Lessons from relational autonomy. Nursing Inquiry, 26(4), p. e12292. doi:10.1111/nin.12292.

Peters, L.A. & Brown, E.M., 2022. The relationship between illness identity and the self-management of inflammatory bowel disease. British Journal of Health Psychology, 27(3), pp. 956–970. doi:10.1111/bjhp.12584.

Petraglia, J., 2007. Narrative intervention in behavior and public health. Journal of Health Communication, 12(5), pp. 493–505. doi:10.1080/10810730701441371.

Pielenz, C., Dragano, N., Kopkow, C. & Nothacker, M., 2022. From conventional to living guidelines – Faster updates for better informed guidance? A scoping review. Zeitschrift Für Evidenz, Fortbildung Und Qualität Im Gesundheitswesen, 174, pp. 20–31. doi:10.1016/j.zefq.2022.08.005.

Pulvirenti, M., McMillan, J. & Lawn, S., 2014. Empowerment, patient centred care and self-management. Health Expectations, 17(3), pp. 303–310. doi:10.1111/j.1369-7625.2011.00757.x.

Qama, E., Diviani, N., Häfliger, C., Jordan, X., Scheel-Sailer, A., Zanini, C. & Rubinelli, S., 2025a. Approaches to self-management integration and influencing factors in everyday life after spinal cord injury: A qualitative narrative analysis. Patient Education and Counseling, 136, p. 108763. doi:10.1016/j.pec.2025.108763.

Qama, E., Diviani, N., Häfliger, C., Jordan, X., Scheel-Sailer, A., Zanini, C. & Rubinelli, S., 2025b. Self-management decision-making in spinal cord injury after initial rehabilitation: A thematic narrative analysis. Patient Education and Counseling, 141, p. 109318.

Qama, E., Rubinelli, S. & Diviani, N., 2022. Factors influencing the integration of self-management in daily life routines in chronic conditions: A scoping review of qualitative evidence. BMJ Open, 12(12), p. e066647. doi:10.1136/bmjopen-2022-066647.

Riegel, B., Jaarsma, T. & Strömberg, A., 2012. A middle-range theory of self-care of chronic illness. Advances in Nursing Science, 35(3), pp. 194–204. doi:10.1097/ANS.0b013e318261b1ba.

Saba, G.W., Chou, C.L., Satterfield, J., Teherani, A., Hauer, K., Poncelet, A. & Chen, H.C., 2014. Teaching patient-centered communication skills: A telephone follow-up curriculum for medical students. Medical Education Online, 19(1), p. 22522. doi:10.3402/meo.v19.22522.

Sadeghi, H., Mohammadi Shahbolaghi, F., Hosseini, M., Fallahi-Khoshknab, M. & Ghaedamini Harouni, G., 2024. Factors associated with self-management in older adults with multiple chronic conditions: A qualitative study. Frontiers in Public Health, 12, p. 1412832. doi:10.3389/fpubh.2024.1412832.

Sadler, E., Wolfe, C.D. & McKevitt, C., 2014. Lay and health care professional understandings of self-management: A systematic review and narrative synthesis. SAGE Open Medicine, 2, p. 2050312114544493. doi:10.1177/2050312114544493.

Siabani, S., Leeder, S.R. & Davidson, P.M., 2013. Barriers and facilitators to self-care in chronic heart failure: A meta-synthesis of qualitative studies. SpringerPlus, 2, p. 320. doi:10.1186/2193-1801-2-320.

Trappenburg, J., Jonkman, N., Jaarsma, T., van Os-Medendorp, H., Kort, H., de Wit, N. & Schuurmans, M., 2013. Self-management: One size does not fit all. Patient Education and Counseling, 92(1), pp. 134–137. doi:10.1016/j.pec.2013.02.009.

Tronto, J.C., 1998. An ethic of care. Generations: Journal of the American Society on Aging, 22(3), pp. 15–20.

Wagner, E.H., Austin, B.T. & Von Korff, M., 1996. Organizing care for patients with chronic illness. The Milbank Quarterly, 74(4), pp. 511–544. doi:10.2307/3350391.

25 Self-Management in Older Adults

Ferhan Tanrıöğer Soyuer

INTRODUCTION

The global elderly population is rapidly increasing. According to the World Health Organization, by 2030, one in six people worldwide will be aged 60 or older. During this period, the share of the population aged 60 and over will rise from 1 billion in 2020 to 1.4 billion. By 2050, the global population aged 60 and over will double (2.1 billion). The population aged 80 and over is expected to triple between 2020 and 2050, reaching 426 million. Aging, the final stage of life, causes individuals to experience biological and physical changes. These changes create difficulties for older individuals to continue their lives and lead to their dependence on others. Due to the influence of external factors, older adults experience more problems in old age than in other periods. These problems can be evaluated as health, social, economic, care, housing, and psychological problems. As these problems are experienced, the expectations of older adults also increase (Barber et al., 2025; Iida et al., 2025). While older adults actively participating in the workforce contribute to economic and social well-being, their increased labor force declines with age, leading to decreased income generation, physical and mental changes, disability, and increased dependency. These developments will increase the need for healthcare services and long-term care, and necessitate a better-educated workforce for older adults (Wu et al., 2024).

The concept of self-management dates back to psychobehavioral therapy in the 1960s. Through self-management, older adults can manage their illnesses, rehabilitate themselves, and maintain their health (Whittaker et al., 2024). Self-management in the elderly emphasizes "person-centered measures" to protect and improve their health by avoiding negative factors and health damage. Today, self-management is used in various fields, particularly in health education programs for chronic diseases such as hypertension, diabetes, and stroke (Kristine et al., 2025; Shao et al., 2025). It has been shown that self-management is more effective than passive participation in disease management (Barlow et al., 2002; Nguyen et al., 2025). Therefore, this section of the book aims to explain the concept of self-management in the older adults in light of current knowledge.

SELF-MANAGEMENT, SELF-MANAGEMENT SUPPORT

Self-management is defined as the ability of an individual to manage disease symptoms, treatment options, and lifestyle changes together with family, community, and health professionals (Buck, 1982; Sajeevanie, 2020). Self-management includes five main skills: 1. decision-making, 2. Problem-solving, 3. using resources, 4. creating consensus between patients and health professionals, 5. taking action (Lorig and Holman, 2003). Self-management support encompasses all educational and supportive interventions systematically provided by healthcare professionals to increase patients' skills and confidence in managing their health problems. This includes regular assessment of progress and problems, goal-setting, and problem-solving support (Dineen-Griffin et al., 2019). The key to self-management support is ensuring a patient/individual-centered approach. The patient-centered approach aims to encourage the elderly to contribute to and manage the process (Barr et al., 2003). In self-management support, decision-making authority rests with the individual. Healthcare professionals support the individual's decision-making process with their

DOI: 10.1201/9781003599074-28

recommendations (Mills et al., 2017). In recent years, many different stakeholders have developed self-management support programs. Self-management programs have been shown to be beneficial in terms of health-related quality of life, self-efficacy, disease-specific self-care behaviors, and cost-effectiveness (Jones et al., 2011). Older adults can benefit from self-management support provided by healthcare professionals, but it has also been shown that these programs are not always aligned with older adults' interests, abilities, and health status (Timmermans et al., 2022). Therefore, it is important to understand more about older adults' physical and mental health, their perspectives on self-management, and their support needs. This can help tailor support programs to their needs.

Self-Management Strategies: While basic self-management skills include five main headings: problem-solving, decision-making, using resources, creating a common idea with the patient and healthcare professionals, and taking action, self-management strategies include focusing on the patient's needs, gaining decision-making and problem-solving skills, and providing emotional and social management along with medical treatment (Dineen-Griffin et al., 2019). In this regard, the most fundamental step of self-management strategies is providing education to the patient and their family (Jonkman et al., 2016). They are gathered under six main headings:

1. **Education and information**: This includes providing education to older adults, their families, and their loved ones. For this purpose, healthcare professionals prepare handbooks, guidelines, and brochures on specific illnesses. The education strategy consists of two main steps: self-management education and patient education.
2. Self-management training includes special training for the elderly, their families, and caregivers to help them adapt to the disease and maintain a normal life.
3. Patient education includes providing older adults with disease-related knowledge and technical skills. This training improves older adults' problem-solving and goal-focused skills. It's important that the training is purposeful and repetitive (Dwarswaard et al., 2016).
4. **Motivational interviewing**: It is an individual-centered approach that helps individuals discover and analyze the ambivalence they experience, thereby developing behavioral change (van Riel et al., 2019). Motivational interviewing has an eight-step strategy: giving advice, removing obstacles, providing choice, increasing desirability, developing empathy, getting feedback, clarifying goals, and active assistance.
5. Peer support and motivation: This includes bringing together individuals with similar challenges and collaborating on healthy lifestyle initiatives, such as participating in support groups.
6. **Symptom diary keeping:** used to help older adults monitor their disease and generate information that can be used in a management plan.
7. **Participating in community-based skills groups:** This includes participating in groups and programs run by NGOs and associations. For example, joining walking groups, fitness, healthy eating, weight loss, etc.
8. **Providing a multidisciplinary approach:** This includes seeking support from different areas of expertise when necessary for the older adult. For example, chronic pain management from an algologist, medication review from a pharmacologist (Glare et al., 2025; Narasimhan and Kapila., 2019). Although self-management strategies are outlined under these six steps, different methods should be included in the program according to the needs of the individual.

SELF-MANAGEMENT AND OLDER ADULTS

Older adults (aged 65 and over) are a highly prevalent group with long-term health problems and multiple illnesses. Much of the long-term health care and daily management is typically handled by the older adult and their close relatives. Individual care needs of older adults constitute a significant portion of their care. Therefore, enabling and supporting older adults to manage their long-term health problems is becoming increasingly important (Steverink, 2009). Self-management is recognized as a fundamental component of living well with a long-term health condition, and adequate self-management support has been shown to lead to better health outcomes and improve quality of life. Self-management can be defined as "the internally controlled ability of an active, responsible, informed, and autonomous individual to live in partnership with healthcare providers and the social structure, with the medical and emotional consequences of their chronic condition(s)" (Barlow et al., 2002). During the aging process, complex and dynamic interactions within changing life circumstances, such as physical changes, loss of family and friends, and disease management, can make self-management increasingly challenging. Many older adults live with multiple morbidities, which can have increasingly complex consequences. Multimorbidity often leads to high treatment burden and conflicting treatment recommendations. Having multiple morbidities is strongly associated with increased healthcare utilization and decreased health-related quality of life. It is clear that multimorbidity and symptom burden negatively impact self-management, and it has been demonstrated (Heid et al., 2020). Furthermore, limited educational attainment, low health literacy, and factors such as anxiety and depression in older adults make self-management more challenging (Okeyo et al., 2024). Health protection and promotion interventions for older adults can help prevent illness and disability and improve their quality of life (Steverink et al., 2005). This can enable older adults to live independently as healthier and more active individuals, strengthening their potential and enhancing their contributions to society.

Chronic Diseases and Self-Management in Older Adults

The aging population worldwide is witnessing an increase in chronic conditions such as diabetes, hypertension, heart disease, and arthritis. According to the World Health Organization, 80% of older adults have at least one chronic disease, and many have more than one (multimorbidity) (Gianfredi et al., 2025). Chronic diseases are long-lasting and irreversible health problems that require long-term treatment, monitoring, and care, and cause physical, mental, and social decline. As such, chronic diseases impose a financial burden on healthcare systems and individuals worldwide (Allegrante et al., 2019). The burden of chronic diseases leads to increased global use of healthcare services and increased medical expenditures. Therefore, the concept of self-management is of great importance (Goldman et al., 2016). Managing chronic diseases is crucial for improving quality of life and reducing healthcare costs. Self-management is defined as engaging in activities that protect and improve health for older adults with chronic illnesses, monitoring and managing the symptoms and signs of the disease, managing the impact of the disease on their emotions and social relationships, and complying with treatment (Peerbolte et al., 2025).

Self-management is one of the most important approaches in geriatrics (Kahe et al., 2018). It is a particularly important strategy for reducing the cost of treatment and care for patients with chronic diseases. The goal of self-management for older adults with chronic diseases is to enable individuals to identify their needs and develop multidimensional strategies to meet their needs in the problems they encounter in daily life related to their illness (Shin et al., 2021). Increasing individuals' self-management of their illnesses is one of the most effective health policies in managing chronic diseases, which require lifelong lifestyle changes. Self-management of chronic illnesses is a multidimensional and dynamic process that includes managing the physiological, psychological, and social problems that arise from the disease, as well as medical treatments, and acquiring coping skills for chronic illnesses (Cong et al., 2024) for older adults with chronic illnesses enable them to develop a sense of responsibility for their own health, better manage their medical treatments, and more easily cope with the effects of the illness on their physical and mental health.

Self-management of chronic diseases includes many daily activities such as health checks, use of medications, and exercise that the older adults uses to control his or her disease (Han, 2020). Most common chronic diseases such as diabetes, hypertension, cardiovascular diseases, and arthritis can be managed with healthy lifestyle behaviors (Hoong et al., 2023). Traditional medical approaches often lead patients to play a passive role in their healthcare choices. It is known that the acquired lifestyles and habits of chronically ill older adults cannot be changed with traditional medical approaches (Shao et al., 2025). Self-management strategies that enable older adults with chronic illnesses to transition from a passive to an active role are important for improving their health and preventing unnecessary healthcare use. Research has shown that self-management strategies for older adults significantly contribute to the successful management of common chronic diseases that lead to disability and death, such as asthma, chronic obstructive pulmonary disease, stroke, diabetes, epilepsy, and cancer (Lawless et al., 2021; Lin et al., 2025). Self-management strategies have emerged as effective tools for older adults to actively participate in healthcare. Self-management in older adults with chronic illnesses refers to the ability to manage the symptoms, treatment, physical and psychosocial consequences of the chronic illness, and lifestyle changes (Glasgow et al., 2019). Educational interventions form the foundation of self-management. Education provides older adults with information about their conditions, treatment options, and healthcare. Programs typically include workshops, printed materials, and online resources providing information. Studies show that educational interventions significantly increase knowledge and self-efficacy in older adults, resulting in better management of chronic conditions (Lanxin et al., 2024). Adherence to prescription medication is crucial for managing chronic conditions. Among strategies for effective medication management, interventions focused on medication management have been shown to significantly increase adherence rates and improve health outcomes among older adults (Peerbolte et al., 2025). Regular physical activity is vital for managing many chronic conditions in older adults. Personalized exercise programs, including strengthening, flexibility exercises, and aerobic activities, can help maintain independence and improve overall health in older adults. Structured exercise programs tailored to older adults have been shown to improve physical function, reduce falls, and improve quality of life. In older adults with chronic illnesses such as diabetes and hypertension, the addition of nutritional programs has shown improved outcomes (Jans et al., 2020). Chronic conditions can have psychological impacts, such as causing anxiety and depression. Self-management strategies include behavioral health support, counseling, and psychotherapy, along with stress management techniques (mindfulness, relaxation exercises). Integrating psychological support into the chronic disease management of older adults has been shown to lead to improved emotional well-being and improved self-management outcomes (Lin et al., 2025). Despite the benefits of self-management, numerous challenges prevent older adults from effectively engaging in these strategies. Cognitive declines, such as dementia and mild cognitive impairment, can hinder older adults' ability to remember their medications, understand educational materials, and follow self-management plans. Mobility problems, chronic pain, and other physical limitations in the elderly can prevent participation in physical activities and hinder the execution of daily self-management tasks (Cong et al., 2024). Social isolation and lack of family support can deter older adults with chronic illnesses from engaging in self-management strategies. A robust support system is essential to promote adherence and provide emotional support. Older adults are at increased risk for low health literacy and are associated with lower cognitive abilities and male gender (Clouston et al., 2017; Ganguli et al., 2021). Those with low health literacy, especially men, are more likely to use more medications (Shebehe et al., 2022). Research on medication burden has shown that older adults receive inadequate or sometimes contradictory medication information (Mohammed et al., 2016). Potential problems associated with this are likely to be exacerbated for those with low health literacy in this group. This barrier can lead to poor self-management practices. Access to healthcare, educational materials, and community programs may be limited, particularly in rural areas (Lu et al., 2021). Transportation issues can further hinder access to necessary resources (Badawoud et al., 2023; Cong et al., 2024). Personalized self-management programs that take into account individual health conditions, cognitive abilities, and social circumstances are crucial in strategies used to improve self-management among older adults with chronic conditions.

Technological applications such as telehealth services and wearable devices can facilitate access to information and resources. Providing training to older adults to use these technologies can increase their ability to effectively manage their health (Garcia Reyes et al., 2023). Self-management strategies are vital for enabling older adults to effectively manage chronic conditions. Educational interventions, goal setting, medication management, physical activity, nutritional support, and psychological support all contribute to improved health outcomes. However, barriers such as cognitive impairment, physical limitations, and lack of support should also be carefully considered to ensure the effectiveness of self-management strategies.

Future efforts should focus on personalized interventions, technology integration, family involvement, and community support to promote successful self-management in older adults with chronic illnesses (Garcia Reyes et al., 2023). By fostering a culture of self-management, older adults' quality of life can be improved, healthcare costs can be reduced, and healthier aging in society can be promoted. The self-management process is dynamic, interactive and iterative. In this process, the with chronic disease is expected to be able to manage lifestyle changes, treatment, and disease symptoms together with his/her family, social environment, and health professionals. For older adults with chronic illnesses, assessment should be planned, implemented, and evaluated based not only on the individual's knowledge but also on their motivation, perception, and readiness to change a specific behavior. A person-centered action plan should be developed. The older adults' goals and obstacles should be identified, progress should be regularly evaluated, and changes should be made to the program as needed to foster and maintain self-management behavior (Almutairi et al., 2025). Self-management is influenced by internal and external factors such as disease knowledge and self-efficacy. Therefore, planning interventions that incorporate these factors will lead to more successful outcomes. Furthermore, the use of motivation and coping strategies, social support, and a high level of health belief are also determinants of this process (Allegrante et al., 2019). The self-management strategy to be used depends on the defined goal(s), the availability of resources, the quality of resources, and the individual's self-management skills. These factors should be considered, and the most appropriate strategy should be determined with a patient-centered approach.

To ensure successful self-management strategies in chronic disease management;

- Individual-oriented, focusing on the needs of the elderly
- Acquiring decision-making and problem-solving skills
- Supporting emotional and social management alongside medical management
- The management skills of the elderly need to be developed and they need to take an active role.

Genetic predisposition, external factors such as accidents and viral diseases, environmental factors, technological developments, a sedentary lifestyle, unhealthy nutrition, excessive alcohol use, smoking, use of tobacco and tobacco products, and excessive sugar consumption also pave the way for the development of a chronic disease. Chronic diseases, a serious problem, leave irreversible scars on human life and significantly increase healthcare costs. Empowering older adults with chronic diseases and equipping them with self-management skills through various programs is crucial for improving quality of life, managing symptoms, preventing complications, and reducing healthcare visits and healthcare costs. Increasing self-management practices will benefit older adults, as well as families, societies, and countries (Nguyen et al., 2022). Each chronic disease presents differences in its self-management process. Chronic kidney disease, a common health problem worldwide, presents a challenging self-management process, and individuals with chronic kidney disease must regularly monitor their disease progress (blood pressure, weight, cholesterol, and blood glucose levels), manage their fluid and dietary intake, engage in regular activity, and adopt and maintain healthy lifestyle behaviors (Friedrich et al., 2025). Self-management in individuals with chronic kidney disease has been found to play a significant role in preserving kidney function and has positive benefits on albuminuria levels, blood pressure control, exercise capacity, and CRP levels. In chronic kidney disease, the number of medications used, socioeconomic status, the individual's environment and culture, the complexity of the treatment regimen, the presence of psychological problems, and the presence of other comorbidities all impact the self-management process (Billany et al., 2023; Lin and Hwang, 2020). It has been determined that self-management practices in chronic obstructive pulmonary disease patients positively affect disease attacks, reduce visits to health institutions and improve the quality of life of individuals (Kukol et al., 2022). It was found that patients with chronic obstructive pulmonary disease who participated in the self-management action plan had higher self-management levels and lower hospitalizations related to respiratory problems, while patients who did not participate had lower self-management levels, more frequent chronic obstructive pulmonary disease exacerbations, and increased respiratory-related mortality rates (Kee et al., 2022).

Diabetes, a disease of significant importance among chronic diseases, is another one that requires self-management. Self-management education provided to patients has been shown to positively impact blood pressure, glycated hemoglobin (HbA1c), lipid levels, and body mass index. Furthermore, this education has been found to improve patients' self-management, disease adaptation, quality of life, and knowledge about the disease (Beck et al., 2021). Although there are studies showing a 0.1–0.8% decrease in HbA1c values in Type 2 diabetes patients following self-management practices (Connelly et al., 2013; Kitsiou et al., 2017). There is also research suggesting that self-management practices have no effect on HbA1c values (Cunningham et al., 2018). In self-management of diabetes, the patient should keep his blood glucose level within the normal range. It is expected that patients maintain a healthy diet and adhere to a disease diet, control their weight, maintain regular and appropriate physical activity, self-measure their blood glucose levels and monitor their results, perform daily diabetes care, monitor foot and skin problems, cope with stress, have regular health checks, and control risk factors for acute and chronic complications. Factors affecting the self-management process in diabetes include the type of disease, the individual's age, duration of diabetes, the presence of depression, knowledge of diabetes, treatment method, social support, and the patient's relationship with healthcare professionals.

In patients with epilepsy, self-management is affected by the severity of the disease, the individual's personal characteristics, previous experiences with the disease, and the individual's health-related beliefs and attitudes (Thuy et al., 2024).

Self-management of epilepsy patients includes regular use of medications and seizure control. These include maintaining adequate and regular nutrition, ensuring adequate sleep, controlling stress, helping patients cope with their problems psychosocially, and developing coping strategies. Self-management and positive behavioral changes in patients with epilepsy have been shown to reduce the number of seizures, increase compliance with medication, and improve social well-being and quality of life (Ernawati et al., 2024).

Methods such as home visits, training in self-management practices, goal setting with the patient, self-monitoring and self-assessment, and tele-counseling regarding medications used have been used to increase self-management in patients with rheumatoid arthritis. Following these interventions, it has been observed that positive improvements, such as maintaining and improving joint mobility in rheumatoid arthritis patients, can be achieved through self-management interventions, and that self-management practices produce positive results (Damgaard et al., 2023; Mollard and Michaud, 2020).

Osteoarthritis and self-management: The most common chronic joint osteoarthritis a major cause of pain and disability. Osteoarthritis is frequently perceived as an inevitable result of aging. Between 60 to 69 years, that prevalence rises to 35% in women and 19% in men. Osteoarthritis can lead to joint pain, muscle weakness, physical disability, and a significant reduction in quality of life, while chronic pain can cause anxiety, depression, and cognitive dysfunction, significantly impacting patients' daily lives and increasing the socioeconomic burden (Lu et al., 2024). The International Osteoarthritis Research Association, Osteoarthritis Research According to the recommendations of the Society International, non-pharmacological therapies, including self-management, should be central to osteoarthritis treatment. Clinical training guidelines and brochures have taken their place as non-pharmacological treatments in osteoarthritis self-management. Clinicians are increasingly interested in the role of self-management interventions in osteoarthritis treatment. Self-management interventions have been shown to improve pain, joint function, physical function, mental health, and quality of life in osteoarthritis patients (Matthias et al., 2024). In recent years, an increasing number of studies have been conducted on osteoarthritis self-management, and the effectiveness of this intervention strategy has been investigated and analyzed (García-Ovejero et al., 2022; Safari et al., 2020). However, the evidence is still insufficient. The importance of wearable technology for osteoarthritis self-management has been demonstrated. Ensuring information sharing between doctor and patient and strengthening this communication through patient monitoring is important (Choi et al., 2019).

Self-management in cardiovascular diseases includes controlling modifiable risk factors (diet, exercise, smoking/alcohol consumption, etc.), monitoring weight and blood pressure by the patient, regularly applying disease treatment, preventing disease complications and making lifestyle changes (Cruz-Ramos et al., 2022; Stamm-Balderjahn et al., 2020).

Chronic Heart Failure and Self-Management: Self-management in patients with chronic heart failure is generally viewed as an active cognitive process that includes medication adherence, fluid and dietary salt restriction, symptom awareness and management, exercise, and regular follow-up. Self-management can significantly contribute to patients addressing the challenges of heart failure, enhancing their capacity to participate in ongoing medical care, and making better lifestyle decisions (Iyngkaran et al., 2022). Increasing research is underway to develop self-care theories for patients with heart failure, and these theories can guide future research (Jobst et al., 2020).

In elderly patients with high self-management, compliance with treatment increases, anxiety, sleep problems, and illness-related stress decrease, the individual uses self-care tools (glucometer, blood pressure monitor, etc.) related to his/her illness more effectively, and manages the symptoms of the illness better. It has been reported that individuals with low self-management are unable to maintain continuity in their care, are unable to manage their illness in collaboration with healthcare professionals, continue to engage in risky behaviors, and experience worsening outcomes (Cong et al., 2024). It has also been emphasized that these elderly patients do not choose effective resources and seek professional care, thus failing to maintain continuity of care. For these reasons, incorporating self-management strategies into the treatment and care of chronic diseases is crucial (Jans et al., 2020). However, in chronic diseases, failure to provide complete treatment, difficulties in integrating lifestyle behaviors, inability to give up habits, lack of social support, and disease control becoming more difficult over time may negatively affect individuals' utilization of health care services. It has also been stated that as the number of medications used decreases, the level of individuals being affected by the disease and perceiving the disease as anxiety decreases (Ibrahim et al., 2023). Having too many medications can lead to frequent drug use in social settings, reduce quality of life, and reduce compliance with treatment. It has been determined that self-management interventions have increased compliance with treatment, a better quality of life, improved stress management, improved sleep quality, and decreased disease complications and hospital admissions (Huang et al., 2024). In order to access easy, practical and fast information about the problems they encounter regarding their illness and general health status, older individuals benefit from the internet, television programs, magazines, and books within the scope of online health-seeking behaviors, and from health professionals and health institutions, as well as from trusted people and people who have had the same disease within the scope of professional health-seeking behaviors (Shao et al., 2025). Given that most individuals with chronic illnesses provide their own care, identifying self-management behaviors and the health-seeking behaviors they employ during this process is crucial. Various models are used for chronic disease management. The most frequently preferred of these models is the chronic care model, which consists of components such as health care organization, self-management support, community resources, and decision-making support. One of the key aspects of this model is the effective interaction between healthcare professionals and the patient (Shao et al., 2025). According to the model, individuals with sufficient knowledge and skills regarding their current condition are expected to take an active role in their own disease management, and chronic disease management can be achieved through the effective interaction of healthcare professionals with the patient (Peerbolte et al., 2025). In the management of chronic diseases, which are a significant public health problem, it is crucial for older individuals to manage their illness together with their families and healthcare professionals, decide on treatment options, and adapt to existing lifestyle changes after the illness. Therefore, in chronic disease management, providing holistic care through teamwork and ensuring continuity of care is crucial. Individuals with high self-management of chronic diseases have shown decreases in the consumption of harmful products such as salt, fat, sugary drinks, tobacco, and alcohol, as well as in stress and depression levels, while increases in physical activity levels and treatment compliance have been observed (Rascón et al., 2023; Sadeghi et al., 2024). Education provided to elderly individuals with chronic illnesses and their families includes specialized training to help patients adapt to life after the illness and embrace their normal lives (Shin et al., 2021). Education and psychosocial support provided to patients in healthcare institutions have been shown to positively improve self-management of chronic diseases such as coronary artery disease, hypertension, and diabetes, help patients manage the disease process and take an active role, and increase care satisfaction (Zhang et al., 2025). It is stated that chronic diseases can be managed successfully with self-management strategies and that the lives of elderly people with chronic diseases can be maintained in better conditions.

Health-Seeking Behaviors in Chronic Diseases

Individuals with chronic illnesses seek solutions to various problems they encounter or potential health issues during their illness. These pursuits are called health-seeking behaviors. Health-seeking behaviors include self-medication, consultation with health professionals, searching for information on the Internet, and information obtained from people around the individual or from people they trust (Changizi and Kaveh, 2017). In other words, health-seeking behavior is when people conduct research on therapeutic actions and gather information from various sources when they are not feeling well. Health-seeking behavior is the process of individuals conducting research and gathering information from various sources regarding therapeutic actions when they are feeling unwell (Maneze et al., 2015). Health-seeking behavior encompasses all of the behaviors an individual believes in and performs to protect, improve, and maintain their health, and to protect themselves from illness (Yang et al., 2020). Health-seeking behaviors were analyzed under three headings: online, professional, and traditional health-seeking behavior methods. It was found that individuals with chronic diseases obtained 62% of their disease information from doctors, 60% from the internet, and 40% from television. When health-seeking behavior and media were examined, the rate of media use for health-related information was found to be 93.8%, with the internet being the most frequently used media tool (71.4%) (Sharma et al., 2020). When the content of individuals' online searches was evaluated, it was observed that individuals with chronic diseases such as lung cancer, breast cancer, diabetes, and chronic obstructive pulmonary diseases engaged in more health-seeking behavior compared to those with other diseases, and their searches increased during disease awareness days (Faiola et al., 2019). Individuals' research about their diseases using mass media such as the internet, television, online magazines, and books is called online health-seeking behavior. Online health-seeking behavior includes conducting disease-related research online, following television programs, communicating with doctors online, learning about medication side effects online, and searching for information about the disease in online magazines and books (Fujii et al., 2022). Online health-seeking behaviors enable individuals to learn about their current health status, diseases, and medications, solve problems caused by the disease, learn healthy lifestyle behaviors, and communicate with healthcare professionals or individuals who have the same disease (Cardoso Barbosa et al., 2021). With online health-seeking behaviors, individuals can easily access information about their health/disease, detect disease symptoms, and make a preliminary diagnosis. They can also communicate with healthcare professionals about their current disease, find solutions to disease-related problems, and help individuals take an active role in decision-making regarding their own health (Xiaoyun et al., 2021). The advantages of online health-seeking behaviors include; While the advantages of accessing information are easy and practical, its disadvantages include overcoming information obtained from health professionals, reliability issues, experiencing feelings such as fear and anxiety, and the emergence of health-related concerns (Farris et al., 2025). Professional health-seeking behaviors are health behaviors that involve individuals seeking medical attention and seeking guidance from healthcare professionals during the illness process. Individuals seek information about the problems they experience during the illness process by seeking support from healthcare professionals (Farris et al., 2025). Traditional health-seeking behavior includes herbal medicines, friends, information obtained from trusted people, and advice from people with the same disease (Allegrante et al., 2019).

Self-Management Levels and Influencing Factors in Chronic Diseases

The self-management is important for the successful treatment and care of chronic diseases in elderly individuals, and that the quality of life of individuals increases with self-management. The World Health Organization has stated that chronic disease management should aim to empower older individuals and communities, and that encouraging patient self-management behaviors is the most effective approach (Sadeghi et al., 2024). Currently, self-management among older adults with chronic illnesses is at a moderate level. Age, gender, duration of illness, psychological state, family support, and resources that make life meaningful are factors that influence self-management (Cong et al., 2024). The multidimensional impact of chronic diseases causes differences in individuals' perceptions of the disease, their reactions to the disease, and their adaptation to the disease process, and affects the self-management process (García-Ovejero et al., 2024). While many factors influence the self-management of chronic diseases, age is the most significant factor influencing self-management. It is generally stated that as age increases, disease treatment, lifestyle changes, protection from the negative effects of the disease, i.e., self-care of the disease, decreases (Cong et al., 2024). Among the reasons for this are the increasing disability associated with chronic illness in older individuals, greater activity restrictions, cognitive impairments, withdrawal from social environments, and an increased need for support from others during the treatment process. This makes self-care and management more challenging with age (Sadeghi et al., 2024).

Gender has been described as an important factor in self-management. Self-management effectiveness levels have been shown to be generally similar between genders, with higher scores in men (Llubes-Arrià et al., 2025; Qama et al., 2022).

Education is the most important factor in individuals' ability to cope with the challenges they face in self-managing chronic illnesses and benefit from effective healthcare. It has been reported that individuals with chronic illnesses and those with lower levels of education have lower levels of disease coping, health responsibility, and self-actualization than those with higher levels of education. It has generally been shown that self-management of chronic illnesses increases with increasing education (Niño de Guzmán Quispe et al., 2021). This may be because, with increasing education levels, individuals become more knowledgeable about their disease, take responsibility, maintain positive lifestyle behaviors, and adopt the disease management process.

Employment status can have both positive and negative effects on individuals with chronic illnesses, it has been found that individuals receiving cancer treatment face discrimination in the workplace. Furthermore, increased socialization and communication with others who share the same illness have been shown to positively impact coping with illness-related challenges experienced by individuals with chronic illnesses (García-Ovejero et al., 2024).

Socioeconomic status is one of the important factors affecting individuals' ability to cope with their problems and effectively utilize healthcare. Among patients with epilepsy, those with lower socioeconomic status have been found to be more affected by the disease (Cong et al., 2024). Generally, individuals with higher income levels have been found to have higher scores for participation in disease care and the disease management process. Individuals with higher socioeconomic status have been shown to have better access to healthcare institutions, greater knowledge of treatment options, and the ability to receive psychological support during the chronic disease management process, which positively impacts the self-management process (Badawoud et al., 2023).

Adopting and maintaining healthy lifestyle behaviors is crucial for self-managing chronic diseases. Smoking and alcohol use negatively impact chronic disease management and increase mortality rates (Liu et al., 2024). Regular health/disease checkups positively impact chronic disease management, while also influencing individuals' ability to take responsibility for their health, cope with illness, and utilize healthcare effectively (Ma et al., 2021). Individuals who do not attend regular checkups have been shown to experience worsening health outcomes. Those who do have regular checkups have been found to have higher healthcare effectiveness scores than those who do not. Regular health/disease checkups in older adults demonstrate that they can manage their own health, gain more knowledge about disease diagnosis and treatment methods, and utilize healthcare more effectively (Thuy Le et al., 2024). The role of health perception in self-management of chronic diseases is important. Individuals with a higher perceived health have been shown to have higher levels of self-efficacy (Hao et al., 2024). Diagnosis time is also among the important factors affecting the quality of life and treatment adherence of individuals with chronic diseases. Patients with a disease duration of 25 months or more were found to not have regular health checkups. Hemodialysis patients with a disease duration of 13 years or more had lower general self-efficacy scores than those with shorter duration. Diabetic patients with a diagnosis duration of 16 years or more had lower general disease prevention and health improvement scores (Sadeghi et al., 2024). Individuals with a long diagnosis period may experience a lack of change in the treatment process, inability to provide complete treatment for chronic diseases, an increased risk of health problems, and more burdensome disease control over time, which may negatively affect individuals' health care services (García-Ovejero et al., 2024; Schiltz, 2022). In individuals with chronic illness, positive psychological well-being is positively associated with stages of self-management. A positive psychological state can reflect strong character traits and increase positive optimism in patients. This can foster a defense mechanism to withstand their chronic illness and improve self-management (Thuy Le et al., 2024). A positive correlation has also been noted between family approach and self-management. Family support has been shown to play a significant role in coping with stressful life events (e.g., chronic illness, etc.) as individuals age. It has been suggested that a supportive family provides positive emotional support to older adults with chronic illnesses, thus benefiting them in terms of happiness, anxiety, and depression, balancing the neuroendocrine system, and promoting healthy behaviors (Ma et al., 2021). The older adults with chronic illnesses become more compassionate and responsible in a harmonious/happy family environment. This increases their awareness of caring for life and enhances their perception of its importance. Situations that provide a source of meaning in life positively impact self-management (Tsamlag et al., 2020). An individual's internal negotiation between self-management and life goals is one of the key factors in self-management.

Cognitive ability in older adults is closely linked to self-management (Sadeghi et al., 2024). Therefore, managing cognitive symptoms in older adults is crucial, as amnesia, memory loss, and inadequate knowledge about dementia can negatively impact self-management.

SUGGESTIONS

- Supporting the disease self-management process in elderly individuals with chronic diseases through counseling and training,
- Ensuring that older adults with chronic diseases use their health-seeking behaviors effectively regarding their health/disease status.

It is crucial for life satisfaction and effective self-management in older adults. Neuroticism is negatively associated with self-management and self-care, while extraversion is positively linked to self-care behaviors. It has been noted that happiness can enhance the personal and social skills of older adults. It has been emphasized that older people are facing retirement, which can lead to financial concerns about paying for medical care (Zhang et al., 2025). Qualified staff caring for older adults contribute significantly to improving self-management by assisting them with planning, decision-making, and problem-solving. Caregiver characteristics and support from family members have been noted to significantly impact the promotion of self-management. The need for adequate and specialized healthcare resources and the importance of insurance coverage for the successful and standardized implementation of self-management have been emphasized (Schiltz, 2022).

Showing respect to older adults can increase their self-esteem, reduce social isolation, and improve their access to care and support (Álvarez-Gálvez et al., 2023). Conversely, discrimination reduces the quality of care, promotes negative attitudes, and discourages older adults from engaging in self-care, ultimately reducing their ability to effectively manage their health.

Self-Management in Older Adults with Multiple Chronic Conditions

As individuals age, the disease burden and the number of people suffering from multiple chronic conditions also increase. Individuals over the age of 60 have at least one chronic disease. Individuals with multiple chronic conditions have two or more coexisting chronic diseases. The prevalence of having two coexisting chronic diseases is 58.2% in the 45–64 age group and 78.9% in those over the age of 65 (Newman et al., 2019). Risk factors for multiple chronic conditions include being over 60 years old, being female, being unemployed, smoking/alcohol or drug use, low education level, physical inactivity, low socioeconomic status, and a high body mass index (Park et al., 2024). Common patterns of multiple chronic conditions include cardiovascular and metabolic diseases, mental health problems, and musculoskeletal disorders (Laxin et al., 2024). Multiple chronic conditions increase the need to use and manage healthcare services appropriately. Multiple chronic conditions represent a significant public health problem with significant needs to control disease complications and treatment costs (Sadeghi et al., 2024). Additionally, they are associated with increased disability, decreased activity levels, increased disease burden, and decreased sense of well-being, all of which impair quality of life and increase the risk of death. Self-management has been shown to be more negative in older adults with multiple chronic conditions. Inadequate responses to treatment and fluctuating health status have been identified as barriers to self-management in older adults with multiple chronic conditions (Smith et al., 2021). Given the growing elderly population, it is important to identify factors related to self-management to develop specific models and practices to maintain and improve health. Self-management in older individuals is influenced by a variety of factors, including families, caregivers, disease complications, the healthcare system, society, culture, and politics. Therefore, a comprehensive approach is essential when planning practices and services for the elderly population (Rascón et al., 2023). Currently, healthcare for multiple chronic conditions focuses primarily on life-threatening conditions and complications, primarily to reduce mortality. However, coordination between care plans, disease management, and self-management is crucial for comprehensive management of multiple chronic conditions in older adults. Therefore, special attention has been paid to self-management of multiple chronic diseases. Findings have revealed that self-management in older adults with multiple chronic conditions is complex and interconnected (Samal et al., 2021). Self-management strategies for individuals with multiple chronic conditions will make significant differences in reducing treatment and care costs by increasing awareness, understanding the disease, increasing compliance with treatment, and improving health. Self-care skills are lower in older adults with multiple chronic conditions. Self-management is higher in older adults who can independently care for themselves (Cajamarca et al., 2023). Long-term treatment of an elderly people with multiple chronic conditions is stressful. It has been shown that a significant portion of elderly individuals with multiple chronic conditions lack the knowledge to manage their medications independently, emphasizing the importance of self-management for appropriate medication management (Baird and Fraser, 2018). Mental health in older adults with multiple chronic conditions is often psychologically focused. Increased anxiety, including stress, can become an obstacle to effective self-management. Furthermore, the time-consuming nature of self-management behaviors can lead to negative emotions and fatigue, which can hinder successful self-management efforts. Maintaining mental health, good sleep quality, coping with illness, engaging in social interactions, and effective communication can increase participation in self-management programs. Barriers to self-management in older adults with multiple chronic conditions include low mood (depression/anxiety), isolation, and loneliness. Strengthening positive psychological attitudes, which are directly related to self-management in older adults with multiple chronic conditions, is recommended (Álvarez-Gálvez et al., 2023). A high number of comorbidities complicates treatment strategies and has a more negative impact on self-management. The need for repeated hospitalization, inappropriate response to treatment, complexity of disease control and treatment, events and fluctuations in health status have an impact on self-management (Park et al., 2024). Medication use, adherence to dietary recommendations, exercise, an active lifestyle, adopting healthy behaviors, taking responsibility, developing conscious, adaptive skills, adjusting lifestyle choices, and paying attention to treatments for chronic diseases can increase self-management in the elderly people with multiple chronic conditions. Providing telephone services for older adults, using web-based sensor devices for treatment and care programs, developing technology centers, successfully implementing patient-specific programs, and adapting standard care programs to meet the needs of older adults with multiple chronic conditions all improve the quality of care and are also cost-effective solutions (Bezerra Giordan et al., 2022 ; Gauthier-Beaupre et al., 2024). To prevent deterioration in functional capacity, participation in physical activities can positively affect the quality of life of older individuals and help maintain independence in basic daily activities. Key factors include maintaining functional abilities, the absence of physical illnesses and psychological problems, and maintaining adequate levels of physical activity (Liu et al., 2024). Frailty in older adults with chronic illnesses reduces their self-management abilities. Disease severity, sudden relapse, disease progression, and mortality risk are all negative factors in self-management (Álvarez-Gálvez et al., 2023). Encouraging self-management in older adults has been shown to reduce hospitalizations, treatment costs, and emergency room visits (by 60%). Conversely, it can lead to higher treatment costs. Individuals with chronic illnesses have a greater need for home care services. The professional competence of healthcare team members is also an important factor in self-management. Qualified personnel better identify the elderly individual's problems and educational needs and can be more helpful in planning, decision-making, and counseling. These factors contribute to improved self-management (Hoong et al., 2023). Cultural factors have been shown to play a significant role in elderly self-management. Elderly individuals are viewed as cultural beings, and media platforms are often used to promote this (Álvarez-Gálvez et al., 2023). This supports the development of cultural services and foundations for elderly care. Adopting a positive cultural perspective on caring for older adults is an important determinant of self-management. Consequently, positive cultural beliefs are present. Traditional approaches to health, a responsible family that sees caring for the elderly as natural, and adherence to traditions and beliefs are important in self-management for older adults with multiple chronic conditions (Álvarez-Gálvez et al., 2023). The overall goals of self-management are to promote informed decision-making, self-care behaviors, problem-solving, and active collaboration with the healthcare team, improving clinical outcomes, health status, and quality of life. To prevent functional capacity deterioration, participation in physical activities can positively impact the quality of life and functional capacity of older adults and help maintain independence in basic daily activities. Furthermore, living alone can impact functional capacity. It is essential to understand the determinants that influence older adults' health and their high level of satisfaction with their health. Key factors include maintaining good functional abilities, the absence of physical illness or psychological problems, and maintaining adequate physical activity. In addition to management and clinical care, it is important to address the self-management needs of older adults with multiple chronic conditions to reduce disease symptoms and maintain their quality of life (Sadeghi et al., 2024). Currently, healthcare providers for this older age group primarily focus on life-threatening conditions and complications to reduce mortality. However, for comprehensive and comprehensive management of multiple chronic conditions in older adults, coordination between care plans, disease management, and self-management is crucial. This coordination depends on the patient's ability and self-care capacity. In recent years, special attention has been paid to self-management strategies, particularly in the management of chronic conditions. Self-management strategies for individuals with chronic illnesses can empower patients to play an active role in disease management, increase awareness, improve disease understanding and adherence to treatment, improve patient health status, and reduce treatment and care costs (Dinh and Bonner, 2023). Because the incidence of multiple chronic conditions is high and its consequences affect self-management more negatively in older adults, it is necessary to analyze the factors related to self-management in this age group. Findings revealed that self-management among older adults with multiple chronic conditions is complex and interconnected (Sadeghi et al., 2024). Self-management ability declines with advancing age. Daily activity levels have been shown to play a significant role in self-management in older adults. There is evidence that decreased activity and performance in older adults lead to an inability to independently perform daily tasks, leading to a decline in self-management. In these situations, older adults often feel more fatigued. Older adults with multiple chronic conditions who experience general fatigue tend to be more dependent on assistance with daily tasks, leading to a further decline in self-management (Dinh and Bonner, 2023). Because the incidence of multiple chronic conditions is high and its consequences affect self-management more negatively in older adults, it is necessary to analyze the factors related to self-management in this age group.

Cognitive ability is closely linked to self-management in older adults with multiple chronic conditions; therefore, managing cognitive symptoms in this population is crucial, as avoidant behaviors, amnesia, memory loss, and poor understanding of dementia can lead to a decrease in self-management (Smith et al., 2021). Self-efficacy has been emphasized to enhance self-management. Furthermore, readiness for change, goal setting, organizing reinforcement meetings, feedback, and problem-solving skills, along with motivational components for self-regulation and problem-solving, have been shown to maintain self-management behavior in older MCCs. Self-care ability is low in older adults with multiple chronic conditions, while self-management is high in older adults with independent self-care. Additionally, adherence to self-care processes, sustainable behavioral changes, and the promotion of empowerment are directly associated with self-management (Smith et al., 2021). Accepting self-care responsibility improves self-management, helping to improve the quality of life of older adults. Behaviors such as self-monitoring medication use, mindfulness, and appropriate diet are associated with self-management in older adults. Self-management is a challenge for older adults with chronic illnesses. Approximately 30 self-management programs are reported, 24 of which are private and six are public (Cajamarca et al., 2023). Older adults with multiple chronic conditions often exhibit decreased self-control when it comes to diet, weight control, and exercise, which reduces self-management. Therefore, older adults should acquire self-management skills. Improving problem-solving skills, health behaviors, and patient activity levels can enhance self-management. These findings suggest that problem-solving ability is an important factor in self-management. Low health literacy in older adults with multiple chronic conditions is inversely related to self-management. Inadequate knowledge about the disease contributes to errors in self-management (Rahman et al., 2020). Education in older adults has been shown to improve treatment adherence and self-care (Delavar et al., 2020; Werfalli et al., 2019; Zhang et al., 2019), increase self-efficacy, and improve treatment outcomes (McGowan, 2012). The importance of knowledge and awareness in self-management has been emphasized. Effective knowledge and skills appear to be limited in caring for older adults with multiple chronic conditions (Chan et al., 2011). Lack of education is a significant barrier to self-management in older adults with chronic illnesses (Werfalli et al., 2019). Knowledge, education, and awareness about the disease contribute to improved self-management, increase self-efficacy, and improve treatment outcomes (Dinh and Bonner, 2023; McGowan, 2012). The important role of mental health in self-management is emphasized. This is particularly true for the elderly population. Elderly people with multiple chronic conditions often struggle with psychological issues; increased anxiety, emotional distress, and stress can impede effective self-management. Furthermore, the time-consuming nature of self-management behaviors, combined with negative emotions, fatigue, and threats to one's identity, can hinder successful self-management efforts (Samal et al., 2021). Maintaining good mental health, coping with illness, engaging in social interactions, and communicating effectively with others can help increase participation in self-management programs. Sleep problems and poor sleep quality have been implicated as factors affecting self-management because they can interfere with daily functioning (Sadeghi et al., 2024). Mental stability in older individuals helps increase the success of self-management programs. Barriers to self-management in older individuals with multiple chronic conditions include low mood, isolation, lack of self-esteem, pain, helplessness, and loneliness. Older adults with mood disorders, anxiety, and depression have lower self-management. Substance abuse, alcoholism, smoking, drug use, and medication overuse impede self-management (Ma et al., 2021). Stress management, the balance between attitudes, beliefs, illness experiences, and life goals are related to self-management and are obstacles to successful self-management in older adults with chronic illness due to the time-consuming nature of self-management behaviors, which can be negative, distressing, distressing, and sometimes identity-threatening (Sadeghi et al., 2024). Older adults with anxiety and depression exhibit lower self-management, and higher self-esteem is directly related to self-management; therefore, strengthening positive psychological attitudes, which are directly related to self-management in older adults with chronic illness, is recommended.

Frailty in older adults with chronic illnesses reduces self-management abilities. Disease severity and symptoms, moderate-to-severe outcomes, sudden relapse, disease progression, and increased mortality risk serve as predictors (Wang et al., 2025). Incurable diseases and the debilitating nature of chronic conditions in older adults create challenges in disease management. Treatment complications include delays in adherence to recommendations and difficulties in accepting recommended treatments, which can hinder self-management and decision-making (Smith et al., 2021). Additionally, complications such as polypharmacy, energy loss from medication consumption, and drug interactions may further reduce self-management abilities. Socioeconomic factors also play a role in self-management. Factors such as high costs of living, economic constraints, low financial income, retirement, and inability to work can negatively impact self-management in individuals with multiple chronic conditions (Llubes-Arrià et al., 2025). Older adults with multiple chronic conditions often face high medical expenses to maintain their health.

Promoting self-management among older adults has been shown to reduce hospitalizations, treatment costs, and emergency room visits. Importantly, individuals with chronic illnesses are increasingly in need of home care services. Promoting self-management can help reduce the cost of care. Research has shown that rising treatment costs directly and indirectly impact self-management (Dinh and Bonner, 2023). Effective self-management has been shown to reduce the frequency of doctor visits, especially in emergencies, by up to 60% (Sadeghi et al., 2024). Conversely, low levels of self-management can lead to higher treatment costs. Findings indicated that consistent social support and support from friends were statistically significantly associated with self-management (Dinh and Bonner, 2023). Failure to adhere to dietary recommendations is often associated with lower levels of self-management. Exercise, maintaining an active lifestyle, adopting healthy behaviors, taking responsibility, making sustainable health behavior changes, being mindful, developing adaptive skills, and adjusting lifestyle choices can contribute to achieving self-management and finding a balance between self-management goals and life goals. The quality of communication with the treatment team, treatment planning, and follow-up care are factors associated with improving self-management (Baird and Fraser, 2018). Effective communication with healthcare professionals plays a key role in implementing self-management programs, increasing older adults' satisfaction, and improving their self-management. Positive therapeutic communication with physicians and specialists enhances self-management, while low levels of counseling and poor communication with physicians diminish self-management. A positive therapeutic relationship between physician and patient has a significant impact on self-efficacy and behavioral outcomes in people with chronic illness (Heid et al., 2018). Quality communication with other members of the treatment team, including increased support from the healthcare team and training in communication with the healthcare team, enhances self-management. Poor communication with treatment personnel, such as physical therapists, psychologists, and occupational therapists, impedes self-management.

Older adults trust formal caregivers and healthcare providers. A heightened sense of security ensures self-management. Furthermore, low levels of trust can prevent older adults from accepting recommended treatment. Increasing healthcare provider support has been shown to improve health and reduce disability in older adults with multiple chronic conditions (Klinedinst et al., 2023). The initial trust older individuals place in healthcare providers has been shown to be associated with promoting self-management. These findings highlight the impact of professional competence among healthcare team members on self-management. Qualified staff can help older adults adapt better, identify problems and educational needs, and provide planning, decision-making, and counseling based on their condition. All of these contribute to improved self-management. Conversely, a lack of knowledge to improve care and staff's failure to utilize specialized geriatric knowledge are negative factors that hinder self-management. Therefore, healthcare and treatment systems need a skilled workforce to address these challenges (Kessler et al., 2023). Empowering elderly care staff is crucial for promoting self-management. One obstacle to promoting self-management among elderly individuals with multiple chronic conditions is insufficient human resources and inadequately trained staff. Therefore, training specialized staff in geriatrics, improving the skills of care staff, and utilizing current/modern methods for training geriatric specialists are essential. This results in staff job satisfaction, encouragement to increase self-management for elderly individuals, and overall improvements in the quality of care (Iida et al., 2025). Current training and treatment guidelines in this area are inadequate, and national action policies are needed to make self-management effective. Governments should be informed about the importance of self-management for chronic diseases, establishing standardized care levels, increasing available resources, and providing financial support to ensure the sustainability of support systems for older adults. Implementing a regular follow-up/monitoring approach for patients, increasing patient knowledge about their current conditions, improving their interactions with healthcare providers, and institutional audits provide a suitable platform for the success of self-management programs. Studies indicate that the lack of regular follow-up and treatment in care is a significant barrier to self-management. It has been noted that older adults have limited access to healthcare resources, and older adults with chronic illnesses often have difficulties communicating with healthcare providers (Lorig et al., 2003). Self-management is considered the cornerstone of chronic disease care and the first step in providing patients with the information they need to care for their health. Self-management of multiple chronic conditions has been defined as the ongoing process of facilitating the knowledge, skills, and abilities necessary for self-care of multiple chronic conditions (Barlow et al., 2002). This process incorporates the needs, goals, and life experiences of the person with multiple chronic conditions and is guided by empirical evidence. The overall goals of self-management are to promote informed decision-making, self-care behaviors, problem-solving, and active collaboration with the healthcare team, and to improve clinical outcomes, health status, and quality of life (Han, 2020). Self-management research have been shown to be inadequate in elderly people with multiple chronic conditions. Given the growing older adult population, it is important to identify factors associated with self-management to develop specific models and interventions to maintain and improve health. Self-management in older individuals is influenced by a variety of factors, including older adults, their families, caregivers, disease complications, the healthcare system, society, culture, and politics (Ko et al., 2025). Therefore, a comprehensive approach is necessary when designing interventions and services for this population.

The Impact of Community Health Coaching

Community health coaching has been shown to be a valuable practice for improving self-management behaviors in older adults with chronic illnesses (Barber et al., 2025). The critical role of patient activity in facilitating adherence to medication, dietary changes, and symptom monitoring in older adults with chronic illnesses has consistently been emphasized. Health coaching provides patients with information, confidence, and motivation, encouraging continued participation in self-care practices and leading to improved chronic disease outcomes (Henry et al., 2025). Despite the overall positive impact, additional approaches for further improvement were identified where patient engagement in the areas of physical activity and symptom monitoring remained inadequate. Coaching strategies that integrate behavioral techniques, goal setting, and personalized support have been shown to further strengthen these aspects of self-management. Integrating health coaching into primary care settings has the potential to support national health policy initiatives aimed at improving chronic disease management, reducing healthcare utilization, and promoting healthier aging (Henry et al., 2025). Future research should investigate the long-term effects, cost implications, and applicability of health coaching in a variety of healthcare contexts, including rural and underserved populations. Additionally, incorporating objective measures of self-management behaviors can further validate the effectiveness of coaching interventions and increase their clinical applicability.

SELF-MANAGEMENT SUPPORT PROGRAMS FOR OLDER ADULTS'S DAILY LIVING ACTIVITIES

The ability of older adults to perform activities of daily living, adapt to their lives, and manage their lives diminishes over time due to age-related physical and cognitive deterioration. Healthcare professionals should support older adults in preventing dependence on activities of daily living and enhancing their ability to adapt to and manage the consequences of living with chronic illness. Life at an advanced age is enjoyable for many older adults, but many older adults also face chronic diseases and other health problems that affect their ability to perform daily living activities (Liu et al., 2024). Older adults are at high risk for decreased mobility and dependency in activities of daily living. Effective interventions aimed at preventing disability in activities of daily living can reduce the burden on older adults, caregivers, and the healthcare system as a whole (Kong et al., 2021).

Effects of self-management support programs on activities of daily living in the older adults—Studies focusing on the effects of self-management support programs on the daily living activities of elderly individuals have shown that the self-management support program generally reduces obstacles in the daily living activities of older adults (DePaul et al., 2020; Kong et al., 2021). A short-term, weekly group support program targeting health promotion and health behavior changes has been shown to lead to significant improvements in physical function. Furthermore, a seven-week self-management group intervention demonstrated significant positive differences in participants' physical function scores from pre- to post-treatment (Connelly et al., 2013; DePaul et al., 2020). Self-management support interventions with a multicomponent structure that includes disease-specific information, knowledge and skills training, health behavior changes, and problem-solving coaching, particularly through a personalized plan, have been shown to result in improvements in physical function and activities of daily living (DePaul et al., 2020). Self-management support programs of all types have shown improvements in activities of daily living in older adults, not only in short-term, weekly group sessions but also in individual, longer-term, less intensive programs (Sahely et al., 2023; Ziv et al., 2024).

CONCLUSION AND RECOMMENDATIONS

Future studies should explore how cognitive factors may influence self-care practices in older adults, allowing for better identification of personalized interventions and support mechanisms. Memory difficulties, common among geriatric individuals, must be effectively addressed in clinical practice. Clinicians should incorporate memory-friendly strategies into older adults' self-management plans. Simplifying medication administration, providing easy-to-understand written instructions, and using phone apps and reminders with caregiver support can significantly improve self-care practices. Family and peer support should not be underestimated. Clinicians should actively involve family members in the care process, as these support networks can play a crucial role in helping geriatric patients adhere to their treatment plans and self-care regimens. Furthermore, establishing a strong physician-patient relationship characterized by trust and collaboration is essential. Clinicians should prioritize effective communication, active listening, and shared decision-making.

By understanding and respecting the values and preferences of geriatric patients, healthcare providers can create treatment plans that align with individual needs, ultimately enhancing patient trust and cooperation. In the psychological arena, individualized support is crucial, including cognitive-behavioral strategies, regular psychological checkups, and coping skills training to manage emotional aspects such as anxiety and depression. Feelings of exclusion and fear of judgment should be mitigated through normalization and peer support groups. From a healthcare perspective, the need to emphasize the fundamental qualities of reassurance and limitations, establish empathic patient relationships, provide clear and accurate information, and address concerns to enhance emotional well-being is crucial.

With technological advancements, web-based training should be prioritized to help older adults access relevant information and maintain their disease management process (Garcia Reyes et al., 2023). The use of web-based and mobile technologies should be increased to support self-management, and providing information and training about diseases online will significantly meet the needs of older adults.

REFERENCES

Allegrante JP, Wells MT, Peterson JC (2019). Interventions to support al self-management of chronic diseases. Annu Rev Public Health. 40(1):127–146. doi:10.1146/annurev-publhealth-040218-044008.

Almutairi M, Almutairi AA, Alodhialah AM (2025). Assessing the impact of community health coaching on self-management of chronic illness among older adults: A cross-sectional approach. Clin Interv Aging. 27(20):231–244. doi:10.2147/CIA.S509637.

Álvarez-Gálvez J, Ortega-Martín E, Carretero-Bravo J, Pérez-Muñoz C, Suárez-Lledó V, Ramos-Fiol B (2023). Social determinants of imorbidity patterns: A systematic review. Front Public Heal. 27(11):1081–518. doi:10.3389/fpubh.2023.1081518.

Badawoud AM, Salgado TM, Lu J, Peron EP, Parsons P, Slattum PW (2023). Medication self-management capacity among older adults living in low-income housing communities. J Am Pharm Assoc. 64(1):88–95. doi:10.1016/j.japh.2023.10.026.

Baird LG, Fraser K (2018). Home care case managers' integrated care of older adults with multiple chronic conditions: A scoping review. Prof Case Manag. 23(4):165–189. doi:10.1097/NCM.0000000000000286.

Barber S, Hayhoe B, Richardson S, Norton J, Karki M, El-Osta A (2025). Drivers and barriers to promoting self-care in individuals living with multiple long-term health conditions: A cross-sectional online survey of health and care professionals. BMC Public Health. 25(1):884. doi:10.1186/s12889-025-21737-0.

Barlow J, Wright C, Sheasby J, Turner A, Hainsworth J (2002). Self-management approaches for people with chronic conditions: A review. Patient Educ Couns. 48:177–187. doi:10.1016/S0738-3991(02)00032-0.

Barr VJ, Robinson S, Marin-Link B, Underhill L, Dotts A, Ravensdale D, et al (2003). The expanded chronic care model: An integration of concepts and strategies from population health promotion and the chronic care model. Hosp Q. 7(1):73–82. doi:10.12927/hcq.2003.16763.

Beck J, Greenwood DA, Blanton L, Bollinger ST, Butcher MK, Condon JE, et al (2021). National standards for self-management education and support. Sci Self Manag Care. 47(1):14–29. doi:10.1177/0145721720987926.

Bezerra Giordan L, Tong HL, Atherton JJ, Ronto R, Chau J, Kaye D, et al. (2022). The use of mobile apps for heart failure self-management: Systematic review of experimental and qualitative studies. JMIR Cardio, 6(1): e33839. doi:10.2196/33839.

Billany RE, Thopte A, Adenwalla SF, March DS, Burton JO, Graham-Brown MPM (2023). Associations of health literacy with self-management behaviours and health outcomes in chronic kidney disease: A systematic review. J Nephrol. 36(5):1267–1281. doi:10.1007/s40620-022-01537-0.

Buck T (1982). Theories of self-management. In: Comparative Industrial Systems. Palgrave, London. doi:10.1007/978-1-349-16701-2_4.

Cajamarca G, Proust V, Herskovic V, Cádiz RF, Verdezoto N, Fernández FJ (2023). Technologies for managing the health of older adults with multiple chronic conditions: A systematic literature review. Healthcare (Basel). 11(21):2897. doi:10.3390/healthcare11212897.

Cardoso Barbosa H, de Queiroz Oliveira JA, Moreira da Costa J, de Melo Santos RP, Gonçalves Miranda L, de Carvalho Torres H, et al. (2021). Empowerment-oriented strategies to identify change in patients with chronic diseases: An integrative review of the literature. Patient Educ Couns. 104(4):689–702. doi:10.1016/j.pec.2021.01.011.

Chan WL, Hui E, Chan C, Cheung D, Wong S, Wong R (2011). Evaluation of chronic disease self-management programme (CDSMP) for older adults in Hong Kong. J Nutr Health Aging. 15:209–214. doi:10.1007/s12603-010-0257-9.

Changizi M, Kaveh MH (2017). Effectiveness of the mHealth technology in improvement of healthy s in an elderly population-a systematic review. Mhealth. 27(3):51. doi:10.21037/mhealth.2017.08.06.

Choi W, Zheng H, Franklin P, Tulu B (2019). mHealth technologies for osteoarthritis self-management and treatment: A systematic review. Health Informatics J. 25(3):984–1003. doi:10.1177/1460458217735676.

Clouston SAP, Manganello JA, Richards M (2017). A life course approach to health literacy: The role of gender, educational attainment and lifetime cognitive capability. Age Ageing. 46(3):493–499. doi:.org/10.1093/ageing/afw229.

Cong Z, Huo M, Jiang X, Yu H (2024). Factors associated with the level of self-management in elderly patients with chronic diseases: A pathway analysis. BMC Geriatr. 24(1):377. doi:10.1186/s12877-024-04956-9.

Connelly J, Kirk A, Masthoff J, MacRury S (2013). The use of technology to promote physical activity in Type 2 management: A systematic review. Med. 30(12):1420–1432. doi: 10.1111/dme.12289.

Cruz-Ramos NA, Alor-Hernández G, Colombo-Mendoza LO, Sánchez-Cervantes JL, Rodríguez-Mazahua L, Guarneros-Nolasco LR (2022). mHealth apps for self-management of cardiovascular diseases: A scoping review. Healthcare (Basel). 10(2):322. doi:10.3390/healthcare10020322.

Cunningham AT, Crittendon DR, White N, Mills GD, Diaz V, LaNoue MD (2018). The effect of self-management education on HbA1c and quality of life in African-Americans: A systematic review and meta-analysis. BMC Health Serv Res. 18(1):367. doi:10.1186/s12913-018-3186-7.

Damgaard AJ, Primdahl J, Esbensen BA, Latocha KM, Bremander A (2023). Self-management support needs of patients with inflammatory arthritis and the content of self-management interventions: A scoping review. Semin Arthritis Rheum. 60:152203. doi:10.1016/j.semarthrit.2023.152203.

Delavar F, Pashaeypoor S, Negarandeh R (2020). The effects of self-management education tailored to health literacy on medication adherence and blood pressure control among elderly people with primary hypertension: A randomized controlled trial. Patient Educ Couns. 103:336–42. doi:10.1016/j.pec.2019.08.028.

DePaul VG, Bosch J, Oczkowski WJ, et al (2020). Promoting independent mobility-related physical activity (IMPACT) in an inpatient stroke rehabilitation unit: A proof-of-concept evaluation of self-management intervention. Disabil Rehabil. 42(22):3172–3181. doi: 10.1080/09638288.2019.1587012.

Dineen-Griffin S, Garcia-Cardenas V, Williams K, Benrimoj SI (2019). Helping patients help themselves: A systematic review of self-management support strategies in primary health care practice. PLoS One. 14(8):e0220116. doi:10.1371/journal.pone.0220116.

Dinh TTH, Bonner A (2023). Exploring the relationships between health literacy, social support, self-efficacy and self-management in adults with multiple chronic diseases. BMC Health Serv Res. 23(1):923. doi:10.1186/s12913-023-09907-5.

Dwarswaard J, Bakker EJ, van Staa A, Boeije HR (2016). Self-management support from the perspective of patients with a chronic condition: A thematic synthesis of qualitative studies. Health Expect. 19:194–208. doi:10.1111/hex.12346.

Ernawati I, Yasin NM, Setyopranoto I, Ikawati Z (2024). Effect of mobile health applications on improving self-management knowledge and seizure control in epilepsy patients: A scoping review. Healthc Inform Res. 30(2):127–139. doi:10.4258/hir.2024.30.2.127.

Faiola A, Papautsky EL, Isola M (2019). Empowering the aging with mobile health: A mhealth framework for supporting sustainable healthy lifestyle. Curr Probl Cardiol. 44(8):232–266. doi:10.1016/j.cpcardiol.2018.06.003.

Farris O, Orbell S, Lamarche VM, Smith R (2025). Promoting self-management in chronic disease: A systematic review and meta-analysis of behaviour change interventions for patients on dialysis. Health Psychol Rev. 19(2):368–408. doi:10.1080/17437199.2025.2471775.

Friedrich NK, Schmitt N, Hruby H, Kugler C (2025). Self-management interventions for adult haemodialysis patients: A scoping review of randomized controlled trials. BMC Nephrol. 26(1):285. doi:10.1186/s12882-025-04229-6.

Fujii M, Nakano J, Tanaka Y, Tonosaki A (2022). Effects of self-management interventions with change support on long-term adherence in patients with chronic respiratory diseases: A systematic review. GHM Open. 2(1):12–24. doi:10.35772/ghmo.2022.01000.

Ganguli M, Hughes TF, Jia Y, Lingler J, Jacobsen E, Chang CH (2021). Aging and functional health literacy: A population-based study. Am J Geriatr Psychiatry. 29(9):972–981. doi:10.1016/j.jagp.2020.12.007

García-Ovejero E, Pisano-González M, Salcedo-Diego I, Serrano-Gallardo P (2024). Impact of chronic disease self-management program on the self-perceived health of people in areas of social vulnerability in Asturias, Spain. Healthcare (Basel). 12(8):811. doi:10.3390/healthcare12080811.

García-Ovejero M, Robinson-Lane SG, Murphy SL, Courser R, Piette JD (2022). A pilot study of a chronic pain self-management program delivered by community health workers to underserved African American older adults. Pain Med 23(12):1965–1978. doi: 10.1093/pm/pnaa468.

Garcia Reyes EP, Kelly R, Buchanan G, Waycott J (2023). Understanding older adults' experiences with technologies for health self-management: Interview study. JMIR Aging. 6:e43197. doi:10.2196/43197.

Gauthier-Beaupré A, Kuziemsky C, Battistini BJ, Jutai JW (2024). Framework for policymaking on self-management of health by older adults using technologies. Health Res Policy Syst. 22(1):32. doi:10.1186/s12961-024-01119-5.

Gianfredi V, Nucci D, Pennisi F, Maggi S, Veronese N, Soysal P (2025). Aging, longevity, and healthy aging: The public health approach. Aging Clin Exp Res. 37(1):125. doi:10.1007/s40520-025-03021-8.

Glare P, Mahendran M, Weiss AD (2025). Update on chronic pain management. Intern Med J. 55(2):200–206. doi:10.1111/imj.16589.

Glasgow RE, Huebschmann AG, Krist AH, Degruy FV (2019). An adaptive, contextual, technology aided support (ACTS) system for chronic illness self-management. Milbank Q. 97(3):669–91. doi:.org/10.1111/1468-0009.12412.

Goldman ML, Spaeth-Rublee B, Nowels AD, Ramanuj PP, Pincus HA (2016). Quality measures at the interface of al health and primary care. Curr Psychiatry Rep. 18(4):39. doi:10.1007/s11920-016-0671-8.

Han Q (2020). A Study on Group Work Intervention Self-Management of Elderly Chronic Patients. Jiang Xi University of Finance and Economics. https://english.jxufe.edu.cn/

Hao Z, Jianrong L, Dongxu J, Linlin H, Weiliang W, Linlin Z (2024). The effect of health literacy on disease management self-efficacy in chronic disease patients: The mediating effects of social support and the moderating effects of illness perception. Patient Prefer Adherence. 18:657–666. doi:10.2147/PPA.S447320.

Heid AR, Gerber AR, Kim DS, Gillen S, Schug S, Pruchno R (2020). Timing of onset and self-management of multiple chronic conditions: A qualitative examination taking a lifespan perspective. Chronic Illn. 16:173–89. doi:10.1177/1742395318792066.

Heid AR, Pruchno R, Wilson-Genderson M (2018). Illness representations of multiple chronic conditions and self-management behaviors in older adults: A pilot study. Int J Aging Hum Dev. 87(1):90–106. doi:10.1177/0091415018771327.

Henry K, El-Osta A, Leedham-Green K (2025). Health coaching for people with long-term conditions and multimorbidity: A mixed methods prospective service evaluation of structured agenda-free coaching conversations (StACC) in UK primary care. BMC Public Health. 25(1):2365. doi:10.1186/s12889-025-23535-0.

Hoong JM, Koh HA, Wong K, Lee HH (2023). Effects of a community-based chronic disease self-management programme on chronic disease patients in Singapore. Chronic Illn. 19(2):434–43. doi:.org/10.1177/17423953221089307.

Huang Y, Li S, Lu X, Chen W, Zhang Y (2024). The effect of self-management on patients with chronic diseases: A systematic review and meta-analysis. Healthcare (Basel). 12(21):2151. doi:10.3390/healthcare12212151.

Ibrahim NA, Wong YY, Lean QY, Ramasamy K, Lim SM, Tan MP, Abdul Majeed AB (2023). Medication self-management among older adults with cognitive frailty. Res Social Adm Pharm. 20(2):172–181. doi:10.1016/j.sapharm.2023.11.001.

Iida K, Ishimaru M, Tsujimura M, Wakasugi A (2025). Community-dwelling older people's experiences of advance care planning with health care professionals: A qualitative systematic review. JBI Evid Synth. 23(1):69–107. doi:10.11124/JBIES-23-00221.

Iyngkaran P, Hanna F, Horowitz JD, de Courten MP (2022). Contextualising evidence based medicine in determining the key root for translational effectiveness for chronic disease self-management and heart failure. Rev Cardiovasc Med. 23(1):37. doi:10.31083/j.rcm2301037.

Jans G, Lenzen S, Van Pottelbergh G, Dobbels F, Daniels R, Lauwerier E (2020). Self-management among community-dwelling people with chronic conditions: Adapting evidence-based group programs using intervention mapping. Patient Educ Couns. 103(3):589–96. doi:.org/10.1016/j.pec.2019.10.001.

Jobst S, Leppla L, Koberich S (2020). A self-management support intervention for patients with atrial fibrillation: A randomized controlled pilot trial. Pilot Feasibility Stud. 6:87. doi:10.1186/s40814-020-00624-y.

Jones MC, MacGillivray S, Kroll T, Psych DA, et al. (2011). A thematic analysis of the conceptualisation of self-care, self-management and self-management support in the long-term conditions management literatüre. J Nurs Health Chronic Illn. 3(3):174–185. doi: 10.1111/j.1752-9824.2011.01096.x

Jonkman NH, Schuurmans MJ, Jaarsma T (2016). Self-management interventions: Proposal and validation of a new operational definition. J Clin Epidemiol. 80:34–42. doi:10.1016/j.jclinepi.2016.08.001.

Kahe M, Vameghi R, Foroughan M, Bakhshi E, Bakhtyari V (2018). The relationships between self-concept and self-efficacy with self-management among elderly of sanatoriums in Tehran. Iran J Ageing. 13:28–37.

Kee D, O'Conor R, Wisnivesky JP, Wolf MS, Federman AD (2022). Patient characteristics associated with retention in an asthma self-management trial for older adults. J Asthma. 59(8):1652–1660. doi:10.1080/02770903.2021.1941090.

Kessler D, McCutcheon T, Rajachandrakumar R, Lees J, Deyell T, Levy M, et al. (2023). Understanding barriers to participation in group chronic disease self-management (CDSM) programs: A scoping review. Patient Educ Couns. 115:107885. doi:10.1016/j.pec.2023.107885.

Kitsiou S, Paré G, Jaana M, Gerber B (2017). Effectiveness of mHealth interventions for patients: An overview of systematic reviews. PLoS One. 12(3):e0173160. doi:10.1371/journal.pone.0173160.

Klinedinst TC, Ciro CA, Kendzor DE (2023). A pilot, randomized, feasibility study to improve health self-management behaviors in older adults with multiple chronic conditions and functional limitations: Protocol for the behavioral activation and occupational therapy trial (BA+OT). J Imorb Comorb. 13:26335565231163037. doi:10.1177/26335565231163037.

Ko G, Song Y (2025). Social network analysis of self-management among older adults. Public Health Nurs. 42(3):1147–1159. doi:10.1111/phn.13537.

Kong D, Zuo M, Chen M (2021). Self-management behaviours of older adults with chronic diseases: Comparative analysis based on the daily activity abilities. Aust J Prim Health. 27(3):186–193. doi:.org/10.1071/PY20159.

Kristine S, Pedersen S, Lillelund Sørensen S, Holm Stabel H, Brunner I, Pallesen H (2025). Effect of self-management support for elderly people post-stroke: A systematic review. Geriatrics. 5:38. doi:10.3390/geriatrics5020038

Kukol LV, Obrezan AG, Pupyshev AV (2022). Motivational interviewing of older patients to participate in self-management programs for chronic obstructive pulmonary disease. Adv Gerontol. 35(2):302–307.

Lanxin W, Yan Z, Yutong T, Lixue M, Li L, Ting Z (2024). Potential profiling of self-management skills in older co-morbid patients. BMC Geriatr. Jun 25 24(1):555. doi:10.1186/s12877-024-05137-4.

Lawless MT, Drioli-Phillips P, Archibald MM, Ambagtsheer RC, Kitson AL (2021). Communicating with older adults with long-term conditions about self-management goals: A systematic review and thematic synthesis. Patient Educ Couns. 104(10):2439–2452. doi:10.1016/j.pec.2021.02.035.

Lin C, Zhu X, Wang X, Wang L, Wu Y, Hu X, Wen J, Cong L (2025). The impact of perceived social support on chronic disease self-management among older inpatients in China: The chain-mediating roles of psychological resilience and health empowerment. BMC Geriatr. 25(1):284. doi:10.1186/s12877-025-05902-z.

Lin CC, Hwang SJ (2020). Patient-centered self-management in patients with chronic kidney disease: Challenges and implications. Int J Environ Res Public Health. 17(24):9443. doi:10.3390/ijerph17249443.

Liu Q, Li X, Hu M, Zhao Y, Wu S, Feng H (2024). Factors influencing the self-management ability among older adults experiencing intrinsic capacity decline: A cross-sectional study. Front Aging Neurosci. 16:1456167. doi:10.3389/fnagi.2024.1456167.

Llubes-Arrià L, Briones-Vozmediano E, Tomás Mateos J, Sol-Cullere J (2025). Gender differences in self-management activation among patients with multiple chronic diseases: A qualitative study. Arch Public Health. 83(1):200. doi:10.1186/s13690-025-01686-1.

Lorig KL, Holman H (2003). Self-management education: History, definition, outcomes, and mechanisms. Ann Behav Med. 26(1):1–7. doi:10.1207/S15324796ABM2601_01.

Lu Q, Zhang D, Li L, Sun H, Wu Y, Zhang W (2024). Factors influencing the self-management stages of older patients with chronic pain: A cross-sectional study. Pain Manag Nurs. 25(6):e411–e419. doi:10.1016/j.pmn.2024.07.012.

Lu R, Li Y, Zheng Z, Yan Z (2021). Exploring factors associated with self-management compliance among rural elders. Inquiry. 58:469580211012491. doi: 10.1177/00469580211012491

Ma YF, Zhang LJ, Liu SC (2021). Promote strategies and influencing factors of health self-management ability among older adults in Hangzhou. J Mod Med Health (Chinese). 37(20):3571–3576. doi:10.3969/j.issn.1009-5519.2021.20.042.

Maneze D, DiGiacomo M, Salamonson Y, Descallar J, Davidson PM (2015). Facilitators and barriers to health-seeking behaviours among Filipino migrants: Inductive analysis to inform health promotion. BioMed Res Int. 2015:506269. doi:10.1155/2015/506269.

Matthias MS, Adams JM, Eliacin J (2024). Volunteer peer support for chronic pain self-management: A qualitative study of benefits and barriers. J Gen Intern Med. 25. doi:10.1007/s11606-024-09217-4.

McGowan PT (2012). Self-management education and support in chronic disease management. Prim Care. 39:307–25. doi:10.1016/j.pop.2012.03.005.

Mills SL, Brady TJ, Jayanthan J, Ziabakhsh S, Sargious PM (2017). Toward consensus on self-management support: The international chronic condition self-management support framework. Health Promot Int. 32(6):942–952. doi:10.1093/heapro/daw030.

Mohammed MA, Moles RJ, Chen TF (2016). Medication-related burden and patients' lived experience with medicine: A systematic review and metasynthesis of qualitative studies. BMJ Open. 6(2):e010035. doi:10.1136/bmjopen-2015-010035.

Mollard E, Michaud K (2020). Self-management of rheumatoid arthritis: Mobile applications. Curr Rheumatol Rep. 23(1):2. doi:10.1007/s11926-020-00968-7.

Narasimhan M, Kapila M (2019). Implications of self-care for health service provision. Bull World Health Organ. 97(2):76–76A. doi:10.2471/BLT.18.228890.

Newman D, Levine E, Kishore SP (2019). Prevalence of multiple chronic conditions in New York state, 2011–2016. PLoS One. 14:e0211965. doi:10.1371/journal.pone.0211965.

Nguyen T, Tang B, Harrison KL, Stadler S, Walter LC, Hoepke K, et al. (2025). Age self care, a program to improve aging in place through group learning and incremental change: Preliminary data. J Am Geriatr Soc. 73(3):920–929. doi:10.1111/jgs.19289.

Nguyen TNM, Whitehead L, Saunders R, Dermody G (2022). Systematic review of perception of barriers and facilitators to chronic disease self-management among older adults: Implications for evidence-based practice. Worldviews Evid Based Nurs. 19(3):191–200. doi:10.1111/wvn.12563.

Niño de Guzmán Quispe E, Martínez García L, Orrego Villagrán C, Heijmans M, Sunol R, Fraile-Navarro D, et al. (2021). The perspectives of patients with chronic diseases and their caregivers on self-management interventions: A scoping review of reviews. Patient. 14(6):719–740. doi:10.1007/s40271-021-00514-2.

Okeyo HM, Biddle M, Williams LB (2024). Impact of the self-management education on A1C levels among black/African Americans: A systematic review. Sci Self Manag Care. 50(1):87–95. doi:10.1177/26350106231213400.

Osteoarthritis Research Society International (OARSI). https://oarsi.org/research

Park GE, Park YH, Kim KG, Park JY, Hwang M, Lee S (2024). Mobile application for digital health coaching in the self-management of older adults with multiple chronic conditions: A development and usability study. Health Inform Res. 30(4):344–354. doi:10.4258/hir.2024.30.4.344.

Peerbolte TF, van Diggelen RJ, van den Haak P, Geurts K, Evers LJ, Bloem BR, et al. (2025). Conversational agents supporting self-management in people with a chronic disease: Systematic review. J Med Internet Res. 27:e72309. doi:10.2196/72309.

Qama E, Rubinelli S, Diviani N (2022). Factors influencing the integration of self-management in daily life routines in chronic conditions: A scoping review of qualitative evidence. BMJ Open. 12(12):e066647. doi:10.1136/bmjopen-2022-066647.

Rahman FI, Aziz F, Huque S, Ether SA (2020). Medication understanding and health literacy among patients with multiple chronic conditions: A study conducted in Bangladesh. J Public Health Res. 9:1792. doi:10.4081/jphr.2020.1792.

Rascón AM, McEwen MM, Slebodnik M (2023). Self-management of chronic disease in Latina Kinship caregivers: An integrative review. J Women Aging. 35(1):65–80. doi:10.1080/08952841.2021.2007827.

Sadeghi H, Mohammadi Shahbolaghi F, Hosseini M, Fallahi-Khoshknab M, Ghaedamini Harouni G (2024). Factors associated with self-management in older adults with multiple chronic conditions: A qualitative study. Front Public Health. 12:1412832. doi:10.3389/fpubh.2024.1412832.

Safari R, Jackson J, Sheffield D (2020). Digital self-management interventions for people with osteoarthritis: Systematic review with meta-analysis. J Med Internet Res. 22(7):e15365. doi:10.2196/15365.

Sahely A, Giles D, Sintler C, Soundy A, Rosewilliam S (2023). Self-management interventions to improve mobility after stroke: An integrative review, Disabil Rehabil. 45(1): 9–26. doi:10.1080/09638288.2022.2028019

Sajeevanie TL (2020). Importance of self-management and future research thoughts: A critical review perspective. Int J Creat Res Thoughts (IJCRT). 8(7):4122–28. doi:10.1093/heapro/daw030.

Samal L, Fu HN, Camara DS, Wang J, Bierman AS, Dorr DA (2021). Health information technology to improve care for people with multiple chronic conditions. Health Serv Res. 56(Suppl 1):1006–1036. doi:10.1111/1475-6773.

Schiltz NK (2022). Prevalence of multimorbidity combinations and their association with medical costs and poor health: A population-based study of U.S. adults. Front Public Heal. 10:953886.

Shao YJ, Duan XC, Xu XJ, Guo HY, Zhang ZY, Zhao S, et al. (2025). Latent profile and determinants of self-management s among older adult patients with chronic diseases: A cross-sectional study. Front Public Health. 13:1506545. doi:10.3389/fpubh.2025.1506545.

Sharma S, Green T, Alexander KE, Bonner A (2020). Educational or behavioural interventions for symptoms and health-related quality of life in adults receiving haemodialysis: A systematic review. J Ren Care. 46(4):233–249. doi:10.1111/jorc.12329.

Shebehe J, Montgomery S, Hansson A, Hiyoshi A (2022). Low health literacy and multiple medications in community-dwelling older adults: A population-based cohort study. BMJ Open. 12(2):e055117. doi:.org/10.1136/bmjopen-2021-055117.

Shin G, et al. (2021). Developing domains and items about self-management among elderly people with chronic disease. Healthcare (Basel). 10(1): 54.

Smith MA, Donelan K, Vaughan-Sarrazin M, Yu M, Vogeli C, Wang X, et al. (2021). Examining the effectiveness of case management programs on preventing hospital stays in older adults with multiple chronic health problems – A PCORnet study. Washington (DC): Patient-centered outcomes. Research Institute (PCORI). J Med Internet Res. 24(6):e29420. doi:10.2196/29420.

Stamm-Balderjahn S, et al. (2020). Correction to: Development and evaluation of a patient passport to promote self-management in patients with heart diseases. BMC Health Serv Res. 716(2019). doi:10.1186/s12913-019-4565-4.

Steverink N (2009). Happy and healthy aging: Well-being, resources and self-management abilities. Tijdschrift voor gerontologie en Geriatrie. 40(6):244–252. doi: 10.1007/BF03088518.

Steverink N, Lindenberg S, Slaets PJ (2005). How to understand and improve older people's self-management of well being. Eur J Ageing. 2(4). doi:10.1007/s10433-005-0012-y.

Thuy Le MA, Quynh Le N, Cong Tran T (2024). Self-management practice of people with epilepsy in Viet Nam and associated factors. Epilepsy Behav. 159:109979. doi: 10.1016/j.yebeh.2024.109979.

Timmermans LD, Boeykens MM, Sirimsi P, Decat V, Foulon A, et al. (2022). Self-management support in Flemish primary care practice: The development of a preliminary conceptual model using a qualitative approach. BMC Prim Care. 23(1):1–13.

Tsamlag L, Wang H, Shen Q, Shi Y, Zhang S, Chang R, et al. (2020). Applying the information-motivation-al model to explore the influencing factors of self-management among osteoporosis patients. BMC Public Health. 20(1):198. doi:10.1186/s12889-020-8292-x.

Van Riel PA, Zuidema RM, Vogel C, et al. (2019). Patient self-management and tracking: A European experience. Rheum Dis Clin North Am. 45(2):187–195. doi:10.1016/j.rdc.2019.01.008.

Wang C, Zhang W, Zhao F, Sun Q, Li D, Li X, Yang J, Ji H (2025). Needs and experiences of older adults with multiple morbidities using health technologies for self-management: A systematic review and meta-synthesis. Worldviews Evid Based Nurs. 22(3):e70030. doi:10.1111/wvn.70030.

Werfalli M, Murphy K, Kalula S, Levitt N (2019). Current policies and practices for the provision of diabetes care and self-management support programmes for older South Africans. Afr J Prim Health Care Fam Med. 11:e1–e12. doi:10.4102/phcfm.v11i1.2053.

Whittaker SL, Brusco NK, Hill KD, Taylor NF (2024). Self-management programs within rehabilitation yield positive health outcomes at a small increased cost compared with usual care: A systematic review and meta-analysis. Arch Phys Med Rehabil. 105(10):1946–1960. doi:10.1016/j.apmr.2024.05.007.

Wu LT, Glass GF Jr, Chew EYH, Ng EJY, Chan EY (2024). Developing a theory of change to guide the design and implementation of a caregiver-centric support service. BMC Health Serv Res. 24(1):1620. doi:10.1186/s12913-024-11931-y.

Xiaoyun J, Yan P, Liangni SL (2021). Online health information seeking behavior: A systematic review. Healthcare (Basel). 9(12):1740. doi:10.3390/healthcare9121740.

Yang J, Bauer BA, Lindeen SA, Perlman AI, Abu Dabrh AM, Boehmer KR, et al. (2020). Current trends in health coaching for chronic conditions: A systematic review and meta-analysis of randomized controlled trials. Medicine (Baltimore). 99(30):e21080. doi:10.1097/MD.0000000000021080.

Zhang R, Lu Y, Shi L, Zhang S, Chang F (2019). Prevalence and patterns of multimorbidity among the elderly in China: A cross-sectional study using national survey data. BMJ Open. 9:e024268. doi:10.1136/bmjopen-2018-024268.

Zhang SQ, Deng M, Xu XJ, Yang Y, Zhao S, Yue J, et al (2025). Social support and self-management activation among older adult chronic disease patients in China: The chain mediating role of acceptance of illness and fatigue. Front Public Health. 13:1637017. doi:10.3389/fpubh.2025.1637017.

Ziv I, Caspi D, CoJocaru D (2024). Self-management elucidates how practicing physical exercises influences the health related quality of life of independently dwelling older adults. Inquiry. 61:469580241271272. doi:10.1177/00469580241271272.

26 Building the Capacity of Children with Disabilities and Their Families to Self-Manage Participation

A Key Goal of Pediatric Rehabilitation

Mats Granlund, Christine Imms, Henrik Danielsson, Magnus Ivarsson, and Jacinta Pennacchia

INTRODUCTION

Recent definitions of health have conceptualized it as being able to manage your own life situation, independent of whether you have impairments or illness (Bickenbach et al., 2023; Huber et al., 2011). This functional approach to understanding health emphasizes the importance of self-management as a mechanism for achieving health. According to Lozano and Houtrow (2018), self-management is the set of management behaviors that people engage in as part of living with a chronic health condition, thus self-management relates to the ability to manage your own life situation over time and over life tasks. Self-management tasks include defining challenges/problems that need to be changed, finding possible solutions to the challenges, defining desired outcomes of changing the problem, planning what to do to change the situation and implementing/executing the change activities that are necessary. How these tasks need to be structured to facilitate self-management will vary, dependent on the age and level of functioning of the child.

Children growing up with disabilities can experience problems with functioning across all three levels functioning described in the International Classification of Functioning, Disability and Health (ICF; WHO, 2001). Therefore, they and their families may need to learn to self-manage problems with body functions, activity performance, and/or participation. These three different types of problems may require different approaches to, or forms of, self-management. Problems with body functions and activity performance (e.g. visual acuity or difficulties reading according to norms) are usually asked about by parents and then investigated by professionals. The professionals identify the difficulties with the help of assessment instruments and then prescribe relevant intervention(s). In these cases, children and families must then self-manage the performance of procedures, or learn strategies, designed by professionals. Most research about self-management relates to these types of problems (Guevara et al., 2003). The focus is on teaching self-management as an intervention (Lindsay et al., 2014).

In contrast to body structures/functions and activity performance, problems with participation in everyday life can only be identified by the child and family or other actors in everyday settings such as preschool or school. Participation problems are not defined based on norms or standards, but rather on what activities the child and family/other care providers consider important to participate in. When addressing participation problems, the professional's primary task is to support the child

DOI: 10.1201/9781003599074-29

and family to generate solutions to the participation problems which were identified by the child and family. Usually, participation problems change with context, age and role expectations. Working in a manner that facilitates self-management is best seen as a useful approach when collaborating with children and families in intervention work. as. In this chapter self-management of improving participation in everyday activities is the focus.

The development of self-management knowledge and skills related to participation problems is a process over time, where the child and family gradually become more skilled and autonomous problem-solvers (Granlund & Imms, 2024). To achieve this, children need the opportunities and support from both family and professionals to build their capacity. Parents/carers raising children with disability have a dual task: to build their own capacity to manage their child's participation challenges, and to support their child to develop capacity for autonomous or inter-dependent self-management. In a survey of parents regarding supporting youth with intellectual disability to use assistive technology for time planning there was a tendency that the youth were not allowed opportunities to use assistive technology to plan their own activities, just to execute the parents' plans (Palmqvist & Danielsson, 2020). This finding suggests the children may have missed an opportunity for learning because the parents did not consider it as an opportunity for self-management. Building capacity for self-management in children with disability focus on problem-solving. It is an opportunity for a collaborative effort between the child, family and professionals: Although the child and people in the proximal environments (i.e., everyday settings) implement interventions, it is not a situation wherein the child and their family must manage problems "by themselves" (Wong Chung et al., 2020).

The development of self-management is influenced by the level of functioning of the child. Problem-solving is a continuum of possibilities for autonomous problem-solving, with very autonomous problem-solving at one end of the continuum to interdependent decision-making with support from relatives of children with severe or profound disabilities, at the other end. With experience and practice of self-management and development of new skills, almost all children with disabilities can become more autonomous problem-solvers to some extent.

The development of self-management is a capacity building process. Ryan, Fathi et al (2025) identified four principles for capacity building, i.e self-management: (1) it needs to have 'real-world application' now and in the future, (2) it cultivates 'youth's' ability to problem-solve through barriers, (3) it empowers youth to take ownership for change, and (4) it is an ongoing process with opportunities for youth to learn and reflect on experiences throughout their life (p. 5187). These principles are particularly salient in the context of three societal transformations that are reshaping pediatric rehabilitation: first a shift from a focus on body function to participation, second a shift from specialized clinics to everyday life settings and third from face-to-face to digital encounters.

Shifting Intervention Focus from Body Function to Participation

Following medical advances, people with chronic conditions are living longer but without being cured. This has shifted the expression of health to one of human functioning rather than absence of disease (Huber et al., 2011) and the focus of pediatric rehabilitation from fixing impairments to supporting children in living a good everyday life with their condition. Thus, the desired outcome of pediatric rehabilitation has expanded from improved body functions and training skills, with typical functioning as the frame of reference, to also include participation interventions with outcomes related to involvement in life situations (Bickenbach et al., 2023). A focus on participation requires changes to intervention content and a shift in power from professionals to children and families. However, studies of desired outcomes of pediatric rehabilitation report that most goals continue to focus on teaching new skills, with only a small proportion of goals focusing on increasing participation Ryan, Miller et al. (2025). These authors also report that although care providers (primarily mothers) contributed to the goal setting process, very few documents (2%) indicated that children were active participants in the process of goal setting. When setting participation goals, however, the active involvement of the children is needed to set goals which have real world application, cultivate children's problem-solving skills and empower children to take ownership for change. Studies report only a low to moderate agreement between parent and child participation goal foci, e.g. Kang et al. (2025). Involvement of children directly in selecting goals for participation interventions is therefore essential, wherever possible.

Moving from Specialized Clinics to Everyday Settings

In the last decade, there has been a transformation of service provision in pediatric rehabilitation from specialized care where children meet with professionals in clinics to professionals coaching of children and families in their natural settings (Anaby et al., 2018; Graham et al., 2019). There is evidence that supporting families and children in their everyday settings is likely to lead to more real-life applications of strategies. In situ learning tends to be generalized and provides more opportunities for problem-solving. Focusing on natural settings lead to empowerment of children and families to take ownership of change (Dunst et al., 2019). Situating learning in everyday settings might lead to parents/carers and children decreasing their contacts with pediatric rehabilitation clinics. However, simply providing the 'usual clinical practice' in an everyday setting is not sufficient to capitalize on the learning opportunities. When talking about everyday settings, professionals are more likely to talk about them as a location, while parents/carers see them as opportunities for learning. Bridging this potential disconnect is important (Ullenhag et al., 2024). Situating the provision of expertise within everyday settings provides the opportunity to focus directly on meaningful participation outcomes in natural settings as opposed to activity competence or body function (Dunst, 2020; Moore et al., 2025).

Moving from Face-To-Face to Digital Encounters

If participation goals, and participation interventions, are set in everyday environments services and professionals need to understand aspects of the everyday setting. Working directly in the everyday setting might be facilitated by digital solutions. Digital solutions can enable children and youth, as well as others, to directly interact with professionals, to show where they are and what they are doing. Thus, professionals and child/care provider may problem-solve together any challenges they experience with implementing a planned intervention or strategy.

The trend toward digital health solutions (Brantnell et al., 2023), has demonstrated benefits. Children with disabilities and their families report reduced stress with digital encounters and that they are more comfortable at home (Gudka et al., 2025; Kodjebacheva et al., 2023). Digital health solutions may also enable people who live remotely to stay in contact with professionals, save time for families with multiple contacts with service systems, and enable professionals to provide more frequent follow-up on progress. While there are digital tools designed for self-management in pediatric rehabilitation, most are focused on supporting and empowering parents/carers (e.g., Mulyana et al., 2023; Wakimizu et al., 2022) rather than children themselves. This is a needed area of development. Gudka et al.'s (2025) review of digital health interventions with healthcare information and self-management resources for young people with ADHD, found that interventions that were co-produced with the target group and contained psychoeducational aspects related to self-managing had the best effects. Co-production supports the individualization and meaningfulness of interventions (Reeve et al., 2016).

Implementing Capacity Building Approaches to Self-Management of Participation

Implementing change takes time, so the question is: how to support pediatric rehabilitation services in tackling the change toward focusing on contextualized problems that are meaningful for children and families? It requires that not only a single intervention is in focus, but the whole intervention process over several interventions. We will discuss self-management in relation to how pediatric rehabilitation organizations as well as professionals within organizations can implement routines and organizational regulations that enhance self-management of participation-related problems. Pediatric rehabilitation ways of working need to have 'real-world applications', to cultivate children and youth's ability to problem-solve through barriers and empower children and youth to take ownership for change. This work needs to be seen as an ongoing process with opportunities for children and youth to learn and reflect on experiences throughout their life. In addition, we will present and discuss some of the instruments/self-reports and procedures that are available for professionals within pediatric rehabilitation to enhance self-management of participation problems in individual encounters with children with disabilities and their families.

ORGANIZATIONAL AND PROFESSIONAL ASPECTS

Pediatric rehabilitation organizations have as their goal to provide children and youth with disabilities and their families with the support necessary for leading a good everyday life. One of the main tasks for the organization is to support and enhance the development of self-management skills in children, such as to identify goals and procedures for managing participation problems. Participation in the ICF is defined as involvement in a life situation (WHO, 2001) and has been operationalized as having two dimensions, attendance and involvement (Imms et al., 2017). Attendance or "being there" in real life or digitally is a prerequisite for being involved in an activity. Pediatric rehabilitation support to self-manage participation interventions requires that the organization structures the intervention work in a manner that provides opportunities for self-management (attendance) and facilitates self-management when the child or youth grasp the opportunity (involvement).

The constructs of attendance and involvement can be used when analyzing if an organization is prepared to support self-management. From an organizational perspective the encounters with a child and family commonly have an intervention cycle as a recurring phenomenon, including six steps: (1) invite the child and family, and preparations before the encounter, (2) identify the current situation and problems/challenges that need to be addressed, (3) explain the identified problems, (4) prioritize among problems to work with and set a goal or desired outcome for intervention, (5) design an intervention and implementing it, and (6) evaluate the outcome.

In all these steps, attendance and involvement aspects of child and family participation in the intervention process are affected by organizational goals and routines. The implicit goal of a series of intervention cycles can be to promote the development of self-management knowledge and skills in the child as well as in other family members. Over time, a series of interventions cycles can be seen as a circular process from being asked to come to the pediatric rehabilitation center/or to see a professional in an everyday setting to evaluate the outcome of one intervention to several interventions. Self-management opportunities and support can therefore be considered in terms of how services are structured to provide or regulate attendance and involvement in each intervention step. Organizations have several goals and regulations fulfilling different purposes that sometimes are difficult to combine.

An intervention process with the goal of enhancing self-management in children and families is one possible task that competes with other organizational goals and tasks regarding resources and time spent in the organization. Reimbursement systems are, for example, designed to steer toward other goals, such as number of children served; teamwork is frequently multi-disciplinary based on a strong profession-specific identity rather than inter- or trans-disciplinary, thus fostering 'silo thinking' (Imms et al., 2024). Considering all these competing tasks and values, an explicit effort to design an intervention process that facilitates children's self-management is necessary. Thus, fostering self-management of participation needs to be an explicitly acknowledged task for the organization.

The organization's main resource is skilled and engaged professionals. However, how these professionals are trained, supervised and deployed will affect how professionals work with an intervention process intended to implicitly enhance self-management of participation problems. The traditional view of focusing on skills development in pediatric rehabilitation is still dominating in practices (Ryan, Miller et al., 2025) and research (Prinsloo et al., 2023). Strong professions defending their professional domain can reinforce this focus on skills-based training goals. Problems to be solved tend to be identified by professionals, using norm referenced tests/questionnaires, who then go on to develop interventions methods to train skills. Assessment is usually seen as the first information collection step in a process where intervention is primarily seen as designing and implementing a method after a goal has been set. Families and children are seen as implementors of the interventions designed by professionals.

If working with participation problems a shift in the power balance is necessary where primarily children and families identify the problems to work with. This identification of participation problems usually starts before meeting the professionals. How children and families are supported at the start of the process is therefore important. When problems to work with are identified, children and families collaborate with professionals in finding strategies to solve the participation challenge. Such a family-centered approach needs to be developed through in-service training within the organization. Illustrations of characteristics of organizational structures and routines for the intervention process that implicitly facilitate self-management in children are presented in Table 26.1.

In step 1, an important question is whether the child attends the meeting where the initial intervention planning takes place. We have unpublished pediatric rehabilitation data about who had participated in habilitation planning over a year, finding that children attended approximately 30% of the meetings. In response to this finding, the staff decided to change the way the family and child were invited to the meeting. The family received the same invitation as before, but the child was personally invited using an invitation letter written with simple text and graphic symbols. In the next six-month period, 70% of planning meetings included the children (Karlsson et al., in prep.).

Step 2 requires that the child is given opportunities to provide information and identifying problems to address. Children can be supported to talk about participation concerns and provide self-report through instruments provided with invitation letter (Liao et al., 2025).

Step 3 is about explaining participation problems. In this step it is important that any assessment of body functions and activity performance is explicitly connected to solving participation problems. That is, the information about impairments and skills deficits can be used by professionals to discuss with the child and family how the environment or activity setting can be adapted to support the child's participation. Participation interventions have successfully focused on supporting youth with disabilities to understand how the environment impacts participation. The students also learned how to adapt the environment after discussing explanations to difficulties with participation (Anaby et al., 2018; Kramer & Schwartz, 2017). The organization needs to acknowledge and support the time that professionals require to collect and analyze information about natural settings for the intervention to be effective.

Step 4 is about prioritizing problems to work with and formulating an explicit desired outcome/goal. There has been a growing focus on helping children and youth with disabilities to formulate goals for participation interventions (e.g., Liao et al., 2025), however it is still uncommon that children actively participate in goal setting. Ryan, Miller et al. (2025) report that in only 2% of rehabilitation goal setting documents analyzed were children explicitly a part of goal setting. Professionals need to have skills in collaborative goal setting strategies with children, families and others in the everyday setting.

Step 5: Designing and implementing intervention requires that professionals have the time and skills necessary for co-constructing feasible interventions in collaboration with child and family. Such interventions need to be followed up with coaching child and parents in implementing method, e.g., solution focused coaching (King et al., 2017).

TABLE 26.1

Characteristics of Organizational Structures and Routines for the Intervention Process that Implicitly Facilitate Self-Management in Children

	Organizational Structure and Routines Enabling Facilitation of Self-management in Child and Caregivers		Tasks of the Professional, Child and Caregiver in Encounters Aimed at Facilitating Self-management	
Step in intervention cycle	Aspects related to attending	Aspects related to involvement	Professional	Child and caregiver
1) Preparing for planning meeting	Forms and procedures used for inviting caregivers and the child to planning meetings can be individually tailored	Child is assigned a support person that can help child and caregivers to identify important activities for change	Individualize invitation letter for child by adapting form and content	Caregivers are asked to support the child in identifying important activities before meeting. Child active part in process
2) Identifying challenge/ problem	Forms and procedures for supporting child self-reported wishes for activities for change are available	Child has a facilitator in planning meetings who supports his/her active participation in meeting	Professional support child with the help of self-rating if possible. Pre-meeting if necessary	Parents/carers support the child in telling about important participation challenges/problems
3) Explaining problem	Routines for assessment include collecting information about body function, activity, as well as environment/context of participation restrictions	Professionals are supported to use a toolbox of participation and environmental measures and procedures to facilitate child/caregiver understanding of participation restriction	Professionals present assessment information in a manner that facilitates discussions with the child and caregiver about links between child impairment and environmental factors	Child and parents generate and validate explanations generated when linking assessment to participation restriction
4) Prioritizing and formulate goal	Child is explicitly supported be a part of the decision-making activity. Adapted material and procedures are available	Professionals are supported to develop knowledge and skills in involving the child and family in the goal setting process	Professionals support the child and family to discuss pros and cons with choosing among the restrictions to focus on. GAS is used as a tool in the process	Child and family formulate concrete description of the desired outcome supported by GAS
5) Designing an intervention and implementing it	Child and family, digitally or in real life, are supported to present the context for challenge/problem to be solved	Professionals are coached in how to facilitate child and family involvement in designing method Time is allowed for professionals to provide digital coaching to families	Professionals provide frequent follow up coaching digitally to facilitate implementing intervention	Child and family are responsible for calibrating the method and evaluating feasibility of method
6) Evaluate outcome	Outcome evaluation is supported by goal documents, e.g., GAS scale	Organizations collect, report and value data on participation outcomes	Child and family are allowed – and supported – to be the primary evaluators of outcome	Child and family both provide evaluation of outcome

Step 6: Outcome evaluation requires that the organization ask professionals to work with goal attainment scales (or other goal instruments) in collaboration with child and caregivers. It is also good if the scales for goal attainment are used in organizational statistics to stress the importance of outcomes and facilitate sustainability.

INSTRUMENTS AND PROCEDURES THAT CAN ENHANCE SELF-MANAGEMENT OF PARTICIPATION PROBLEMS

A key step to self-management of participation problems is learning to self-assess participation. This would include the reconceptualization of everyday challenges as participation restrictions: that is too little or too much attendance, too much or too little involvement in one life situation or in the pattern of participation across life situations. Lundy's model of child participation (Lundy, 2007) conceptualizes Article 12 of the UN Convention of the Rights of the Child. It provides an understanding of participation in decision-making. It is a crucial aspect of learning self-management of participation. The model is conceptualized through four interrelated elements: space, voice, audience, and influence.

Space

The first step for children and young people to learn the skills needed to self-manage their own participation is to include them in relevant conversations and decision-making processes. For children and young people to be involved, the first questions you might ask yourself are: Is the child present? Does the child know that he/she is allowed to share views? Does the child feel comfortable and safe in this space? Has the child been given the information he/she needs to form a view?

Voice

Children and young people need to be given voice, that is they should be 'facilitated to express their views' (Lundy, 2007). Facilitating children and young people's voices can be achieved through access to materials, procedures, and information that are communicatively, cognitively, and physically accessible. Tools or procedures used to achieve this will depend on the access needs of the child. This section will provide some examples of tools and procedures.

There are two main paths for professionals and organizations seeking to increase accessibility in assessments: (i) to choose alternatives specifically developed for children with accessibility needs or (ii) to adapt their standard instruments and procedures.

Choose Alternatives Specifically Developed for Children with Accessibility Needs

In the context of patient-reported outcome measures, cognitively accessible assessment design has been defined as a "design that anticipates respondent variability in cognitive abilities and reduces cognitive demands and/or supports cognitive processes to enable respondents to interpret and respond to assessment items as intended" (Kramer & Schwartz, 2017, p. 1707). Consequently, identifying and lowering cognitive and communicative demands in procedures, layout, and content is essential not only for accessibility in the short term but also for fostering involvement and supporting children's ability to manage their own participation over time.

Picture My Participation (PMP) (Arvidsson et al., 2019) is an example of a participation self-rating instrument where accessibility was considered in the development phase through different strategies, such as basing it on a Talking Mats (Murphy & Cameron, 2008) approach with pictorial support for both activities and response options. It is designed to assess children's attendance and involvement across 20 broad activity domains. In addition, it enables the child to identify and prioritize personally meaningful activities, as well as to describe perceived barriers and facilitators to participation. PMP has been successfully administered both in person and remotely via video conferencing (Ivarsson et al., 2023). It is a guided interview, rather than a questionnaire or scale, to ensure its flexibility.

Children – AAC-users or not – could use Talking Mats™ (Murphy & Cameron, 2008) to engage in decision-making around their participation. Talking Mats™ (Murphy & Cameron, 2008) is a visual communication and thinking tool that can support people to weigh up options and prioritize them to inform future decision-making. For instance, it can be used to accommodate goal setting. For people with disabilities, sometimes there are several allied health members involved in their care who might each have their own discipline-specific priorities. Talking Mats might support children and families to prioritize where they want to spend their time and effort across a potentially large range of goals. For people with severe to profound disability, clinicians can learn from standard 'Supported decision making' practices (Shogren et al., 2019).

Adapt Standard Instruments and Procedures

There is little guidance from quantitative data on which specific types of adaptations to standard assessment procedures and instruments that will increase their accessibility the best. Typically, strategies from the augmentative and alternative communication (AAC) field are used to support both expressive and receptive communication. Providing a range of ways to respond is essential for all children, but especially for those with communication disabilities.

Children with different conditions (e.g., autism, cerebral palsy, intellectual disability, genetic syndromes, others) may use AAC. Using AAC does not mean a child has a cognitive impairment: they might be using AAC for a speech purpose like dysarthria. If a child has an established AAC system of preference, they must be allowed, encouraged, and supported to use it to participate in self-management.

Other strategies aiming at lowering cognitive and communicative demands include, but are not limited to (Ivarsson et al., 2025; Kramer & Schwartz, 2017): written information in easy-to-read language, pictorial support, providing information in written form with time to think about it before making decisions, having a familiar person facilitate communication between the child and the health professional, providing real-life examples of potential consequences of a decision relative to the individual, rather than vague, non-specific information

When a child does not have an established AAC system or preference, the strategies that most efficiently bridge the gap between the child's specific cognitive and/or communicative challenge(s) and the demands in the assessment situation are chosen (Ivarsson et al., 2025). Establishing which specific adaptations are the best is typically an iterative process. Essential for this process is first ensuring there is sufficient time to test and adapt specific instruments and procedures. Secondly to pay attention to identifying signs that could indicate that the cognitive and communicative demands do not match the child's needs.

In summary, there are many ways of facilitating children and young people to self-manage their participation. By analyzing different aspects of accessibility in assessment and by using strategies to reduce inherent cognitive and communicative demands, children and families are supported to self-manage participation. Participation is complex to discuss. In a study investigating the use of spontaneous adaptations in different interview-administered PROMs, the instrument in need of the most adjustment to ensure accessibility was the PMP (Ivarsson et al., 2025). This finding may seem unexpected, given the intended accessibility of the instrument compared with the other measures used to assess outcomes such as life satisfaction. This likely reflects that some constructs, such as involvement and barriers/facilitators for participation, which are measured with PMP, are inherently more abstract or complex than others (e.g., what activities that are fun).

Audience

Next, we should consider who is receiving the views of the child. Who is listening? The audience should be someone with a responsibility to listen, and someone who has the power to take on the child's view to aggregate with other information to make decisions about next steps. In the intervention planning process, and with the goal of self-management of participation, children need to learn to voice their needs, and parents/carers and others in the situation need to learn how to listen.

Influence

Teaching children with disabilities to self-manage participation is unlikely to be a quick or easy process: environmental and personal barriers/facilitators are abstract concepts, and families may be unaccustomed to viewing everyday challenges through a participation lens. Investing time in this process may save time and resources over time and lead to better long-term outcomes. Something that will help with teaching children and young people to have ownership over their support is when they can see and feel the influence of their views. This means that children's views are 'given due weight' (Lundy, 2007). Children will not independently make all the decisions, but their view needs to be considered alongside parents' and health professionals' views for them to develop agency. This learning needs to start early—as it too requires changes on the part of the child/youth as well as others in the situation to respond to the views of children and youth. As children become older or become more developmentally mature, it is essential that the weight given to their preferences also grows.

CONCLUSIONS

Self-management is a learned skill, requiring opportunity for trial and error, and practice. Parents and professionals can support the development of self-management in children growing up with a disability, by providing structured opportunities for learning within the intervention process. This approach requires that assessment is seen as a learning process, not only an information collection process. How professionals work is, however, also dependent on the importance that service organizations assign to self-management and how the organizational rules and regulations support it.

At the level of the organization, it is fundamental to ensure that reimbursement systems align with the shift toward teaching self-management of participation. This requires a shift in how reimbursement systems are designed, with a stronger emphasis on encounters with families outside traditional face-to-face visits in clinical settings. Organizations will also require appropriate quality indicators for participation interventions. Specific quality indicators are needed, as organizational metrics that focus on counting "face-to-face patient visits" tends to bias practice toward interventions that require less individual tailoring (e.g., child ability or function training). Organizations need to explicitly value participation goals. Organizations will also need to develop ways of motivating their staff to do new things that may seem less efficient in the short term (e.g., asking the child instead of the carer/parent about some participation-related questions may take more time).

The role of professions is complex. Some professions have embraced a shift toward teaching self-management of participation problems as a key outcome for pediatric rehabilitation more quickly than others. Variation in the uptake of this approach may be dependent on professionals' attitudes toward promoting child and family influence over decisions, the different areas of expertise of the professions and the focus of interventions. A key issue is how to support professionals to change their perspective from primarily working with body functions and training skills toward including working toward participation as a main professional task. Consequently, tools and procedures used in collaboration with children and families need to be adapted in both form and content to facilitate the development of self-management, not only for the carers but also for the child.

Children's skills in self-management are dependent on opportunities provided by the service organization to learn self-management and on the child's motivation and ability to learn considering their cognitive and communicative ability and skills. Thus, children's self-management is best seen as a continuum from autonomous problem solving to interdependent problem solving with support from carers and other people important to the child. Children are dependent on their caregivers, and those raising children want what is best for their children. Part of this is realizing that through their actions, caregivers can explicitly support children to become more autonomous in managing their life situation.

REFERENCES

Anaby, D, Law, M., Feldman, D., et al. (2018). The effectiveness of the pathways and resources for engagement and participation (PREP) intervention: Improving participation of adolescents with physical disabilities. *Developmental Medicine & Child Neurology*, *60*(5), 513–519.

Arvidsson, P., Dada, S., Granlund, M., Imms, C., Bornman, J., Elliott, C., & Huus, K. (2019). Content validity and usefulness of picture my participation for measuring participation in children with and without intellectual disability in South Africa and Sweden. *Scandinavian Journal of Occupational Therapy*, *27*(5), 336–348. https://doi.org/10.1080/11038128.2019.1645878

Bickenbach, J., Rubinelli, S., Baffone, C., & Stucki, G. (2023). The human functioning revolution: Implications for health systems and sciences. *Frontiers in Science*, *1*, 1118512.

Brantnell, A., et al. (2023). Barriers to and facilitators of the implementation of digital mental health interventions as perceived by primary care decision makers: Content analysis of structured open-ended survey data. *JMIR Human Factors*, *10*, e44688.

Dunst, C. J. (2020). Everyday learning opportunities of young children with and without developmental disabilities or delays. *International Journal of Early Childhood Environmental Education*, *7*(3), 23–41.

Dunst, C. J., Hamby, D. W., & Raab, M. (2019). Modeling the relationships between practitioner capacity-building practices and the behavior and development of young children with disabilities and delays. *Educational Research and Reviews*, *14*(9), 309–319.

Graham, F., King, G., Schwellnus, H., Servais, M., & Baldwin, P. (2019). Solution-focused coaching in pediatric rehabilitation: Investigating transformative experiences and outcomes for families. *Physical & Occupational Therapy in Pediatrics*, *39*(1), 16–32.

Granlund, M., & Imms, C. (2024). Participation as a means: Implications for interventions. *Frontiers in Rehabilitation Sciences*, *5*, 1399818.

Gudka, R., McGlynn, E., Lister, K., Shaw, N., Pitchforth, E., Mughal, F., French, B., Headly Ward, J., Newlove-Delgado, T., & Price, S. (2025). Digital health interventions with healthcare information and self-management resources for young people with ADHD: A mixed-methods systematic review and narrative synthesis. *European Child and Adolescent Psychiatry*, *24*, 1817–1835.

Guevara, J. P., Wolf, F. M., Grum, C. M., & Clark, N. M. (2003). Effects of educational interventions for self management of asthma in children and adolescents: Systematic review and meta-analysis. *BMJ*, *326*(7402), 1308–1309.

Huber, M., Knottnerus, J. A., Green, L., Van Der Horst, H., Jadad, A. R., Kromhout, D., & Smid, H. (2011). How should we define health? *BMJ*, *343*, d4163.

Imms, C., Granlund, M., Wilson, P., Steenbergen, B., Rosenbaum, P., & Gordon, A. (2017). Participation – Both a means and an end. A conceptual analysis of processes and outcomes in childhood disability. *Developmental Medicine and Child Neurology*, *59*(1), 16–25. https://doi.org/10.1111/dmcn.1323732

Imms, C., Moore, T., Luscombe, D., SNAICC, Wilson, M., & Knight, S. (2024). *Review of best practice in early childhood intervention: Review report*. The University of Melbourne, funded by and provided to the Commonwealth of Australia's Department of Social Services. https://healthy-trajectories.com.au/eci-framework/development-of-the-framework/

Ivarsson, M., Andersson, A. K., & Almqvist, L. (2023). Self-rating via video communication in children with disability – A feasibility study. *Frontiers in Psychology, 14*, 1130675. https://doi.org/10.3389/fpsyg.2023.1130675

Ivarsson, M., Danielsson, H., Almqvist, L., & Imms, C. (2025). Enhancing cognitive accessibility in assessments for children with neurodisability: Development and implementation of an adaptation tracking questionnaire. *Disability and Rehabilitation, 47*(18), 4830–4839. https://doi.org/10.1080/09638288.2025.2455532

Kang, L.-J., Granlund, M., Dada, S., & Huus, K. (2025). Perceived activity competence and participation in everyday activities of children with and without neurodevelopmental disorders. *Physical and Occupational Therapy in Pediatrics, 45*(4), 498–516.

Karlsson, C., Granlund, M., & Augustine, L. (in prep.). *You Have to Attend an Activity to Be Involved in It*. Jönköping University.

King, G., Schwellnus, H., Servais, M., & Baldwin, P. (2017). Solution-focused coaching in pediatric rehabilitation: Investigating transformative experiences and outcomes for families. *Physical & Occupational Therapy in Pediatrics, 39*(1), 16–32. https://doi.org/10.1080/01942638.2017.1379457

Kodjebacheva, G. D., Culinski, T., Kawser, B., & Amin, S. (2023) Satisfaction with pediatric telehealth according to the opinions of children and adolescents during the COVID-19 pandemic: A literature review. *Frontiers in Public Health, 11*, 1145486. https://doi.org/10.3389/fpubh.2023.1145486

Kramer, J. M., & Schwartz, A. (2017). Reducing barriers to patient-reported outcome measures for people with cognitive impairments. *Archives of Physical Medicine and Rehabilitation, 98*(8), 1705–1715. https://doi.org/10.1016/j.apmr.2017.03.011

Liao, H. F., Liao, Y.-T., Chen, L.-C., Wu, Y.-T., Kang, L.-J., Granlund, M., & Björck, E. (2025). Collaborative goal-setting approaches to support participation of children with special educational needs. *Pediatric Physical Therapy, 37*(3), 336–344.

Lindsay, S., Kingsnorth, S., Mcdougall, C., & Keating, H. (2014). A systematic review of self-management interventions for children and youth with physical disabilities. *Disability and Rehabilitation, 36*(4), 276–288.

Lozano, P., & Houtrow, A. (2018). Supporting self-management in children and adolescents with complex chronic conditions. *Pediatrics, 141*(Supplement_3), S233–S241.

Lundy, L. (2007). 'Voice' is not enough: Conceptualising article 12 of the United Nations Convention on the Rights of the Child". *British Education Research Journal, 33*(6), 927–942. https://doi.org/10.1080/01411920701657033

Moore T., Imms, C., Luscombe, D., SNAICC, Bonyhady, B., Dimmock, K., Deane, K, D'Aprano, A., & Kakoschke-Moore, S. (2025). National best practice framework for early childhood intervention. The University of Melbourne. Commissioned by the Commonwealth of Australia's Department of Social Services. https://healthy-trajectories.com.au/eci-framework/

Mulyana, A. M., Rakhmawati, W., Wartakusumah, R., Fitri, S. Y. R., & Juniarti, N. (2023). The efficacy of internet-based interventions in family-centered empowerment among children with chronic diseases: A mixed-methods systematic review. *Journal of Multidisciplinary Healthcare, 16*, 3415–3433. https://doi.org/10.2147/JMDH.S440082

Murphy, J., & Cameron, L. (2008). The effectiveness of talking mats® for people with intellectual disability. *British Journal of Learning Disability, 36*(4), 232–241.

Palmqvist, L., & Danielsson, H. (2020). Parents act as intermediary users for their children when using assistive technology for cognition in everyday planning: Results from a parental survey. *Assistive Technology, 32*(4), 194–202. https://doi.org/10.1080/10400435.2018.1522523

Prinsloo, P., Dada, S., Bastable, K., Raghavendra, P., & Granlund, M. (2023). The application of the family of participation-related constructs (fPRC) framework to AAC intervention outcomes in children with complex communication needs: A scoping review. *Augmentative and Alternative Communication, 40*(3), 182–195. https://doi.org/10.1080/07434618.2023.2276701

Reeve, J., Cooper, L., Harrington, S., et al. (2016). Developing, delivering and evaluating primary mental health care: The co-production of a new complex intervention. *BMC Health Services Research, 16*, 470. https://doi.org/10.1186/s12913-016-1726-6

Ryan, A. K., Miller, M., MacDonald, M., & Johnston, L. (2025). How do we capture child and family goals? Examining the goal setting practices used by community-based allied health professionals. *Disability and Rehabilitation*. https://doi.org/10.1080/09638288.2025.2454974

Ryan, M., Fahti, N., Phoemix, M., Granlund, M., Graham, F., & Anaby, D. (2025). Capacity building for youth with disabilities: Principles and key ingredients identified through a scoping review. *Disability and Rehabilitation*. https://doi.org/10.1080/09638288.2025.2471572

Shogren, W., Martinis, & Blanck. (2019). https://www.supportfordecisionmakingresource.com.au/

Ullenhag, A., Imms, C., Anaby, D., Kramer, J., Girdler, S., Gorter, J., Ketelaar, M., Elliot, C., & Granlund, M. (2024). How can we reach long-lasting inclusive participation for all? A vision for the future. *Child: Care, Health and Development*, *50*(2):e13249.

Wakimizu, R., Sasaki, K., Yoshimoto, M., Miyazaki, A., & Saito, Y. (2022). Multidisciplinary approach for adult patients with childhood-onset chronic disease focusing on promoting pediatric to adult healthcare transition interventions: An updated systematic review. *Frontiers in Pediatrics*, *10*, 919865.

Wong Chung, R., Willemen, A., Voorman, J., Ketelaar, M., Becher, J., Verheijden, J., & Schuengel, C. (2020). Managing oneself or managing together? Parents' perspectives on chronic condition self-management in Dutch pediatric rehabilitation services. *Disability and Rehabilitation*, *42*(23), 3348–3358. https://doi.org/10.1080/09638288.2019.1594396

World Health Organization. (2001). *International Classification of Functioning, Disability and Health.*

27 Health Coaching as a Tool for Self-Management in Rehabilitation

John Naylor

THE CONSEQUENCES OF UNHEALTHY BEHAVIOURS

The fact that unhealthy behaviours and related lifestyle choices can be linked with numerous preventable health conditions is, by now, widely understood. Yet, it appears that knowing something is *probably* bad for your health is rarely sufficient impediment for doing exactly that. The lag between *cause and effect* with most health 'decisions' means that even those motivated to change might be unsuccessful without some appropriate support. Effective and sustained behaviour change is not an easy process.

In situations where chronic disease or long-term illness is already a person's reality, this effective transition to the status of *patient* should, one would have thought, make it more difficult to dismiss health behaviours that are so consequential to the management and progression of their condition. Yet rather than dispassionately weighing up and acting on the best way forward for their future health, a lifelong 30-a-day smoker with newly diagnosed chronic obstructive pulmonary disease (COPD) might, for example, still question the purpose of quitting when the damage is already done – staking *healthier life years* on this continuing behaviour. Individuals' health decisions are, therefore, not always necessarily as logical as one might expect.

HEALTH INEQUALITY

We all know harmful behaviours such as smoking or unhealthy eating can be tough habits to break but ignoring best practice guidelines for medical conditions is surely more irresponsible, right? In recent years, however, much has been made of the influence on health inequality of *social determinants of health*, namely, unfair and avoidable differences in health status based on one's access to power, money and resources (WHO, 2025). For example, women living in the poorest areas of England can expect to experience around 19 fewer years of good health compared to the wealthiest neighbourhoods (Health Foundation, 2025). Furthermore, the average English adult life expectancy is reportedly worse by seven years in those poorer areas (Marmot, 2010). Therefore, the well-educated and well-paid professional who passes judgement on the dietary choices of a single mother-of-five may not have considered the unseen forces amounting to health dice stacked against her and her family. Still, according to a leading coalition of health and social care charities in England, "the strongest correlation to ill health – stronger than education level, deprivation, age or ethnicity" is in actual fact, *health literacy* (National Voices, 2017).

HEALTH LITERACY

The term *Health literacy* is often used to explain how people access, comprehend and utilise information to make decisions about their own health. Lower health literacy, common among socially and economically disadvantaged groups, when unaddressed, risk widening the existing health inequalities (NHSE, 2025a). The reality is that patients across health literacy and socioeconomic

DOI: 10.1201/9781003599074-30

spectra, for their own personal reasons, don't always make logical decisions in following what is *best* for their future health or an existing health condition; effectively exercising their freedom of personal choice. Humanistic concerns aside, the question of why an individual's poor health decisions should even matter tends to come into sharper focus when the resulting impact is being felt by other healthcare users. It is at this fault line where the conviction of a purported *live-and-let-live* philosophy can be tested.

Health Service Challenges

There is a growing burden on health care services, internationally, from non-communicable diseases. Musculoskeletal conditions, such as arthritis and chronic pain, for example, affect a staggering 20 million adults in the UK – equating to around 30% of the population (Versus Arthritis, 2024). Broader demographic changes in the West have led to the situation where more people are living longer while suffering from multiple long-term health conditions. Given the increased demands on health services that include additional clinical contact time, medications and expensive hospital admissions, the health and social care costs, footed by the taxpayer here in the UK, are as eye-watering as they are unsustainable.

Health Policy Challenges

Rolling UK news footage of ambulances queuing to transfer patients into hospital; case studies of work absences due to delayed waits for surgery and reports of elderly patients being nursed on busy corridors provide but a few vignettes of a healthcare model in crisis. Faced with this bleak picture and ominous future, health policy makers find themselves in a relentless hunt for panaceas without the commensurate budgets to fund such improvement. A recent example in the UK being the Labour Government's pivot towards NHS app-based service-delivery model as part of their new *10-year plan* (Department of Health and Social Care, 2025), where innovations on a digital platform promise both improved patient experience and access. Whether or not this will have the desired impact stands to be seen, but innovative ways to offer something different from the *business-as-usual* approach are now, more than ever, necessary and welcome.

Self-management: Part of a Social Contract?

The healthcare approach of *supported self-management*, central to the UK Government's *NHS long term plan* (2019), is re-emphasised in the *10-year plan* (Department of Health and Social Care, 2025). And expecting more in terms of better self-management from those with existing health conditions would seem a sensible way of reducing health service pressures including costly hospital admissions.

Despite the renewed optimism being placed on self-management as a health strategy, it is important to recognise that this is not a new concept and successful implementation *en masse* is fraught with practical and ethical challenges. When implementing a self-management strategy – one that attempts to redirect patients away from poorer health trajectories, as we have seen, effective patient education becomes an essential element. But if well-educated individuals with high levels of health literacy can make decisions that are bad for their health, then health education alone is surely insufficient.

Within a nationalised healthcare system, like here in the UK, there exists a *social contract* of sorts between citizens and *their* NHS. With this comes a tacit responsibility for individuals to do their bit to stay healthy as not to overburden a service funded through taxation. However, not everyone will see things through a societal lens, feeling entitled to consume as much healthcare as they need *because* of their national insurance contributions. Whether employed or not, the *NHS Constitution* enshrines all citizens' rights of access to health services, good quality of care and to be treated by appropriately qualified and experienced staff, among other key tenets (Department of Health, 2013). Accusations could be made that the promotion of self-management presents a convenient delegation of health service responsibility for those patients it purports to serve. The challenge, therefore, is in finding the sweet spot of empowered personal health responsibility which lies somewhere between the extremes of 'nanny state' and Governmental dereliction of duty for its citizens' health.

Nudge Theory

With such self-management goals in mind, the UK Coalition Government of 2010 adopted principles of gentle persuasion, applying behavioural science to public policy through a 'Behavioural Insights Team', colloquially referred to as the "Nudge Unit" (Institute for Government, 2020). Based on research challenging conventional ideas of *rational economic actors* – this supposedly led to the creation of *choice architecture* for making better changes within individuals' own self-interest (Thaler and Sunstein, 2008). With a similar focus on personalisation, positive reinforcement and encouragement – as well as 'option talk' equivalents to *choice architecture* that uphold autonomy, a practical application of this theory already existed in the form of health coaching (HC).

Health Coaching as a Person-Centred Approach

Putting aside the obvious limitations of *expecting* all patients to do what is best for them, the other extreme of attempting to *make* patients do what is best for them is, at best, controversial and, at worst, disturbing – harking back to a paternalistic biomedical model long-rejected by modern healthcare professionals. To enlightened proponents of person-centred practice – who espouse principles of individualised care and shared decision-making, corollary notions of *patient compliance* are an anathema to the principled stance of *patient as a partner.*

Supported self-management for musculoskeletal conditions, on the other hand, has been described as "what the health and social care system can put in place to help people's confidence, ability and capability to manage" (ARMA, 2024). While self-management is, of course, not limited to musculoskeletal issues, this serves as a useful focus given the author's area of expertise. It is fortunate then that HC constitutes a middle ground where person-centred clinicians can support self-management.

An Introduction to the Concept of Health Coaching

HC describes a therapeutic, person-centred behaviour change intervention - orchestrated by health care professionals from various backgrounds, with the explicit aim of improving a patient's health outlook (Sforzo et al., 2018). It is through its ability to improve individuals' health by changes in their health behaviours and, thus, prevent non-communicable diseases (James et al., 2018) that has led to calls for *all* healthcare professionals to receive training in HC (ARMA, 2024). Many health professionals, including in the author's own speciality of physiotherapy, have embraced this tool for empowering patients to achieve self-determined goals – as part of their ultimate attempts to support patient self-management.

Theoretical Models that Underpin Health Coaching

HC, as an approach, is theoretically underpinned by several well-known models of behaviour change, most notably the *social cognitive theory* of Albert Bandura (1977); Prochaska and Velicer's *stages of (transtheoretical) change model* (1997); and the *motivational interviewing method of* Rollnick and Miller (1995).

SOCIAL COGNITIVE THEORY

Bandura's *social cognitive theory* is centred around the concept of self-efficacy, namely, an individual's belief in their innate ability to achieve goals (Bandura, 1977). Self-efficacy's supposed influence on whether a task is attempted, the level of effort put in, and perseverance when faced by challenges hold obvious relevance here and, thus, have become a foundational tenet of HC.

TRANSTHEORETICAL CHANGE MODEL

The *transtheoretical change model* (Prochaska and Velicer, 1997) frameworks how people change their (health) behaviours through distinct stages of *precontemplation* (i.e., no intention to change); *contemplation* (i.e., considering the possible change); *preparation* (i.e., planning for change in the coming month); *action* (i.e., changes made in the last six months); and *maintenance* (i.e., for at least six months and attending to possible relapses), with the ever-present chance of a *relapse* (i.e., return to unhealthy behaviour). Importantly, *relapse* here is not considered a failure but rather a normal part of a change process that can be resumed, hence allowing for the back and forward movement with this non-linear model.

MOTIVATIONAL INTERVIEWING (MI)

Motivational interviewing (MI) adopts a more structured counselling style of communication to aid individuals to explore their *ambivalence to change* and strengthen their resolve in attaining this (Rollnick and Miller, 1995). With MI, the practitioner attempts to tap into individuals' inherent desire and capacity for change while respecting their autonomy and not simply trying to persuade them to change. MI practitioners adopt core principles that *express empathy; develop discrepancy; roll with resistance; and support self-efficacy*, which are, in turn, supported by the key skills of open-ended questioning; affirmations; reflective listening; and summarising. With MI and HC constituting complementary, person-centred approaches, the former might be considered a specific tool within a broader HC approach.

A Brief History of Coaching: from Humanistic to Person-Centred

Emergence of the contemporary model of HC, and the associated structured models of coaching such as '*GROW*' (Whitmore, 1992), are better understood through brief discussion of its origins. *The hidden history of coaching* (Wildflower, 2013) lists various interwoven influences on coaching that include therapy, humanistics, self-help, success case studies and biographies.

The history of western philosophy holds *Socratic questioning* as an early precursor to modern coaching – albeit in group rather than a one-to-one interaction. Jumping to the end of the 19th century onwards, advances in psychology, from Freud's *psychoanalysis* to Skinner's *behaviourism*, produced the more optimistic branch of *Humanistic Psychology* that, in turn, sparked interest in the concept of *Positive Psychology*; a field strongly associated with HC. It was the work of psychologist Carl Rogers, originator of the humanistic '*person-centred approach*', that provided the foundations of HC.

Development of the 'GROW' Model: a Universal Coaching Framework

During the 1960s, the influential coaching trio of Carl Rogers, Timothy Gallwey and John Whitmore spent time at the counter-cultural Californian retreat of '*Esalen*' nurturing exploration of inner feelings and human potential (Wildflower, 2013). It was prior to this that Gallwey reportedly began developing his '*Inner Game Theory*'; a coaching approach concerned with the unlocking of potential to maximise client performance (Gallwey, 1974). Inspired by Gallwey's work, Whitmore brought these ideas back to the UK, popularising the now ubiquitous '*GROW model of coaching*'. This model, initially developed by Graham Alexander, was first published by Whitmore in his *Coaching for Performance* (Whitmore, 1992). The focus here being on helping a coachee to address a specific issue or skills deficit to achieve improved performance within a particular area.

'GROW' itself is an acronym for a simple coaching framework commonly used to structure coaching conversations that aim to help individuals achieve their goals:

Goal – i.e. *what do you want?*
Reality – i.e. *where are you now?*
Options – i.e. *what could you do?*
Wrap-up/Way forward – i.e. *what will you do?*

(Performance Consultants, n.d.)

There are many sample questions that can be used to yield answers beneath each area e.g. for Goal – *what will achieving this goal give you?* in a process of "unlocking a person's potential to maximise their own performance helping them to learn as opposed to teaching them" (Whitmore, 1992). 'GROW' is a non-linear framework that allows for some *back-and-forward* as the coach helps to untangle convoluted thinking (Grant, 2011). Various adaptations e.g., 'T-GROW' (with the prefixing of 'T' for topic: the specific area of focus for the session) as well as alternative frameworks, such as the 'CLEAR' model, are available beside the standard 'GROW' model.

Whitmore's commercial website lists the proposed benefits and impacts of employing his famous model including its simplicity, practicality, ability to raise awareness and generate responsibility - with claims that "some of the world's most successful companies, including Google, teach their managers to use GROW" (Performance Consultants, n.d.). The essential premise of using this model to structure a coaching session is that the *coachee already has the potential solutions within themselves* with the coaching session serving to facilitate these discoveries.

Applying Principles of Coaching to Health: 'coaching Not Fixing'

Having rejected outdated paternalistic notions of *clinician knows best,* HC facilitates patient engagement with their health issues through the setting of goals as a motivational partner. By stepping out of 'expert mode' and renouncing the unspoken power gradient that exists between clinician and their patient, the HC philosophy becomes a partnering process of behaviour change towards self-generated health goals. Consequently, rather than having notions of 'fixing' patients, the effective health coach should guide their patients (and their significant others) to come up with the solutions for themselves, while considering the complexities of their individual situated lifeworld. Exploring patient perceptions, attitudes and beliefs elucidates the potential barriers to the desired behaviour change. There is, after all, a big difference in, for example, a physiotherapist simply providing a sheet of exercises for shoulder pain versus their attempting to understand how the problem is affecting what is important in the patient's life. The latter allows for motivating more situated goals – and this is the essence of HC.

Health Coaching and Long-Term Conditions

While the roots of coaching run deep, the modern HC movement only really got started in the 1990s before gaining greater attention in the early 2000s (Health Coaching Institute, 2025). The author, himself, recalls HC visibility within his own physiotherapy profession in the second decade of the new millennium, when its utility for supporting self-management in patients with long-term conditions and multimorbidity was promoted. HC has since entered the wider consciousness: from undergraduate teaching to the array of post-graduate clinical HC training courses, including those offered by the personalised care institute, and its delivery by non-clinical health and wellbeing coaches/social prescribers.

In 2002, a report to examine the future demands on the NHS and to recommend ways of improving public health and reduce health inequalities was commissioned by the UK Treasury (Wanless, 2002). Following the Wanlass report, and its allusion to patients as independent agents of their own health, HC was touted as a possible route for sustainability through targeting patient engagement, specifically. Following this reasoning, *patient activation* – akin to self-efficacy, and health *ownership* – a proxy for empowerment, become essential prerequisites for success (Henry et al., 2025).

Scientific Evidence for Health Coaching

There are some high-quality studies that provide evidence for HC's effectiveness in supporting self-management for a range of long-term illnesses that include respiratory and cardiovascular conditions, as well as for improving weight management, diet and activity levels (NHSE, 2025b). Common long-term conditions linked to HC include COPD; diabetes mellitus (DM); cardiovascular and kidney disease. For example, a systematic review and meta-analysis of 22 randomised controlled trials (RCT) employed HC as a strategy to self-manage type 2 DM, reporting favourable impact on blood sugar (Hb1Ac) levels at several interval periods up to 18 months (Pirbaglou et al., 2018). Another meta-analysis of 30 RCTs on HC's effectiveness for chronic condition care found improvements in quality of life (QoL), self-efficacy and depression across illness populations (Boehmer et al., 2023).

Individual RCTs, too, have reported improvements resulting from a HC intervention that include a 12-week intervention for older adults demonstrating improved self-efficacy and blood pressure maintained at three-month follow-up (Chung et al., 2026). A nine-month trial of HC intervention versus usual care, completed by 158 adults with moderate to severe COPD, demonstrated no significant difference in primary or secondary outcomes, but reported better quality of care, less episodes of depression and fewer COPD related hospitalisation events (Thom et al., 2018). Finally, in a single-centre, parallel group RCT of 108 patients with early stage (CKD1-3a) kidney disease, a HC intervention demonstrated improvements in QoL and self-management and a raising of self-efficacy and activation levels through which self-management and QoL can further improve (Lin et al., 2021).

Mode of Delivery for Health Coaching

As we have seen, HC combines elements from life-coaching, behaviour change and clinical communication skills. According to NHS England's supported self-management guide, HC can be delivered as either a standalone service or an embedded approach across a service or pathway (NHSE, 2023). Examples provided here include dedicated health and wellbeing coaches in primary care. While these would tend to be practitioners from non-clinical backgrounds, i.e., the SP model, in the authors' experience, this might also be delivered by clinicians in the same setting e.g. first contact practitioner (FCP). While HC constitutes a rather heterogeneous approach, whichever format is adopted, this is always based on an underlying person-centred and empowering philosophy, with the common aim of unlocking the individual's potential for better health outcomes.

HC has been traditionally delivered as an in-person intervention – typically one-to-one, but sometimes within a group. However, in the post-pandemic era, there has been a normalisation of remote clinical interactions with patients ranging from basic telephone conversations to technology-supported digital video platform, mobile apps and wearable devices. The explosion in wellness tech and healthcare platforms, combined with a rapid acceptance of the important role that artificial intelligence (AI) will play, has opened promising possibilities for digital health interventions (DHI). In fact, the HC field has already begun to explore state-of-the-art, AI-powered HC approaches.

A recent systematic and narrative synthesis of 35 studies examining DHIs and HC approaches highlighted three key coaching modalities: digital human coaching, artificial intelligence coaching and hybrid (human-AI) coaching – with all of these modalities demonstrating acceptability and feasibility (Loughnane et al., 2025). In-keeping with the challenges from the heterogeneity of approach, this review also highlighted the importance of standardising how methods are measured and contextualised in order to build an evidence-base for digital HC.

With HC not being formularised by a single specific method, this flexibility can also be its *Achilles' heel.* A lot of this will come down to the type and extent of HC training. A systematic review of outcomes from different pharmacist-delivered HC modalities (i.e., face-to-face, telephone or electronic), for example, was unable to recommend any superiority of approach due to reporting inconsistencies on the training received by the health coach (Singh et al., 2020).

Issues of Training for Health Coaching

The HC concept appears in many UK policy documents and reports and thus constitutes a strategic pillar of personalised care aspects for supported self-management (NHS, 2019; Department of Health and Social Care, 2025). As already reported, HC can be particularly effective in supporting self-management of musculoskeletal conditions with behavioural or lifestyle risk factors (NHSE, 2023). The arthritis and musculoskeletal alliance, therefore, recommend ensuring all healthcare professionals receive at least some training in HC, alongside that of health inequalities and health behaviour change (ARMA, 2024). However, effective workforce training in HC presents assorted challenges to employers from issues related to programme quality, standardisation and accreditation; departmental costs and time needed for HC training; and the capacity and interpersonal skills for delivery – including unpreparedness to venture into domains of psychology or mental health that might exceed the scope of practice. Even after training is complete, for embedded models, there remains an issue of providing clearer guidance on how to successfully incorporate HC into clinicians' existing roles (Carter et al., 2015; Davies et al., 2020).

Health Coaching across the Health Ecosystem

Having journeyed through its origins, while outlining the principles of HC, the following section is structured in such a way as to take the reader through the NHS healthcare ecosystem (primary, secondary, tertiary and community healthcare) from the perspective of a musculoskeletal physiotherapist. Practical applications of HC, alongside real-world considerations, are discussed at each level.

PRIMARY CARE

First Contact Practitioners

As part of its *supporting self-management* initiative, the *NHS long term plan* included a provision for all adults in England to access specialist musculoskeletal physiotherapists within general practice, without a referral, by 2024 (NHS, 2019). It is possible that the lack of reference to this first-contact practitioner (FCP) model in the subsequent *10-year plan* (Department of Health and Social Care, 2025) reflects successful roll-out within this short, intervening period. Given the significant burden afflicted on the available workforce by treatable musculoskeletal conditions like low back pain, such early access is invaluable for expediting recovery, as well as reducing the incidence of chronicity.

Alongside their provision of expert assessment, diagnosis and management of musculoskeletal conditions – including referrals for imaging and specialist opinion, the FCP model provides wider access to the health promotion and HC skill sets these experienced musculoskeletal clinicians have at their disposal. In their '...*roadmap to practice*' capability framework, for example, HC features within a 'condition management, interventions and prevention' domain as 'coaching support' (HEE,

2021). The author currently works as an FCP and strongly endorses HC embedded in clinical practice.

Let's take the hypothetical example of an older, overweight person who presents to an FCP with reduced activity due to chronic knee pain. Rather than just providing a sheet of knee exercises, a HC approach here would attempt to address the bigger picture of the negative effects of a sedentary lifestyle by perhaps exploring:

> What is most important to you about your health right now?

...and attempting to elicit patient motivation, using scaling to address ambivalence:

> On a scale of 1 to 10, how ready are you to start exercising regularly?
>
> ...and what would help make this a 7?.

While identifying and problem-solving barriers with questions which might include:

> What is stopping you from doing the exercises?
>
> What would make the exercises easier to fit in?

This might reveal unplaced fears of exercise causing joint damage; something that could be immediately addressed by the FCP. Depending on the level of health literacy present, varying levels of health education will be indicated, alongside broader empowerment and health promotion strategies that might include, for example, weight management. Where self-management is unsatisfactory or insufficient, there is the option of diagnostic imaging, combined with shared decision making on interventions like prescribed medications or corticosteroid injection. Perhaps, even, a referral to an appropriate weight management service or social prescription. In the case of social prescribing, in particular, a full programme from a specialised (health) coaching service, i.e., something the embedded FCP model is unable to provide, can be delivered over multiple recurrent sessions or as necessary.

The overall point about HC in this case is that the patient is afforded the opportunity for a catharsis of sorts; to process personal barriers and facilitators that open the door to meaningful behaviour change that addresses their knee issue. It is the author's stance that provision of such a clear self-realised action plan would not be achievable by a sheet of exercises alone.

Social Prescribers: 'non-clinical' Health Coaching in Primary Care

While it is important to acknowledge that health and wellbeing coaches are often core components of primary care networks and available in general practice, it is the intention of the author to discuss this in the later community care setting.

SECONDARY CARE

The Musculoskeletal Physiotherapy Outpatient Department

Despite some well-publicised shortfalls in patient access to rehabilitation provision nationally, UK physiotherapy departments based in secondary care hospital settings continue to provide facilities for ongoing, specialist physiotherapy. However, in contrast to the numerous face-to-face sessions required for a post-trauma or post-operative rehabilitation protocol e.g., external fixator frames or anterior cruciate ligament reconstruction (ACL), a typical clinical interaction within a musculoskeletal outpatient department in 2025 might amount to a single, or limited number of, sessions before patient-initiated follow-up or discharge.

During this time, in both larger urban *and* smaller community hospitals, contemporary outpatient musculoskeletal physiotherapy will tend to prioritise screening, diagnosis and treatment based on a *self-management where possible* approach. This might even involve a telehealth interaction rather than traditional face-to-face consultation. Despite this constituting *secondary care* – by virtue of referral from another clinician to a hospital-based service, considering the use of space, equipment and general delivery method here, this format may actually be more akin to primary care models such as FCP.

Limited follow-ups reduce the total clinical contact time and, by extension, the opportunity to use HC methods compared with, say, an ACL gym-based rehabilitation that might span nine months. Attempts to deliver comprehensive new patient consultations – with screening, diagnosis and treatment plans, inclusive of the 50 minutes suggested for a standalone HC programme (NHSE, 2023) are clearly not feasible in this setup. As in the FCP example, a more general, as opposed to condition-specific, HC-informed method might loosely employ the GROW model as part of an embedded approach. This would allow for exploration of psychosocial factors leading to meaningful goals, incorporating patient realities such as potential barriers to success, option talk and clear *next steps* on the way forward.

For HC to be successfully embedded and implemented by all, rather than just some of the physiotherapists within a given outpatient department, managers must first identify the necessary skill gaps and support staff development in these areas. This is important as the emphasis to affect positive behaviour change in all patients aligns perfectly with the *making every contact count* initiative; originally promoted by Health Education England and Public Health England, and now part of the standard contract for NHS England.

One would expect a clinician who was in possession of stronger HC skills to exhibit heightened communication abilities including active listening, paraphrasing and summarising, alongside a keen awareness of patient cues and their own non-verbal communication. Additionally, it is important to ensure the patients' clinical records reflect that HC methods were employed to allow for resumption and continuity of this person-centred approach in future visits with other clinicians.

Emergency Departments

The past decade has seen significant growth in the number of physiotherapists managing patients with undifferentiated musculoskeletal presentations who attend frontline emergency departments (ED). Given ED's focus on stabilising injuries and illness through one-off clinical interactions, as well as the requirement for efficient onward transit to maintain a patient throughflow, unsurprisingly, this is not somewhere one naturally associates with HC.

With no EDs in England meeting the target to have admitted, transferred, or discharged 95% of patients within four hours for the last decade (RCEM, 2023), emergency care has become a very challenging environment in which to deliver optimised care. Political austerity of 2010s, the COVID-19 pandemic at the end of the decade followed by ongoing industrial action post-COVID-19 has left a legacy of long waits for clinical treatment in, and ward transfers from, ED; such that we find ourselves in the era of the *12-hour ED wait.* While these problems are much bigger than HC alone can solve, the author wishes to demonstrate the utility and application of embedded HC skills in such high pressure, acute settings.

Using the example of a patient with acute severe low back pain who was brought in by ambulance to ED majors and who is now reportedly unwilling to move off the bed due to fear of pain or harm – an ED musculoskeletal physiotherapist can deploy HC to good effect here. With strong medication already administered by the medics, and an MRI reporting nothing that explains this extreme, acute pain presentation – the pressure is now on the ED physiotherapist to *get this patient up and home.* It is important to remember that the strong medication and medic's reassurance about their scan, here, were insufficient to get the patient moving. The physiotherapist must therefore take a different approach, namely, taking time to engage the patient on their problem and actively listen to receive their full narrative. It is only through such person-centred approaches, that encompass empathy and interest, that an individual can feel genuinely heard and their ideas truly understood. This, in turn, allows the physiotherapist to unravel the psychosocial aspects so central to complex multifactorial presentations like back pain.

As always, the body language really matters here, as standing with a clipboard or tablet looking down on a person in the bed will not engender rapport. Getting down to their level, making good eye contact rather than repeatedly looking away at a screen, and using affirmative nods will make all the difference. After validating the patient's pain and decision to attend ED, the physiotherapist might open with:

> So, what do you believe is going on with your back?

Such an approach aligns with the person-centred *ideas, concerns and expectations (ICE) framework* (Matthys et al., 2009); something with good utility for unravelling what it was in the patient's mind that could be bad enough to call an ambulance. Moreover, this can reveal unhelpful beliefs such as pain erroneously being equated to harm – rendering non-movement a sensible decision. Patients commonly talk in terms of backs "crumbling" and discs "slipping" - recognised nocebo terms that are able to conjure distressing visions, particularly for those with poor health literacy.

Before being able to reach the point of promoting self-management, the physiotherapist must first take the time to focus on reducing the crippling fear, even in the fast-paced, acute setting of ED. It might be the case that this presentation is a culmination of previous worsening episodes that have, thus far, not been appropriately addressed leading to their desperation in calling the ambulance. The education and explanation provided by the physiotherapist, in this case, is different from what they know, or may have already been told in ED, precisely *because* they received the full patient narrative. This enabled the building of trust and affirmation that this wasn't just some standard physiotherapeutic *spiel* but, rather, something more personalised to their current situation: nothing is dismissed, however odd it might seem, as this is the patient's current reality.

In many cases, the ED attendance reflects shortcomings upstream at the primary care level that leave emergency care the provider of last resort, even when inappropriate. It is even more important therefore, to spend the time in avoiding reattendance attributable to unfulfilled patient needs or expectations – another *make every contact count* moment. The health coach, here, must allow the patient to self-actualise an active empowered mindset in terms of what they can do to address an ongoing issue. Some appropriate coaching questions might focus on meaningful activity before using this to connect movement in the present as a small step towards this goal:

> Is there something you want to get back to that this back pain is preventing?

It is of course important to break down such goals into practical steps that, in this case, might amount to the gradual exposure of small movements in the bed, with a reframing of the resulting discomfort as *normal*, rather than damaging. A framing and emphasis on movement to commence healing or to achieve their goal, as opposed to just getting the patient out of hospital, is important but requires mutual trust.

TERTIARY CARE

The Neurosurgical Unit

Tertiary care refers to highly specialist treatment including, for example, that which is provided by a regional hospital-based neurosurgery unit. A scenario involving a person with a spinal cord injury (SCI) here provides the opportunity to discuss how a specialist neurosurgical physiotherapist might enact HC skills alongside their specialist rehabilitative role.

In the hypothetical, but not uncommon, example of a person in their twenties, involved in a car accident that resulted in a complete SCI – one can only imagine what might be going through their mind after finding themselves in an acute hospital – on a medically complex neurosurgical ward, awaiting rehabilitation, before they are well enough for transfer to a rehabilitation centre. However, this would most likely include some level of shock and uncertainty about what the future holds for them.

As with the other acute hospital setting of ED, building trust between patient and clinician will be vital here, but unlike all other examples, they might be working together daily for a protracted period of time. So, when the physiotherapist initially appears to "start the rehab", there will be much more going on than meets the eye in terms of how they deploy their HC skills alongside traditional rehabilitative focus. The clinician's experience of similar patients will have taught them that a HC mindset requires them to quickly establish rapport and psychological safety. After introductions are done, their HC conversation might thus commence with an exploration of their health literacy:

> What do you understand about what's going on so far?

While consideration of cognitive and emotional states will dictate whether or not the person is ready for such coaching, there should be an expectation of emotional reactions. Whether this manifests as anger or sadness, despite them not being a psychologist as such, the coach must be emotionally available to offer reassurance in validating and normalising these feelings:

> it's totally normal for you to feel overwhelmed right now

> I am going to help you

> Don't worry, we are going to take this day by day

The next step might involve setting some rehabilitation goals, such as being able to sit with support, through to something more meaningful to the person, like to leave the ward with a family member for half an hour. Starting with, and demonstrating achievement of, such small and clear goals here will allow the patient to realise their ability to influence outcomes – restoring some feeling of control over the situation.

As the weeks on the ward pass by and the person gradually comes to terms with, and adapts to, their condition, HC questions might naturally shift to more of a focus on self-efficacy, for example:

> What is most important to your recovery right now?

> What would make you feel like you have achieved something today?

Following SCIs, alongside the necessary physical support, is the pressing need to facilitate significant psychological adjustments within the person. While goal setting to achieve patient empowerment must of course be realistic – based on the level of injury, there remains the important power of hope which is something that mustn't be snuffed out by unnecessarily harsh truths delivered with good intentions. Even though some patients may never walk again, a delicate balance must still be struck in the early days if the patient's hope is not to be collateral damage for the dispelling of unrealistic ideas of recovery. The use of HC must therefore set out to support more proximal 'SMART' goals that allow for a self-realisation of what is possible and what will occur over time. Adjustment to the new reality will be key, goals will likely straddle the regaining of independence and autonomy that was taken away, albeit a new and different version of independence.

Commonalities with previous examples would include the focus on education and motivation toward patient empowerment, universal to HC. At any, or all, stages the health coach mindset is framed to move the person away from thinking of themselves as a patient and more towards a self-managing individual.

As must be true with all physiotherapy examples of HC, this scenario constitutes an embedded rather than stand-alone approach. Having said that, the extent and ongoing nature of the HC in this scenario will depend on how soon before the person is transferred to a specialist SCI rehabilitation centre. Since they might be swiftly transferred or remain on the neurosurgical ward for weeks, the ongoing and developing coaching interaction in the latter may share more features with a standalone HC service.

COMMUNITY HEALTH

All examples, thus far, have positioned physiotherapists somewhere along a spectrum that is based on an *embedded model*: from one-off FCP interaction to more involved and recurrent delivery with a neurosurgical inpatient. Such embedded approaches will, of course, differ greatly from stand-alone services that are set up purely for coaching. Due to the specific professional activities and standards required when working under the registered title of 'physiotherapist', HC can only ever be an adjunctive part of their primary clinical responsibilities; that for a musculoskeletal consultation, for example, would include the screening and onward referral for identified red flags. While specialised coaching services that are run by clinicians for specific cohorts will exist, there is a well-established role for *non-clinicians* in which HC can be delivered as a stand-alone service generally referred to as social prescription.

The social prescriber model is, fundamentally, the same as that already discussed but, without the professional duty of care that might constrain a physiotherapist, allows for adoption of a purer coaching style. The principles of HC in this model are, otherwise, unchanged, with this remaining a person-centred approach that supports individuals to improve their general health and wellbeing – in particular, those with long-term conditions, potential complex social needs or mental health issues.

Patients can access social prescriber services directly via self-referral or indirect referral by their GP; other members of the primary care team, as well as other community or secondary care professionals. Depending on the level of patient engagement, this particular HC model might typically occur once or twice weekly, continuing anywhere from six-to-12 weeks; either in person, online or over the phone.

As before, the social prescriber model here is based on coaching to support behaviour change through goal setting, using familiar structures based on MI or 'GROW' model frameworks. As a holistic approach, with the end goal of empowerment for self-management, this will require the coach to address any pertinent physical, social and emotional factors, while considering and integrating lifestyle choices such as smoking, exercises, diet, etc.

As outlined in the earlier section on MI, the core aspects here will be around skilful deployment of open questioning, active listening, use of scaling questions, 'SMART' goal setting, affirmations and summarising. In the case of a person who reports putting on weight due to lack of motivation, poor sleeping and a generally flat mood, the coach might paraphrase back with:

> So, listening to what you just said there, it sounds like you are wanting to feel a bit more energised, and you feel that might come from better sleep, and perhaps feeling more comfortable in your own body. Are these the things that you'd like us to work towards?

The author has tried to demonstrate in this community context, HC need not be limited to hospital or primary care settings, and it does not necessarily need to be delivered by a clinician. In fact, social prescribers might be better placed to offer more time and repeated coaching sessions to support lasting improvements in a person's health and wellbeing.

CONCLUSION

This chapter started by introducing the idea of health behaviour change for self-management within the current sociopolitical context, discussing barriers such as health inequality, health literacy and the growing burden of non-communicable diseases and long-term conditions. Through nudge theory, we arrived at the main topic of '*health coaching to support self-management*', providing an overview of the history, philosophy and theory on which HC is based. After introducing common frameworks like the 'GROW' model, the discussion moved on to issues of training and modes of delivery while highlighting studies that support HC. Finally, attempts were made to place HC within a real-world healthcare ecosystem, with hypothetical examples at each *level*, based on the author's physiotherapeutic lens.

While it is clear that some areas may be more suitable than others for employing HC, the author has attempted to demonstrate the versatility and applicability of HC across the broad healthcare system. The hope is that this chapter might encourage and help support fellow health professionals to embed at least some aspects of HC within their current practice. This is based on a belief that this is a much-underutilised tool. However, for HC to become more widely adopted and effectively delivered by clinicians, they must be encouraged and supported, through HC training, to become competent and confident in using this potent method. There is also a need for more specific studies that support its efficacy in the different contexts in which clinicians are currently practising.

REFERENCES

ARMA. (2024). *Musculoskeletal Health Inequalities and Deprivation Act Now: Musculoskeletal Health Inequalities and Deprivation Report of Arthritis and Musculoskeletal Alliance's (ARMA) inquiry*. Available: https://arma.uk.net/wp-content/uploads/2024/03/Musculoskeletal-Health-Inequalities-and-Deprivation-report_v07.pdf. Accessed 24 July 2025.

Bandura, A. (1977). Self-efficacy: Toward a unifying theory of behavioral change. *Psychological Review*, 84(2), 191–215.

Boehmer, K. R., Alvarez-Villalobos, N. A., Barakat, S., de Leon-Gutierrez, H., Ruiz-Hernandez, F. G., Elizondo-Omana, G. G., Vaquera-Alfaro, H., Ahn, S., Spencer-Bonilla, G. & Gionfriddo, M. R. (2023). The impact of health and wellness coaching on patient-important outcomes in chronic illness care: A systematic review and meta-analysis. *Patient Education and Counseling*, 117, 107975.

Carter, A., Tamkin, P., Wilson, S. & Miller, L. (2015). *The Case for Health Coaching. Lessons Learned from Implementing a Training and Development Intervention for Clinicians Across the East of England*. Institute for Employment Studies.

Chung, E. K. H., Leung, H. H., Yeung, D. Y., Leung, E. Y., Wong, E. L., Yeoh, E. K. & Chen, F. Y. (2026). Health coaching enhanced older adults' self-efficacy in managing their chronic diseases: A randomized controlled trial. *Journal of Applied Gerontology*, *45*(2), 213–224

Davies, F., Wood, F., Bullock, A., Wallace, C. & Edwards, A. (2020). Training in health coaching skills for health professionals who work with people with progressive neurological conditions: A realist evaluation. *Health Expectations*, 23(4), 919–933.

Department of Health. (2013). *The NHS Constitution for England*. Department of Health.

Department of Health and Social Care. (2025). *Fit for the Future: 10 Year Health Plan for England*. Available: https://www.gov.uk/government/publications/10-year-health-plan-for-england-fit-for-the-future/fit-for-the-future-10-year-health-plan-for-england-executive-summary. Accessed 01 July 2025.

Gallwey, W. T. (1974). *The Inner Game of Tennis*. Random House.

Grant, A. M. (2011). Is it time to REGROW the GROW model? Issues related to teaching coaching session structures. *The Coaching Psychologist*, 7(2), 118–126.

Health Coaching Institute. (2025). *Health Coach: The History of Health Coaching*. Available: https://www.healthcoachinstitute.com/articles/history-of-health-coaching/. Accessed 24 July 2025.

Health foundation. (2025). *Inequalities in Life Expectancy and Healthy Life Expectancy*. Available: https://www.health.org.uk/evidence-hub/health-inequalities/inequalities-in-life-expectancy-and-healthy-life-expectancy. Accessed 25 June 2025.

HEE. (2021). *First Contact Practitioners and Advanced Practitioners in Primary Care: (Musculoskeletal) A Roadmap to Practice*. Available: https://www.hee.nhs.uk/sites/default/files/documents/MSK%20July21-FILLABLE%20Final%20Aug%202021_2.pdf. Accessed 01 July 2025.

Henry, K., El-Osta, A. & Leedham-Green, K. (2025). Health coaching for people with long-term conditions and multimorbidity: A mixed methods prospective service evaluation of structured agenda-free coaching conversations (StACC) in UK primary care. *BMC Public Health*, 25, 2365.

Institute for Government. (2020). *Explainer Topics "Nudge Unit"*. Available: https://www.instituteforgovernment.org.uk/article/explainer/nudge-unit. Accessed 25 June 2025.

James, S. L., Abate, D., Abate, K. H., Abay, S. M., Abbafati, C., Abbasi, N., Abbastabar, H., Abd-Allah, F., Abdela, J., Abdelalim, A. & Abdollahpour, I. (2018). Global, regional, and national incidence, prevalence, and years lived with disability for 354 diseases and injuries for 195 countries and territories, 1990–2017: A systematic analysis for the global burden of disease study 2017. *The Lancet*, 392(10159), 1789–1858.

Lin, M. Y., Cheng, S. F., Hou, W. H., Lin, P. C., Chen, C. M. & Tsai, P. S. (2021). Mechanisms and effects of health coaching in patients with early-stage chronic kidney disease: A randomized controlled trial. *Journal of Nursing Scholarship*, 53(2), 154–160.

Loughnane, C., Laiti, J., O'Donovan, R. & Dunne, P. J. (2025). Systematic review exploring human, AI, and hybrid health coaching in digital health interventions: Trends, engagement, and lifestyle outcomes. *Frontiers in Digital Health*, 7, 1536416.

Marmot. (2010). *Fair Society, Healthy Lives: The Marmot Review*. Available: https://www.instituteofhealthequity.org/resources-reports/fair-society-healthy-lives-the-marmot-review/fair-society-healthy-lives-full-report-pdf.pdf. Accessed 25 June 2025.

Matthys, J., Elwyn, G., Van Nuland, M., Van Maele, G., De Sutter, A., De Meyere, M. & Deveugele, M. (2009). Patients' ideas, concerns, and expectations (ICE) in general practice: Impact on prescribing. *British Journal of General Practice*, 59(558), 29–36.

National Voices. (2017). *A New Relationship with People and Communities: Actions for Delivering Chapter 2 of the NHS Five Year Forward View*. Available: https://www.nationalvoices.org.uk/publication/new-relationship-people-and-communities. Accessed 25 June 2025.

NHS. (2019). *The NHS Long Term Plan*. Available: https://webarchive.nationalarchives.gov.uk/ukgwa/20250506042016/https://www.longtermplan.nhs.uk/publication/nhs-long-term-plan/

NHSE. (2023). *Supported self-management: Health Coaching Guide*. Available: https://www.england.nhs.uk/long-read/health-coaching/#how-is-health-coaching-delivered. Accessed 29 June 2025.

NHSE. (2025a). *Personalised Care – Workforce Training: Health and Wellbeing Coaches*. Available: https://www.england.nhs.uk/personalisedcare/workforce-and-training/health-and-wellbeing-coaches/. Accessed 29 June 2025.

NHSE. (2025b). *Enabling People to Make Informed Health Decisions: Health Literacy*. Available: https://www.england.nhs.uk/personalisedcare/health-literacy. Accessed 25 June 2025.

Performance consultants. (n.d.). Available: https://www.performanceconsultants.com/solutions/grow-essentials/. Accessed 25 June 2025.

Pirbaglou, M., Katz, J., Motamed, M., Pludwinski, S., Walker, K. & Ritvo, P. (2018). Personal health coaching as a type 2 diabetes mellitus self-management strategy: A systematic review and meta-analysis of randomized controlled trials. *American Journal of Health Promotion*, 32(7), 1613–1626.

Prochaska, J. O. & Velicer, W. F. (1997). The transtheoretical model of health behavior change. *American Journal of Health Promotion*, 12(1), 38–48.

RCEM. (2023). *RCEM Performance Tracker*. Available: https://rcem.ac.uk/nhs-performance-tracker/. Accessed 03 August 2025.

Rollnick, S. & Miller, W. R. (1995). What is motivational interviewing? *Behavioural and Cognitive Psychotherapy*, 23(4), 325–334.

Sforzo, G. A., Kaye, M. P., Todorova, I., Harenberg, S., Costello, K., Cobus-Kuo, L., Faber, A., Frates, E. & Moore, M. (2018). Compendium of the health and wellness coaching literature. *American Journal of Lifestyle Medicine*, 12(6), 436–447.

Singh, H., Kennedy, G. A. & Stupans, I. (2020). Does the modality used in health coaching matter? A systematic review of health coaching outcomes. *Patient Preference & Adherence*, 14, 1477–1492.

Thaler, R. H. & Sunstein, C. R. (2008). *Nudge: Improving Decisions About Health, Wealth, and Happiness*. Yale University Press.

Thom, D. H., Willard-Grace, R., Tsao, S., Hessler, D., Huang, B., DeVore, D., Chirinos, C., Wolf, J., Donesky, D. & Garvey, C. (2018). Randomized controlled trial of health coaching for vulnerable patients with chronic obstructive pulmonary disease. *Annals of the American Thoracic Society*, 15(10), 1159–1168.

Versus Arthritis. (2024). *The State of Musculoskeletal Health 2024: Arthritis and Other Musculoskeletal Conditions in Numbers*. Available: https://versusarthritis.org/media/tffdkiax/va_state-of-msk-report-nov2024-1.pdf. Accessed 24 July 2025.

Wanless, D. (2002). *Securing Our Future Health: Taking a Long-term View*. Final report. HM Treasury.

Whitmore, J. (1992). *Coaching for Performance*. Nicholas Brealey.

WHO. (2025). *Social Determinants of Health – Overview*. Available: https://www.who.int/health-topics/social-determinants-of-health#tab=tab_1. Accessed 25 June 2025.

Wildflower, L. (2013). *The Hidden History of Coaching*. McGraw-Hill Education (UK).

28 Opening Pandora's Box on Supported Self-Management within Rehabilitation

Meredith Perry, Leigh Hale, Lizz Carrington, Bernadette Jones, Tristram Ingham, and Elijah Areli

INTRODUCTION

Self-management, a prominent strategy in rehabilitation aimed at empowering individuals with long-term conditions and disabled people to actively manage their health (Morgan et al. 2017; Taylor et al. 2014), is often perceived as straightforward. However, closer critical examination reveals a complex and contested concept, underpinned by divergent philosophies and expectations (Francis et al. 2018; Holland et al. 2024; Orpwood et al. 2026; Taylor et al. 2014). In this chapter, we aim to critically interrogate these concepts within the rehabilitation context, thereby intentionally opening up "Pandora's box" to provoke debate.

Despite being promoted as a panacea for the growing challenge of long-term conditions the language of self-management is marked by terminological slippage. Terms such as "self-management", "self-management support", and "supported self-management" are often used interchangeably; yet, when unpacked, they carry distinct meanings and entail different assumptions about agency, responsibility, and support. Clarifying these distinctions is not merely semantic: it has philosophical and clinical implications for how rehabilitation goals are set, how decisions are made, and how support is organised.

The concept of self-management has evolved significantly since its inception. Lorig and Holman's (2003) seminal work established core principles emphasising problem-solving, resource utilisation, and partnership with healthcare providers. However, Kendall et al. (2011) argue that self-management initiatives have often been co-opted by neoliberal policy agendas, privileging individual responsibility over addressing structural determinants of health. This reinforces problematic assumptions inherent in what Greenhalgh (2009) identified as the "expert patient" model.

Definitions of "self-management" typically underscore individual agency. Barlow (Barlow et al. 2002, p. 178), for instance, defines it as "an individual's ability to manage the symptoms, treatment, physical and psychological consequences, and lifestyle changes inherent in living with a chronic condition". Similarly, the US Institute of Medicine states, "Self-management is defined as the tasks that individuals must undertake to live with one or more chronic conditions. These tasks include having the confidence to deal with medical management, role management and emotional management of their conditions" (Corrigan et al. 2004). These definitions clearly place the responsibility of the "self" squarely on the individual and their personal agency, with the explicit expectation that the person possesses the confidence and control to execute these actions (Morgan et al. 2017).

However, for many people, a wide array of disadvantageous factors renders this individual responsibility untenable. Such factors include, for example, geography, culture, ethnicity, language, physical or cognitive limitations, literacy, communication, and socio-economic status, all of which can perpetuate inequities in healthcare access and outcomes (Hale et al. 2022b). This strongly suggests that many individuals require support to self-manage, and that this support must be provided through various tailored modes of delivery and formats, adapting to needs and circumstances that may fluctuate over time.

DOI: 10.1201/9781003599074-31

We adopt the perspective that "self-management support" specifically refers to the utilisation of educational resources, such as brochures, pamphlets, website information, books, and programmes aimed at teaching people how to self-manage, *rather than* "people" resources (Hale et al. 2024; McConnell & Hale 2024). Although these materials are helpful, and may be sufficient for some individuals, particularly those with higher education, literacy, and socio-economic advantage, they are generally considered to have low efficacy in improving overall self-management ability (de Silva 2011).

Crucially, self-management carries assumptions about the self, independence, and responsibility that are deeply shaped by neoliberal discourses and Western ideals of autonomy. In contrast, rehabilitation practice often unfolds within relationships of trust, dependence, and reciprocity, spaces that reflect collective, family, and community values. Recent empirical and theoretical work (Devan et al. 2018; Hale et al. 2025; Monk et al. 2023) consistently demonstrates that while policy often frames self-management as a route to independence, the lived experience is far more relational, fluid, and culturally grounded.

SUPPORTED SELF-MANAGEMENT AS A RELATIONAL CONCEPT

The dominant discourse in self-management literature has long privileged individualistic approaches, positioning people with long-term conditions and disabled people as primarily responsible for their own health. Increasingly, however, research challenges this paradigm, arguing that self-management is fundamentally relational, embedded in social, cultural, and environmental contexts, and sustained through interpersonal connections. This relational understanding extends across diverse populations and conditions, offering a unifying theoretical framework for supported self-management.

Entwistle et al. (2018) proposed a 'broader-than-autonomy' framework that recognises how self-management capabilities are shaped by social relationships and environmental factors. Similarly, Morgan et al. (2017) critiqued narrow, task-focused interventions that isolate self-management from the relational contexts in which it occurs. Both perspectives challenge the individualistic assumptions embedded in traditional approaches and highlight that effective supported self-management depends not only on developing skills and knowledge but also on strengthening social networks and supportive environments.

This reconceptualisation aligns with broader theoretical frameworks in disability studies and care ethics. Tronto's (1998) foundational work situates care as a practice embedded in relationships, while Wendell's critique of independence in disability discourse exposes how rehabilitation's focus on autonomy often obscures the interdependence that characterises all human life (Wendell 1997). When applied to rehabilitation and long-term condition management, these insights reposition supported self-management as a collaborative, contextually responsive practice that evolves through ongoing relationships.

While Western relational frameworks often operate within health system hierarchies, Indigenous worldviews offer more holistic understandings of wellbeing that emphasise interconnection between people, land, spirit, and community. For example, Māori, the indigenous people of Aotearoa, New Zealand, place relationships (whanaungatanga) and collective responsibility at the centre of wellbeing. Abel et al. (2018) identified whanaungatanga as central to Māori experiences of diabetes management, while Kyoon Achan et al. (2022) demonstrated that community-based supported self-management approaches in First Nations contexts produced better outcomes than individualised interventions. These culturally grounded approaches illustrate how self-management is shaped by collective identity and social obligation.

Translating these worldviews into practice requires whānau-centred design (including telehealth and digital services), co-governance through structures that honour Te Tiriti o Waitangi (the Treaty of Waitangi) and environmental stewardship, so that relational accountability is embedded in everyday care (Ingham et al. 2023; Pene et al. 2023; Perry et al. 2022; Wilson et al. 2021).

Māori-centred models of health also foreground the socio-political determinants of wellbeing. Wilson et al. (2021) identified key dimensions of health, including whanaungatanga (connectedness) and whakawhanaungatanga (relationship-building), situated within the contexts of colonisation, urbanisation, racism, and marginalisation. Pene et al. (2023) emphasised the responsibilities of healthcare professionals in upholding cultural safety, effective communication, and relational partnership.

Extending this analysis, Māori disability scholars highlight the compounding effects of disconnection from whakapapa (line of descent or genealogy), te reo Māori (Māori language), mātauranga Māori (Māori knowledge, understanding), and whenua (land), and argue that Western disability models fail to acknowledge Māori epistemologies and ontologies of care (Ingham et al. 2023; Jones et al. 2023). These perspectives reveal how systemic neglect of relational worldviews perpetuates inequities and limits access to whānau-based approaches.

Pacific understandings of health similarly centre collective wellbeing and relational interdependence. The concept of *vā,* "the space between, not that which separates but that which relates" (Wendt 1999), captures the relational fabric binding individuals, families (aiga, kainga), and communities. Within this worldview, health management involves shared responsibility, spiritual connection, and social obligation.

Research with Pacific communities in Aotearoa, New Zealand, highlights how collective support networks sustain motivation and adherence to management plans (Mila-Schaaf & Hudson 2009; Tamasese et al. 2005). Consequently, culturally aligned supported self-management for Pacific peoples emphasises relational accountability, shared decision-making, and the integration of spiritual and communal care (Mila-Schaaf 2006; Teariki & Leau 2024). These Indigenous and Pacific paradigms offer holistic, culturally responsive alternatives to Western individualist models.

Relationality is also evidenced across the life-course and is present in the lives of people with different clinical conditions. Research involving disabled people and those with complex needs further demonstrates how self-management is enacted relationally. Studies of diabetes management among people with learning disabilities identified 'negotiated autonomy', a process of ongoing collaboration with support workers and health professionals (Whitehead et al. 2016). Similarly, individuals with learning disabilities and epilepsy relied on networks of family members, paid carers, and healthcare providers (Karakis et al. 2025). Parallel patterns are evident in Hammel et al.'s (2015) work with people with spinal cord injury, which showed that accessible environments and supportive relationships are essential for effective supported self-management. Across these contexts, supported self-management emerges as a collective rather than purely individual endeavour.

For children and young people, supported self-management is similarly relational and developmental. Franklin and Sloper (2009) demonstrated how supported participation in decision-making enables children to build self-management capacity as parents and professionals adjust levels of support over time. This perspective aligns with Family-Centred Care principles, where mutual trust and shared knowledge underpin responsive partnerships (Kuo et al. 2012). Within paediatric rehabilitation, relationships are dynamic, requiring continual renegotiation of roles to balance autonomy with support as children's abilities evolve.

Persistent pain management has also moved beyond biomedical frameworks towards relational and psychosocial models. Reviews by Devan et al. (2018, 2019a) emphasise the value of empathy, personalised education, and sustained relational support alongside technical interventions. Interventions that promote psychological flexibility and social participation produce greater improvements in pain-related disability than those focused solely on physical outcomes (Ashton-James et al. 2022). By foregrounding social outcomes, connection, role participation, and relational wellbeing, these accounts substantiate the shift from symptom control to relational, psychosocial supported self-management (Ashton-James et al. 2022; Eccleston et al. 2023).

Co-designed programmes such as iSelf-help (Hale et al. 2025; Perry et al. 2022) exemplify this approach by integrating cultural adaptation, collaborative design, and peer support. The value of iSelf-help rests on enabling interaction, participation, and context fit, not on information provision alone. Conceptually, this reframes effective persistent pain self-management as a socially embedded practice shaped by relational, cultural, and environmental factors (Eccleston et al. 2023).

Beyond clinical settings, the relational nature of self-management extends into community spaces and everyday environments. Access to green spaces has been shown to enhance motivation and wellbeing for people with long-term conditions (Buckley et al. 2020). Social (family relationships and peer support) networks and healthcare interactions likewise shape supported self-management practices among people with long-term conditions (Audulv et al. 2021; Vassilev et al. 2014).

Longitudinal research further underscores the dynamic and non-linear nature of supported self-management. Audulv et al. (2019) identified multiple self-management patterns that shifted in response to changing relationships and life circumstances. Similar non-linear trajectories were found among people recovering from anterior cruciate ligament reconstruction (Scott et al. 2018) and older adults with cognitive impairment (Mesbah et al. 2023a), suggesting that relational and temporal dimensions of supported self-management may be universal across conditions. Taken together, across diverse populations and research traditions, evidence converges on supported self-management as a relational practice shaped by social, cultural, and environmental interactions, with autonomy and wellbeing sustained through relationships among individuals, families, communities, and healthcare providers.

As a consequence, autonomy is strengthened, not diminished, by shared decision-making and ongoing relational support (Boland et al. 2018). Recognising supported self-management as relational reframes rehabilitation and long-term condition management. The task is not merely to equip individuals with knowledge and skills, but to cultivate supportive networks, foster collaboration, and design accessible environments. Integrating Indigenous and relational approaches offers a pathway towards more equitable, holistic, and culturally responsive health systems (Moewaka Barnes & McCreanor 2019).

THE NEOLIBERAL SELF AND COLLECTIVE REALITIES

The concept of "self-management" is deeply embedded in neoliberal ideologies that privilege individual responsibility and minimise collective obligations for health and wellbeing (Ould Brahim 2019; Pickett & Wilkinson 2015). These ideologies position self-management as a moral imperative, a responsibility that "good citizens" fulfil to reduce their burden on healthcare systems and society. Such framing reflects what Rose (2001) terms "ethopolitics", where health becomes a site of ethical self-governance and individuals are expected to actively manage risks and demonstrate responsible personhood to minimise their dependence on state resources.

This neoliberal underpinning has significant implications for how self-management is conceptualised and implemented in rehabilitation. Nicholls and Gibson (2010) have demonstrated how neoliberal governmentality has shaped physiotherapy practice towards emphasising individual responsibility and self-discipline, often at the expense of acknowledging structural determinants of health. Their Foucauldian analysis reveals how seemingly neutral *'empowerment'* approaches can function as forms of surveillance and control that reinforce rather than challenge health inequities. This critical perspective helps explain why many self-management interventions, despite their empowerment rhetoric, may inadvertently reinforce existing power imbalances and health disparities. As Kendall et al. (2011) argue, self-management initiatives often emphasise individual behaviour change while neglecting structural determinants of health such as poverty, discrimination, and inadequate access to resources.

This narrow focus can inadvertently shift responsibility and blame individuals for circumstances beyond their control while obscuring how social, economic, and environmental factors enable or constrain self-management capabilities. Research with healthcare professionals further reveals how neoliberal assumptions shape clinical practice. Monk et al. (2023) found that physiotherapists' beliefs about self-management varied widely, with some uncritically reproducing neoliberal ideals of individual responsibility while others sought more nuanced, person-centred approaches.

Similarly, Mudge et al. (2015) identified tensions between health professionals' desire to promote patient autonomy and their recognition of structural barriers that limit patients' capacity for self-management. These findings highlight how neoliberal discourses create contradictions for practitioners who recognise the relational and contextual nature of health management but work within systems that emphasise individual responsibility.

For many Indigenous and minority groups, the Western concept of "self" that underlies self-management discourse is fundamentally incongruent with collective worldviews. As Realo (2003) explains, in cultures prioritising collectivism, the individual self is less prominent than group identity and interconnectedness. This creates a fundamental mismatch between individualistic self-management approaches and how many people understand health and identity, often leading to ineffective interventions and cultural alienation when Western models are imposed without adaptation (Basurrah et al. 2022; Wilson et al. 2022). Indigenous perspectives, in particular, offer powerful counter-narratives to neoliberal individualism. For instance, Ingham et al. (2023) and Jones et al. (2023) demonstrate that Māori concepts of health and wellbeing (hauora) are grounded in collective identity and self-determination. Here, the self exists through relationships with whānau (family/extended family), *hapū* (sub-tribe), *iwi* (tribe), *whenua* (land), and *tupuna* (ancestors). Similarly, Drysdale et al. (2022) describe how Pacific caregivers emphasise communal engagement and cultural connection as essential to wellbeing and rehabilitation, sharply contrasting with individual-focused approaches. These relational ontologies challenge the foundation of individualistic self-management discourse by positioning health as inherently collective.

Further challenging these individualistic assumptions are the experiences of people with learning disability or cognitive impairments, who are often excluded from self-management discourse based on perceived cognitive capacity. Yet, research consistently challenges these assumptions. Studies by Hale et al. (2011), House et al. (2018), and Trip et al. (2016) demonstrate that people with learning disabilities can successfully engage in supported self-management programmes when provided with appropriate support. Whitehead et al.'s (2016) concept of "negotiated autonomy" further illustrates how people with learning disabilities actively participate in managing their health through collaborative relationships rather than independently, thus challenging the false binary between dependence and independence that underpins neoliberal approaches to self-management.

The COVID-19 pandemic starkly exposed the limitations of individualistic approaches to health and self-management. Perry et al. (2020) documented how expectations of independence during the pandemic overlooked systemic inequities and placed additional burdens on disabled people. Russell et al. (2023) further demonstrated that self-management capacity was fundamentally tied to environmental enablers and relational supports, which were significantly compromised during lockdowns. These disruptions exposed what disability scholars have long argued: independence is produced through accessible environments, supportive relationships, and available resources, revealing our fundamental interdependence (Perry et al. 2020; Russell et al. 2023).

The pandemic's impact on chronic condition management further challenged individualistic models. Jesus et al. (2021) found that even those with well-established self-management routines experienced significant deterioration when regular healthcare contacts, community resources, and social supports were unavailable. Similarly, personal responsibilities for health maintenance were rendered impossible without collective infrastructures of care and access (Shakespeare & Watson 2023). An intersectional lens further demonstrates how individualist approaches exacerbated inequities across disability, race, and socioeconomic status.

As Bowleg (2020) demonstrates in her intersectional analysis, individualistic approaches to health not only failed to address but actively exacerbated existing health inequities based on disability, race, and socioeconomic status. These pandemic-era findings substantiate what disability justice advocates have long maintained: independence is not freedom from need or support but rather sufficient access to resources that enable choice and agency. When systems of support were disrupted during COVID-19, the myth of independent self-management was exposed, revealing our fundamental interdependence (Jesus et al. 2021; Russell et al. 2023). As Jesus et al. (2021) argues, the pandemic created an opportunity to reimagine self-management beyond individualistic frameworks towards models that acknowledge the social, environmental, and relational foundations upon which all health practices depend.

Collectively, these critiques reveal how neoliberal constructions of self-management conflict with the lived realities of many people, particularly those from collectivist cultures, disabled people, and others whose experiences challenge Western or Global North concepts of individualism. This discourse underscores the need for approaches to self-management that acknowledge collective identities, recognise structural determinants of health, and value diverse ways of being and knowing.

DEPENDENCE, INDEPENDENCE, AND COLLECTIVE CAPACITY

Rehabilitation has traditionally valorised independence as its primary goal, often casting dependence as a deficit to be overcome rather than a normal aspect of human life. This independence-focused paradigm underpins many self-management approaches that seek to reduce reliance on health services and professionals. In contrast, disability scholarship and research on collective capacity reconceptualise the relationship between dependence, independence, and capacity. Shakespeare (2000) challenges the false binary, arguing that all humans live in states of interdependence, giving and receiving support throughout our lives. Fine and Glendinning (2005) similarly recast dependency as relational and reciprocal rather than a deficit, while Kittay's (2011) ethics of care positions dependency as universal and maintains that acknowledging interdependence produces more just and responsive care systems than those founded on myths of autonomous selfhood. Extending beyond humanist framings, Nicholls et al. (2024) propose a posthumanist approach to rehabilitation that decentres the autonomous individual and understands health as emerging through assemblages of human and non-human actors; on this view, capacity is distributed across networks of people, technologies, environments, and systems, aligning with a focus on collective rather than solely individual capacity.

Building on this reframing, ecological accounts locate supported self-management within multi-level relationships. Greenhalgh and Papoutsi (2019) propose a micro (individual), meso (organisational), macro (policy/system) model that integrates individual factors with organisational practices and policy environments, challenging narrow conceptualisations focused on individual behaviour change. Empirical analyses of social networks confirm that capacity is co-produced within social ecologies rather than residing solely within individuals.

Across diverse systems, the configuration and resources of social networks shape self-management capacity, underscoring that practices are co-produced within social ecologies rather than residing solely within individuals (Audulv et al. 2021; McKinlay et al. 2019; Timmermans et al. 2024; Vassilev et al. 2014; Vassilev et al. 2016). The concept of "collective efficacy" described by Vassilev et al. (2014) offers a particularly useful framework for rehabilitation practice. Their research demonstrated how the capacity for self-management was distributed across social networks rather than residing solely within individuals (Vassilev et al. 2013). Consistent with this, McKinlay et al. (2019) highlighted how the configuration of patients' social networks significantly shaped their capacity for managing multimorbidity. This perspective shifts attention from individual deficits to collective resources and suggests that interventions should aim to strengthen networks of support rather than focusing exclusively on individual skills development.

Capacity is also conditioned by environments and structures. Inaccessible settings diminish participation regardless of individual skills (Hammel et al. 2015), and successful use of adaptive equipment depends on appropriate technology within supportive contexts (Boland et al. 2018). Environmental resources matter too: nature-based and outdoor activities improve mental and physical health by fostering stress reduction, social connection, and physical activity (Coventry et al. 2021), while urban green-space interventions can enhance health equity and collective self-management capacity (Hunter et al. 2019). However, access to these benefits is uneven, reflecting and reinforcing broader social inequities (Zuniga-Teran et al. 2021). More broadly, social determinants including socioeconomic status, neighbourhood resources, and racial discrimination shape the capacity for self-management, creating barriers that cannot be addressed through individual skills training alone (Allen et al. 2016; Hale et al. 2021; Hale et al. 2022b). An ecological approach to self-management, therefore, requires attention to environmental and structural justice alongside individual and relational factors.

Indigenous and culturally diverse perspectives further expand these insights by centring collective resources. Ingham et al. (2023) demonstrate that Māori concepts of health and disability foreground social and cultural determinants and understand health as emerging through collective capacity and interconnectedness, contrasting sharply with individualistic models of self-management. Yoshikawa et al. (2020) similarly show how sociocultural brokerage and cultural safety enable equitable participation in rehabilitation for culturally and linguistically diverse communities, strengthening collective capacity.

The relationship between capacity and healthcare engagement is dynamic and mutually shaping. Limited health literacy constrains people's ability to navigate systems, access appropriate services, and implement self-management strategies (Levasseur et al. 2023). Conversely, targeted interventions that build capacity, aligned to everyday decision contexts, improve utilisation and outcomes for older adults with long-term conditions (Cramm & Nieboer 2017).

For people with learning disability, deficit-focused assessments have often underestimated the potential for supported decision-making. Research shows that when assessments prioritise everyday decision contexts rather than abstract reasoning, they can enable rather than constrain participation (Casey et al. 2025; Douglas et al. 2015; Geukes et al. 2019). Complementary digital literacy initiatives also enhance engagement when they build on existing capacities and preferences rather than assuming deficits (Chadwick et al. 2023).

These principles translate into practice through models that embed collective capacity within rehabilitation. Family-centred approaches, such as the relate–know–respond framework, position families as partners in decision-making and support, with reciprocal "knowing each other" aligning actions with the realities of family life and strengthening family capacity (Carrington et al. 2021, 2025). Such approaches foster genuinely collaborative relationships between professionals, children, and family systems, and are associated with improved outcomes for disabled children, particularly when interventions build family capacity rather than focusing exclusively on child functioning (Smith et al. 2015).

Across these diverse approaches, collective capacity emerges as a crucial and often overlooked dimension of rehabilitation. By recognising how capacity exists not just within individuals but also within families, communities, and systems, rehabilitation can move beyond individualistic models of self-management towards approaches that acknowledge our fundamental interdependence and work with, rather than against, existing networks of support (Audulv et al. 2021; McKinlay et al. 2019; Vassilev et al. 2014). Together, these perspectives reconceptualise capacity as emergent, contextual, and collective rather than fixed, individual, and binary. The implication for rehabilitation is clear: effective self-management support should strengthen family and community resources, redesign environments, and address structural inequities, not merely develop individual skills or motivation.

THE ESSENTIAL ROLE OF TRUST AND SUSTAINED PERSONAL INTERACTION

At the heart of effective supported self-management lies a productive paradox: the capacity for "self"-management frequently emerges through meaningful relationships with others, particularly healthcare professionals. Qualitative studies across diverse long-term conditions consistently show that sustained, trusting relationships provide the foundation for developing and maintaining self-management capabilities, challenging instrumental approaches that foreground information transfer or discrete skills training while neglecting the quality of therapeutic relationships.

Trust operates as a precondition for effective supported self-management. It is built through professionals' demonstrated competence, reliability, and genuine concern for patients' wellbeing, which in turn increases engagement with self-management strategies and re-engagement during periods of difficulty (Hale et al. 2022a; Jesus et al. 2022). Relationship quality is further enhanced when practitioners acknowledge preferences, encourage autonomy, and provide tailored guidance, which are all practices associated with greater confidence and active involvement (Jesus et al. 2022; van Dongen et al. 2020). These mechanisms are evident in our work on the Blue Prescription intervention for people with multiple sclerosis, where participants valued autonomy-supportive guidance delivered over time, "*somebody's kindly following you along the line*", more than brief, didactic education (Hale et al. 2018; Smith et al. 2013, p. 1178). This exemplar shows that pairing autonomy-supportive guidance with relational continuity and the building of trust can sustain behaviour change over time. Similarly, in the Diabetes Community Exercise Programme (DCEP), participants identified person/whānau-centredness and a relational social environment as the "glue" sustaining commitment and participation (Hale et al. 2022a). Here, person/collective-centred interactions cultivated trust and validated participants' preferences, enacting autonomy-support through culturally safe communication (Hale et al. 2022a).

For disabled people and those living with long-term conditions, needs fluctuate in intensity and form, necessitating ongoing, flexible support rather than time-limited contacts. Continuity of care is associated with improved self-management outcomes for people with multimorbidity (Liddy et al. 2014). More broadly, principles of supported self-management emphasise dignity, compassion, and personalised support (de Longh et al. 2015), aligning with our synthesis that support requirements evolve over time as people navigate changing circumstances (Francis et al. 2018; Hale et al. 2024; Holland et al. 2024; Mesbah et al. 2023a). In our co-creative research with people with multiple sclerosis, participants wanted physiotherapy expertise to be available while retaining autonomy over their activities and the pace of their engagement, with their choices respected and encouragement sustained over time (Hale et al. 2012). Taken together, these findings position continuity and responsiveness not as adjuncts but as core clinical work in supported self-management.

Digital platforms and telehealth can expand access and flexibility, but their effectiveness rests on intentional relational work rather than content delivery alone. In the Internet-delivered Self-help programme for Persistent Pain (iSelf-help), participants valued interactive sessions with healthcare professionals and peer facilitators, underscoring that engagement was sustained by human connection (Hale et al. 2025; Perry et al. 2022). A rural telehealth intervention for people with multiple sclerosis reinforced this finding: "*She listened to what I was looking for and… gave me desire to do it*" (Sangelaji 2018). These observations align with the concept of "relational work" in digital health, the often invisible labour required to build and maintain therapeutic relationships through technology (Mair et al. 2012). Digital and telehealth solutions, therefore, augment rather than replace relational care and are most effective when paired with autonomy-supportive, tailored practice (Devan et al. 2019; Hale et al. 2012b).

Peer support provides a complementary form of relational assistance that differs from, but strengthens, professional relationships. In iSelf-help, peer facilitators with lived experience of persistent pain offered distinctive insights and encouragement valued by participants (Hale et al. 2025; Perry et al. 2022). This mirrors broader evidence that shared experience generates forms of knowledge and support that complement professional expertise in diabetes and severe mental illness (Davidson et al. 2012; Heisler 2010). Consistent with these findings, participants in the DCEP emphasised that relationships among participants, as well as with professionals, were central to sustained engagement (Hale et al. 2021).

Efficiency-focused healthcare models that prioritise brief, standardised encounters risk undermining the relational foundations of supported self-management (Jesus et al. 2022). Effective interventions are "underpinned by a collaborative/communicative relationship between the patient and healthcare professional within the context of a healthcare organisation that actively promotes self-management" (Taylor et al. 2014, p. 5). Realising this requires organisational support for time, continuity, and collaboration across professional and peer roles, alongside service designs that value relational labour, whether delivered in person, digitally, or via telehealth.

In practical terms, supported self-management should be enacted as relationship-centred clinical work, with healthcare services resourced for continuity and follow-up and clinicians prioritising autonomy-supportive, preference-sensitive, and tailored guidance to build trust, confidence, and capability (Hale et al. 2022a; Jesus et al. 2022; Timmermans et al. 2024; van Dongen et al. 2020). Digital and telehealth provision ought to be designed around intentional "relational work" and interactive contact, rather than one-way content delivery, thereby harnessing technology to augment, not replace, therapeutic relationships across modalities (Hale et al. 2025; Mair et al. 2012; Perry et al. 2022). Integrating peer and community components can provide distinctive, yet complementary forms of support that sustain engagement alongside professional input (Davidson et al. 2012; Hale et al. 2022a; Heisler 2010).

More broadly, supported self-management should be treated as person- and relationship-centred practice rather than primarily a mechanism to reduce healthcare utilisation, aligning with evidence that effective interventions are embedded within organisations that explicitly promote collaborative self-management (Taylor et al. 2014). In sum, supported self-management is most effective when healthcare systems and practitioners create the relational, temporal, and organisational conditions through which people can develop and sustain self-management practices over time, working with, rather than against, the human relationships that make "self"-management possible.

THE IMPORTANCE OF SUPPORTED DECISION-MAKING FOR SUPPORTED SELF-MANAGEMENT

Supported decision-making reframes autonomy as a relational, rights-based practice. Rather than resorting to substituted judgment when "capacity" is questioned, it proceeds from a presumption that all people can make decisions affecting their lives when provided with tailored support that reflects their needs and preferences. This approach is codified in international law through the United Nations Convention on the Rights of Persons with Disabilities (UNCRPD), particularly Article 12, which affirms equal recognition before the law and the right to support in exercising legal capacity (United Nations 2006). Translating this mandate into everyday rehabilitation requires shifts from guardianship models and substitute decision-making to enabling supported decision-making (Dinerstein 2012). Its salience in healthcare is evident for people with intellectual and cognitive disabilities (Kripke 2016) and aligns with human rights frameworks that respect autonomy while acknowledging the inherently relational character of decision-making (Flynn & Arstein-Kerslake 2014).

Realising these rights in practice requires moving beyond binary tests of capacity towards spectrum-based, enabling models. Bach and Kerzner (2010) conceptualise decision-making capability across three statuses: legally independent, supported, and facilitated, each retaining the person's central role while calling for different forms of assistance. This spectrum approach accommodates the reality that capacity fluctuates across contexts and over time, mandating flexible supports rather than all-or-nothing determinations. Accordingly, contemporary scholarship positions assessment as a process for identifying strengths and support needs, not a gatekeeping exercise aimed at establishing incapacity (Douglas et al. 2015; Gurbai et al. 2020). This reframing shifts clinical attention from abstract cognitive performance to the relational, communicative, and environmental conditions under which individuals can express preferences and participate meaningfully (Browning et al. 2021).

Evidence from mental health and learning disability services indicates that supported decision-making improves participation and outcomes. When people with mental health conditions were supported to make treatment decisions, they reported greater satisfaction, adherence, and a stronger sense of agency (Douglas et al. 2015), findings consistent with broader accounts of recovery that foreground personal agency and with normative arguments that supported decision-making enhances autonomy and wellbeing (Gooding 2015). In healthcare for people with learning disabilities, supported decision-making enables the articulation of preferences and participation in decisions previously made on their behalf (Watson 2016). Parallel evidence in diabetes self-management shows how "negotiated autonomy" facilitates engagement and shared responsibility in everyday care (Whitehead et al. 2016). Collectively, studies demonstrate that aligning assessment and support with individuals' communicative styles and contexts generates meaningful gains in agency, participation, and clinical engagement.

These principles translate directly into rehabilitation practice. In the context of assistive technologies, involving stroke survivors in equipment-related decisions enhances ownership, satisfaction, and actual use, thereby operationalising supported decision-making through collaborative processes (Boland et al. 2018). Similarly, tailoring exercise delivery modes to participant preference among people with cognitive impairment improves engagement, demonstrating that supported decision-making can be woven into routine intervention design and delivery (Mesbah et al. 2023b). In both cases, the locus of clinical value shifts from professional prescription to structured collaboration that honours the person's preferences, priorities, and life context in how they choose to 'manage' their health.

Family-centred approaches provide practical routes for implementing supported decision-making, particularly for children and people with complex needs. Carrington et al.'s (2025) relate–know–respond model offers a structured method for engaging families in healthcare decisions that respects both individual autonomy and family systems. The model builds transparent communication, trust, and "knowingness" of values, capacities, and constraints, recognising that family capacity fluctuates with changing child needs, health events, and external pressures. This dynamic understanding enables providers to recalibrate expectations and roles over time, sustaining realistic, compassionate shared decision-making. Crucially, the model acknowledges organisational conditions, such as continuity, time, and coordination, that can enable or constrain relational practice, and it demonstrates how supported decision-making can operate simultaneously at the level of individuals within families and families within healthcare systems.

Implementing supported decision-making also entails system-level reform. Findings from the Royal Commission of Inquiry into Historical Abuse in State Care and in the Care of Faith-based Institutions, alongside related scholarship, document routine assumptions of incapacity and the paradox that the more complex the decision, the less support is available (Harding & Taşcıoğlu 2018; Mirfin-Veitch 2016; Mirfin-Veitch et al. 2022). Addressing these historical and ongoing deficits requires services that both empower individuals and families and build organisational capability to provide appropriate supports.

Proportionate safeguards in advance care planning illustrate how rights can be balanced with protection without reverting to substitution. For example, contemporary frameworks maximise participation while acknowledging vulnerability (McKenzie et al. 2017, 2024). Such approaches recalibrate, rather than remove, protections and thus respond to legitimate concerns about exposure to risk without reverting to substitute decision-making.

Authentic enactment of supported decision-making depends on practitioner capabilities and the relational labour of care. Key practices include deeply knowing the person, creating tailored communication methods, respecting identity and preferences, remaining reflexive about professional influence, and investing time in relationship-building (Bigby et al. 2017; Browning et al. 2021). These competencies anchor a shift from tokenistic involvement to genuine collaboration and require organisational support for continuity and reflective practice.

Taken together, this body of work positions supported decision-making as both the ethical and operational foundation for supported self-management in healthcare. By replacing binary capacity judgements with enabling assessments, prioritising relational and contextual supports, and embedding family and system-level responsiveness, rehabilitation can move beyond prescriptive models towards authentic collaboration. Accordingly, goal-setting, intervention planning, and outcome evaluation become processes that are co-produced with individuals and those who support them, aligning strategies with people's values, life contexts, and evolving capacities.

PRACTICE IMPLICATIONS FOR REHABILITATION

Reconceptualising supported self-management as relational, culturally situated, and co-produced through collaborative decision-making shifts rehabilitation beyond knowledge transfer, discrete skills training, and individual responsibility. Nicholls et al. (2016) propose "connectivity" as a guiding principle for physiotherapy, foregrounding how health emerges through dynamic connections among people, environments, and systems rather than through isolated, body-focused interventions. This principle provides a foundation for the relational supported-self-management practices advocated here, reorienting practitioners to strengthen connections between people, places, and services, rather than focusing solely on building individual capabilities within clinic walls. It positions clinicians as facilitators of relationship-centred care that links clinical encounters with everyday environments, including, green and community spaces (Buckley et al. 2020; Cleland et al. 2015), and aligns support with local assets and age-friendly policies that foster participation (Levasseur et al. 2023).

Operationalising connectivity requires shifts in professional identity and capabilities. Physiotherapists commonly navigate tensions between prescriptive expertise and collaborative partnering, highlighting the need to move from "fixing" towards facilitation and partnership (Mudge et al. 2015) and to interrogate assumptions about independence, expertise, and self-management (Monk et al. 2023). Core competencies in supported decision-making include knowing the person well, tailoring communication, respecting preferences and identity, and remaining reflexive about professional influence (Bigby et al. 2017), alongside relational goal-setting that enables rather than constrains meaningful involvement (Kayes et al. 2015).

Crucially, upskilling in cultural competence, cultural humility, and sociocultural brokerage is essential; without it, inequities in access, participation, and outcomes will persist because dominant cultural norms continue to shape rehabilitation encounters and marginalise diverse ways of knowing and doing (Abel et al. 2018; Yoshikawa et al. 2020). In Aotearoa, New Zealand, equitable practice entails culturally grounded approaches. For Māori, Te Tiriti-based and decolonising approaches to cultural safety remain central to equitable practice (Ingham et al. 2023; Jones et al. 2023; Pene et al. 2023). For Pacific peoples, practice anchored in relational ethics and the vā, and enacted through dialogic methods such as talanoa, provides a culturally coherent basis for care (Mila-Schaaf 2006; Mila-Schaaf & Hudson 2009; Teariki & Leau 2024).

Professional education must therefore develop relational skills, cultural responsiveness, and critical reflection on power and responsibility. Current curricula often underplay these domains and leave beliefs about patient capability and responsibility unexamined, thereby perpetuating inequities if not addressed (McConnell & Hale 2024; Mudge et al. 2015; Orpwood et al. 2026; Synnott et al. 2015).

Relational supported self-management extends beyond clinical encounters into the places where people live, work, and participate. Incorporating green and community spaces into rehabilitation supports everyday self-management, requiring practitioners to develop skills in environmental assessment and modification, and knowledge of local assets (Buckley et al. 2020; Cleland et al. 2015). Community engagement strategies via peer support can amplify these effects by aligning support with local contexts and social participation opportunities (Jesus et al. 2022; Timmermans et al. 2024). Age-friendly municipal components further foster social participation for ageing populations (Levasseur et al. 2023), while design resources such as the Can I Get There? Can I Play? Can I Stay? (Bringolf & Carnemolla 2022) offer practical guidance for inclusive outdoor environments that support health management across the life course.

Governance approaches that welcome diverse voices are necessary to embed these ecological perspectives into service design and commissioning, including Te Tiriti-accountable structures and

Māori, Pacific and disabled people leadership in decision-making (Ingham et al. 2023; Jones et al. 2023; Kuper et al. 2025; Mila-Schaaf 2006; Mila-Schaaf & Hudson 2009; Pene et al. 2023). Without inclusive design and participatory governance, environmental barriers and resource inequities will continue to constrain self-management, even when individual skills are strong.

Digital health and telehealth can expand access, particularly for rural or underserved populations, but they must augment, rather than replace, human relationships. Implementation is most effective when technology is paired with relational support and follow-up (Boland et al. 2018; Mesbah et al. 2023b). In iSelf-help, interactive sessions with healthcare professionals and peer facilitators were particularly valued, underscoring the centrality of human connection in digital programmes (Hale et al. 2025; Perry et al. 2022). Virtual environments can enhance or undermine self-management depending on accessibility, usability, culturally responsive content, and how well they integrate with offline supports and networks (Kalantari et al. 2023; Yin et al. 2025). Equity-by-design is imperative: culturally anchored communication, co-design with Māori and Pacific communities, and attention to digital inclusion are required to prevent the entrenchment of disparities.

Family-centred frameworks offer practical routes for embedding relational supported self-management in everyday decision-making. The relate–know–respond model provides structured guidance for engaging families as partners, respecting individual preferences within family systems and acknowledging family knowledge and expertise (Carrington et al. 2025). Strengthening family resources shifts power dynamics, enhances collective capacity, and is associated with improved outcomes for children with disabilities (Smith et al. 2015). Embedding cultural competence within family-centred work is critical to avoid reproducing inequities in how preferences are elicited, interpreted, and acted upon across diverse cultural contexts. This is particularly important when working with whānau and aiga, as these concepts of "family" represent the living, relational, and spiritually grounded system of belonging, collective obligation, identity, and care, in which decision-making is inherently communal rather than individual (Abel et al., 2018; Ingham et al., 2023; Jones et al., 2023; Mila-Schaaf, 2006; Mila-Schaaf & Hudson, 2009; Pene et al., 2023; Yoshikawa et al., 2020).

Relational supported self-management depends on organisational conditions that enable continuity, flexible scheduling, and team-based care (Liddy et al. 2014). Effective interventions are situated within healthcare organisations that "actively promote self-management" through supportive policies and resourcing, rather than relying solely on individual practitioner effort (Taylor et al. 2014). System-wide commitment to equity requires dedicated investment in workforce upskilling in cultural competence, routine access to culturally responsive resources, and accountability for distributional impacts; without these enablers, relational approaches remain aspirational and inequities endure.

Outcome frameworks should move beyond narrow indicators of functional change or adherence to professional recommendations. Broader conceptualisations include quality of life, autonomy, and relational wellbeing (Entwistle et al. 2018), alongside measures that capture collective capacity within families and communities rather than exclusively individual functioning (Audulv et al. 2019; Audulv et al. 2021). Practically, collective capacity can be operationalised through indicators such as whānau/aiga involvement in decision-making and care planning, social network characteristics (for example, size, diversity, reciprocity, and perceived availability of support), environmental accessibility measures (for example, access to transport and green space, step-free routes, and availability of culturally safe services), and digital inclusion (for example, device/data access and usability of telehealth).

Equity-sensitive evaluation should also consider who benefits and who is left behind across cultural and socioeconomic groups; aligning measurement with relational, contextual, and cultural understandings of supported self-management ensures evaluation reflects what matters to those receiving support.

Embedding relational supported self-management involves reorienting practice around interdependence and the ethics of care, strengthening networks of support and recognising the moral significance of therapeutic relationships (Fine & Glendinning 2005; Kittay 2011). This stance resonates with disability ethics, which frames dependence as a human norm

(Shakespeare 2000; Wendell 1997) and positions care as fundamentally relational and politically situated (Tronto 1998).

Operationally, this requires workforce upskilling in cultural competence, ecological design (including digital), family partnership, and organisational support. Rehabilitation can move beyond compliance-focused models towards practices that more effectively and ethically enhance wellbeing, capacity, and identity. Without targeted upskilling and equity-centred system design, inequities in participation and outcomes will endure, regardless of advances in self-management techniques.

CONCLUSION

Our critical examination of supported self-management reveals the need to fundamentally reconceptualise this approach within rehabilitation. Family, whānau, and community capacity must be recognised as integral to effective self-management, not merely adjuncts to individual capacity.

Positioning interdependence as the human norm reframes goals, processes, and system design towards culturally inclusive, relationship-centred rehabilitation. This relational understanding is supported by converging evidence from co-designed programmes, family-centred approaches, Indigenous perspectives, ecological frameworks, and analyses of environmental influences on health management. Across these diverse sources, wellbeing consistently emerges through interdependence and connection, shaped by broader social, environmental, and political contexts that determine what forms of self-management are possible for different individuals and communities.

By situating supported self-management within lived experiences and ecological contexts, rehabilitation can more effectively support wellbeing, capacity, and identity through sustained relationships, supported decision-making, and attention to structural enablers and barriers. Acknowledging interdependence as the human norm rather than a deficit transforms how we conceptualise rehabilitation goals and processes. Reconceptualising supported self-management as fundamentally relational, culturally situated, and collectively sustained, embodying an ethics of care, has transformative potential for professional practice and for health systems designed to promote wellbeing rather than merely manage disease.

REFERENCES

Abel, S., Whitehead, L. C., & Coppell, K. J. (2018). Making dietary changes following a diagnosis of prediabetes: A qualitative exploration of barriers and facilitators. *Diabetic Medicine*, *35*(12), 1693–1699. https://doi.org/10.1111/dme.13796

Allen, C. G., Brownstein, J. N., Satsangi, A., & Escoffery, C. (2016). Community health workers as allies in hypertension self-management and medication adherence in the United States, 2014. *Preventing Chronic Disease*, *13*, E179. https://doi.org/10.5888/pcd13.160236

Ashton-James, C. E., Anderson, S. R., Mackey, S. C., & Darnall, B. D. (2022). Beyond pain, distress, and disability: The importance of social outcomes in pain management research and practice. *Pain*, *163*(3), e426–e431. https://doi.org/10.1097/j.pain.0000000000002404

Audulv, Å, Ghahari, S., Kephart, G., Warner, G., & Packer, T. L. (2019). The taxonomy of everyday self-management strategies (TEDSS): A framework derived from the literature and refined using empirical data. *Patient Education and Counseling*, *102*(2), 367–375. https://doi.org/10.1016/j.pec.2018.08.034

Audulv, Å., Hutchinson, S., Warner, G., Kephart, G., Versnel, J., & Packer, T. L. (2021). Managing everyday life: Self-management strategies people use to live well with neurological conditions. *Patient Education and Counseling*, *104*(2), 413–421. https://doi.org/10.1016/j.pec.2020.07.025

Bach, M., & Kerzner, L. (2010). *A New Paradigm for Protecting Autonomy and the Right to Legal Capacity*. Law Commission of Ontario. https://www.lco-cdo.org/wp-content/uploads/2010/11/disabilities-commissioned-paper-bach-kerzner.pdf

Barlow, J., Wright, C., Sheasby, J., Turner, A., & Hainsworth, J. (2002). Self-management approaches for people with chronic conditions: A review. *Patient Education and Counseling*, *48*(2), 177–187. https://doi.org/10.1016/S0738-3991(02)00032-0

Basurrah, A. A., Al-Haj Baddar, M., & Di Blasi, Z. (2022). Positive psychology interventions as an opportunity in Arab countries to promoting well-being. *Frontiers in Psychology, 12*, 793608. https://doi.org/10.3389/fpsyg.2021.793608

Bigby, C., Whiteside, M., & Douglas, J. (2017). Providing support for decision making to adults with intellectual disability: Perspectives of family members and workers in disability support services. *Journal of Intellectual & Developmental Disability, 42*(4), 324–341. https://doi.org/10.3109/13668250.2017.1378873

Boland, P., Levack, W. M., Graham, F. P., & Perry, M. A. (2018). User perspective on receiving adaptive equipment after stroke: A mixed-methods study. *Canadian Journal of Occupational Therapy, 85*(4), 297–306. https://doi.org/10.1177/0008417418800834

Bowleg, L. (2020). We're not all in this together: On COVID-19, intersectionality, and structural inequality. *American Journal of Public Health, 110*(7), 917. https://doi.org/10.2105/AJPH.2020.305766

Bringolf, J., & Carnemolla, P. (2022). I get there? Can I play? Can I stay? Creating an inclusive playspace guide in Australia. *Studies in Health Technology and Informatics, 2*(297), 103–110. https://doi.org/10.3233/SHTI220827

Browning, M., Bigby, C., & Douglas, J. (2021). A process of decision-making support: Exploring supported decision-making practice in Canada. *Journal of Intellectual & Developmental Disability, 46*(2), 138–149. https://doi.org/10.3109/13668250.2020.1789269

Buckley, A., Brownlie, K., Hill, K., Hallamore, R.-R., Vijan, N., & Perry, M. (2020). Health professionals' inclusion of green space in the management of long term conditions: A scoping review. *Physical Therapy Reviews*, 1–12. https://doi.org/10.1080/10833196.2020.1832715

Carrington, L., Hale, L., Freeman, C., & Perry, M. (2025). The development of the relate-know-respond model to enhance family-centred care. *Disabilities, 5*(3). https://doi.org/10.3390/disabilities5030071

Carrington, L., Hale, L., Freeman, C., Qureshi, A., & Perry, M. (2021). Family-centred care for children with biopsychosocial support needs: A scoping review. *Disabilities, 1*, 301–330. https://doi.org/10.3390/disabilities1040022

Casey, H., Trayer, Á, Desmond, D., & Coffey, L. (2025). Experiences and perceptions of everyday decision-making in the lives of adults with intellectual disabilities, their care partners and direct care support workers. *Journal of Intellectual Disabilities, 29*(3), 683–705. https://doi.org/10.1177/17446295231189020

Chadwick, D., Richards, C., Molin, M., & Strnadová, I. (2023). Digital inclusion and people with learning disabilities. *British Journal of Learning Disabilities, 51*(2), 119–124. https://doi.org/10.1111/bld.12530

Cleland, V., Hughes, C., Thornton, L., Squibb, K., Venn, A., & Ball, K. (2015). Environmental barriers and enablers to physical activity participation among rural adults: A qualitative study. *Health Promotion Journal of Australia, 26*(2), 99–104. https://doi.org/10.1071/HE14115

Corrigan, J. M., Greiner, A. C., & Adams, K. (Eds.). (2004). *The 1st Annual Crossing the Quality Chasm Summit: A Focus on Communities: Report of a Summit*. National Academies Press.

Coventry, P. A., Brown, J. E., Pervin, J., Brabyn, S., Pateman, R., Breedvelt, J., Gilbody, S., Stancliffe, R., McEachan, R., & White, P. L. (2021). Nature-based outdoor activities for mental and physical health: Systematic review and meta-analysis. *SSM - Population Health, 16*, 100934. https://doi.org/https://doi.org/10.1016/j.ssmph.2021.100934

Jones, B., King, P. T., Baker, G., & Ingham, T. (2020). COVID-19, intersectionality, and health equity for Indigenous peoples with lived experience of disability. American Indian Culture and Research Journal, 44(2), 71–88. https://doi.org/10.17953/aicrj.44.2.jones

Cramm, J. M., & Nieboer, A. P. (2017). Self-management abilities and quality of life among frail community-dwelling individuals: The role of community nurses in the Netherlands. *Health & Social Care in the Community, 25*(2), 394–401. https://doi.org/10.1111/hsc.12318

Davidson, L., Bellamy, C., Guy, K., & Miller, R. (2012). Peer support among persons with severe mental illnesses: A review of evidence and experience. *World Psychiatry, 11*(2), 123–128. https://doi.org/10.1016/j.wpsyc.2012.05.009

de Longh, A., Fagan, P., Fenner, J., & Kidd, L. (2015). *A Practical Guide to Self-management Support: Key Components for Successful Implementation*. The Health Foundation. https://www.health.org.uk/resources-and-toolkits/quick-guides/a-practical-guide-to-self-management-support

de Silva, D. (2011). *Helping People Help Themselves: A Review of the Evidence Considering Whether It is Worthwhile to Support Self-management*. The Health Foundation. https://www.health.org.uk/reports-and-analysis/reports/evidence-helping-people-help-themselves

Devan, H., Godfrey, H. K., Perry, M. A., Hempel, D., Saipe, B., Hale, L., & Grainger, R. (2019a). Current practices of health care providers in recommending online resources for chronic pain self-management. *Journal of Pain Research, 12*, 2457–2472. https://doi.org/10.2147/JPR.S206539

Devan, H., Hale, L., Hempel, D., Saipe, B., & Perry, M. A. (2018). What works and does not work in a self-management intervention for people with chronic pain? Qualitative systematic review and meta-synthesis. *Physical Therapy*, *98*(5), 381–397. https://doi.org/10.1093/ptj/pzy029

Devan, H., Perry, M. A., van Hattem, A., Thurlow, G., Shepherd, S., Muchemwa, C., & Grainger, R. (2019b). Do pain management websites foster self-management support for people with persistent pain? A scoping review. *Patient Education and Counseling*, *102*(9), 1590–1601. https://doi.org/10.1016/j.pec.2019.04.009

Dinerstein, R. D. (2012). Implementing legal capacity under article 12 of the UN convention on the rights of persons with disabilities: The difficult road from guardianship to supported decision-making. *Human Rights Brief*, *19*(2), 8–12.

Douglas, J., Bigby, C., Knox, L., & Browning, M. (2015). Factors that underpin the delivery of effective decision-making support for people with cognitive disability. *Research and Practice in Intellectual and Developmental Disabilities*, *2*(1), 37–44. https://doi.org/10.1080/23297018.2015.1036769

Drysdale, D., Carrington, L., Sanerivi, O., Smith, D., & Perry, M. (2022). Perceptions of Pasifika caregivers on a pacific community playgroup and implications for paediatric physiotherapists. *New Zealand Journal of Physiotherapy*, *50*(2), 72–81. https://doi.org/https://doi.org/10.15619/NZJP/50.2.04

Eccleston, C., Begley, E., Birkinshaw, H., Choy, E., Crombez, G., Fisher, E., Gibby, A., Gooberman-Hill, R., Grieve, S., & Guest, A. (2023). The establishment, maintenance, and adaptation of high-and low-impact chronic pain: A framework for biopsychosocial pain research. *Pain*, *164*(10), 2143–2147. https://doi.org/10.1097/j.pain.0000000000002951

Entwistle, V. A., Cribb, A., & Owens, J. (2018). Why health and social care support for people with long-term conditions should be oriented towards enabling them to live well. *Health Care Analysis*, *26*(1), 48–65. https://doi.org/10.1007/s10728-016-0335-1

Fine, M., & Glendinning, C. (2005). Dependence, independence or inter-dependence? Revisiting the concepts of 'care' and 'dependency'. *Ageing and Society*, *25*(4), 601–621. https://doi.org/10.1017/S0144686X05003600

Flynn, E., & Arstein-Kerslake, A. (2014). Legislating personhood: Realising the right to support in exercising legal capacity. *International Journal of Law in Context*, *10*(1), 81–104. https://doi.org/10.1017/S1744552313000384

Francis, H., Carryer, J., & Wilkinson, J. (2018). Self-management support? Listening to people with complex co-morbidities. *Chronic Illness*, *16*(3), 161–172. https://doi.org/10.1177/1742395318796176

Franklin, A., & Sloper, P. (2009). Supporting decision-making of disabled young people: A review. *Children & Society*, *23*(1), 3–15. https://doi.org/10.1111/j.1099-0860.2007.00131.x

Geukes, C., Bröder, J., & Latteck, Ä. D. (2019). Health literacy and people with intellectual disabilities: What we know, what we do not know, and what we need: A theoretical discourse. *International Journal of Environmental Research and Public Health*, *16*(3). https://doi.org/10.3390/ijerph16030463

Gooding, P. (2015). Navigating the 'flashing amber lights' of the right to legal capacity in the United nations convention on the rights of persons with disabilities: Responding to major concerns. *Human Rights Law Review*, *15*(1), 45–71. https://doi.org/10.1093/hrlr/ngu045

Greenhalgh, T. (2009). Patient and public involvement in chronic illness: Beyond the expert patient. *BMJ*, *338*, b49. https://doi.org/10.1136/bmj.b49

Greenhalgh, T., & Papoutsi, C. (2019). Spreading and scaling up innovation and improvement. *BMJ*, *365*, l2068. https://doi.org/10.1136/bmj.l2068

Gurbai, S., Fitton, E., & Martin, W. (2020). Insight under scrutiny in the court of protection: A case law survey. *Frontiers in Psychiatry*, *11*, 560329. https://doi.org/10.3389/fpsyt.2020.560329

Hale, L., Higgs, C., Keen, D., & Smith, C. (2021). Long term exercise engagement of adults living with type two diabetes is enhanced by a person-centred care approach delivered by knowledgeable, well trained health care professionals. *Frontiers in Rehabilitation Sciences*, *2*. https://doi.org/10.3389/fresc.2021.692311

Hale, L., Higgs, C., Keen, D., & Smith, C. (2022a). It is 'all about relationships' in lifestyle programmes for adults living with type two diabetes underpinned by a person/whānau-centred care approach. *Frontiers in Rehabilitation Sciences*, *3*. *https://doi.org/10.3389/fresc.2022.829542*

Hale, L., Perry, M., Gray, A. R., Leung, W., Dean, S. G., Hempel, D., Davies, C., Dowell, A., Grainger, R., Ingham, T., Jones, B., Saipe, B., Dassanayake, S., & Devan, H. (2025). A group-based, online-delivered pain management programme (iSelf-help) is not inferior to a group-based, in-person programme in reducing pain-related disability for people with persistent pain: A non-inferiority randomised, two-arm, parallel, open-label trial. *Journal of Pain*, *32*, 105447. https://doi.org/10.1016/j.jpain.2025.105447

Hale, L., Trip, H. T., Whitehead, L., & Conder, J. (2011). Self-management abilities of diabetes in people with an intellectual disability living in New Zealand. *Journal of Policy and Practice in Intellectual Disabilities*, *8*(4), 223–230. https://doi.org/10.1111/j.1741-1130.2011.00314.x

Hale, L., Wilkinson, A., Pilusa, S., & Stewart, A. (2024). Supported self-management in long-term conditions in an African context. *South African Journal of Physiotherapy*, *80*(1), 1978. https://doi.org/10.4102/sajp.v80i1.1978

Hale, L. A., Oosman, S., & Stewart, A. V. (2022b). Challenging the concept of self-management support in unique and diverse populations. *Frontiers in Rehabilitation Sciences*, *3*, 999528. https://doi.org/10.3389/fresc.2022.999528

Hale, L. A., Smith, C., Mulligan, H., & Treharne, G. J. (2012). Tell me what you want, what you really really want….": Asking people with multiple sclerosis about enhancing their participation in physical activity. *Disability and Rehabilitation*, *34*(22), 1887–1893. https://doi.org/10.3109/09638288.2012.670037

Hale, L. A., Smith, C. M., Mulligan, H. F., Adhia, D., Siew, B., & Treharne, G. J. (2018). Exploring the blue prescription intervention to promote physical activity in people with long-term conditions. *International Journal of Therapy & Rehabilitation*, *25*(7), 365–376. https://doi.org/10.12968/ijtr.2018.25.7.365

Hammel, J., Magasi, S., Heinemann, A., Gray, D. B., Stark, S., Kisala, P., Carlozzi, N. E., Tulsky, D., Garcia, S. F., & Hahn, E. A. (2015). Environmental barriers and supports to everyday participation: A qualitative insider perspective from people with disabilities. *Archives of Physical Medicine and Rehabilitation*, *96*(4), 578–588. https://doi.org/10.1016/j.apmr.2014.12.008

Harding, R., & Taşcıoğlu, E. (2018). Supported decision-making from theory to practice: Implementing the right to enjoy legal capacity. *Societies*, *8*(2). https://doi.org/10.3390/soc8020025

Heisler, M. (2010). Different models to mobilize peer support to improve diabetes self-management and clinical outcomes: Evidence, logistics, evaluation considerations and needs for future research. *Family Practice*, *27*(Suppl 1), i23–i32. https://doi.org/10.1093/fampra/cmq003

Holland, E., Matthews, K., Macdonald, S., Ashworth, M., Laidlaw, L., Cheung, K. S. Y., Stannard, S., Francis, N. A., Mair, F. S., & Gooding, C. (2024). The impact of living with multiple long-term conditions (multimorbidity) on everyday life–a qualitative evidence synthesis. *BMC Public Health*, *24*(1), 3446. https://doi.org/10.1186/s12889-024-20763-8

House, A., Latchford, G., Russell, A. M., Bryant, L., Wright, J., Graham, E., Stansfield, A., Ajjan, R., & On behalf of the OK Diabetes team. (2018). Development of a supported self-management intervention for adults with type 2 diabetes and a learning disability. *Pilot and Feasibility Studies*, *4*(1), 106. https://doi.org/10.1186/s40814-018-0291-7

Hunter, R. F., Cleland, C., Cleary, A., Droomers, M., Wheeler, B. W., Sinnett, D., Nieuwenhuijsen, M. J., & Braubach, M. (2019). Environmental, health, wellbeing, social and equity effects of urban green space interventions: A meta-narrative evidence synthesis. *Environment International*, *130*, 104923. https://doi.org/10.1016/j.envint.2019.104923

Ingham, T. R., Jones, B., Perry, M., von Randow, M., Milne, B., King, P. T., Nikora, L. W., Sporle, A., & Group, T. A. M. S. (2023). Measuring Māori health, wellbeing, and disability in Aotearoa using a web-based survey methodology. *International Journal of Environmental Research and Public Health*, *20*(18), 6797. https://doi.org/10.3390/ijerph20186797

Jesus, T. S., Bhattacharjya, S., Papadimitriou, C., Bogdanova, Y., Bentley, J., Arango-Lasprilla, J. C., Kamalakannan, S., The Refugee Empowerment Task Force, & International Networking Group of the American Congress of Rehabilitation Medicine. (2021). Lockdown-related disparities experienced by people with disabilities during the first wave of the covid-19 pandemic: Scoping review with thematic analysis. *International Journal of Environmental Research and Public Health*, *18*(12), 6178. https://doi.org/10.3390/ ijerph18126178

Jesus, T. S., Papadimitriou, C., Bright, F. A., Kayes, N. M., Pinho, C. S., & Cott, C. A. (2022). Person-centered rehabilitation model: Framing the concept and practice of person-centered adult physical rehabilitation based on a scoping review and thematic analysis of the literature. *Archives of Physical Medicine and Rehabilitation*, *103*(1), 106–120. https://doi.org/10.1016/j.apmr.2021.05.005.

Jones, B., King, P. T., Baker, G., Nikora, L. W., Hickey, H., Perry, M., Pouwhare, R., & Ingham, T. R. (2023). Karanga rua, karanga maha: Māori with lived experience of disability self-determining their own identities. *Kōtuitui: New Zealand Journal of Social Sciences Online*, 1–20. https://doi.org/10.1080/1177083X.2023.2224422

Kalantari, S., Xu, T. B., Mostafavi, A., Kim, B., Dilanchian, A., Lee, A., Boot, W. R., & Czaja, S. J. (2023). Using immersive virtual reality to enhance social interaction among older adults: A cross-site investigation. *Innovation in Aging*, *7*(4), igad031. https://doi.org/10.1093/geroni/igad031

Karakis, I., Flesler, S., Ghorpade, S., Pineda, R. C., Joshi, K., Cooper, J., Patkar, S., Schulz, A., Anand, S. B., & Barnes, N. (2025). Caregiver burden and healthcare providers perspectives in epilepsy: An observational study in China, Taiwan, and Argentina. *Epilepsy & Behavior Reports*, *30*, 100736. https://doi.org/10.1016/j.ebr.2024.100736

Kayes, N. M., Mudge, S., Bright, F. A. S., & McPherson, K. M. (2015). Whose behavior matters? Rethinking practitioner behavior and its influence on rehabilitation outcomes. In K. M. McPherson, B. E. Gibson & A. Leplege (Eds.), *Rethinking Rehabilitation: Theory and Practice* (pp. 249–271). CRC Press. https://doi.org/10.1201/b18118-18

Kendall, E., Ehrlich, C., Sunderland, N., Muenchberger, H., & Rushton, C. (2011). Self-managing versus self-management: Reinvigorating the socio-political dimensions of self-management. *Chronic Illness*, *7*(1), 87–98. https://doi.org/10.1177/1742395310380281

Kittay, E. F. (2011). The ethics of care, dependence, and disability. *Ratio Juris*, *24*(1), 49–58. https://doi.org/10.1111/j.1467-9337.2010.00473.x

Kripke, C. (2016). Supported health care decision-making for people with intellectual and cognitive disabilities. *Family Practice*, *33*(5), 445–446. https://doi.org/10.1093/fampra/cmw060

Kuo, D. Z., Houtrow, A. J., Arango, P., Kuhlthau, K. A., Simmons, J. M., & Neff, J. M. (2012). Family-centered care: Current applications and future directions in pediatric health care. *Maternal and Child Health Journal*, *16*(2), 297–305. https://doi.org/10.1007/s10995-011-0751-7

Kuper, H., Mpanju-Shumbusho, W., & Shakespeare, T. (2025). Building leadership in disability inclusion in health. *The Lancet*, *406*(10511), 1452–1453. https://doi.org/10.1016/S0140-6736(25)00006-6

Kyoon Achan, G., Eni, R., Phillips-Beck, W., Lavoie, J. G., Kinew, K. A., & Katz, A. (2022). Canada First Nations strengths in community-based primary healthcare. *International Journal of Environmental Research and Public Health*, *19*(20). https://doi.org/10.3390/ijerph192013532

Levasseur, M., Dubois, M. F., Généreux, M., Naud, D., Trottier, L., Menec, V., Roy, M., Gabaude, C., Couturier, Y., & Raina, P. (2023). Key age-friendly components of municipalities that foster social participation of aging Canadians: Results from the Canadian longitudinal study on aging. *Journal of Urban Health*, *100*(5), 1032–1042. https://doi.org/10.1007/s11524-023-00762-7

Liddy, C., Blazkho, V., & Mill, K. (2014). Challenges of self-management when living with multiple chronic conditions: Systematic review of the qualitative literature. *Canadian Family Physician*, *60*(12), 1123–1133.

Lorig, K., & Holman, H. (2003). Self-management education: History, definition, outcomes, and mechanisms. *Annals of Behavioral Medicine*, *26*(1), 1–7. https://doi.org/10.1207/S15324796ABM2601_01

Mair, F. S., May, C., O'Donnell, C., Finch, T., Sullivan, F., & Murray, E. (2012). Factors that promote or inhibit the implementation of e-health systems: An explanatory systematic review. *Bulletin of the World Health Organization*, *90*, 357–364. https://doi.org/10.2471/BLT.11.099424

McConnell, L., & Hale, L. (2024). Undergraduate physiotherapy students' perspectives on optimising the curriculum for supported self-management education. *New Zealand Journal of Physiotherapy*, *52*(1), 17–25. https://doi.org/10.15619/nzjp.v52i1.359

McKenzie, N., Mirfin-Veitch, B., Conder, J., & Brandford, S. (2017). I'm still here": Exploring what matters to people with intellectual disability during advance care planning. *Journal of Applied Research in Intellectual Disabilities*, *30*(6), 1089–1098. https://doi.org/10.1111/jar.12355

McKenzie, N., Mirfin-Veitch, B., Trip, H., & Conder, J. (2024). My plan for a good life, right to the end: An accessible approach to advance care planning. *Journal of Intellectual & Developmental Disability*, *49*(4), 475–487. https://doi.org/10.3109/13668250.2024.2362979

McKinlay, E., McDonald, J., Darlow, B., & Perry, M. (2019). The social networks of New Zealand patients with multimorbidity and the work of those nominated as their 'significant supporters': An exploratory study. *Health & Social Care in the Community*, *27*(2), 392–399.

Mesbah, N., Perry, M., Hale, L., Hill, K. D., & Wilkinson, A. (2023a). Perspectives of people with mild to moderate cognitive impairment and their caregivers about physical activity and exercise for fall prevention: A qualitative study. *Disabilities*, *3*(2), 255–268. https://doi.org/10.3390/disabilities3020017

Mesbah, N., Perry, M., Hill, K. D., Manlapaz, D., & Hale, L. (2023b). The experiences of older adults with dementia of "balance wise"—an individual or group-delivered exercise programme: A qualitative study. *Disabilities*, *4*(1), 11–26. https://doi.org/10.3390/disabilities4010002

Mila-Schaaf, K. (2006). Vā-centred social work: Possibilities for a Pacific approach to social work practice. *Social Work Review*, *18*(1), 8–13.

Mila-Schaaf, K., & Hudson, M. (2009). The interface between cultural understandings: Negotiating new spaces for Pacific mental health. *Pacific Health Dialog*, *15*(1), 113–119.

Mirfin-Veitch, B. (2016). *Exploring Article 12 of the United Nations Convention on the Rights of Persons with Disabilities: An integrative Literature Review.* Donald Beasley Institute Report. https://www.donaldbeasley.org.nz/publications/uncrpd

Mirfin-Veitch, B., Tikao, K., Asaka, U., Tuisaula, E., Hilary Stace, H., Francis Watene, R., & Frawley, P. (2022). *Tell Me About You: A Life Story Approach to Understanding Disabled people's Experiences in Care (1950–1999).* Donald Beasley Institute. https://www.donaldbeasley.org.nz/our-projects/tell-me-about-you-a-life-story-approach-to-understanding-disabled-peoples-experiences-in-care-1950-1999

Moewaka Barnes, H., & McCreanor, T. (2019). Colonisation, hauora and whenua in Aotearoa. *Journal of the Royal Society of New Zealand*, *49*(S1), 1–33. https://doi.org/10.1080/03036758.2019.1668439

Monk, C., Sole, G., & Perry, M. (2023). Physiotherapists' attitudes and beliefs about self-management as part of their management for low back pain. *Musculoskeletal Science and Practice*, *64*. https://doi.org/10.1016/j.msksp.2023.102727

Morgan, H. M., Entwistle, V. A., Cribb, A., Christmas, S., Owens, J., Skea, Z. C., & Watt, I. S. (2017). We need to talk about purpose: A critical interpretive synthesis of health and social care professionals' approaches to self-management support for people with long-term conditions. *Health Expectations*, *20*(2), 243–259. https://doi.org/10.1111/hex.12453

Mudge, S., Kayes, N., & McPherson, K. (2015). Who is in control? Clinicians' view on their role in self-management approaches: A qualitative metasynthesis. *BMJ Open*, *5*(5), e007413. https://doi.org/10.1136/bmjopen-2014-007413

Nicholls, D. A., Ahlsen, B., Bjorbaekmo, W., Dahl-Michelsen, T., Hoppner, H., Rajala, A. I., Richter, R., Hansen, L. S., Sudmann, T., Sviland, R., & Maric, F. (2024). Critical physiotherapy: A ten-year retrospective. *Physiotherapy Theory and Practice*, *40*(11), 2617–2629. https://doi.org/10.1080/09593985.2023.2252524

Nicholls, D. A., Atkinson, K., Bjorbaekmo, W. S., Gibson, B. E., Latchem, J., Olesen, J., Ralls, J., & Setchell, J. (2016). Connectivity: An emerging concept for physiotherapy practice. *Physiotherapy Theory and Practice*, *32*(3), 159–170. https://doi.org/10.3109/09593985.2015.1137665

Nicholls, D. A., & Gibson, B. E. (2010). The body and physiotherapy. *Physiotherapy Theory and Practice*, *26*(8), 497–509. https://doi.org/10.3109/09593981003710316

Orpwood, B., Wilkinson, A., Perry, M., Keen, D., & Hale, L. (2026). Understanding New Zealand physiotherapy scholars' philosophies and practices of supported self-management: A qualitative study. *Disability and Rehabilitation*, 1–16. https://doi.org/10.1080/09638288.2026.2632938

Ould Brahim, L. (2019). Reconsidering the 'self' in self-management of chronic illness: Lessons from relational autonomy. *Nursing Inquiry*, *26*(3), e12292. https://doi.org/10.1111/nin.12292

Pene, B.-J., Gott, M., Clark, T. C., & Slark, J. (2023). Conceptualising relational care from an indigenous Māori perspective: A scoping review. *Journal of Clinical Nursing*, *32*, 6879–6893. https://doi.org/10.1111/jocn.16794

Perry, M. A., Devan, H., Davies, C., Hempel, D., Ingham, T., Jones, B., Reid, S., Saipe, B., & Hale, L. (2022). iSelf-help: A co-designed, culturally appropriate, online pain management programme in Aotearoa. *Research Involvement and Engagement*, *8*(1), 1–15. https://doi.org/10.1186/s40900-022-00339-9

Perry, M. A., Ingham, T., Jones, B., & Mirfin-Veitch, B. (2020). At "risk" and "vulnerable"! Reflections on inequities and the impact of COVID-19 on disabled people. *New Zealand Journal of Physiotherapy*, *48*(3), 107–116. https://doi.org/10.15619/NZJP/48.3.02

Pickett, K. E., & Wilkinson, R. G. (2015). Income inequality and health: A causal review. *Social Science & Medicine*, *128*, 316–326. https://doi.org/10.1016/j.socscimed.2014.12.031

Realo, A. (2003). Comparison of public and academic discourses: Estonian Individualism and collectivism revisited. *Culture & Psychology*, *9*(1), 47–77. https://doi.org/10.1177/1354067X03009001004

Rose, N. (2001). The politics of life itself. *Theory, Culture & Society*, *18*(6), 1–30. https://doi.org/10.1177/02632760122052020

Russell, A., Filec, S., Serper, M., Opsasnick, L., Batio, S., O'Conor, R. M., Curtis, L., Kwasny, M., Benavente, J. Y., Wismer, G., Bonham, M., Zheng, P., Lovett, R., Arvanitis, M., Ladner, D. P., McCaffery, K., Linder, J. A., Bailey, S. C., & Wolf, M. S. (2023). Impact of COVID-19 on the capacity to self-manage health and chronic conditions. *PEC Innovation*, *2*, 100163. https://doi.org/10.1016/j.pecinn.2023.100163

Sangelaji, B. (2018). Developing an intervention to promote physical activity engagement for people with multiple sclerosis living in rural settings. Doctor of Philosophy - PhD, University of Otago. Handle: https://hdl.handle.net/10523/8371

Scott, S. M., Perry, M. A., & Sole, G. (2018). Not always a straight path": Patients' perspectives following anterior cruciate ligament rupture and reconstruction. *Disability and Rehabilitation*, *40*(19), 2311–2317. https://doi.org/10.1080/09638288.2017.1335803

Shakespeare, T. (2000). *Help.* Venture Press.

Shakespeare, T., & Watson, N. (2023). Frameworks, models, theories, and experiences for understanding disability. In R. L. Brown, M. Maroto & D. Pettinicchio (Eds.), *The Oxford Handbook of the Sociology of Disability* (pp. 17–37). Oxford University Press. *https://doi.org/10.1093/oxfordhb/9780190093167.013.1*

Smith, C., Hale, L. A., Mulligan, H., & Treharne, G. J. (2013). Participant perceptions of a novel physiotherapy approach ('Blue Prescription') for increasing levels of physical activity in people with multiple sclerosis: A qualitative study following intervention. *Disability and Rehabilitation*, *35*(14), 1174–1181. https://doi.org/10.3109/09638288.2012.723792

Smith, J., Swallow, V., & Coyne, I. (2015). Involving parents in managing their child's long-term condition—A concept synthesis of family-centered care and partnership-in-care. *Journal of Pediatric Nursing*, *30*(1), 143–159. https://doi.org/10.1016/j.pedn.2014.10.014

Synnott, A., O'Keeffe, M., Bunzli, S., Dankaerts, W., O'Sullivan, P., & O'Sullivan, K. (2015). Physiotherapists may stigmatise or feel unprepared to treat people with low back pain and psychosocial factors that influence recovery: A systematic review. *Journal of Physiotherapy*, *61*(2), 68–76. https://doi.org/10.1016/j.jphys.2015.02.016

Tamasese, K., Peteru, C., Waldegrave, C., & Bush, A. (2005). Ole Taeao Afua, the new morning: A qualitative investigation into Samoan perspectives on mental health and culturally appropriate services. *Australian & New Zealand Journal of Psychiatry*, *39*(4), 300–309. https://doi.org/10.1080/j.1440-1614.2005.01572.x

Taylor, S. J. C., Pinnock, H., Epiphaniou, E., Pearce, G., Parke, H. L., Schwappach, A., Purushotham, N., Jacob, S., Várnai, Z., & Sheikh, A. (2014). A rapid synthesis of the evidence on interventions to support self-management for people with long-term conditions: PRISMS – Practical systematic review of self-management support for long-term conditions. *Health Services and Delivery Research*, *2*(53). https://doi.org/10.3310/hsdr02530

Teariki, M. A., & Leau, E. (2024). Understanding Pacific worldviews: Principles and connections for research. *Kōtuitui: New Zealand Journal of Social Sciences Online*, *19*(2), 132–151. https://doi.org/10.1080/1177083X.2023.2292268

Timmermans, L., Boeykens, D., Sirimsi, M. M., Van de Velde, D., De Vriendt, P., Decat, P., Foulon, V., Van Hecke, A., Vermandere, M., Schoenmakers, B., & the Primary Care Academy. (2024). Self-management support (SMS) in primary care practice: A qualitative focus group study of care professionals' experiences. *BMC Primary Care*, *25*(1), 76. https://doi.org/10.1186/s12875-024-02317-4

Trip, H. T., Conder, J., Hale, L., & Whitehead, L. (2016). The role of key workers in supporting people with intellectual disability in the self-management of their diabetes: A qualitative New Zealand study. *Health & Social Care in the Community*, *24*(6), 789–798. https://doi.org/10.1111/hsc.12262

Tronto, J. C. (1998). An ethic of care. *Generations: Journal of the American Society on Aging*, *22*(3), 15–20. http://www.jstor.org/stable/44875693

United Nations. (2006). *Convention on the rights of persons with disabilities.* Retrieved 29 November 2020 from https://www.ohchr.org/en/instruments-mechanisms/instruments/convention-rights-persons-disabilities

van Dongen, S. I., de Nooijer, K., Cramm, J. M., Francke, A. L., Oldenmenger, W. H., Korfage, I. J., Witkamp, F. E., Stoevelaar, R., van der Heide, A., & Rietjens, J. A. (2020). Self-management of patients with advanced cancer: A systematic review of experiences and attitudes. *Palliative Medicine*, *34*(2), 160–178. https://doi.org/10.1177/0269216319883976

Vassilev, I., Rogers, A., Blickem, C., Brooks, H., Kapadia, D., Kennedy, A., Sanders, C., Kirk, S., & Reeves, D. (2013). Social networks, the 'work' and work force of chronic illness self-management: A survey analysis of personal communities. *PLoS One*, *8*(4), e59723.

Vassilev, I., Rogers, A., Kennedy, A., & Koetsenruijter, J. (2014). The influence of social networks on self-management support: A metasynthesis. *BMC Public Health*, *14*(1), 719.

Vassilev, I., Rogers, A., Kennedy, A., Wensing, M., Koetsenruijter, J., Orlando, R., Portillo, M. C., & Culliford, D. (2016). Social network type and long-term condition management support: A cross-sectional study in six european countries. *PLoS One*, *11*(8), e0161027. https://doi.org/10.1371/journal.pone.0161027

Watson, J. (2016). Assumptions of decision-making capacity: The role supporter attitudes play in the realisation of article 12 for people with severe or profound intellectual disability. *Laws*, *5*, 6. https://doi.org/10.3390/laws5010006

Wendell, S. (1997). *The Rejected Body: Feminist Philosophical Reflections on Disability* (1st ed.). Routledge. https://doi.org/10.4324/9780203724149. E book ISBN 9780203724149.

Wendt, A. (1999). Afterword: Tatauing the post-colonial body. In V. Hereniko & R. Wilson (Eds.), *Inside Out: Literature, Cultural Politics, and Identity in the New Pacific* (pp. 399–412). Rowman & Littlefield.

Whitehead, L. C., Trip, H. T., Hale, L. A., & Conder, J. (2016). Negotiated autonomy in diabetes self-management: The experiences of adults with intellectual disability and their support workers. *Journal of Intellectual Disability Research*, *60*(4), 389–397. https://doi.org/10.1111/jir.12257

Wilson, D., Moloney, E., Parr, J. M., Aspinall, C., & Slark, J. (2021). Creating an indigenous Māori-centred model of relational health: A literature review of Māori models of health. *Journal of Clinical Nursing, 30*(23–24), 3539–3555. https://doi.org/10.1111/jocn.15859

Wilson, L., Wilkinson, A., & Tikao, K. (2022). Health professional perspectives on translation of cultural safety concepts into practice: A scoping study. *Frontiers in Rehabilitation Sciences, 3*, 891571. https://doi.org/10.3389/fresc.2022.891571

Yin, C., McIntosh, J., & Marques, B. (2025). Integrating digital health technologies and place attachment: Theoretical foundations and practical implications. *Exploration of Digital Health Technologies, 3*, 101160. https://doi.org/10.37349/edht.2025.101160

Yoshikawa, K., Brady, B., Perry, M. A., & Devan, H. (2020). Sociocultural factors influencing physiotherapy management in culturally and linguistically diverse people with persistent pain: A scoping review. *Physiotherapy, 107*, 292–305. https://doi.org/10.1016/j.physio.2019.08.002

Zuniga-Teran, A. A., Gerlak, A. K., Elder, A. D., & Tam, A. (2021). The unjust distribution of urban green infrastructure is just the tip of the iceberg: A systematic review of place-based studies. *Environmental Science & Policy, 126*, 234–245. https://doi.org/https://doi.org/10.1016/j.envsci.2021.10.001

29 The Hidden Side of Self-Management Among Children with Disabilities and Their Families

Kinga Pozniak, Elizabeth Chambers, Genevieve Currie, and Olaf Kraus de Camargo

INTRODUCTION

The philosophy and operational practices of self-management in health care and rehabilitation are generally accepted as desirable and optimal. In this chapter we examine how this philosophy and practices play out in the lives of children living with disabilities and their parents, who are the principal agents charged with the task of managing both their children's care and self-management. We explore discourses and practices related to self-management, showing it to be a "double-edged sword" that may be empowering in principle but in practice is experienced as largely burdensome and at times exploitative of parents.

Our thinking about these issues is informed by our long-standing work with parents and caregivers on numerous research studies and other initiatives, combined with our own lived experiences. We are a team of researchers and parents affiliated with a Canadian research centre for childhood-onset disability. KP is a socio-cultural anthropologist; GC is a nurse researcher; EC is an educator and advocate; and OKDC is a developmental paediatrician. In addition to our professional roles, we all have personal experiences with navigating the paediatric health care and rehabilitation systems on behalf of our own children who have complex medical conditions. In this chapter we draw from our existing research studies with parents and youth to explore the experience of self-management in the lives of children/youth with disabilities and their families. All parents' and children's names used throughout the chapter are pseudonyms.

SELF-MANAGEMENT IN HEALTHCARE AND CHILD HEALTH

The concept of self-management in healthcare refers to the activities that individuals and families undertake to maximize or improve their health, well-being, and quality of life (Barlow et al. 2002). This can encompass activities such as adhering to medication and treatment programs; dealing with fatigue, stress and depression; eating healthy and exercising; communicating with healthcare providers; and navigating the healthcare system (e.g. finding and accessing relevant services and supports). It is argued that engaging in these self-care activities and behaviours can "augment medical treatments, improve health outcomes, quality of life, self-efficacy, reduce morbidity, emergency visits, and costs of care" (Lindsay et al. 2014).

The concept of self-management is related to other concepts such as patient education, goal-setting, person-centred care, and shared decision-making (Audulv 2026). Philosophically, it is underpinned by diverse (and perhaps incompatible) values, including, on the one side, rights-based approaches such as self-determination, patient involvement, independence and empowerment, and on the other, market-related values such as efficiency in healthcare spending, and minimizing

DOI: 10.1201/9781003599074-32

people's reliance on the state by having them assume individual responsibility for their outcomes (Fletcher et al. 2019).

In child health, the concept of self-management takes on an additional dimension because of the role of parents and other caregivers in meeting their children's care needs (Modi 2012). Here, "self-management" encompasses activities related to medical management (e.g. monitoring symptoms, administering medication, delivering therapy, managing medical technology); lifestyle modifications (e.g. eating, exercising, socializing with others); general parenting, empowerment and self-efficacy; psycho-education and behaviour training (Modi 2012). Initially, the primary responsibility for this work falls to primary caregivers (commonly parents, but depending on the family, could also include siblings, grandparents, or others). As children grow and develop, and especially as they transition out of paediatric healthcare, they are increasingly expected to assume greater responsibility for managing their own care (Nguyen et al. 2023). However, as many as 50-75% of children with chronic conditions experience challenges with adhering to their self-management activities because of developmental or medical conditions, and thus still need to be supported by parents (Betz 2017; Modi 2012; Nightingale et al. 2022).

In clinical practice, activities from providers oriented towards enabling and supporting self-management among families include: providing information (e.g. written visit summaries and care plans); peer supports (e.g. parent groups, mentors); coaching (e.g. practicing treatment skills); asking families about their concerns and preferences for medical care; offering multiple modes of communication between patient and providers; and family management (e.g. stress management programs) (Henry and Schor 2015). Many of these activities align with other organizing principles in child health, including Family-Centred service (Pozniak et al. 2024). For example, key premises of Family-Centred Service state that parents know their children best, and that parents and healthcare providers should work together on healthcare plans (Rosenbaum et al. 1998).

UNPACKING AND PROBLEMATIZING THE PHILOSOPHY

The philosophy of self-management – along with its accompanying practices – is generally accepted as desirable and an end goal: *of course* it's a good thing for parents to support their children to become more independent! *Of course* it's good for children to learn to look after their own health! However, in this chapter we seek to unpack how these taken-for-granted assumptions actually can be detrimental for families. We suggest that one of the reasons these assumptions are accepted as optimal is because they align with other dominant societal values prevalent in contemporary capitalist states. These include independence, individual responsibility, and a model of citizenship in which individuals have a moral obligation to minimize their dependence on society and its resources, by taking an active role in managing their health, and making "informed decisions" that comply with medical advice (Ellis et al. 2017; Polzer and Power 2016). In effect, people's demands for entitlements are transformed into "privatized solutions and 'choices' that download responsibilities onto individuals and families" (Polzer and Power 2016). In a critical analysis of the concept of self-care (which is a key element of self-management), Ward (2015) argued that it "obscures the responsibility of the state to adequately provide for its citizens" and "has been used by policymakers to dismantle public welfare systems and shift responsibility for care onto individual citizens" (Ward 2015).

While the concept of self-management is fairly entrenched in healthcare, it has received some critique. For example, Ellis et al. (2017) note that the idea of "choice" is a façade when the only permissible "choices" are those that comply with the directives of healthcare providers. Furthermore, this discourse overlooks the socio-economic barriers that limit some people's ability to make the choices that are deemed to be the correct ones (Ellis et al. 2017; Francis et al. 2020).

Furthermore, the notion that fostering "independence" should be the ultimate goal of healthcare and rehabilitation has also been problematized (McClure and Leah 2021; Ould Brahim 2019). McClure and Leah, distinguish between "independence, whereby people can accomplish tasks on their own, that is, without support from others" and "autonomy", where they "may require others to help implement the task, but they control their life goals and living situation" (2021). They point out that complete "independence" is unattainable for many people and instead recommend that the goal of rehabilitation should be autonomy.

Next, scholars have noted that self-management is a Western concept and may not be relevant in more collectively oriented cultures "where family and community are more valued" (Hale et al. 2024). And last – most prescient to the discussion that will follow – while activities related to "self-management" are framed as "responsibilities", they in fact constitute *work* – care work that is "unpaid and most often unrecognized" (Katzman 2016).

We now examine these ideas in the context of children's health and rehabilitation. We draw on several of our research studies that address the experiences of families with healthcare (and other) services, and their needs for support. These studies include: developing a new measure of Family-Centred Service; exploring support needs of children with disabilities and their families following the COVID-19 pandemic; transitioning from paediatric to adult care among youth with a rare condition (Duchenne Muscular Dystrophy); and the caregiving experiences of parents of adult children with lifelong care needs. We will synthesize several themes from these research studies and will highlight some of the hidden costs and consequences associated with self-management practices.

SELF-MANAGEMENT AMONG PARENTS

Parents Are Required to Self-Manage ALL Aspects of Their Children's Care

A consistent finding across our research studies is a pervasive lack of adequate supports across all domains of life (healthcare, education, social services), which requires parents to "self-manage" all areas of their children's and families' care. While one could argue that this is the case for ALL parents (not just parents of children with disabilities or health conditions), it is worth highlighting the multitude of tasks parents with children with complex needs perform in addition to "regular" parenting duties. They are therapists, care coordinators, care navigators, nurses (sometimes performing complicated medical procedures), and advocates. Some parents reported to the need to train medical professionals (e.g. nurses, respite workers) in performing procedures on their children, and parents of children who have rare conditions reported having to inform physicians about these conditions.

> I definitely have to be the Momager or CEO.... I feel so much pressure to not let the ball drop anywhere. To not forget something. Am I accessing everything I can here through our system? Am I getting everyone who needs to be involved, involved with him?
>
> **('Sarah', speech language pathologist and mother of a two-year old with a rare condition)**

Some parents reported the extraordinary lengths they went to support their children. For example, one mother, who previously had no background in healthcare, reported getting a job at her local children's hospital to ensure that her daughter's care was properly coordinated among over eighty providers and multiple organizations.

Self-management Takes Extraordinary Time and Energy

Parents described the amount of time, energy and effort entailed in engaging in self-management activities. One particularly poignant example of this is a self-managed system of care which in the province of Ontario, Canada is called "family managed home care". Under this arrangement, families who are approved for this program (i.e. children with medical complexity requiring 24/7 care), hire the support staff to meet their child's care needs, whose wages are then paid for by the ministry. Many families prefer this arrangement to the alternative model of agency-delivered care, where the agency is contracted by the government. Parents explain that there are multiple problems with agency-delivered care, including a chronic shortage of staff, unreliable supports (e.g. workers who do not show up for shifts) and poorly trained or unprofessional workers (e.g. who sleep on their shift, leave child unattended while they smoke outside, or even steal from the family). For parents who have had these negative experiences with agency-delivered care, family-managed home care is an opportunity to have some control over who they have in their homes. This, however, requires parents to hire, train, and potentially fire, their own workers, coordinate workers' schedules, manage paperwork such as medical charts for liability reasons, keep accurate financial records of hours worked and money paid, and submit these documents within the required timeframe to a certified bookkeeper or accountant. For parents, these tasks can be extremely burdensome. Such is the case for 'Lilly', mother of a teenager with muscular dystrophy, who "chose" to self-manage the staffing of her son's school-based and home-based supports because her agency could not find careworkers:

> [W]e were forced into that [family managed health care] because they were finding us zero nursing. And I have about 400 hours a month of nursing that I have to sort out plus another 300 hours of personal support workers on top of that. So, when you think about that, it's like a little job for me... You're basically taking over somebody else's job for absolutely nothing. I have a staff of over 10 to 12 people at any time that I need to hire and fire and schedule.... All of my nurses work somewhere else, because you can never get anybody full-time, they're all working at hospitals...they're all just sort of doing part-time in my house. I basically have to take what I can get. When I have people who aren't good, I have to figure out how to fire them, I have to hire new ones, it takes months to train, and then I have to pay weekly.... it is insane in my house, that family-managed home care. There is nothing family about it... I've tried to work with the [provincial health network] and they don't care, they're just happy that I'm doing it and they're not.... I'm not an accountant... I'm always making mistakes and they're not nice and helpful about it, they send in jargon that I don't even know what they're talking about. They threaten to stop my funding if I don't correct my mistakes.
>
> **('Lilly', retired teacher and mother of a teenager with a neuromuscular condition)**

For Lilly, while family-managed care may be better than the alternative of having no nursing/ personal care worker support at all, it is nonetheless onerous and overwhelming. She also feels it is punitive in that she is threatened with withdrawal of funding if she makes any mistakes in managing the care workers.

Self-management Is Not Properly Supported

Parents reported not receiving support from health, education and social systems to meet their child's care needs. They shared that they received practical assistance not from professionals, but from other parents. Most support they received from professionals was in the form of advice as to what they should be doing, which was not responsive to their circumstances, nor considerate of their existing workload.

> [T]heir focus plan is on parent training. When they come, they train me how to work with my son, but I just find it is so overwhelming with everything that is already going and all the care that I already have to provide for him. To become his therapist is adding so much to the pile.... [W]hen the therapist comes to my home I want you to take him and work with him during this hour please and do the best job you can. For me personally, that is an hour break where I don't have even think about what you are doing - I can relax and enjoy how he is progressing. But instead as a parent we are being taught how to do this therapy at home and given this pressure of, "okay, at the next check-in we are going to see how well you did it"
>
> **("Vicky", mother of a three-year old child with a rare condition)**

Instead of training and advice, many parents wished they would receive practical, tangible help. These activities included performing hands-on tasks such as programming a speech device;

filling out government forms; delivering therapy (instead of teaching the parent how to do it); and arranging and coordinating services and appointments for the family (rather than expecting the parent to do it).

Parents also reported that they received little emotional support or understanding from their children's healthcare providers. For example, parents shared that healthcare providers rarely asked parents how they were feeling, showed concern about family members' well-being, or acknowledged the challenges the parents were trying to manage. One mother whose daughter spent a month in the hospital after a transplant, noted that she was expected to perform most of her daughter's nursing tasks. During this time, the only person who asked her how *she* was doing was the custodian:

> [I]f they could just remember that I am a mom and ask me, 'how are you doing as a mom?' The only person who asked me that was a person who came to clean our room every single morning.
>
> **('Dina', nurse and mother of a teenage daughter with a chronic progressive condition)**

Self-management Is Enforced through Judgement and Blame

Parents want to have a major role in supporting their children's care. However, they relayed that professionals shifted too many responsibilities to them, so that meeting these responsibilities became unmanageable. Parents also reported feeling blamed and judged by healthcare providers who conveyed to them that they were not doing enough to help their children reach their potential:

> There was the unrealistic expectations of… you need to brush him for 10 minutes every hour for 10 hours (to increase sensory input)… And then the physios would be like, you need to do this, and this, and this, and they make you feel like if you don't, you're in big trouble. Like your child will never reach their potential
>
> **('Samantha', child life specialist and mother of a teenager with a rare condition)**

"Self-managing" Takes a Physical, Emotional and Mental Toll

Parents' extraordinary self-management comes at a cost. It is well-documented that caregivers of children with disabilities experience elevated levels of stress, anxiety, and depression (Çolak and Kahriman 2023; King et al. 2025; Li et al. 2024). Across our various studies, parents reported being overwhelmed, stressed and exhausted – experiences they attributed not to the child's health condition, but rather to the magnitude of responsibilities, lack of appropriate supports, and inconsiderate and disrespectful treatment on the part of professionals. In effect, many primary caregivers (most often mothers) either scaled back on, or entirely abandoned, their professional goals and aspirations, which negatively impacted not only their household financial stability, but also their sense of identity and self-worth (Pozniak and Gorter 2024).

> Society expects mothers to be superheroes when you have a child with disabilities, and I think it's because no one knows how to help you, or no one knows what to do. No one really wants to burden themselves. There's not enough money. There's not enough help. And so, if you want your child to live with you and to have a certain quality of life, then you have to sacrifice yourself. And there's no empathy about that…. It's just you're supposed to do it.
>
> **(Gina, mother of two teenage boys, one of whom lives with a rare condition)**

Parents also reported the physical toll associated with untenable caregiving responsibilities. This included musculoskeletal problems from lifting and carrying their children, chronic exhaustion from years of sleep deprivation, and other conditions related to stress and exhaustion, such as migraines or chronic pain.

> I was recently diagnosed with a chronic pain syndrome, which has been going on for more than ten years. It took ten years to finally get to the point where somebody actually would look at me. It's similar to fibromyalgia. But the doctor did point out that there have been legitimate research studies that have directly linked chronic sleep deprivation to these developments
>
> **('Kate', mother and full-time caregiver to 25-year old son with complex care needs)**

Excelling at Self-Management Leads to More Self-Management

Parents also noted the reward for doing a good job of managing their child's care was being given more responsibilities. One mother shared that her provincial government program tasked her to be her son's therapist because they were not able to find qualified staff for the role:

> They actually called me in and said, 'You're actually more skilled than any of our staff. So we're going to have to let you work with him'
>
> **('Kate', mother and full-time caregiver to 25-year old son with complex care needs)**

Self-management Blurs Roles

Parents also felt that taking on health care professionals' tasks and roles interfered with their primary role as parents and adversely affected their relationship with their child.

> I hate that sometimes I am the administrator of medications he doesn't want, or therapies, and I have to be the bad guy a lot of the time.... I would like to be more mom, but I think things would fall apart unfortunately.
>
> **('Amanda', mother of three elementary school children, the oldest of whom has a rare condition)**

> I was forced to be a therapist for [son] before we could secure funding for therapy, and it very negatively affected our relationship. Every interaction we had became a therapeutic one out of necessity.... As parents of disabled children, we already are tasked with significantly more on our plate, this was not helpful and disallowed a normal parent/child bond.
>
> **('Ruth', mother of two children in middle school, one of whom has behavioural, sensory and learning challenges)**

'Ruth' went on to question the ethics of downloading certain self-management tasks (such as carrying out therapies), to parents:

> It is actually against most professional colleges code of ethics for family members to deliver therapy to close contacts such as their own children... yet parents are still being asked/forced to do this? We should be looking for ways to increase, not diminish, our standard of care.

SELF-MANAGEMENT FOR YOUTH

As children with disabilities grow older, the health care system increasingly expects them to take on more responsibility for their own care. In theory, this is a reasonable expectation. However, in practice, the ways in which independence and responsibility are fostered among youth with disabilities can be problematic for these youth and families. In child health, there is a robust body of research and clinical work related to the topic of "transition" from paediatric to adult care. There are numerous resources for both parents and youth to support this process. However, when young people with disabilities turn the age of majority, their parent(s) and themselves often feel lost, forgotten and unsupported (Li et al. 2024). Why is this happening?

Self-Management Initiatives for Youth Reflect Priorities of the Health Care System and Healthcare Providers

Many of the transition initiatives described by healthcare providers in our study were oriented towards preparing youth and parents for the decline of quality of care in adult care. While Canadian healthcare, rehabilitation and social assistance systems for children are plagued by problems, it is widely acknowledged that adult systems are even more fragmented and under resourced (Toulany et al. 2022). For example, youth with disabilities and their parents/caregivers need and value centralized and coordinated care, with different specialties located in one place, different healthcare providers communicating with each other, and a designated point-person to provide assistance with activities such as referrals and making appointments (Ghotane et al. 2024). This type of wraparound care is generally only available to youth with complex care needs. However, transition activities often prepare these youth and their families that this wraparound care will be taken away. In one of our studies, paediatric healthcare providers who provided these supports described them as "holding hands", insinuating that youth and families are privileged to receive this practical assistance, but that it renders them unprepared to face the "real world" of adult care:

> [I]n peds we're so good at holding hands, a little bit too good…
>
> **('Michelle', nurse in a neuromuscular clinic)**

> I think having the child be a strong advocate for themselves is really important, because when you… are moving from a pediatric world into an adult, it's going to be a lot different…There might not be as much hand-holding at different facilities as they get here, and then they have to be prepared to mark these things down and attend their appointments and take their medication when there are less checks and balances… Some [healthcare providers] can be quite fast and maybe a bit rude or not understand their condition the same way, and so that's why we need to make sure they have their own voice, so that they know when to speak up for themselves.
>
> **('Eleanor', exercise testing technician at neuromuscular clinic)**

The Parameters of Self-Management Are Determined by Healthcare Providers – but the Work Is Done by Parents

Parents are tasked with the responsibility of preparing and supporting their children's self-managed care. They are instructed on skills they need to work on with their children and are given checklists and guidelines to gauge their own and their children's "readiness" for tasks that the healthcare system deems to be indicative of "independence". At the same time, healthcare providers and organizations have their own criteria and practices regarding the extent to which parent involvement is desired and allowed. For example, some parents noted that the health information system in their hospital automatically shuts off parents' access to their children's records once the child turns 16, and some healthcare providers disallowed parents' presence at appointments. One mother described being excluded from her teenage daughter's care when her daughter was receiving a liver transplant:

> The professional came out and said, "she is now 16 and you have to prepare her for transition and so you can stay here in the waiting room, and we are going to take her.
>
> **('Dina', mother of a teenage daughter with a rare condition)**

Activities such as restricting parents' access to their children's health information was understandably intended to enable children's independence and respect their privacy. However, the reality for many families is that these youth often still need their parents' support – as indeed is the case with many adult healthcare users, especially those undergoing complicated procedures such as transplants or taking vital medications. In effect, such practices only make it more challenging for parents to perform the roles that are still socially (and sometimes legally) expected of them. Dina, for example, noted that her daughter, unbeknownst to her, stopped taking her medication: "What I found out later is that there was a lot of non-adherence to some of the medications because she wanted to feel normal, and so I found all these pills that she said she was taking, in a bag".

Parents are often depicted by healthcare providers and researchers as being unwilling or unprepared to let go of control and to assign their growing children greater responsibility. They are also judged and criticized for being too enabling or doing too much "hand-holding". However, our research findings were more nuanced. For example, in our study on Family-Centred Service, even parents of young children expressed that they wished that healthcare providers engaged more with their children, asked for the children's opinions, and took those opinions into consideration. Furthermore, while transition discourses promote having youth advocate for themselves, the reality is that they are not always taken seriously when they do so, a fact noted by one of the youths in our study:

> At one point I was dealing with... mental health issues and I was bringing it up to my medical team, and it didn't seem like any of them were really understanding.... until my father went with me to the appointment and it took him having to say exactly what I just told them for them to take it seriously.
>
> **(23-year-old man living with a rare condition)**

In our work on healthcare transition among youth with Duchenne Muscular Dystrophy, we observed that the healthcare system is particularly concerned with self-management of youth in narrowly defined areas. For example, healthcare providers wanted youth to bring their own health card to appointments, know what medications they were taking, make their own healthcare appointments, and attend appointments alone without parents. However, these providers were not fully cognizant of organizational and societal barriers that hampered youth's ability to self-manage in ways that were actually important to *them*. For example, youth and their parents noted that due to lack of accessible transportation where they lived, the youth still needed their parents to drive them to healthcare appointments (which in turn required the parent to coordinate these appointments around their other work and family commitments). Youth also reported that not all medical clinics have accessible examination rooms and washrooms, thus causing them to rely on their parents' assistance. There is thus a disconnect between the goals of "independence" in theory, and the reality of inadequate social support systems and structural barriers that prevent individuals with disabilities from exercising autonomy in ways that are meaningful to them.

DISCUSSION

Our research demonstrates that self-management techniques in children's healthcare and rehabilitation are increasing the care work performed by parents. Parents of children with disabilities are extraordinary "self-efficacious" at managing their children's care to optimize their child's health and social outcomes. Their unpaid labour provides a significant subsidy to the healthcare system; in Canada, caregivers are estimated to contribute $24 billion in cost savings by performing informal care giving annually to the care system (Shearkhani et al. 2025). But what are the hidden costs of these savings? Our goal in this chapter was to bring attention to some of the lesser-known outcomes and hidden costs of self-management practices.

The parents in our studies reported a significant burden associated with adhering to self-management practices. However, the majority of parents who take part in child health research studies represent the most structurally privileged sectors of the population: in Canada, they are more likely to be university-educated, white, Canadian-born, and speak English as a first language. In addition, many of the parents who participated in our own research studies were also themselves healthcare providers. We can anticipate that parents who lack structural privileges are facing additional challenges that we have not captured here (for example, challenges related to not having their own transportation or navigating the healthcare system in a language that is not their first).

More broadly, the philosophy of self-management makes us question some of the fundamental principles of healthcare, for example: what are the responsibilities of people to the system, and of the system to the people? At present, what constitutes appropriate and desirable self-management for children/youth with disabilities or chronic care needs and their parents, is defined by the healthcare system, largely for its own benefit. Patients' and caregivers' unmet care needs and the need for services and support become channelled into interventions which become the responsibility of parents (and the youth, when they reach a certain age/developmental stage). This serves the already under resourced and taxed healthcare system because it shifts the work (and the associated costs) to patients and caregivers. But is this how we as citizens actually want our care systems to operate?

Having said that, we do not want to characterize self-management as unequivocally bad. A consistent theme that runs through our research studies is that parents want to be actively involved in their children's care. Parents also want their children to be involved in their own care, as much as is developmentally appropriate. Youth themselves also want to be listened to and taken seriously and make decisions about their care when they want to do so. All of the above are central tenets of Family-Centred Service (Pozniak et al. 2024). It appears, then, that the philosophy of self-management aligns, at least in part, with concepts of Family-Centred Service. However, just as the concept of Family-Centred Service can be misapplied in practice, the same can be true of self-management.

In order for self-management initiatives to be empowering, they need to be oriented towards helping people define and achieve their own goals, rather than leaving families unsupported by shifting responsibilities from the system to individuals. Instead of trying to build "capacity" and "self-efficacy", we can shift the focus to providing, and advocating for, the things that youth and families are telling us are actually helpful (Hale et al. 2022). Authentic capacity, self-efficacy and independence may be better developed by asking families what they need to live lives that are as healthy and meaningful as possible – and then helping bring these about through research, clinical practice and advocacy. If we can agree that the purpose of healthcare is to help people be at their best, we need to manage systems and services so that they work for their users, rather than managing people so that they can bolster failing systems.

REFERENCES

Audulv, Å, Packer, T., Hutchinson, S., Roger, K.S. and Kephart, G., 2026. Coping, adapting or self-managing–what is the difference? A concept review based on the neurological literature. Journal of Advanced Nursing, 72(11), pp. 2629–2643.

Barlow, J.H., Sturt, J. and Hearnshaw, H., 2002. Self-management interventions for people with chronic conditions in primary care: Examples from arthritis, asthma and diabetes. Health Education Journal, 61(4), pp. 365–378.

Betz, C.L., 2017. Self-management and health care transition: Trials, tribulations and triumphs. Journal of Pediatric Rehabilitation Medicine, 10(3–4), pp. 177–183.

Çolak, B. and Kahriman, I., 2023. Evaluation of family burden and quality of life of parents with children with disability. The American Journal of Family Therapy, 51(2), pp. 113–133.

Ellis, J., Boger, E., Latter, S., Kennedy, A., Jones, F., Foster, C. and Demain, S., 2017. Conceptualisation of the 'good' self-manager: A qualitative investigation of stakeholder views on the self-management of long-term health conditions. Social Science & Medicine, 176, pp. 25–33.

Fletcher, S., Kulnik, S.T., Demain, S. and Jones, F., 2019. The problem with self-management: Problematising self-management and power using a Foucauldian lens in the context of stroke care and rehabilitation. PloS One, 14(6), p. e0218517.

Francis, H., Carryer, J. and Wilkinson, J., 2020. Self-management support? Listening to people with complex co-morbidities. Chronic Illness, 16(3), pp. 161–172.

Ghotane, S., Hirve, R., Forman, J., Tan, D., Achercouk, Z. and Wolfe, I., 2024. Integrated care for children and young people with special health and care needs: A systematic review. Archives of Disease in Childhood, 109(11), pp. 924–931.

Hale, L., Oosman, S. and Stewart, A.V., 2022. Challenging the concept of self-management support in unique and diverse populations. Frontiers in Rehabilitation Sciences, 3, p. 999528.

Henry, H.K. and Schor, E.L., 2015. Supporting self-management of chronic health problems. Pediatrics, 135(5), pp. 789–792.

Katzman, E., 2016. Self-management and the government of disability: Reinforcing normalcy through the construction of able-disabled subjectivities. Neoliberal Governance and Health: Risks and Vulnerabilities. Montreal: McGill-Queen's University Press, pp. 307–329.

King, G., Pozniak, K., Teplicky, R. and Earl, S., 2025. The experiences of parents of children with disabilities receiving healthcare services: Negative emotions and associated situations. Research in Developmental Disabilities, 156, p. 104896.

Li, L., Carter, N., Gorter, J.W., Till, L., White, M. and Strachan, P.H., 2024. Surviving transition: A qualitative case study on how families adapt as their youth with medical complexity transitions from child to adult systems of care. Health Care Transitions, 2, p. 100035.

Lindsay, S., Kingsnorth, S., Mcdougall, C. and Keating, H., 2014. A systematic review of self-management interventions for children and youth with physical disabilities. Disability and Rehabilitation, 36(4), pp. 276–288.

McClure, J. and Leah, C., 2021. Is independence enough? Rehabilitation should include autonomy and social engagement to achieve quality of life. Clinical Rehabilitation, 35(1), pp. 3–12.

Modi, A.C., Pai, A.L., Hommel, K.A., Hood, K.K., Cortina, S., Hilliard, M.E., Guilfoyle, S.M., Gray, W.N. and Drotar, D., 2012. Pediatric self-management: A framework for research, practice, and policy. Pediatrics, 129(2), pp. e473–e485.

Nguyen, L., Dawe-McCord, C., Frost, M., Arafeh, M., Chambers, K., Arafeh, D., Pozniak, K., Thomson, D., Mosel, J., Cardoso, R., Galuppi, B., Strohm, S., Via-Dufresne Ley, A., Cassidy, C., McCauley, D., Doucet, S., Alazem, H., Fournier, A., Marelli, A. and Gorter, J. W. 2023. A commentary on the healthcare transition policy landscape for youth with disabilities or chronic health conditions, the need for an inclusive and equitable approach, and recommendations for change in Canada. Frontiers in Rehabilitation Sciences, 4, p. 1305084. https://doi.org/10.3389/fresc.2023.1305084

Nightingale, R., McHugh, G.A., Swallow, V. and Kirk, S., 2022. Shifting responsibilities: A qualitative study of how young people assume responsibility from their parents for self-management of their chronic kidney disease. Health Expectations, 25(4), pp. 1919–1929.

Ould Brahim, L., 2019. Reconsidering the 'self' in self-management of chronic illness: Lessons from relational autonomy. Nursing Inquiry, 26(3), p. e12292.

Polzer, J. and Power, E., 2016. The governance of health in neoliberal societies. Neoliberal Governance and Health: Duties, Risks, and Vulnerabilities. Montreal: McGill-Queen's University Press, pp. 3–42.

Pozniak, K. and Gorter, J.W., 2024. Caregiver identity in health research: Mothers of children with disabilities share their experiences with partnering on health research studies. International Journal of Care and Caring, pp. 1–18.

Pozniak, K., King, G., Chambers, E., Martens, R., Earl, S., Kraus de Camargo, O., McCauley, D., Teplicky, R. and Rosenbaum, P., 2024. What do parents want from healthcare services? Reports of parents' experiences with pediatric service delivery for their children with disabilities. Disability and Rehabilitation, 46(12), pp. 2670–2683.

Rosenbaum, P., King, S., Law, M., King, G. and Evans, J., 1998. Family-centred service: A conceptual framework and research review. Physical & Occupational Therapy in Pediatrics, 18(1), pp. 1–20.

Shearkhani, S., Bai, Y.Q., Kuluski, K., Anderson, G.M. and Wodchis, W.P., 2025. Informal caregiving: Health system cost implications. Western Journal of Nursing Research, 47(3), pp. 140–148.

Toulany, A., Gorter, J.W. and Harrison, M., 2022. A call for action: Recommendations to improve transition to adult care for youth with complex health care needs. Paediatrics & Child Health, 27(5), pp. 297–309. https://doi.org/10.1093/pch/pxac047

Ward, L., 2015. Caring for ourselves? Self-care and neoliberalism. Ethics of Care. Bristol: Policy Press, pp. 45–56.

30 Role of Self-Management Interventions in the Rehabilitation of Patients with Chronic Neurological Conditions

Ahmad Sahely and Sheeba Rosewilliam

INTRODUCTION

One in six people live with a chronic neurological condition (CNC) worldwide and that includes people with acquired brain injury, stroke, multiple sclerosis, Parkinson's disease, Epilepsy, Alzheimer's and Dementia. A chronic neurological condition presents with a myriad of consequences in the physical, psychological, and cognitive realms; overall well-being and quality of life due to social limitations suffer therefore, following CNC (Fakolade et al., 2020). Chronic neurological conditions could either be illnesses with a sudden onset that stabilise in the long term or conditions that could progressively worsen. Due to the progressive nature of CNCs such as multiple sclerosis and Parkinson's disease, it is key to integrate self-management support (SMS) for all patients with CNCs rather than offer programmes for selective self-motivated patients (Davies et al, 2017; Grady and Gough, 2014).

THE CONCEPT OF SELF-MANAGEMENT IN NEUROREHABILITATION

Several definitions have been used to describe self-management, a majority of which advocate the role of an individual in the management of their chronic condition (Corbin and Strauss, 1988; Hinder and Greenhalgh, 2012; Lenzen et al., 2017, p. 2; Parke et al., 2015; Sadler et al., 2017; Wilkinson and Whitehead, 2009). However, the definitions seem to focus more on the medical management of the conditions and focus lightly on dealing with functional, emotional, or psychological issues which are vital to the community integration of a person with a CNC. Further, SMS in chronic neurological conditions would fluctuate depending upon the progress of the disease and hence it is not a time limited process, and this is not captured in many definitions.

Encompassing a biopsycho-social model, self-management in CNC could be defined as an *"individual's ability, in conjunction with family, community, and the appropriate healthcare professionals to manage the symptoms, treatment, physical, psychosocial, cultural, and spiritual consequences and inherent lifestyle changes required for living with a chronic disease"* (Wilkinson and Whitehead, 2009, p. 1145). Working within such a model would require the collaboration of several stakeholders within the individual context of patients with CNC. Therefore, considering the chronic nature, the variations in progression and the complexity of the consequences for people with CNC, the focus of self-management should be broad enough to include psychosocial aspects, self-resilience, self-efficacy in addition to the traditional medical and symptom management (Kılınc et al., 2022).

DOI: 10.1201/9781003599074-33

NEUROPHYSIOLOGICAL ASPECTS OF SMS

In patients with central neurological conditions the frontal cortex that functions to process choice, cost benefit, task difficulty, effort and anticipated reward could be affected. Planning and identifying alternatives that are important to achieve success in attaining goals in SMS are affected in the central nervous system pathologies. If executive functions are affected due to central nervous system lesions, patients find it hard to adhere to behavioural change strategies and hence complete self-management tasks (Dobkin, 2016). In acquired brain lesions, cognitive decline needs to be intervened to improve memory, planning and execution skills to support self-management. The self-management tasks that incorporate behaviour change techniques such as receiving instructions, rehearsal, and repeated practice lead to development of knowledge and skill for implementing self-management in line with repetitive task theory (Ahmed et al., 2021; Fakolade et al., 2020). These task-specific, goal-directed practices engage neural circuits involved in motor control and drive experience-dependent neuroplasticity, strengthening synaptic connectivity through repetition and intensity. According to motor learning and task-oriented training frameworks, such high dose, functionally meaningful practice through SMS promotes cortical reorganisation and expansion of motor maps, thereby enhancing lasting behavioural changes (Grady and Gough, 2014; Piccoli et al., 2018). SMS training and carrying out tasks can in turn improve executive function through feedback to nervous system (Devittori et al., 2024). Feedback and self-monitoring feed forward to improve problem solving and planning to carry out SMS tasks; however, these strategies are being employed to a lesser extent in self-management interventions in neurological conditions.

PERSPECTIVES OF PATIENTS WITH CNC

The perspectives of people with CNC about what self-management experience meant to them was explored and built into a framework represented by the diagram below by Kılınç et al. (2022). People with CNC suggested that they wanted their life to be meaningful and purposeful. They wanted to

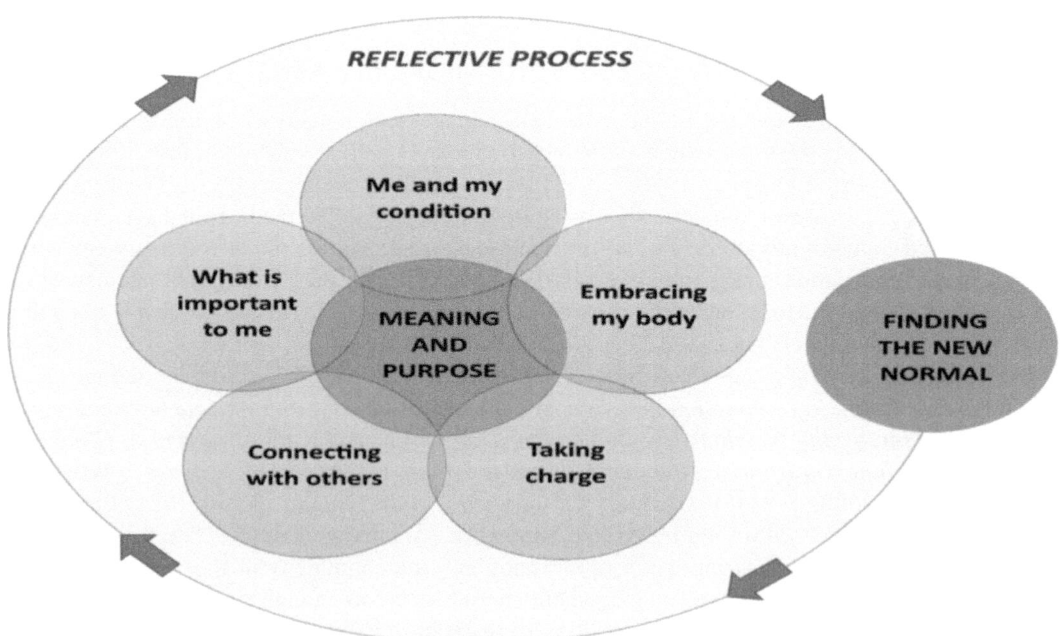

FIGURE 30.1 Framework for the self-management of neurological conditions. (Kılınc et al., 2022.)

move away from their identity as patients and rebuild their sense of self, develop connections with others and live life to full, with resilience and active learning. Achieving goals that were relevant to them kept them engaged. To aid the above, the process of self-managing should involve developing an awareness about themselves, their needs/priorities, their body and condition. These elements are interconnected and could influence each other. The authors suggest that identifying which element needed support would improve the delivery and effectiveness of SMS. Strategies for people with neurological conditions should incorporate working with others for connections and help develop a sense of control. Ultimately, SMS must be an ongoing reflective process due to the fluctuating and chronic nature of neurological conditions (Figure 30.1).

CHALLENGES TO IMPLEMENTATION OF SELF-MANAGEMENT IN NEUROLOGICAL CONDITIONS

1. Providers reported that they lack basic knowledge and awareness about neurological conditions and the principles of self-management (Jaglal et al., 2014).
2. There is a lack of instruction on how to manage symptoms and information on support services after discharge which makes SMS a primary challenge for patients with neurological conditions living in the community (Pugh et al., 2019).
3. Cognitive deficits such as memory, confusion, communication problems along with emotional issues of fear of re-stroking, fear of falling, trying to avoid negative perceptions and stigma, feeling of guilt about not doing enough and becoming demotivated are other patient reported challenges.
4. Other psychological and physical issues such as depression, fatigue and co-morbidities are patient related challenges (Coulter and Ellins, 2006; Sadler et al., 2017).
5. Certain perspectives of patients were extreme, such as, patients feeling that SMS meant that they were taking care of themselves. They felt they were losing rights to receiving supervised care since they believed therapists were shifting a part of their responsibility to patients (Sahely et al., 2023).
6. Mismatch in goals between professionals or misunderstanding of recovery prospects between professionals has been reported as a major challenge for goal-setting within SMS.
7. Professional workload, staffing and organisational barriers such as financial limitations and leadership support have also been identified as limiting implementation of SMS.
8. Lack of mentoring or support after initiating SMS, after providing education can lead to participants misunderstanding information or over confidence leading to risky behaviours and safety issues such as falling (Ward et al., 2004).
9. Not identifying who could benefit from the programme or readiness to engage (Boger et al., 2015) could lead to more wastage of resources if patients did not adhere and benefit from the SMS (Newman et al., 2004).
10. Participants included in research routinely had mild to moderate impairments and people with severe impairments (physical, cognitive, or aphasia) were excluded thus having less opportunities within community-based SMS (Sahely et al., 2023). Further, it might be challenging for survivors to engage in SMS in the early stages after stroke due to the above reasons (Laver et al., 2010; Satink et al., 2015).
11. Considering the long-term nature of chronic neurological conditions SMS should have impactful outcomes for the long term; however, there is limited evidence around SMS in the long term.
12. The biomedical approach to treatment and organisational policies (i.e., early discharge) in the acute care settings, were considered by physiotherapist as barriers to supporting SM at this stage (Sadler et al., 2017).

TAILORING OF SM INTERVENTIONS

Patients prefer tailored interventions and view them as being more relevant to their needs (Kreuter et al., 2013; Plow et al., 2016). Patients may be more likely to think about and adhere to tailored interventions if these are tailored to their needs. Tailoring SMS could involve altering the information provided, the delivery strategies such as choice of remote or in person (clinical tailoring), and/or dosing (i.e., the frequency or amount of contacts) based on an assessment of an individual's specific characteristics such as the mental status, biomarkers, and environment (Fanning et al., 2012; Free et al., 2013).

In patients with stroke, tailoring of self-management interventions can be done either through one to one, in-person meetings, online or over the phone based on patients' preferences, their impairments, what barriers they faced, risks, and psychosocial constraints. Written material can then be used to deliver tailored self-management interventions based on current behaviour, psychosocial constraints and barriers using computerised algorithms. In addition to computer algorithms, individual's judgement can be used to decide the interventions, the dose catering to outcomes relevant to risk management, physical function, fun activities, medication adherence, and nutrition.

For effective tailoring and monitoring of delivery plans, innovations within mobile technology, incorporating artificial intelligence, using biomarkers such as an indicator of cardiovascular risk can be used in addition to the routinely used self-report questionnaires.

TECHNOLOGY IN SM

Increasingly apps are being used to facilitate self-management to improve health outcomes for patients. Patients with neurological diseases commonly use emails, social media, and search engines for health resources. They suggest that the use of apps helps them take control of health through monitoring their health, disease progression and impairments (Winberg et al., 2021). Patients with CNCs used Apps to monitor life-style factors such as food, medication, exercise and sleep. The Apps helped them through feedback when they worked towards their goals. Contrarily, sometimes the feedback from Apps could be demotivating for patients and may not be disease specific (Winberg et al., 2021). Generally, Apps need to be less complicated to use, and App makers should ensure that the Apps were trustworthy, safe and relevant to users. Currently not many Apps have been developed collaboratively with health professionals, despite their potential to help communicate and share health information with patients.

OUTCOME MEASURES

The most commonly used measures to assess self-management are Patient Activation Measure (PAM), the Partners in Health scale (PIH), and the Self-efficacy for Managing Chronic Disease scale (SEMCD). These three measures are used commonly in clinical practice and research and are based on the social cognitive theory (Kephart et al., 2019).

The PAM measures the factors required for a patient to be activated for self-management such as the knowledge, skills, beliefs, and behaviours to manage a chronic condition. It has an interval level scale based on difficulty, for 13 items in the shorter version and has been shown to be a reliable and valid scale (Hibbard et al., 2005).

The PIH can be used to measure patient's self-management knowledge, skills, and ability along with impact of the chronic condition on physical activities, emotions, social life, and patient's empowerment. Twelve items are scored from 0-8 and produce a single score (Battersby et al., 2003).

The SEMCD scale is a unidimensional measure consisting of six items designed to assess an individual's confidence in managing various aspects of chronic disease (Lorig et al., 1989). The items are adapted from the original Self-Efficacy to Manage Symptoms and Self-Efficacy to Manage Disease scales developed by Lorig et al. (1989). The SEMCD focuses on a person's perceived ability to handle symptoms, health problems, and disease-related tasks, making it a widely used tool in chronic condition self-management research.

These scales are composite scales of self-management, with each scale summarising different dimensions of self-management. In patients with chronic neurological conditions these common measures were found to not have structural validity. The best fit for a measurement model was found to be with the SEMCD (Kephart et al., 2019). However, disease specific multidimensional scales that capture the complexity of self-management interventions are required.

PROGRESSIVE NEUROLOGICAL CONDITIONS

The SMS strategies from literature for various neurological conditions will be discussed briefly in the following sections. This discussion has been grouped under progressive and non-progressive conditions even though there are similarities for both groups in SMS for management of symptoms and complications; however, differences in delivery could arise considering rate of progression in conditions and around options for secondary prevention.

Progressive neurological conditions (PNCs) refer to disorders marked by the gradual deterioration of the central or peripheral nervous system, leading to cumulative impairments in motor, cognitive, emotional, and functional domains (Anestis et al., 2020). Common examples include multiple sclerosis (MS), Parkinson's disease (PD), and motor neurone disease (MND), which together significantly reduce quality of life and independence over time. Empirical evidence supports the effectiveness of self-management strategies and task-oriented training in enhancing motor and cognitive outcomes, particularly when systematically embedded into rehabilitation regimens (Clare et al., 2019; Tickle-Degnen et al., 2010). Ultimately, personalised, sustained rehabilitation is essential to mitigate decline, foster adaptation, and support long-term well-being among individuals with PNCs.

Multiple Sclerosis (MS) and Parkinson's Disease

MS is a chronic progressive, immune-mediated disorder of the central nervous system characterised by inflammation, demyelination, and subsequent neurodegeneration. It leads to a wide range of neurological symptoms, including motor weakness, sensory disturbances, fatigue, and cognitive impairment, which often fluctuate over time (Dobson and Giovannoni, 2019). MS typically starts between the ages of 20–40 years; women are affected twice more than men and is a leading cause of non-traumatic disability in this population.

Parkinson's disease (PD) is a progressive neurodegenerative disorder primarily affecting the dopaminergic neurons in the substantia nigra region of the brain. It is clinically characterised by motor symptoms such as bradykinesia, resting tremor, rigidity, and postural instability, as well as a variety of non-motor symptoms including cognitive decline, mood disorders, and autonomic dysfunction (Kalia et al., 2015). PD predominantly affects adults older than 50 years but can be seen in younger adults less frequently. PD significantly impacts quality of life as the disease advances.

Preparation for SMS

As a first, step patients need to be self-motivated to join programmes that are slightly longer and have multiple interventions. This readiness for change should be assessed before enrolling to SMS. Personalised input for a patient from various MDT members along with customised information leaflet about condition should be shared. Educational packages even from the point of diagnosis have been found to improve well-being in patients with MS (Rakhshani et al., 2024).

Interventions for SMS

Motivational interviewing and goal-setting could be used to motivate and determine next steps in SMS. Action plans including condition specific exercise programmes, medication adherence, smoking and alcohol reduction, fatigue, stress, pain and cognitive management could be part of

home-based SMS interventions (Rae-Grant et al., 2011). Exercise programmes involving dexterity, functional activities, use of visual and auditory cues, and arts and craft making have been tried as a part of home-based SMS (Taylor et al., 2014).

Other than the above home-based programme, a **professionally guided self-care programme** using an information booklet to discuss self-care based on client priorities showed improvement in mental health and independence in daily activities (Taylor et al., 2014). Workshop sessions discussing stress, time management, social support, relationships, and physical care have been shown to reduce perceived stress and improved mental health in patients with PNCs (Rae-Grant et al., 2011).

In a **community-based programme,** weekly sessions led by lay tutors who led discussion around exercise, pain, fatigue, relaxation, depression, nutrition, communication, and SMART goal-setting improved self-efficacy, physical functioning, and better self-management skills (Taylor et al., 2014). Everyday self-care decision making around managing urinary incontinence and cognitive training are some other interventions that have been included in SMS for people with MS (Rae-Grant et al., 2011). Additionally, information about self-help organisations has been found to be useful for these patients (Rakhshani et al., 2024).

Mode of Delivery

Intensive outpatient programmes, home-based exercises, and community-based led by lay persons, and internet-based programmes have been delivered (Taylor et al., 2014). The programmes could be in a group or individualistic using online and telephone support. An eight-week class with bimonthly telephone follow-up for three months focusses on education, skills for goal setting and achieving them, improved overall health behaviours, self-efficacy, mental health, and pain scales (Rae-Grant et al., 2011). Telephone counselling and encouragement for health promotion over 12 weeks resulted in self-reported health promotion activities such as physical activity, spiritual growth, and stress management (Grady and Gough, 2014).

Follow-Up

Relevant contact information should be given once SMS has been set up. Fortnightly, follow-up should be in place to reinforce information and action plan. Once a month, follow-up on the phone has been shown to reduce falls in patients with PD (Tickle-Degnen et al., 2010).

NON-PROGRESSIVE NEUROLOGICAL CONDITIONS

Stroke

Stroke is a sudden-onset neurological condition caused by an interruption of blood supply to the brain, either due to a blockage (ischaemic stroke) or bleed (haemorrhagic stroke), leading to rapid loss of brain function. It results in a wide range of physical, cognitive, and emotional impairments depending on the location and extent of brain damage (Plow et al., 2016). Stroke is a leading cause of adult disability worldwide, with the majority of cases occurring in individuals over 60 years of age, although it can affect younger adults as well. SMS has shown the potential to improve the quality of life for people with chronic conditions like stroke and is considered to work in parallel with the Early Support Discharge programmes (Pearce et al., 2015).

Preparation

Patient education and reflection about their conditions should be the first step. Stroke specific education and increasing patients' understanding of their condition and challenges can improve their feelings of personal confidence and empowerment, especially when provided with peer support (Roman, 2008). Education also enables skills to proactively problem-solve. Information provision, particularly when provided in a way that actively involves patients and carers, has beneficial effects on mood and QoL (Taylor et al., 2014).

Interventions

Goals for the patient's self-management can be set and actions can be planned collaboratively with their therapists based on what is important to the patient (Lenzen et al., 2017). For successful formation of goals and action plans, it might be useful for therapists to start with an exploration of patients' beliefs and values so they can consider them in the process (Bodenheimer et al.,2002, 2). Also, it is important to develop goals that are SMART (specific, measurable, achievable, realistic, and time-framed) as they can provide a powerful plan for SMS post-stroke (Bovend'Eerdt et al., 2009; Rehman et al., 2014). Goal-setting skills enable autonomy, control and empowerment which are vital for self-management. Setting goals and following up on the extent to which the goals are achieved is the next step in SMS.

The interventions that have been used and tested in people with stroke are problem-solving skills, decision making, remediation training; support with adaptive equipment and ADL training (Taylor et al., 2014). Problem-solving interventions facilitated survivors' reintegration into their communities (Parke et al., 2015). In addition, proactive self-monitoring and encouraging people to monitor their symptoms and know when to take appropriate action and follow-up have been used in SMS for patients with stroke.

If self-management can be supplementary to therapy at all stages of rehabilitation rather than leaving it till the community phase, that can help in increasing the volume and intensity of training even in the acute phase. Further, SM initiated in the early stages of recovery and rehabilitation improved basic and extended activities of daily living (Parke et al., 2015) and helps to prepare patients for transition to the community.

Mode of Delivery

Most often SMS was carried out at home and sometimes in outpatient facilities. Technologies such as telerehabilitation, smartphones, videoconferencing, and online resources can be used as useful tools that implementation of SM programmes for survivors who live away from the areas of services or cannot physically attend their sessions (Sahely et al., 2024).

Opportunities to share and learn from other service users should be built within the SMS programmes (de Silva, 2011). SM interventions delivered in groups in the community can be more effective in reducing the feeling of isolation felt by survivors and increasing their self-efficacy as it allows them to share and exchange experiences and coping strategies with other stroke survivors (Pearce et al., 2015; Warner et al., 2015).

Stroke liaison workers have provided multifaceted services including social support, liaison with other services, education, and information provision within SMS. Often OTs also play a key role in delivering SMS. SM interventions can lead to better outcomes if carers are involved in the process to help stroke survivors in improving their SM skills (Kalra et al., 2004)

Follow-Up

Though SMS skills include self-monitoring, having a point of contact has been found to be helpful for patients living with stroke in the community. Follow-up can be done using apps, e-health, telerehabilitation, and other online services to have continuity in care through contact with their therapists remotely (Laver et al., 2020; Simpson et al., 2018).

SMS Outcomes in People with Stroke

SMS has also been shown to play a role in reducing the length of stay in hospitals and other poor outcomes such as death and patient dependence (Lorig et al., 1999; Parke et al., 2015). Interventions in both studies had applied patient education, self-monitoring, and personalised care plans in managing chronic diseases and improving patient outcomes. For example, a systematic review of the studies that examined the effectiveness of SMS programmes for stroke rehabilitation has confirmed the positive role of SM in improving function and participatory outcomes in several contexts (Warner et al., 2015). Likewise, the findings of Lennon et al. review (2013) confirmed the positive outcomes of SM programmes on measures of disability, confidence in recovery, the stroke-specific quality of life, and the physical component scale of the short form (SF-36) score.

Models for SMS in Stroke

There are two examples of SMS following stroke evidenced in the literature:

1. The BRIDGES programme, which was delivered for the patients in the community to increase their SM skills (McKenna et al., 2015). BRIDGES is a six-week community-based self-management programme designed to help stroke survivors take control of their recovery. It supports participants in setting personalised goals, developing problem-solving skills, and building confidence to manage the challenges of daily life after stroke. The programme encourages collaboration with healthcare professionals and peers, empowering individuals to actively engage in their recovery and improve their independence and quality of life. Feasibility for implementation in practice is limited due to the costs of training therapists and the programme lacked some of the self-efficacy principles such as peer-support and vicarious experiences.
2. The Re-Train programme, focusing on mobility in the community following a stroke, was found to be feasible to integrate into community rehabilitation (Dean et al., 2018). The programme includes a group exercise programme for people recovering from a stroke that helps them take control of their own recovery. It combines practical physical exercises with self-management skills like goal-setting, problem-solving, and building confidence to stay active and independent long-term. The programme supports ongoing recovery and encourages participants to manage their health in everyday life after formal rehabilitation ends. However, it was criticised for using a high number of supervised therapy sessions and lack of clarity about the theoretical construct that underpinned the SM intervention.

SMS Intervention to Help Stroke Survivors' Mobility Training in the Community

Work was undertaken to develop a self-management intervention that focused on mobility training in the community (SIMS). The SIMS was developed based on evidence from a systematic review of the literature about self-management for mobility rehabilitation following stroke (Sahely et al., 2022) and in consultation with senior stroke survivors and NHS clinicians as an effort for knowledge translation into practice (Sahely et al., 2024). The mobility outcomes that showed improvement in descriptive analysis were functional mobility, walking ability (speed, distance, and endurance), and an increase in number of steps per day (Sahely et al., 2024). The various stages of this programme were set up over a period of 12 weeks.

Preparation:
Week 1:

- Education about impact of stroke, improving gait, self-management and safety and a baseline assessment for groups.

Intervention:
Week 1:

- Self-management strategies were set up for individuals including goal-setting for mobility goals in the first meeting followed by action-planning using exercises from a booklet with a selection of appropriate exercises for strengthening, balance and endurance training.
- A leaflet on how to do exercises at home safely on zoom was provided prior to the start of group exercise classes.

- Patient were taught home exercises using the same exercise booklets and given a recording diary for self-monitoring adherence and an activity log.

Week 2, 4, 6, 8, and 10 (in Groups)

- One group session per week for 10–12 people where participants were taught exercises for strengthening, balance, and mobility from the exercise booklets. They did this as a group in their homes but watched by therapists from a room with zoom conferencing facilities.
- To improve safety in zoom classes, a junior therapist and a senior therapist were both present to deliver the classes.
- An online meeting was held every two weeks where peer support was provided by an experienced stroke patient.
- At week 12, a reiteration of safety, review of mobility-training and positive reinforcement was discussed with each participant for long-term sustainability.

Mode of delivery:

Interventions such as goal-setting and action planning were delivered in their homes when they were visited by the research team and education through online zoom meetings over a period of 12 weeks.

Follow-up:

Week 3, 5, 7, 9, and 11:

A follow-up call was made by the therapist to each individual for reviewing goals, updating exercise plan and reviewing patient's progress in the programme every fortnight. Self-monitoring was done by participants using a pedometer and a recording diary to record their daily training and number of steps.

Challenges for delivering SIMS:

- Lack of technology or limited knowledge to use zoom.
- The COVID protocols limited face to face contact with patients.
- Stress and confusion that stroke survivors and their families experienced at the time of discharge from acute care due to lack of smooth transition to community.

Spinal Cord Injury (SCI)

Spinal cord injury (SCI) leads to sensory, motor and autonomic dysfunctions that can affect multiple systems and as a chronic neurological condition presents with secondary complications such as fractures, spasticity, ulcers, urinary tract infection, bowel problems, and depression (Ahuja et al., 2017). SMS could help to reduce the negative impact of these complications on the quality of life, mental health, independence, and productivity of the person (Munce et al., 2014). Psychological benefits include an improved positive outlook, acceptance of situation, and perception of control.

Preparation

Preparation for SMS programmes for SCI patient should include information sharing about complications, risks prevention, social support, and management for complications.

Intervention

In patients with spinal cord injuries self-management can be facilitated through support given by caregivers for activities of daily living, support for basic functions, monitoring and management of complications (Munce et al., 2014). Caregivers also seem to support self-management through encouragement and advocacy. Caregivers are taught these SMS skills; however, ageing and physical fatigue challenges the support offered by them.

Peer support seemed to help reduce fears, share experiences, and should be arranged at the time when the person is ready to access peer support after injury.

Epilepsy and Migraine

Epilepsy

Epilepsy is a chronic neurological disorder characterised by recurrent, unprovoked seizures resulting from abnormal electrical activity in the brain. The condition presents with a wide spectrum of seizure types and associated symptoms, which may include motor disturbances, altered awareness, and sensory changes (Fisher et al., 2014). Epilepsy can develop at any age, with peaks in early childhood and older adulthood. It often affects quality of life due to the unpredictability of seizures and associated psychosocial impacts, including stigma, anxiety, and reduced independence.

Self-management education and strategies to improve adherence to drug treatment for epilepsy include education about the effects of drugs, intensive patient reminders for appointments and prescription refills and a discussion group involving mothers. Further, to improve adherence to medication, patients were asked to complete a worksheet linking their intention to take drugs to a routine daily activity, indicating time and place. Cognitive behavioural therapy (CBT) has been shown to be effective in reducing dysphoria and depression, self-reported anxiety, stress and anger. Support offered by specialist nurses to people with epilepsy showed improved quality of life (Bradley et al., 1996).

Migraine

Migraines presenting with headaches lasting more than three months or episodic migraines can affect relationships, work, financial, and general health (Buse et al., 2019). Despite drug treatment, many people continue to suffer with migraine and may require self-management strategies, such as the psychological therapies to prevent migraine (Sharpe et al., 2019). Behavioural changes that include sleep modification and CBT for insomnia, psychological education around migraine combined with mindfulness over six weeks and mindfulness-based CBT for ten weeks have been shown to reduce frequency of headache or reduction in head ache days, headache related disability, severity of symptoms and improve migraine related quality of life. Consumption of medication for headaches could also reduce with psychological and educational therapies (Hailston et al., 2025).

Fatigue in Neurological Conditions

Up to 95% of people with chronic neurological conditions report having secondary fatigue with physical, cognitive and psycho-social effects (Ghahari and Packer, 2012). Fatigue in neurological conditions is not easily relieved and worsens over a day. Memory, attention, and information processing is affected due to fatigue in these patients. Apathy and reduced participation in activities of daily living can occur.

Self-management for fatigue involved a six-week course (seven weeks online). It included activities and discussion around rest, body mechanics, rearranging activity stations, prioritising, and balancing a schedule (Ghahari and Packer, 2012). A trained facilitator with knowledge of self-efficacy and self-management theory checked in online (for the online programme) with patients daily to answer queries and encouraged patients to continue self-management. Previous programme participants were involved to share experiences and support patients to facilitate behaviour change. The physical aspects of fatigue and personal wellbeing index were improved following the use of this self-management programme online (Ghahari and Packer, 2012).

Remote Delivery of SMS

In-person self-management rehabilitation requires resources that are costly and have pragmatic challenges such as geographical and financial barriers. However, following COVID, telehealth and remote rehabilitation have been resourceful for better access to digital self-management interventions that are effective in improving depression, anxiety, fatigue and self-efficacy among people with neurological disorders (Lau et al., 2022). It has been proposed that SMS interventions modulate the self-regulatory mechanisms and change maladaptive thoughts that are disrupted in neuropsychiatric illnesses (Lau et al., 2022).

SM interventions can be started in the hospitals settings and continued using remote technology for monitoring, supervision and updating the programme based on the fluid needs of the patient (Lau et al., 2022). Wearable sensors linked to smart phones and blue tooth devices are being used in stroke patients for remote SMS (Lau et al., 2022).

CBT-based digital interventions yielded larger effects in improving depression, anxiety, fatigue, and self-efficacy. CBT focuses on changing negative and self-destructive thoughts and teaches skills to enhance motivation and willpower, reliance on memory (Lau et al., 2022; Plow et al., 2016). Problem solving, goal-setting, exercise, and education are the key elements of CBT-based digital interventions that can include online education on disease-specific information, self-assessment of symptoms, self-reporting of activities, and web conferencing (Lau et al., 2022).

Strategies to Consider for Implementation of SMS

1. SMS should be developed collaboratively with the professionals. Theoretically, combining more strategies in one intervention is seen to be more effective in improving recovery outcomes (Parke et al., 2015).
2. Providers must decide the aims and feasibility of integration of SMS into routine practice. SMS should be integrated to formal therapy plans not as a separate intervention (Boger et al., 2015; Rudd et al., 2016; Sahely et al., 2023).
3. Introduction and endorsement of SMS programme should be routinely carried out by authorities such as the consultant or rehabilitation lead even when patients are still in the hospital or during a general physician visit.
4. Successful integration of SMS by health professionals would require professionals to be trained in general person-centred skills, behaviour change skills, organisational knowledge, and time management skills.
5. Competencies related to use of SMS strategies, protocols and interventions are required (Jaglal et al., 2014). Professionals need to be trained in skills for group facilitation, problem solving, and goal-setting during their education or as CPD as they report lack of training.
6. Involvement of the family and carers would enable patients to set realistic goals relevant to the patient, to manage challenges at home, and for reintegration in the community after discharge from hospital (Lawler et al., 2019; Warner et al., 2015). A clear description of a carer role in the SMS process has been suggested to facilitate patient's independence and avoid extra support from family/carers that might limit patient's skills for SM (Satink et al., 2018).
7. Patients suggest offering services very early in the rehabilitation process, to improve knowledge of progression of the condition, coping strategies and support services for physical, social and psychological aspects from the very beginning. However, readiness for SMS should be assessed individually.
8. A key identified person such as a community neurological nurse with a specialist knowledge of neurological conditions (Kirton et al., 2012) or an occupational therapist at the point of discharge should be identified. This key person provides continuity, acts as a link between the hospital, the family, and the community to identify, advocate and support with referrals.
9. Safety assurance is very important for the delivery of any SMS intervention, especially when there is minimal supervision of formal therapists. This warrants a home visit to assess patients in the environment in which they will carry out their SM training (Mayo, 2016)

10. Some eligible patients for SM might be reluctant to participate in SM programmes because of conceptual misunderstanding of SM concept (Sadler et al., 2017). For these patients, patient education is an essential step to increase their awareness and knowledge in preparation for SM prior to discharge from hospital or outpatient services.
11. Patients' competence to engage in remote rehabilitation using technology should be assessed prior to delivering self-management technology. Future clinical practice should consider the digital divide and improve opportunities for Information Technology education.

CONCLUSION

This chapter has shown that self-management support is a practical, adaptable tool for managing chronic neurological conditions. By outlining specific elements from targeted education to collaborative goal-setting and patient's engagement in care delivery, we have provided a clear framework for their use in diverse clinical and community settings. This shift from a purely medical model to one that empowers patients to take an active role in their care is crucial for improving long-term outcomes and enhancing their quality of life. The path forward, as we have seen, will require a concerted effort from researchers and healthcare professionals to fully integrate these practices into standard care protocols.

REFERENCES

Ahmed, S., Heaven, A., Lawton, R., Rawlings, G., Sloan, C., & Clegg, A. (2021). Behaviour change techniques in personalised care planning for older people: A systematic review. British Journal of General Practice, 71(703), e121–e127. https://doi.org/10.3399/bjgp20X714017

Ahuja, C. S., Wilson, J. R., Nori, S., Kotter, M. R. N., Druschel, C., Curt, A., & Fehlings, M. G. (2017). Traumatic spinal cord injury. Nature Reviews Disease Primers, 3, 17018. https://doi.org/10.1038/nrdp.2017.18

Anestis, E., Eccles, F., Fletcher, I., French, M., & Simpson, J. (2020). Giving and receiving a diagnosis of a progressive neurological condition: A scoping review of doctors' and patients' perspectives. Patient Education and Counseling, 103(9), 1709–1723.

Barr, V., Robinson, S., Marin-Link, B., Underhill, L., Dotts, A., Ravensdale, D., & Salivaras, S. (2003). The expanded chronic care model. Hospital Quarterly, 7(1), 73–82.

Battersby, M. W., Ask, A., Reece, M. M., Markwick, M. J., & Collins, J. P. (2003). The partners in health scale: The development and psychometric properties of a generic assessment scale for chronic condition self-management. Australian Journal of Primary Health, 9(3), 41–52.

Bodenheimer, T., Lorig, K., Holman, H., &Grumbach, K. (2002). Patient self-management of chronic disease in primary care. JAMA, 288(19), 2469–2475. https://doi.org/10.1001/jama.288.19.2469

Boger, E. J., Demain, S. H., & Latter, S. M. (2015). Stroke self-management: A focus group study to identify the factors influencing self-management following stroke. International Journal of Nursing Studies, 52(1), 175–187.

Bovend'Eerdt, T. J. H., Botell, R. E., & Wade, D. T. (2009). Writing SMART rehabilitation goals and achieving goal attainment scaling: A practical guide. Clinical Rehabilitation, 23(4), 352–361.

Bradley, P., & Lindsay, B. (2001). Specialist epilepsy nurses for treating epilepsy. Cochrane Database of Systematic Reviews, (4), CD001907. https://doi.org/10.1002/14651858.CD001907. Update in: Cochrane Database Syst Rev. 2008 Jan 23;(1):CD001907.

Buse, D. C., Murray, S., Dumas, P. K., Adams, A. M., Reed, M. L., Fanning, K. M., & Lipton, R. B. (2019). Life with migraine, effect on relationships, career and finances, and overall health and well-being: Results of the chronic migraine epidemiology and outcomes (CaMEO) study (S59. 002). Neurology, 92(15_supplement), S59–002.

Clare, L., Teale, J. C., Toms, G., Kudlicka, A., Evans, I., Abrahams, S., & Thompson-Coon, J. (2019). Cognitive rehabilitation, self-management, psychotherapeutic and caregiver support interventions in progressive neurodegenerative conditions: A scoping review. NeuroRehabilitation, 43(4), 443–471.

Corbin, J. M., & Strauss, A. (1988). Unending Work and Care: Managing Chronic Illness at Home. Jossey-Bass.

Coulter, A., & Ellins, J. (2006). Patient-Focused Interventions: A Review of the Evidence. Health Foundation London.

Davies, F., Wood, F., Bullock, A., Wallace, C., & Edwards, A. (2017). Interventions to improve the self-management support health professionals provide for people with progressive neurological conditions: Protocol for a realist synthesis. BMJ Open, 7(3), e014575. https://doi.org/10.1136/bmjopen-2016-014575

Dean, S. G., Poltawski, L., Forster, A., Taylor, R. S., Spencer, A., James, M., & Calitri, R. (2018). Community-based rehabilitation training after stroke: Results of a pilot randomised controlled trial (ReTrain) investigating acceptability and feasibility. BMJ Open, 8(2), e018409.

de Silva, D. (2011). Helping People Help Themselves: A Review of the Evidence Considering Whether It Is Worthwhile to Support Self-Management. Health Foundation.

Devittori, G., Akeddar, M., Retevoi, A., Schneider, F., Cvetkova, V., Dinacci, D., & Lambercy, O. (2024). Towards RehabCoach: Design and preliminary evaluation of a conversational agent supporting unsupervised therapy after stroke. In: 2024 10th IEEE RAS/EMBS International Conference for Biomedical Robotics and Biomechatronics (BioRob) (pp. 569–574). IEEE.

Dobkin, B. H. (2016). Behavioral self-management strategies for practice and exercise should be included in neurologic rehabilitation trials and care. Current Opinion in Neurology, 29(6), 693–699.

Dobson, R., & Giovannoni, G. (2019). Multiple sclerosis–a review. European Journal of Neurology, 26(1), 27–40.

Fakolade, A., Walters, A. J., Cameron, J., Latimer-Cheung, A. E., & Pilutti, L. A. (2020). Healthy together: A systematic review of theory and techniques used in health interventions for persons with chronic neurological conditions and their caregivers. Patient Education and Counseling, 103(4), 788–803.

Fanning, J., Mullen, S. P., & McAuley, E. (2012). Increasing physical activity with mobile devices: A meta-analysis. Journal of Medical Internet Research, 14(6), e2171.

Fisher, R. S., Acevedo, C., Arzimanoglou, A., Bogacz, A., Cross, J. H., Elger, C. E., & Wiebe, S. (2014). ILAE official report: A practical clinical definition of epilepsy. Epilepsia, 55(4), 475–482.

Free, C., Phillips, G., Galli, L., Watson, L., Felix, L., Edwards, P., & Haines, A. (2013). The effectiveness of mobile-health technology-based health behaviour change or disease management interventions for health care consumers: A systematic review. PLoS Medicine, 10(1), e1001362.

Ghahari, S., & Packer, T. (2012). Effectiveness of online and face-to-face fatigue self-management programmes for adults with neurological conditions. Disability and Rehabilitation, 34(7), 564–573.

Grady, P. A., & Gough, L. L. (2014). Self-management: A comprehensive approach to management of chronic conditions. American Journal of Public Health, 104(8), e25–e31. https://doi.org/10.2105/AJPH.2014.302041

Hailston, A., Davies, N., Ratna, M. B., Matharu, M., & Underwood, M. (2025). The effectiveness of educational, behavioural, and cognitive self-management support interventions for chronic migraine: A systematic review. Primary Health Care Research & Development, 26, e98.

Hibbard, J. H., Mahoney, E. R., Stockard, J., & Tusler, M. (2005). Development and testing of a short form of the patient activation measure. Health Services Research, 40(6p1), 1918–1930.

Hinder, S., & Greenhalgh, T. (2012). "This does my head in". Ethnographic study of self-management by people with diabetes. BMC Health Services Research, 12(1), 83.

Jaglal, S. B., Guilcher, S. J., Bereket, T., Kwan, M., Munce, S., Conklin, J., & Riopelle, R. (2014). Development of a chronic care model for neurological conditions (CCM-NC). BMC Health Services Research, 14(1), 409.

Kalia, L. V., Lang, A. E., Hazrati, L. N., Fujioka, S., Wszolek, Z. K., Dickson, D. W., & Marras, C. (2015). Clinical correlations with Lewy body pathology in LRRK2-related Parkinson disease. JAMA Neurology, 72(1), 100–105.

Kalra, L., Evans, A., Perez, I., Melbourn, A., Patel, A., Knapp, M., & Donaldson, N. (2004). Training carers of stroke patients: Randomised controlled trial. BMJ, 328(7448), 1099.

Kephart, G., Packer, T. L., Audulv, Å, & Warner, G. (2019). The structural and convergent validity of three commonly used measures of self-management in persons with neurological conditions. Quality of Life Research, 28(2), 545–556.

Kılınç, S., Erdem, H., Healey, R., & Cole, J. (2022). Finding meaning and purpose: A framework for the self-management of neurological conditions. Disability and Rehabilitation, 44(2), 219–230. https://doi.org/10.1080/09638288.2020.1764115. Epub 2020 May 14.

Kirton, J. A., Jack, B. A., O'Brien, M. R., & Roe, B. (2012). Care of patients with neurological conditions: The impact of a generic neurology nursing service development on patients and their carers. Journal of Clinical Nursing, 21(1–2), 207–215.

Kreuter, M., Farrell, D., Olevitch, L., Brennan, L., & Rimer, B. K. (2013). Tailoring Health Messages: Customizing Communication with Computer Technology. Taylor and Francis. https://doi.org/10.4324/9781315045382

Lau, S. C., Bhattacharjya, S., Fong, M. W., Nicol, G. E., Lenze, E. J., Baum, C., Hardi, A., & Wong, A. W. (2022). Effectiveness of theory-based digital self-management interventions for improving depression, anxiety, fatigue and self-efficacy in people with neurological disorders: A systematic review and meta-analysis. Journal of Telemedicine and Telecare, 28(8), 547–558. https://doi.org/10.1177/1357633X20955122

Laver, K., Halbert, J., Stewart, M., & Crotty, M. (2010). Patient readiness and ability to set recovery goals during the first 6 months after stroke. Journal of Allied Health, 39(4), 149E–154E.

Laver, K. E., Adey-Wakeling, Z., Crotty, M., Lannin, N. A., George, S., & Sherrington, C. (2020). Telerehabilitation services for stroke. Cochrane Database of Systematic Reviews, 1(1), CD01025.

Lennon, S., McKenna, S., & Jones, F. (2013). Self-management programmes for people post stroke: A systematic review. Clinical Rehabilitation, 27(10), 867–878.

Lenzen, S. A., Daniëls, R., van Bokhoven, M. A., van der Weijden, T., & Beurskens, A. (2017). Disentangling self-management goal setting and action planning: A scoping review. PloS One, 12(11), e0188822.

Lorig, K., Chastain, R. L., Ung, E., Shoor, S., & Holman, H. R. (1989). Development and evaluation of a scale to measure perceived self-efficacy in people with arthritis. Arthritis & Rheumatism: Official Journal of the American College of Rheumatology, 32(1), 37–44.

Lorig, K. R., Sobel, D. S., Stewart, A. L., Brown, B. W. Jr, Bandura, A., Ritter, P., & Holman, H. R. (1999). Evidence suggesting that a chronic disease self-management program can improve health status while reducing hospitalization: A randomized trial. Medical Care, 37(1), 5–14.

Mayo, N. E. (2016). Stroke rehabilitation at home: Lessons learned and ways forward. Stroke, 47(6), 1685–1691.

McKenna, S., Jones, F., Glenfield, P., & Lennon, S. (2015). Bridges self-management program for people with stroke in the community: A feasibility randomized controlled trial. International Journal of Stroke, 10(5), 697–704.

Munce, S. E., Webster, F., Fehlings, M. G., Straus, S. E., Jang, E., & Jaglal, S. B. (2014). Perceived facilitators and barriers to self-management in individuals with traumatic spinal cord injury: A qualitative descriptive study. BMC Neurology, 14(1), 48.

Newman, S., Steed, L., & Mulligan, K. (2004). Self-management interventions for chronic illness. The Lancet, 364(9444), 1523–1537.

Parke, H. L., Epiphaniou, E., Pearce, G., Taylor, S. J., Sheikh, A., Griffiths, C. J., & Pinnock, H. (2015). Self-management support interventions for stroke survivors: A systematic meta-review. PLoS One, 10(7), e0131448.

Pearce, G., Pinnock, H., Epiphaniou, E., Parke, H. L., Heavey, E., Griffiths, C. J., & Taylor, S. J. (2015). Experiences of self-management support following a stroke: A meta-review of qualitative systematic reviews. PLoS One, 10(12), e0141803.

Piccoli, A., Rossettini, G., Cecchetto, S., Viceconti, A., Ristori, D., Turolla, A., & Testa, M. (2018). Effect of attentional focus instructions on motor learning and performance of patients with central nervous system and musculoskeletal disorders: A systematic review. Journal of Functional Morphology and Kinesiology, 3(3), 40.

Plow, M., Mangal, S., Geither, K., & Golding, M. (2016). A scoping review of tailored self-management interventions among adults with mobility impairing neurological and musculoskeletal conditions. Frontiers in Public Health, 4, 165.

Pugh, J. D., Williams, A. M., Bentley, B., Pienaar, C. A., McCoy, K., & Monterosso, L. (2019). Neurological patients' and caregivers' post-discharge challenges explored in a world café. Collegian, 26(5), 528–533.

Rae-Grant, A. D., Turner, A. P., Sloan, A., Miller, D., Hunziker, J., & Haselkorn, J. K. (2011). Self-management in neurological disorders: Systematic review of the literature and potential interventions in multiple sclerosis care. Journal of Rehabilitation Research & Development, 48(9), 1087–1100.

Rakhshani, T., Afroozeh, S., Kashfi, S. M., Kamyab, A., & Khani Jeihooni, A. (2024). The effect of education of self-care behaviors on the quality of life and resilience of multiple sclerosis patients. BMC Neurology, 24(1), 264.

Rehman, A., Berry, J., & Siddiqui, M. A. (2014). Post stroke rehabilitation based on SMART goals: A case study. Journal of Experimental and Integrative Medicine, 4(1), 71.

Roman, M. W. (2008). Lessons learned from a school for stroke recovery. Topics in Stroke Rehabilitation, 15(1), 59–71.

Rudd, T., Browen, A., James, M., & Kilbride, C., & National Clinical Guideline Centre. (2016). National Clinical Guideline for Stroke: Prepared by the Intercollegiate Stroke Working Party (5th ed.). Royal College of Physicians.

Sadler, E., Wolfe, C. D., Jones, F., & McKevitt, C. (2017). Exploring stroke survivors' and physiotherapists' views of self-management after stroke: A qualitative study in the UK. BMJ Open, 7(3), e011631.

Sahely, A., Giles, D., Sintler, C., Soundy, A., & Rosewilliam, S. (2023). Self-management interventions to improve mobility after stroke: An integrative review. Disability and Rehabilitation, 45(1), 9–26. https://doi.org/10.1080/09638288.2022.2028019. Epub 2022 Jan 22.

Sahely, A., Sintler, C., Soundy, A., & Rosewilliam, S. (2024). Feasibility of a self-management intervention to improve mobility in the community after stroke (SIMS): A mixed-methods pilot study. PLoS One, 19(8), e0286611.

Satink, T., et al. (2015). Self-management: Challenges for allied healthcare professionals in stroke rehabilitation–a focus group study. Disability and Rehabilitation, 37(19), 1745–1752.

Satink, T., Cup, E. H., de Swart, B. J., & Nijhuis-van der Sanden, M. W. (2018). The perspectives of spouses of stroke survivors on self-management–a focus group study. Disability and Rehabilitation, 40(2), 176–184.

Sharpe, L., Dudeney, J., de C Williams, A. C., Nicholas, M., McPhee, I., Baillie, A., & McGuire, B. (2019). Psychological therapies for the prevention of migraine in adults. Cochrane Database of Systematic Reviews, 7(7), CD012295.

Simpson, D., Schmidt, M., Bird, M. L., Smith, S., & Callisaya, M. (2018, August). Increasing intensity of practice after stroke using apps, internet and sensors to connect patients and therapists remotely: A feasibility study. International Journal of Stroke, 13, 3. 1 Olivers Yard, 55 City Road, London Ecly 1sp, England: Sage Publications Ltd.

Taylor, S. J., Taylor, S., Pinnock, H., Epiphaniou, E., Pearce, G., Parke, H. L., & Sheikh, A. (2014). A rapid synthesis of the evidence on interventions supporting self-management for people with long-term conditions: PRISMS–Practical systematic review of self-management support for long-term conditions. Health Services and Delivery Research, 2(53), 1–580.

Tickle-Degnen, L., Ellis, T., Saint-Hilaire, M. H., Thomas, C. A., & Wagenaar, R. C. (2010). Self-management rehabilitation and health-related quality of life in Parkinson's disease: A randomized controlled trial. Movement Disorders, 25(2), 194–204. https://doi.org/10.1002/mds.22940

van Hooft, S. M., Been-Dahmen, J. M., Ista, E., van Staa, A., & Boeije, H. R. (2017). A realist review: What do nurse-led self-management interventions achieve for outpatients with a chronic condition? Journal of Advanced Nursing, 73(6), 1255–1271.

Wade, D. T. (2009). Goal setting in rehabilitation: An overview of what, why and how. Clinical Rehabilitation, 23(4), 291–295.

Wade, D. T., & Halligan, P. W. (2017). The biopsychosocial model of illness: A model whose time has come. Clinical Rehabilitation, 31(8), 995–1004.

Ward, C. D., Turpin, G., Dewey, Fleming, S., Hurwitz, B., Ratib, S., von Fragstein, M. & Lymbery, M. (2004). Education for people with progressive neurological conditions can have negative effects: Evidence from a randomized controlled trial. Clinical Rehabilitation, 18(7), 717–725.

Warner, G., Packer, T., Villeneuve, M., Audulv, A., & Versnel, J. (2015). A systematic review of the effectiveness of stroke self-management programs for improving function and participation outcomes: Self-management programs for stroke survivors. Disability and Rehabilitation, 37(23), 2141–2163. https://doi.org/10.3109/09638288.2014.996674.

Whitehead, L., & Seaton, P. (2016). The effectiveness of self-management mobile phone and tablet apps in long-term condition management: A systematic review. Journal of Medical Internet Research, 18(5), e6009.

Wilkinson, A., & Whitehead, L. (2009 Aug). Evolution of the concept of self-care and implications for nurses: A literature review. The International Journal of Nursing Studies, 46(8), 1143–1147. https://doi.org/10.1016/j.ijnurstu.2008.12.011

Winberg, C., Kylberg, M., Pettersson, C., Harnett, T., Hedvall, P.-O., Mattsson, T., & Månsson Lexell, E. (2021). Feeling controlled or *being in control*? Apps for self-management among older people with neurological disability. Disability and Rehabilitation: Assistive Technology, 16(6), 603–608. https://doi.org/10.1080/17483107.2019.1685017

31 Self-Management for People with Chronic Conditions

Lauren Winterbottom

INTRODUCTION

Self-management refers to activities that individuals engage in to optimize their health and wellbeing when living with a chronic health condition (Pearce et al., 2016). This includes management of medical needs, management of meaningful life roles, and management of emotions related to changes caused by the condition (Lorig & Holman, 2003; Pearce et al., 2016). While self-management is similar to self-care, it is a narrower concept. Self-management involves behaviors related to a specific health condition, whereas self-care refers to activities that individuals engage in to maintain their health and wellbeing in general (Lawless et al., 2021; Pearce et al., 2016). Self-management involves self-regulation, or the ability to control one's behavior and make decisions that positively impact one's health and participation. This involves the way a person perceives and responds to their own behavior (Mol et al., 2022). People with chronic health conditions have identified insight into one's strengths and impairments, coping ability, and active use of strategies to optimize life functioning as important self-regulation abilities (Mol et al., 2022). Self-management is also strongly influenced by the environment, including the physical, social, and cultural factors that impact participation.

Self-management is a dynamic process that involves carrying out goal-directed behaviors to fulfill self-care needs, maintain heath, and participate in meaningful roles for people with chronic health conditions (Lorig & Holman, 2003). Successful performance of these behaviors is influenced by a dynamic interaction between a person's cognitive, psychosocial, and sensorimotor abilities and the environment. Performance is also influenced by a person's motivation or drive to carry out self-management behaviors (Schulman-Green et al., 2016). Development of habits and routines that support self-management is important for acquiring and maintaining healthy behaviors related to personal wellbeing and role expectations (Phillips et al., 2016; Schulman-Green et al., 2016; Stone et al., 2023; Youngson, 2019). As individuals with chronic conditions encounter challenges related to their health or life situation, they often need to adapt their behavior to new conditions, which may involve acquiring new knowledge or skills, developing new habits and routines, and maintaining supportive behaviors even when environmental challenges are encountered (Lorig & Holman, 2003). These changes can place new demands on the individual's underlying capacities, requiring motivation and daily practice to successfully adapt, as well as additional support from the environment (Fisher et al., 2005).

In healthcare and rehabilitation settings, interventions for individuals with chronic health conditions have become increasingly focused on supporting self-management (Dobkin, 2016; Whittaker et al., 2024). Self-management interventions are often focused on enhancing the processes of self-management, so that people with chronic conditions can actively engage in activities that support their health and wellbeing. Self-management processes include taking ownership of one's health and engaging in behaviors to support health condition-related needs, such as medication management, diet, and physical activity (Lorig & Holman, 2003; Schulman-Green et al., 2012). Additionally, actively seeking out support and resources in the healthcare system and community as well as learning how to access reliable information to support informed decision-making are also important for self-management (Lorig & Holman, 2003; Schulman-Green et al., 2012). In rehabilitation settings, self-management can also involve active engagement in activities to improve functional abilities

DOI: 10.1201/9781003599074-34

such as mobility and arm use (Da-Silva, Moore & Price, 2018; Sahely et al., 2023). Other important processes related to living with a chronic illness include emotional processing, adjustment, lifestyle modification, and creating personal meaning in life as changes caused by the condition can have a negative impact on a person's participation in their valued life roles (Schulman-Green et al., 2012). Using strategies such as problem-solving, goal setting, and action planning can help people with chronic conditions navigate these changes and increase successful engagement in self-management activities (Allegrante, Wells & Peterson, 2019; Lorig & Holman, 2003). Providers can help support self-management by forming a partnership with their patients and taking on the role of teacher and coach (Lorig & Holman, 2003; Rethorn, Bezner & Pettitt, 2022). This can help empower people with chronic conditions to make informed choices regarding their care and develop skills that enable successful self-management.

A number of factors can influence engagement in self-management, which are important for providers to consider when implementing self-management interventions. Schulman-Green and colleagues (2016) conducted a metasynthesis of factors that impact self-management of chronic health conditions. These factors include a person's knowledge, beliefs, psychological distress, motivation, and life patterns, such as habits and routines. In addition, a person's health status, their access to resources, the characteristics of their environment, and the support offered by their health care system can all influence self-management (Schulman-Green et al., 2016). Awareness of these factors can help practitioners better identify and address potential barriers for self-management and provide care that addresses individual needs.

THEORIES THAT INFORM SELF-MANAGEMENT INTERVENTIONS

Many theories of behavior and behavior change have been applied to self-management interventions (Davis et al., 2015; Lau et al., 2022; Lawless et al., 2021). These theories help identify the determinants of behavior change as well as the processes through which that change occurs. A few key theories used in self-management interventions are presented here. For a more comprehensive list and analysis, please see work by Hale and colleagues (2020).

Social Cognitive Theory

Albert Bandura's social cognitive theory is one of the most widely used theories for self-management interventions (Lau et al., 2022; Lawless et al., 2021). *Self-efficacy* is a central construct in social cognitive theory and involves a person's beliefs about their ability to meet specific goals (Bandura, 1977, 2004, 1997). This theory suggests that self-efficacy interacts with barriers and facilitators in the environment to influence motivation, behavior, and wellbeing (Bandura, 2004). Social cognitive theory proposes that a person's core beliefs influence their ability to change their behavior and develop healthy habits, as well as their ability to maintain healthy behaviors and recover from relapses. It also acknowledges the importance of the social environment in health promotion and the crucial need for social systems to support healthy behavior change (Bandura, 2004). Bandura identifies the core determinants for health promotion as having adequate *knowledge* of healthy behaviors, having *self-efficacy* to be able to develop and maintain healthy habits, understanding positive and negative consequences of engaging in different behaviors (*outcome expectations*), engaging in individualized *goal setting* and *action planning* to achieve one's goals, and also acknowledging *barriers* and *facilitators* in the social environment that can either inhibit or support behavior change (Bandura, 2004). Social cognitive theory also recognizes the power of collective action to implement broad changes in health promotion, which then supports individual behavior change (Bandura, 2004). Indeed, research has found that the environment has a strong impact on self-management behaviors. For example, people may have difficulty maintaining self-management behaviors after self-management interventions end, and so interventions that are longer in duration and offer continued support are more likely to be effective (Fisher et al., 2005; Norris et al., 2002). Many self-management interventions are based on social cognitive theory. For example, the Stanford Chronic Disease Management Program is a widely implemented intervention for people with chronic conditions and has been used to support self-management with a variety of populations (Franek, 2013; Lorig, 2014; Lorig et al., 1999).

Self-Determination Theory

Self-determination theory, developed by Edward Deci and Richard Ryan, is another influential theory used in self-management interventions (Deci & Ryan, 2008; Lawless et al., 2021; Ng et al., 2012; Ryan & Deci, 2000). The primary proposal of this theory is that all people have a basic psychological need for *competence*, *autonomy*, and *relatedness* to others (Ryan & Deci, 2000). When these needs are supported by the social context, people will have optimal motivation and activity, leading to better psychological, developmental, and behavioral outcomes (Deci & Ryan, 2008; Ryan & Deci, 2000). This theory is focused not only on the *amount* of motivation a person has but also the *type* of motivation. Self-Determination Theory differentiates *autonomous motivation*, or motivation resulting from one's own volition and choice, from *controlled motivation*, or motivation resulting from external pressures and demands. This theory assumes that people have natural desire for success and that creating a social environment at supports autonomous motivation can improve outcomes (Deci & Ryan, 2008). Autonomous motivation has been associated with increased persistence, improved performance, and better psychological wellbeing (Deci & Ryan, 2008). Interventions based on self-determination theory have been used in numerous healthcare contexts (Ng et al., 2012). These interventions have demonstrated improvements in health behaviors, and autonomous motivation has been shown to have a positive association with health behavior change (Ntoumanis et al., 2021).

Capability, Opportunity, Motivation – Behavior (COM-B) Model

The capability, opportunity, motivation – behavior (COM-B) model, developed by Susan Michie and colleagues, aims to explain the mechanisms of behavior so as to support the development of behavior change interventions (Michie, van Stralen & West, 2011). The components of this model include *capability*, *opportunity*, and *motivation*, which interact to produce *behavior. Capability* involves the physical and psychological capacity or skill needed to perform a behavior. *Opportunity* refers to affordances provided by a person's physical and social environment. *Motivation* is broadly defined as all neurologic processes that prompt and direct behavior; these processes can be *reflective*, involving intentional thoughts related to beliefs and planning, or *automatic*, involving emotional or habitual processes related to associative learning (Michie, van Stralen & West, 2011). This model has been used to explain engagement in physical activity and effectiveness of physical activity interventions (Paterson et al., 2024; Webb et al., 2022; Willmott, Pang & Rundle-Thiele, 2021).

SELF-MANAGEMENT INTERVENTIONS

Self-management interventions are designed to support participation in activities needed to manage chronic health conditions in the context of daily life (Lorig & Holman, 2003). In rehabilitation, these interventions generally involve programs that are completed outside of medical appointments or therapy sessions within a person's daily life to elicit engagement in activities that support health, wellbeing, and functioning, and can be administered in both inpatient and outpatient settings (Whittaker et al., 2024, 2025). Self-management interventions are focused on promoting behavior change and encourage people with chronic conditions to play an active role in the management of their condition (Foster et al., 2007; Fryer et al., 2016; Lorig & Holman, 2003; Whittaker et al., 2024). Often, they involve forming a partnership with healthcare providers and emphasize problem solving, goal setting, decision-making, and coping to aid in the management of the condition (Whittaker et al., 2024). Self-management interventions can also focus on skill acquisition to improve daily life function and health management. Please see the Practice Reviews in Self-Management Support (PRISMS) taxonomy for a classification of key intervention components that are used to support self-management behaviors (Pearce et al., 2016).

Behavior Change Techniques and Mechanisms of Action

Behavior change techniques are considered the "active ingredients" of complex interventions that are focused on changing behavior (Marques et al., 2023; Michie et al., 2013). These techniques have been comprehensively classified by the Behavior Change Technique Taxonomy v1 (Michie et al., 2013) and more recently in the Behavior Change Technique Ontology (Marques et al., 2023). These techniques are defined as the smallest components of behavioral interventions and include common strategies such as goal setting, self-monitoring, and social support (Michie et al., 2013). *Mechanisms of action* are the processes through which a behavior change technique is thought to impact behavior. Mechanisms of action influence the effects of an intervention and can be characteristics of the person, such as self-efficacy, or characteristics of the environment, such as the healthcare system (Carey et al., 2019). Mechanisms of action help to explain *why* a given intervention technique may or may not be effective for addressing a specific behavioral goal or outcome. Carey and colleagues (2019) explored the relationship between behavior change techniques and mechanisms of action in behaviors such as physical activity, diet, alcohol use, and smoking. They found that common behavior change techniques included "instruction on how to perform a behavior" and "problem solving," and the most common mechanisms of action were "beliefs about capabilities" and "intention" (Carey et al., 2019). While this work is ongoing, determining the relationships between behavior change techniques and mechanisms of action has the potential to make future self-management interventions more effective and efficient.

Key Considerations for Self-Management Interventions

According to Lorig and Holman (2003), self-management interventions should be client-centered, focusing on a person's individual concerns and problems. Numerous complex interventions have been implemented to support the development of self-management skills and help individuals maintain self-management behaviors. This section identifies key considerations for the development and implementation of self-management interventions.

Enhancing Utilization of Healthcare Resources

Resource utilization is a core self-management skill that involves teaching individuals with chronic conditions how to navigate the healthcare system and seek out information and resources from reliable sources (Lorig & Holman, 2003). The healthcare system can either support or inhibit self-management depending on access and ease of navigating the system. For example, the availability of self-management programs, healthcare specialists, and educational resources can influence self-management in a community (Schulman-Green et al., 2016). Patients may also face challenges when navigating health care systems, including difficulty making appointments and confusing communication from providers, such as conflicting or inconsistent advice (Schulman-Green et al., 2016). Self-management interventions can help to overcome these barriers by providing patients with contact information and easy access to advice regarding the management of their condition (Pearce et al., 2016). Additionally, access to resources such as financial support can also influence self-management. Lack of financial resources, health insurance, and affordable health care can limit self-management due to inability to afford medication, healthy food, and therapies (Lyu et al., 2025;

Schulman-Green et al., 2016). Offering patients information on how to obtain financial support can help them access the resources they need for self-management (Pearce et al., 2016; Schulman-Green et al., 2016).

Creating a Partnership Between Patient and Provider

In order to support self-management for people with chronic conditions, providers can adopt the role of teacher, coach, and partner (Lorig & Holman, 2003; Rethorn, Bezner & Pettitt, 2022). This can help patients feel comfortable reporting their symptoms and experiences and empower them to take an active role in their treatment (Lorig & Holman, 2003). Stroke survivors have reported that barriers in rehabilitation settings such as depersonalized care or lack of time can negatively impact their adherence to self-directed practice outside of therapy time (Vadas et al., 2022). On the other hand, satisfaction with the therapist's ability to answer questions and provide support, encouragement, and supervision may promote adherence to home-based therapy programs (Essery et al., 2017). Self-management interventions emphasize the need for healthcare providers to collaborate with people with chronic conditions and provide ongoing support (Pearce et al., 2016). This involves providing personalized care with adequate time and frequency as well as developing relationships built on trust. Client-centered approaches that involve active listening acknowledge the patient's experience and can help support the development of collaborative goals. These approaches require sufficient time and attention on the part of the provider (Schulman-Green et al., 2016). Providers can support self-management by conducting regular clinical visits where they offer key information on the condition and discuss its management, as well as lifestyle recommendations, such as physical activity and diet (Pearce et al., 2016; Schulman-Green et al., 2016). Supportive relationships with knowledgeable providers help to develop trust so that individuals can share their concerns. This may help patients develop communication skills to increase collaboration with healthcare providers and encourage shared decision-making (Lorig & Holman, 2003; Pearce et al., 2016).

Providing Knowledge to Support Informed Decision-Making

Knowledge about a health condition, how it is treated, and how that knowledge is applied in everyday life is critical for self-management (Schulman-Green et al., 2016). This information is needed for patients to make informed decisions about their care and choose appropriate self-management strategies (Lorig & Holman, 2003). When insufficient information is provided or the information is not tailored to ensure the patient's understanding, the patient may not engage in important self-management activities due to lack of awareness. For example, stroke survivors' recovery may be limited by a lack of knowledge of the importance of self-directed practice and exercise to reacquire skills and abilities (Vadas et al., 2022). On a similar note, a study of people who underwent hip arthroscopy found a positive correlation between perceived importance of the home exercise program and positive outcomes related to activities of daily living and satisfaction with the hip. This suggests that patients who believed that the home exercise program was important may have been more likely to complete the prescribed exercises, resulting in better outcomes (Amar et al., 2021). Another study of men with prostate cancer found that belief in the importance of exercise facilitates self-management, while believing that exercise is not important was a barrier (Fox et al., 2019). *Thus, it is important for providers not only to emphasize the importance of self-management activities but also to link behaviors with expected outcomes.* When people perceive that their effort will lead to positive outcomes or that lack of a behavior will contribute to a poor prognosis, they may be more likely to engage in self-management behaviors (Bandura, 2004). For example, stroke survivors may be more likely to engage in daily practice if they believe it is needed to maintain improvements in function (Vadas et al., 2022). As such, discussing the potential health consequences related to self-management activities, such as the consequences of not taking medication as prescribed or the benefits of exercising, can help promote self-management.

Promoting Skill Acquisition

Self-management of chronic conditions often involves the acquisition of new skills or the reacquisition of previously learned skills that were negatively impacted by the individual's health condition (Lorig & Holman, 2003). These skills may be related to the medical management of the condition, such as managing medications or taking one's blood pressure. They can also involve skills that support participation in daily activities, such as walking and arm use (Da-Silva, Moore & Price, 2018; Pearce et al., 2016; Sahely et al., 2023). Self-management interventions can focus on teaching these skills and may also provide equipment, such as self-care items and medical equipment (Pearce et al., 2016). Behavior change techniques such as practice and rehearsal of skills can be implemented within self-management interventions to help support skill acquisition and mastery (Lorig & Holman, 2003; Michie et al., 2013). Consideration of the individual's knowledge of how to perform a task and well as their physical and cognitive abilities is important for ensuring the individual is set up for success.

Skill acquisition approaches can involve compensatory methods in which the requirements of task are adapted to meet the needs of the individual. For example, stroke survivors with severe upper limb hemiparesis may benefit from adaptive equipment and one-handed techniques to successfully complete daily activities (Goldberg et al., 2021). Alternatively, approaches can focus on improving underlying capacities within the context of functional task practice. For example, constraint-induced movement therapy is a treatment approach for stroke survivors with less severe upper limb hemiparesis that uses a behavioral technique called shaping to improve functional upper limb use. Shaping involves breaking a task down into small achievable steps; task difficulty is gradually increased to ensure just-right challenge and to maintain the learner's perceptions of competence (Taub, 2012). This approach relies on repetitive practice of the skill with the affected upper limb to support learning and enhance adaptive neuroplasticity (Kleim & Jones, 2008). Cognitive problem-solving strategies can also be used to improve performance of meaningful activities and may encourage generalization. For example, the cognitive orientation to daily occupational performance (CO-OP) approach demonstrated improved performance in not only trained tasks but also untrained tasks for individuals with subacute stroke (McEwen et al., 2015). Recently, this approach was combined with constraint-induced movement therapy in a home-based telerehabilitation intervention for stroke survivors that showed promise for improving performance of meaningful activities as well as perceived arm use (Rowe et al., 2025). Thus, skill acquisition approaches have the potential to improve both functional performance as well as underlying abilities.

Encouraging Habit Formation

Daily habits and routines that support the implementation of self-management behaviors are important (Schulman-Green et al., 2016; Youngson, 2019). Management of chronic conditions can require changes to habits and routines, such as avoiding unhealthy behaviors, taking medication, or engaging in exercise. These changes can be challenging for people with chronic conditions (Lyu et al., 2025). Habits, which are behaviors that are repeated automatically without the need for conscious self-regulation and attention, are important for the maintenance of self-management behaviors (Gardner, Lally & Wardle, 2012). Studies of diabetes management have found an association between habit strength and performance self-management behaviors (Stone et al., 2023). In fact, one study of patients with Type 2 diabetes found that the strength of one's habits predicted adherence to self-management behaviors better than one's beliefs (Phillips et al., 2016).

Formation of new habits requires repetition of the activity within the real-world context (Stone et al., 2023). Habit formation is supported by months of consistent daily practice to develop automaticity of the behavior. Planning when and where the behavior will occur, repeating the action with consistency, and keeping a daily record of the behavior can help new habits to form (Gardner, Lally & Wardle, 2012). For example, constraint-induced movement therapy is an intervention for individuals with upper limb hemiparesis after stroke that includes a set of behavioral techniques called a "transfer package." These techniques, which include a daily home dairy, self-assessment of arm use, problem solving, and consistent upper limb practice in specified tasks at home, are focused on increasing habitual, spontaneous arm use during real-world daily activities (Taub et al., 2013). Previous experiences can also influence willingness to engage in self-management behaviors, depending on whether positive or negative outcomes were experienced (Bandura, 2004; Schulman-Green et al., 2016). For example, previous adherence to home-based physical therapy programs may increase likelihood that one will adhere to current programs (Essery et al., 2017). In addition, disruptions to one's routine and busy schedules can negatively impact habits and routines, so additional supports and reminders may be needed (Schulman-Green et al., 2016). As such, it is important for providers to discuss barriers and facilitators to habit formation with their patients and collaborate with them to encourage consistent engagement in self-management activities.

Developing Goal Setting, Action Planning, and Problem-Solving Skills

Many behavioral interventions rely on behavior change techniques such as goal setting, action planning, problem solving, and behavior contracts to help support behavior change (Lorig & Holman, 2003; Michie et al., 2013; Pearce et al., 2016). These interventions can be used to support achievement of behavioral goals as well as to manage clinical symptoms (Pearce et al., 2016). In *goal setting* interventions, an agreement is made on a given action that the individual will complete (Michie et al., 2013). Collaboration with patients during goal setting is important to ensure that patients have a sense of ownership of their goals and that goals are adapted to their individual needs (Alanko et al., 2019; Scobbie et al., 2013). *Action planning* involves creating a plan with specific steps to carry out the goal and identifies the context, frequency, duration, and intensity of the actions to be taken (Michie et al., 2013). Lorig and Holman (2003) recommend having patients rate their confidence in their ability to carry out an action plan (i.e. self-efficacy). If the rating is 6 out of 10 or lower, the provider should re-evaluate the plan with the client and problem-solve to address barriers (Lorig & Holman, 2003). Clinical action plans for symptom management are important for individuals with chronic health conditions (Lyu et al., 2025; Pearce et al., 2016; Schrijver et al., 2022). For example, clinical action plans for acute exacerbation of chronic obstructive pulmonary disease have been shown to improve health-related quality of life and decrease probability of hospital admissions related to respiratory distress (Schrijver et al., 2022). *Problem solving* is another core self-management skill that involves defining the problem or goal, generating solutions and a plan, implementing the plan, and then evaluating the result (Lorig & Holman, 2003; McEwen et al., 2015; Missiuna et al., 2001). Problem solving interventions may help with generalization so that clients can implement problem solving skills in new contexts or activities (McEwen et al., 2015; Missiuna et al., 2001). Finally, a *behavior contract*, which is written plan that is agreed upon by both the patient and provider, may also be helpful to elicit commitment for performing behaviors such as daily exercise (Michie et al., 2013). For example, a behavior contract is used in constraint-induced movement therapy to increase real-world arm use for stroke survivors (Taub et al., 2013). Thus, goal setting, action planning, problem solving, and behavior contracts are all behavior change techniques that providers can consider when designing and implementing self-management interventions.

Offering Feedback and Encouraging Self-Monitoring

Providers can also offer *feedback* on performance and encourage *self-monitoring* of self-management behaviors to support learning and behavior change (Pearce et al., 2016). For example, stroke survivors have reported a need for adequate feedback, supervision, and accountability from the therapist to facilitate engagement in self-directed practice (Vadas et al., 2022). Self-management interventions can offer patients ways to monitor their own symptoms and behaviors and receive feedback from providers, which may help with accountability. For instance, digital interventions may be used to track progress and offer feedback to patients (Akinosun et al., 2021). Behavioral supports such as activity logs, diaries, reminders, and check-in calls can also be implemented to help support adherence to self-management activities. This may include providing specific equipment for self-monitoring (Pearce et al., 2016). For example, accelerometers, wearable trackers, and smartphone apps can collect data and offer feedback on physical activity (Fedorchenko et al., 2024; Gebruers et al., 2010; Lau et al., 2025). Thus, feedback and self-monitoring can be incorporated into complex self-management interventions to help show progress and potentially increase adherence.

Enhancing Self-Efficacy

Self-efficacy is an important mechanism for improving health-related behavior as changes in self-efficacy have been positively associated with changes in health status (Lorig & Holman, 2003). When individuals believe their actions will have a positive impact on their quality of life and have confidence in their ability to successfully perform self-management behaviors, they are more likely to be successful in self-management (Schulman-Green et al., 2016). For example, self-efficacy has been shown to predict physical activity and exercise adherence and can mediate improvements in functional performance (Caetano et al., 2020; Essery et al., 2017; Nott et al., 2021; Williams & French, 2011). On the other hand, low self-efficacy can impede engagement in self-management behaviors. For example, if stroke survivors believe that their impairments are unlikely to improve even with practice, then they may be unwilling to expend the energy needed to engage in self-directed exercises (Vadas et al., 2022). A number of factors can influence self-efficacy. Because self-efficacy is influenced by one's mastery of a given skill, interventions that focus on skill acquisition as well as behavior change techniques such as goal setting, action planning, and problem solving can help to enhance self-efficacy (Lorig & Holman, 2003; McEwen et al., 2015; Williams & French, 2011). Additional strategies to increase self-efficacy can include modeling a behavior as well as the use of peer teaching and social persuasion. For example, seeing someone else receive a positive outcome from a behavior can increase a person's confidence and belief that they may also have a positive outcome (Lorig & Holman, 2003). Self-efficacy is often an outcome in self-management interventions and can be measured by having the individual rate their confidence in successfully performing a behavior (Bandura, 2006).

Supporting Motivation

Motivation can influence an individual's willingness to persist with self-management. This is influenced by self-efficacy, as well as a personal sense of autonomy or control (Bandura, 2004; Deci & Ryan, 2008; Schulman-Green et al., 2016). Motivation is also influenced by the perceived outcomes of behaviors. For example, stroke survivors report needing to see improvements that are linked to their daily life to support their motivation for self-directed practice (Vadas et al., 2022). Likewise, individuals may be motivated to engage in self-management in order to avoid perceived negative consequences, such as needing accommodations or devices (Schulman-Green et al., 2016). Personal values and interests can also influence motivation for self-management and may be barriers; for example, individuals with diabetes may find it difficult to manage their diet if it makes it challenging to participate in valued and enjoyable social events involving food (Youngson, 2019). Self-management interventions may help support motivation by incorporating achievable goals, enjoyable activities that provide an optimal level of challenge, and feedback that demonstrates improvement (Vadas et al., 2022). Motivation is important to address as it can increase adherence to self-management behaviors and help support habit formation (Essery et al., 2017; Gardner & Lally, 2013).

Reducing Psychological Distress

Psychological distress, such as stress, anxiety, and negative mood, can have an unfavorable impact on self-management (Schulman-Green et al., 2016). For example, stroke survivors report that the experience of failure and other negative emotions can limit engagement in home-based practice activities (Vadas et al., 2022). The experience of negative emotions such as anxiety, depression, and sadness has also been identified as a self-management barrier for people with head and neck cancer who may view themselves as a burden, leading to reduced motivation to engage in self-management (Lyu et al., 2025). Self-management interventions may include mindfulness training, relaxation techniques, coping skills, or cognitive restructuring interventions to address these concerns (Kayser et al., 2023; Pearce et al., 2016; Van Helm et al., 2022; Whittaker et al., 2024).

Addressing Social and Environmental Support

Positive social support is an important facilitator for self-management. Support from family and peers can be empowering and help individuals manage their health conditions, such as physical activity, medication management, nutrition, and medical appointments; however, lack of support with important lifestyle changes can have a negative impact on self-management (Gallant, 2003; Lyu et al., 2025; Schulman-Green et al., 2016). For example, social support from family and friends can help support adherence to home exercise programs (Essery et al., 2017). For individuals with stroke, this support is important because they may require assistance to complete recommended exercises (Vadas et al., 2022). On the other hand, the home environment can present challenges for self-management. For example, different dietary preferences in the home may increase the challenge of following a recommended diet. In addition, focusing on the needs of other family members may make it more difficult for an individual to prioritize the management of their condition (Schulman-Green et al., 2016). Engaging family members in self-management interventions may help to increase support and understanding.

Self-management interventions can intentionally address social support by connecting individuals with support groups and peer mentoring (Franek, 2013; Pearce et al., 2016). Peers who share a health condition can be an important source of support, community, and information sharing (Schulman-Green et al., 2016). Peer-led self-management interventions have demonstrated improvements in exercise frequency, management of cognitive symptoms, self-efficacy, and self-reported health (Foster et al., 2007). These programs can be condition specific. For example, peer support interventions for people with coronary heart disease have demonstrated improvements in self-management behaviors, self-efficacy, and risk of hospital readmission (Weddell et al., 2025).

Evaluation of the community environment can also help identify potential barriers to self-management. The environmental characteristics of the community such as support at a person's workplace and factors such as transportation, access to healthy food, and social context also influence an individual's ability to successfully participate in self-management activities (Schulman-Green et al., 2016). For example, cultural beliefs and practices may influence acceptance of self-management recommendations if they conflict with cultural norms, and providers can support self-management by providing recommendations that are sensitive to a person's culture and preferences (Schulman-Green et al., 2016; Youngson, 2019). Other factors such as work stressors, lack of transportation, unhealthy food in the community, and poor public awareness of a health condition can also be barriers (Schulman-Green et al., 2016). These factors can be addressed in self-management interventions by problem-solving and connecting people with resources to support their needs (Lorig & Holman, 2003; Pearce et al., 2016).

Providing Access to Technology and Equipment

Self-management interventions may also provide technology and equipment to support engagement in self-management behaviors (Pearce et al., 2016). For example, interventions such as telehealth can be helpful for self-management and may lead to improvements in outcomes such as quality of life, self-care, and blood pressure (Lee et al., 2022). However, technology and equipment may present both supports and barriers for self-management. For example, individuals may use the internet to learn about their health condition and access peer support. However, the internet can also be unreliable or may offer too much information, making it difficult to know what is most important (Schulman-Green et al., 2016). In another example, technologies such as telerehabilitation can help individuals with stroke engage in self-directed practice in their home environment and can allow for flexible scheduling. However, the use of such technologies may be limited by space, malfunctions, or need for assistance (Vadas et al., 2022).

In spite of potential challenges, technology has been successfully used to support self-management. For example, an internet-based self-management program was found to reduce fatigue and improve mental health and sleep quality for people with cancer (Huang et al., 2020). In another example, an app-based exercise program for people with multiple sclerosis demonstrated significant reductions in spasticity (Amatya et al., 2024; Ehling et al., 2017). Technology has also been used to support management of cardiovascular conditions through interventions delivered on personal devices and other digital technologies; these interventions may help improve physical activity, diet, and medication adherence (Akinosun et al., 2021). Thus, technology-based interventions have promise for improving self-management, and the acceptability of these technologies should be tested to ensure that they are user-friendly and that adequate support is provided to ensure success.

Considering Health Status and Adapting Care to Meet Individual Needs

An individual's health status, including their illness severity, fatigue, cognitive and sensorimotor impairments, comorbidities, and symptoms, can have a strong impact on self-management, and self-management interventions should be individualized to ensure that these factors are considered (Schulman-Green et al., 2016). For example, walking ability is one factor that predicts exercise adherence after stroke, suggesting that the degree of functional impairment can impact ability and desire to engage in exercise (Caetano et al., 2020). Sensorimotor impairments and experience of fatigue are common after stroke and can limit participation in home-based exercise. The severity of these impairments can impact a person's beliefs about how much recovery is possible and may limit willingness to engage in practice (Vadas et al., 2022). Similarly, men with prostate cancer report that factors such as fatigue and incontinence can be barriers for self-management (Fox et al., 2019), while symptoms such as shortness of breath increase difficulty of engaging in exercise for people with chronic obstructive pulmonary disease (Qin et al., 2025; Schulman-Green et al., 2016). Cognitive impairment also leads to difficulties with self-management due to reduced awareness of symptoms, difficulty remembering to take medications, and reduced problem-solving ability (Schulman-Green et al., 2016; Świątoniowska-Lonc et al., 2021). Thus, personalized assessment and treatment planning from disciplines such as occupational therapy are often needed to help tailor interventions that optimize successful participation in self-management based on individual strengths and challenges.

EFFECTIVENESS OF SELF-MANAGEMENT INTERVENTIONS

Self-management interventions have demonstrated effectiveness in improving a number of outcomes, including improved *quality of life* for individuals with chronic conditions (Lee et al., 2022; Whittaker et al., 2024). Improvements in quality of life have been found for a number of specific populations, including stroke (Fryer et al., 2016), cancer (Rimmer et al., 2023), chronic obstructive pulmonary disease (Schrijver et al., 2022), amputation (Van Helm et al., 2022), and knee osteoarthritis (Wu et al., 2022). *Self-efficacy* is another common focus of self-management interventions, and a number of studies have found significant increases in self-efficacy for individuals with chronic conditions (Foster et al., 2007), including stroke (Lau et al., 2022), cancer (Rimmer et al., 2023), and cardiovascular disease (Weddell et al., 2025). Improvements in *functional ability* and *self-management skills*, such as mobility and performance of daily activities, can also be seen in populations with chronic conditions (Foster et al., 2007; Lee et al., 2022), including older adults (Hunter & Kearney, 2018), stroke (Sahely et al., 2023; Toh, Chia & Fong, 2022), amputation (Van Helm et al., 2022), diabetes (Asmat et al., 2022), cardiovascular disease (Akinosun et al., 2021; Weddell et al., 2025), and chronic pain/fibromyalgia (Geraghty et al., 2021).

Self-management interventions can also increase *physical activity* for people with chronic conditions, such as in populations with stroke (Sahely et al., 2023), diabetes (Asmat et al., 2022), cardiovascular disease (Akinosun et al., 2021), amputation (Van Helm et al., 2022), and knee osteoarthritis (Wu et al., 2022). Other potential benefits of self-management interventions may include reduced *pain* (Foster et al., 2007; Geraghty et al., 2021; Wu et al., 2022), improved *mental health* (Foster et al., 2007; Huang et al., 2020; Witzig Brändli et al., 2023; Wu et al., 2022), reduced *hospital readmissions* (Schrijver et al., 2022; Weddell et al., 2025), improved *disease management* (Asmat et al., 2022; Lee et al., 2022), reduced *fatigue* (Foster et al., 2007; Huang et al., 2020), and improved *sleep quality* (Huang et al., 2020). While self-management interventions may help a number of areas of self-management for people with a variety of chronic conditions, more research is needed to determine the most important components of these interventions for bringing about change.

CONCLUSION

Self-management is important for providers to address with people with chronic health conditions to help them access resources, gain knowledge about the treatment of their condition, learn self-management skills, and develop new habits and routines that support maintenance of self-management behaviors. This chapter reviewed the concept of self-management, including core self-management skills and theories that guide self-management interventions. In addition, factors that influence self-management and key considerations for self-management interventions were covered. Self-management interventions have demonstrated effectiveness for outcomes such as improved quality of life, self-efficacy, and functional performance, but future work is needed to determine which aspects of these interventions are most important for bringing about change.

REFERENCES

Akinosun AS, Polson R, Diaz-Skeete Y, De Kock JH, Carragher L, Leslie S et al (2021). Digital technology interventions for risk factor modification in patients with cardiovascular disease: Systematic review and meta-analysis. JMIR Mhealth Uhealth. 9(3):e21061. doi:10.2196/21061.

Alanko T, Karhula M, Kröger T, Piirainen A, Nikander R (2019). Rehabilitees perspective on goal setting in rehabilitation – A phenomenological approach. Disabil Rehabil. 41(19):2280–2288. doi:10.1080/09638288.2018.1463398.

Allegrante JP, Wells MT, Peterson JC (2019). Interventions to support behavioral self-management of chronic diseases. Annu Rev Public Health. 40:127–146. doi:10.1146/annurev-publhealth-040218-044008.

Amar E, Martin RL, Tudor A, Factor S, Atzmon R, Rath E (2021). Midterm outcomes and satisfaction after hip arthroscopy are associated with postoperative rehabilitation factors. Orthop J Sports Med. 9(1):2325967120981888. doi:10.1177/2325967120981888.

Amatya B, Khan F, Song K, Galea M (2024). Effectiveness of non-pharmacological interventions for spasticity management in multiple sclerosis: A systematic review. Ann Rehabil Med. 48(5):305–343. doi:10.5535/arm.240064.

Asmat K, Dhamani K, Gul R, Froelicher ES (2022). The effectiveness of patient-centered care vs. usual care in type 2 diabetes self-management: A systematic review and meta-analysis. Front Public Health. 10:994766. doi:10.3389/fpubh.2022.994766.

Bandura A (1977). Self-efficacy: Toward a unifying theory of behavioral change. Psychol Rev. 84(2):191–215. doi:10.1037/0033-295X.84.2.191.

Bandura A (1997). *Self-Efficacy: The Exercise of Control*. New York: W. H. Freeman and Company.

Bandura A (2004). Health promotion by social cognitive means. Health Educ Behav. 31(2):143–164. doi:10.1177/1090198104263660.

Bandura A (2006). Guide for constructing self-efficacy scales. In: Pajares F, Urdan T, editors. *Self-Efficacy Beliefs of Adolescents* (pp. 307–337). Greenwich: Information Age Publishing.

Caetano LCG, Pacheco BD, Samora GAR, Teixeira-Salmela LF, Scianni AA (2020). Self-efficacy to engage in physical exercise and walking ability best predicted exercise adherence after stroke. Stroke Res Treat. 2020:1–6. doi:10.1155/2020/2957623.

Carey RN, Connell LE, Johnston M, Rothman AJ, de Bruin M, Kelly MP et al (2019). Behavior change techniques and their mechanisms of action: A synthesis of links described in published intervention literature. Ann Behav Med. 53(8):693–707. doi:10.1093/abm/kay078.

Da-Silva RH, Moore SA, Price CI (2018). Self-directed therapy programmes for arm rehabilitation after stroke: A systematic review. Clin Rehabil. 32(8):1022–1036. doi:10.1177/0269215518775170.

Davis R, Campbell R, Hildon Z, Hobbs L, Michie S (2015). Theories of behaviour and behaviour change across the social and behavioural sciences: A scoping review. Health Psychol Rev. 9(3):323–244. doi:10.1080/17437199.2014.941722.

Deci EL, Ryan RM (2008). Facilitating optimal motivation and psychological well-being across life's domains. Can Psychol. 49(1):14–23. doi:10.1037/0708-5591.49.1.14.

Dobkin BH (2016). Behavioral self-management strategies for practice and exercise should be included in neurologic rehabilitation trials and care. Curr Opin Neurol. 29(6):693–699. doi:10.1097/WCO.0000000000000380.

Ehling R, Edlinger M, Hermann K, Dröge K, Seidinger Y, Miller U et al (2017). Successful long-term management of spasticity in patients with multiple sclerosis using a software application (APP): A pilot study. Mult Scler Relat Disord. 17:15–21. doi:10.1016/j.msard.2017.06.013.

Essery R, Geraghty AWA, Kirby S, Yardley L (2017). Predictors of adherence to home-based physical therapies: A systematic review. Disabil Rehabil. 39(6):519–534. doi:10.3109/09638288.2016.1153160.

Fedorchenko Y, Zimba O, Sagtaganov Z, Yessirkepov M (2024). Enhancing chronic disease management through physical activity and pedometry-based health monitoring. Rheumatol Int. 44(12):2737–2743. doi:10.1007/s00296-024-05738-7.

Fisher EB, Brownson CA, O'Toole ML, Shetty G, Anwuri VV, Glasgow RE (2005). Ecological approaches to self-management: The case of diabetes. Am J Public Health. 95(9):1523–1535. doi:10.2105/AJPH.2005.066084.

Foster G, Taylor SJC, Eldridge SE, Ramsay J, Griffiths CJ (2007). Self-management education programmes by lay leaders for people with chronic conditions. Cochrane Database Syst Rev. (4):CD005108. doi:10.1002/14651858.CD005108.pub2.

Fox L, Wiseman T, Cahill D, Beyer K, Peat N, Rammant E et al (2019). Barriers and facilitators to physical activity in men with prostate cancer: A qualitative and quantitative systematic review. Psychooncology. 28(12):2270–2285. doi:10.1002/pon.5240.

Franek J (2013). Self-management support interventions for persons with chronic disease: An evidence-based analysis. Ont Health Technol Assess Ser. 13(9):1–60. http://www.ncbi.nlm.nih.gov/pubmed/24194800

Fryer CE, Luker JA, McDonnell MN, Hillier SL (2016). Self management programmes for quality of life in people with stroke. Cochrane Database Syst Rev. 2016(8):CD010442. doi:10.1002/14651858.CD010442.pub2.

Gallant MP (2003). The influence of social support on chronic illness self-management: A review and directions for research. Health Educ Behav. 30(2):170–195. doi:10.1177/1090198102251030.

Gardner B, Lally P (2013). Does intrinsic motivation strengthen physical activity habit? Modeling relationships between self-determination, past behaviour, and habit strength. J Behav Med. 36(5):488–497. doi:10.1007/s10865-012-9442-0.

Gardner B, Lally P, Wardle J (2012). Making health habitual: The psychology of 'habit-formation' and general practice. Br J Gen Pract. 62(605):664–666. doi:10.3399/bjgp12X659466.

Gebruers N, Vanroy C, Truijen S, Engelborghs S, De Deyn PP (2010). Monitoring of physical activity after stroke: A systematic review of accelerometry-based measures. Arch Phys Med Rehabil. 91(2):288–297. doi:10.1016/j.apmr.2009.10.025.

Geraghty AWA, Maund E, Newell D, Santer M, Everitt H, Price C et al (2021). Self-management for chronic widespread pain including fibromyalgia: A systematic review and meta-analysis. PLoS One. 16(7):e0254642. doi:10.1371/journal.pone.0254642.

Goldberg C, Winterbottom L, Ryan PA, Sullivan JW, Gillen G (2021). Adaptations for managing daily activities with hemiparesis. In: Gillen G, Nilsen D, editors. *Stroke Rehabilitation: A Function-Based Approach* (5th ed., Vol. 2021, pp. 120–137). Philadelphia: Elsevier.

Hale J, Hastings J, West R, Lefevre CE, Direito A, Bohlen LC et al (2020). An ontology-based modelling system (OBMS) for representing behaviour change theories applied to 76 theories. Wellcome Open Res. 5:177. doi:10.12688/wellcomeopenres.16121.1.

Huang J, Han Y, Wei J, Liu X, Du Y, Yang L et al (2020). The effectiveness of the internet-based self-management program for cancer-related fatigue patients: A systematic review and meta-analysis. Clin Rehabil. 34(3):287–298. doi:10.1177/0269215519889394.

Hunter EG, Kearney PJ (2018). Occupational therapy interventions to improve performance of instrumental activities of daily living for community-dwelling older adults: A systematic review. Am J Occup Ther. 72(4):7204190050p1–7204190050p9. doi:10.5014/ajot.2018.031062.

Kayser J, Hu RX, Rosenscruggs D, Li L, Xiang X (2023). A systematic review of the impact of select mindfulness interventions on psychological outcomes among older adults with chronic health conditions. Clin Gerontol. 46(3):302–314. doi:10.1080/07317115.2022.2076636.

Kleim JA, Jones TA (2008). Principles of experience-dependent neural plasticity: Implications for rehabilitation after brain damage. J Speech Lang Hear Res. 51(1):39–S225. doi:10.1044/1092-4388(2008/018).

Lau SCL, Bright L, Connor LT, Baum CM (2025). Experiences with mobile health-enabled ambulatory monitoring among stroke survivors: A qualitative study. OTJR (Thorofare N J). 45(2):232–240. doi:10.1177/15394492241238948.

Lau SCL, Judycki S, Mix M, DePaul O, Tomazin R, Hardi A et al (2022). Theory-based self-management interventions for community-dwelling stroke survivors: A systematic review and meta-analysis. Am J Occup Ther. 76(4). doi:10.5014/ajot.2022.049117.

Lawless MT, Tieu M, Feo R, Kitson AL (2021). Theories of self-care and self-management of long-term conditions by community-dwelling older adults: A systematic review and meta-ethnography. Soc Sci Med. 287:114393. doi:10.1016/j.socscimed.2021.114393.

Lee AYL, Wong AKC, Hung TTM, Yan J, Yang S (2022). Nurse-led telehealth intervention for rehabilitation (telerehabilitation) among community-dwelling patients with chronic diseases: Systematic review and meta-analysis. J Med Internet Res. 24(11):e40364. doi:10.2196/40364.

Lorig K (2014). Chronic disease self-management program: Insights from the eye of the storm. Front Public Health. 2(APR):253. doi:10.3389/fpubh.2014.00253.

Lorig KR, Holman H (2003). Self-management education: History, definition, outcomes, and mechanisms. Ann Behav Med. 26(1):1–7. doi:10.1207/S15324796ABM2601_01.

Lorig KR, Sobel DS, Stewart AL, Brown BW, Bandura A, Ritter P et al (1999). Evidence suggesting that a chronic disease self-management program can improve health status while reducing hospitalization: A randomized trial. Med Care. 37(1):5–14. doi:10.1097/00005650-199901000-00003.

Lyu J, Yin L, Zhang H, Xu L, Yang Q, Wang A (2025). Striving to integrate self-management into daily life: A qualitative meta-synthesis of the perspectives and experiences from head and neck cancer survivors. BMJ Open. 15(6):e094440. doi:10.1136/bmjopen-2024-094440.

Marques MM, Wright AJ, Corker E, Johnston M, West R, Hastings J et al (2023). The behaviour change technique ontology: Transforming the behaviour change technique taxonomy v1. Wellcome Open Res. 8:308. doi:10.12688/wellcomeopenres.19363.2.

McEwen S, Polatajko H, Baum C, Rios J, Cirone D, Doherty M et al (2015). Combined cognitive-strategy and task-specific training improve transfer to untrained activities in subacute stroke: An exploratory randomized controlled trial. Neurorehabil Neural Repair. 29(6):526–536. doi:10.1177/1545968314558602.

Michie S, Richardson M, Johnston M, Abraham C, Francis J, Hardeman W et al (2013). The behavior change technique taxonomy (v1) of 93 hierarchically clustered techniques: Building an international consensus for the reporting of behavior change interventions. Ann Behav Med. 46(1):81–95. doi:10.1007/s12160-013-9486-6.

Michie S, van Stralen MM, West R (2011). The behaviour change wheel: A new method for characterising and designing behaviour change interventions. Implement Sci. 6(1):42. doi:10.1186/1748-5908-6-42.

Missiuna C, Mandich AD, Polatajko HJ, Malloy-Miller T (2001). Cognitive orientation to daily occupational performance (CO-OP): Part I–theoretical foundations. Phys Occup Ther Pediatr. 20(2–3):69–81. http://www.ncbi.nlm.nih.gov/pubmed/11345513).

Mol TI, van Bennekom CAM, Scholten EWM, Visser-Meily JMA, Reneman MF, Riedstra A et al (2022). Self-regulation as rehabilitation outcome: What is important according to former patients? Disabil Rehabil. 44(24):7484–7490. doi:10.1080/09638288.2021.1998663.

Ng JYY, Ntoumanis N, Thøgersen-Ntoumani C, Deci EL, Ryan RM, Duda JL et al (2012). Self-determination theory applied to health contexts: A meta-analysis. Perspect Psychol Sci. 7(4):325–340. doi:10.1177/1745691612447309.

Norris SL, Lau J, Smith SJ, Schmid CH, Engelgau MM (2002). Self-management education for adults with type 2 diabetes: A meta-analysis of the effect on glycemic control. Diabetes Care. 25(7):1159–1171. doi:10.2337/diacare.25.7.1159.

Nott M, Wiseman L, Seymour T, Pike S, Cuming T, Wall G (2021). Stroke self-management and the role of self-efficacy. Disabil Rehabil. 43(10):1410–1419. doi:10.1080/09638288.2019.1666431.

Ntoumanis N, Ng JYY, Prestwich A, Quested E, Hancox JE, Thøgersen-Ntoumani C et al (2021). A meta-analysis of self-determination theory-informed intervention studies in the health domain: Effects on motivation, health behavior, physical, and psychological health. Health Psychol Rev. 15(2):214–244. doi :10.1080/17437199.2020.1718529.

Paterson S, Dawes H, Winward C, Bartram E, Dodds E, McKinon J et al (2024). Use of the capability, opportunity and motivation behaviour model (COM-B) to understand interventions to support physical activity behaviour in people with stroke: An overview of reviews. Clin Rehabil. 38(4):543–557. doi:10.1177/02692155231224365.

Pearce G, Parke HL, Pinnock H, Epiphaniou E, Bourne CLA, Sheikh A et al (2016). The PRISMS taxonomy of self-management support: Derivation of a novel taxonomy and initial testing of its utility. J Health Serv Res Policy. 21(2):73–82. doi:10.1177/1355819615602725.

Phillips LA, Cohen J, Burns E, Abrams J, Renninger S (2016). Self-management of chronic illness: The role of 'habit' versus reflective factors in exercise and medication adherence. J Behav Med. 39(6):1076–1091. doi:10.1007/s10865-016-9732-z.

Qin H, Jia P, Yan Q, Li X, Zhang Y, Jiang H et al (2025). Barriers and facilitators to pulmonary rehabilitation in COPD: A mixed-methods systematic review. BMC Pulm Med. 25(1):314. doi:10.1186/s12890-025-03769-9.

Rethorn ZD, Bezner JR, Pettitt CD (2022). From expert to coach: Health coaching to support behavior change within physical therapist practice. Physiother Theory Pract. 38(13):2352–2367. doi:10.1080/09593985.2021.1987601.

Rimmer B, Brown MC, Sotire T, Beyer F, Bolnykh I, Balla M et al (2023). Characteristics and components of self-management interventions for improving quality of life in cancer survivors: A systematic review. Cancers (Basel). 16(1):14. doi:10.3390/cancers16010014.

Rowe VT, Wilcox EA, Chatto CA, Carrick RM (2025). Remotely delivered task-oriented training and evaluation (reTOTE) for stroke rehabilitation. Arch Rehabil Res Clin Transl. 7(3):100491. doi:10.1016/j.arrct.2025.100491.

Ryan RM, Deci EL (2000). Self-determination theory and the facilitation of intrinsic motivation, social development, and well-being. Am Psychol. 55(1):68–78. doi:10.1037/0003-066X.55.1.68.

Sahely A, Giles D, Sintler C, Soundy A, Rosewilliam S (2023). Self-management interventions to improve mobility after stroke: An integrative review. Disabil Rehabil. 45(1):9–26. doi:10.1080/09638288.2022.2028019.

Schrijver J, Lenferink A, Brusse-Keizer M, Zwerink M, van der Valk PD, van der Palen J et al (2022). Self-management interventions for people with chronic obstructive pulmonary disease. Cochrane Database Syst Rev. 1(1):CD002990. doi:10.1002/14651858.CD002990.pub4.

Schulman-Green D, Jaser S, Martin F, Alonzo A, Grey M, McCorkle R et al (2012). Processes of self-management in chronic illness. J Nurs Scholarsh. 44(2):136–44. doi:10.1111/j.1547-5069.2012.01444.x.

Schulman-Green D, Jaser SS, Park C, Whittemore R (2016). A metasynthesis of factors affecting self-management of chronic illness. J Adv Nurs. 72(7):1469–89. doi:10.1111/jan.12902.

Scobbie L, McLean D, Dixon D, Duncan E, Wyke S (2013). Implementing a framework for goal setting in community based stroke rehabilitation: A process evaluation. BMC Health Serv Res. 13(1):190. doi:10.1186/1472-6963-13-190.

Stone JY, Mayberry LS, Clouse K, Mulvaney S (2023). The role of habit formation and automaticity in diabetes self-management: Current evidence and future applications. Curr Diab Rep. 23(4):43–58. doi:10.1007/s11892-023-01499-y.

Świątoniowska-Lonc N, Polański J, Tański W, Jankowska-Polańska B (2021). Impact of cognitive impairment on adherence to treatment and self-care in patients with type 2 diabetes mellitus. Diabetes. Metab Syndr Obes. 14:193–203. doi:10.2147/DMSO.S284468.

Taub E (2012). The behavior-analytic origins of constraint-induced movement therapy: An example of behavioral neurorehabilitation. Behav Anal. 35(2):155–178. doi:10.1007/BF03392276.

Taub E, Uswatte G, Mark VW, Morris DM, Barman J, Bowman MH et al (2013). Method for enhancing real-world use of a more affected arm in chronic stroke. Stroke. 44(5):1383–1388. doi:10.1161/STROKEAHA.111.000559.

Toh SFM, Chia PF, Fong KNK (2022). Effectiveness of home-based upper limb rehabilitation in stroke survivors: A systematic review and meta-analysis. Front Neurol. 13:964196. doi:10.3389/fneur.2022.964196.

Vadas D, Prest K, Turk A, Tierney S (2022). Understanding the facilitators and barriers of stroke survivors' adherence to recovery-oriented self-practice: A thematic synthesis. Disabil Rehabil. 44(22):6608–6619. doi:10.1080/09638288.2021.1968512.

Van Helm S, Krops LA, Dekker R, Vrieling AH (2022). Effectiveness of (active) lifestyle interventions in people with a lower limb amputation: A systematic review. Arch Rehabil Res Clin Transl. 4(4):100207. doi:10.1016/j.arrct.2022.100207.

Webb J, Baker A, Palmer T, Hall A, Ahlquist A, Darlow J et al (2022). The barriers and facilitators to physical activity in people with a musculoskeletal condition: A rapid review of reviews using the COM-b model to support intervention development. Public Health Pract. 3:100250. doi:10.1016/j.puhip.2022.100250.

Weddell J, Shi W, Redfern J, Buckley T, Gallagher R (2025). Effectiveness of coronary heart disease peer support interventions: A systematic review and meta-analysis. Eur J Prev Cardiol. 1–17. doi:10.1093/eurjpc/zwaf241.

Whittaker SL, Brusco NK, Hill KD, Taylor NF (2024). Self-management programs within rehabilitation yield positive health outcomes at a small increased cost compared with usual care: A systematic review and meta-analysis. Arch Phys Med Rehabil. 105(10):1946–1960. doi:10.1016/j.apmr.2024.05.007.

Whittaker SL, Brusco NK, Hill KD, Ekegren CL, Taylor NF (2025). A self-management program increases the dosage of inpatient rehabilitation by 26 minutes per day: A process evaluation. Disabil Rehabil. 47(2):425–434. doi:10.1080/09638288.2024.2339533.

Williams SL, French DP (2011). What are the most effective intervention techniques for changing physical activity self-efficacy and physical activity behaviour–and are they the same? Health Educ Res. 26(2):308–322. doi:10.1093/her/cyr005.

Willmott TJ, Pang B, Rundle-Thiele S (2021). Capability, opportunity, and motivation: An across contexts empirical examination of the COM-B model. BMC Public Health. 21(1):1014. doi:10.1186/s12889-021-11019-w.

Witzig Brändli V, Lange C, Kobleder A, Kohler M (2023). Effectiveness and content components of nursing counselling interventions on self- and symptom management of patients in oncology rehabilitation-A systematic review. Nurs Open. 10(5):2757–2769. doi:10.1002/nop2.1545.

Wu Z, Zhou R, Zhu Y, Zeng Z, Ye Z, Wang Z et al (2022). Self-management for knee osteoarthritis: A systematic review and meta-analysis of randomized controlled trials. Pain Res Manag. 2022:2681240. doi:10.1155/2022/2681240.

Youngson B (2019). Understanding diabetes self-management using the model of human occupation. Br J Occup Ther. 82(5):296–305. doi:10.1177/0308022618820010.

32 Harnessing Technologies for Self-Management in Rehabilitation

Jiali He, Ziwei Li, Yiling Tang, and Alex W. K. Wong

EVOLUTION OF SELF-MANAGEMENT IN REHABILITATION

Despite advances in the healthcare system that have allowed more people to live with disabilities for longer periods, they still face major challenges physically, mentally, and socially during their recovery. People with disabilities have significantly poorer health compared to their able-bodied peers. Long-term disabilities require ongoing attention to preserve patients' independence and quality of life throughout their entire journey. However, hospital or institutional rehabilitation services cannot always meet these needs. As a result, rehabilitation is shifting from the traditional provider-patient relationship – where the healthcare provider is regarded as an expert and the patient is a passive recipient of care – to a new model that empowers patients to navigate their care in collaboration with healthcare providers (Allegrante et al., 2019; Newman et al., 2004).

Patients engaged in managing their own care are referred to as self-management, which has been defined as "the day-to-day management of chronic conditions by individuals over the course of an illness" (Grady and Gough, 2014). Self-management for patients involves three distinct but related sets of goals: medical or behavioral management of the disease, role management, and emotional management (Lorig and Holman, 2003). For self-management to be successful, it must encompass six key self-management skills: problem-solving, decision-making, resource utilization, forming and maintaining a patient–provider partnership in the long term, action planning, and self-tailoring. Self-management is increasingly seen as a key part of rehabilitation programs because it helps patients with disabilities reach their full potential in life.

Self-management interventions are typically provided through peer-led or co-led small group sessions. (Lorig and Holman, 2003). It is based on the idea that patients facing similar health and social issues can act as partners in managing their condition. Small health-related group sessions offer participants face-to-face interaction, fostering peer support and social connection within a community setting. Although this format benefits health care outcomes, attendance and completion rates may decrease because patients need to physically attend scheduled sessions. For those who are unwilling or unable to join face-to-face group meetings, mailed printed materials might serve as an alternative intervention method (Lorig et al., 2015). However, since neither the classroom sessions nor the distribution of printed materials are site-specific or labor-intensive, scaling the delivery of the self-management program efficiently remains challenging.

Over the past decade, rapid advancements in information and communication technologies have significantly transformed health service delivery and broadened the reach of self-management programs (Oldenburg et al., 2015). Technology-based interventions now leverage a wide range of tools – including the internet, mobile applications, social media, advanced wearable sensors (e.g., accelerometers, gyroscopes, pedometers, heart rate monitors), robotics, artificial intelligence, and virtual reality – to design, develop, and deliver health content and strategies aimed at improving physical or psychological health outcomes for target users (Su et al., 2021). These tools enhance self-management by extending the treatment reach to larger populations, reducing administrative costs, enabling real-time monitoring and adaptive feedback, and increasing fidelity through

DOI: 10.1201/9781003599074-35

the integration of core therapeutic components into digital formats. Such technology-driven programs have demonstrated effectiveness across various neurological conditions (e.g., stroke, spinal cord injury, dementia) and chronic illnesses (e.g., chronic pain, chronic obstructive pulmonary disease [COPD], diabetes), offering accessible, affordable, convenient, and user-friendly solutions (Glueckauf and Lustria, 2008; Oldenburg et al., 2015).

KEY FACTORS FOR DEVELOPING TECHNOLOGY-BASED INTERVENTIONS

The increasing integration of technology into self-management represents a promising advancement in rehabilitation. To ensure the success of technology-based interventions, it is essential to address key factors for development. These factors encompass both user-related and technological considerations. On the user side, key factors include condition-specific needs, digital literacy, and support from healthcare providers and caregivers. Concurrently, technological aspects such as accessibility, affordability, user experience, and seamless integration with existing healthcare services play a vital role in promoting the long-term adoption and sustainability of self-management solutions.

The Users

Condition-Specific Issues

To successfully implement technology-based interventions, it is essential to consider the specific needs associated with a patient's health condition. For example, individuals with neurological conditions, such as stroke, spinal cord injury, and Alzheimer's disease, often face barriers to technology use due to mobility impairments and cognitive challenges. To enhance engagement, self-management platforms should incorporate adaptive features like voice input and biometric authentication. For patients with chronic illnesses, such as diabetes or chronic kidney disease, tools must support critical tasks like self-monitoring and dietary management. Additionally, co-morbidities and age-related functional limitations, such as fatigue, reduced manual dexterity, or vision impairments, must be considered during development (Moody et al., 2022). Providing daily support that enables patients to integrate condition-specific needs into their routines is a key consideration for designing effective technology-based interventions.

Personalization

Research demonstrates that user-centered technological interventions – those that allow individuals to customize tools based on their personal preferences and daily routines – can significantly enhance technology adoption rates (Moody et al., 2022). Many patients value the ability to adjust the level and complexity of tasks, such as gradually increasing difficulty in alignment with their physical skills. Preferences for using various tools and resources vary across areas, including financial planning, health screening, and well-being support. In other cases, simpler technologies are more easily integrated into everyday life. Conversely, interventions that fail to align with a patient's needs or preferences may lead to disengagement or abandonment (Tadas and Coyle, 2020). Therefore, effective technology-based interventions should be grounded in comprehensive, individualized assessments that are continuously updated to reflect changes throughout the rehabilitation process.

Digital Literacy

With the growing complexity of technologies, digital literacy has become a critical factor in the effective use of self-management tools. Digital literacy refers to the knowledge, skills, and attitudes required to navigate and utilize technology proficiently, and is shaped by variables such as age, education, socioeconomic status, and cultural background (Pangrazio et al., 2020). It has been identified as one of the "super social determinants of health" in today's digital healthcare landscape (Van Kessel et al., 2022). Individuals who lack awareness of technology's role in healthcare or the skills to use digital tools are less likely to adopt self-management technologies, placing them at a disadvantage in accessing essential health resources. Moreover, low digital literacy is often associated with fear and anxiety when encountering unfamiliar technologies (Boyle et al., 2022). To mitigate the impact of the digital divide on health outcomes, tailored strategies must be implemented to equip patients with the necessary competencies and confidence to engage with technology. Evidence-based approaches include offering education resources, such as online courses, technology demonstrations, and hands-on practice sessions, as well as providing social support from tech-savvy healthcare professionals, family members, and peers (Arias López et al., 2023).

Healthcare Providers and Caregivers

Users of technology-based self-management interventions include not only patients but also healthcare providers, such as physical and occupational therapists, along with informal caregivers. In Australia, for example, nearly half of occupational therapists reported not prescribing assistive technologies or telecare solutions due to limited awareness of available options, resource constraints, and the additional workload associated with integrating new technologies into their busy routines. These challenges often require providers to acquire new skills and maintain ongoing communication with patients. (Jarvis et al., 2017). Meanwhile, caregivers are increasingly assuming extended roles in supporting patients after discharge from medical settings. Despite often lacking formal training or compensation, these caregivers play a significant role in promoting adherence to long-term self-management strategies and providing daily assistance. Evidence suggests that equipping caregivers with appropriate training, user-friendly technologies, self-installation options, and robust support packages can vastly improve the long-term success of technology-based self-management interventions (Forducey et al., 2012).

The Technology

Accessibility and Affordability

Accessibility and affordability are critical considerations in the adoption of technology-based interventions, particularly among patients with diverse medical conditions, and these concerns extend beyond low- and middle-income countries (Egan and Pot, 2016). Accessibility refers to when and where users can engage with technology and has become increasingly important as rehabilitation services shift from hospital-based care to community settings to support ongoing recovery. Despite this shift, innovative health technologies remain under-integrated in many countries, especially in underserved regions. To address this gap, providing free foundational resources, such as Internet access and mobile platforms, is essential.

Affordability also plays a pivotal role. Even when patients have the financial means to purchase healthcare technologies, they may lack the resources for ongoing maintenance, leading to hesitation around upfront investments. To mitigate this barrier, alternative payment models, such as trial periods or rental options, should be considered to make these technologies more accessible and sustainable.

Reminders and Monitoring

Self-management is a long-term commitment for patients, and technology plays a vital role in sustaining motivation and driving behavioral changes in daily life. Automated reminders, such as text messages and mobile app notifications, have proven effective in helping individuals stay aligned with their health goals. In addition to prompting action, technology should support real-time health monitoring and provide feedback, which can reinforce positive behaviors and enhance engagement (Tadas and Coyle, 2020).

User Experience

User experience is a critical factor in enabling access to technology for self-management. Key facilitators include a simple login process, clear and intuitive instructions, and rapid familiarization with the system. Technical features such as stability, reliability, and consistent performance further enhance usability. Importantly, some patients prefer portable and discreet technology, as wearing visible or non-inclusive trackers and sensors may contribute to stigma and increase feelings of vulnerability within the community (Moody et al., 2022).

Integrate with Existing Services

Technology serves as a valuable complement to traditional rehabilitation therapy, but it is widely acknowledged that it should enhance – not replace – face-to-face interactions with healthcare providers. Research shows that patients' perceptions of the benefits of technology-based interventions in supporting their recovery are central to successful adoption (Sauerzopf et al., 2024). Ideally, these interventions should leverage digital tools to help patients set meaningful goals and be tailored to their individual needs and contexts. Incorporating elements, such as gamified designs (Papastergiou, 2009) can enhance motivation and engagement, making the intervention both effective and personally relevant.

FRAMEWORKS FOR DESIGNING AND EVALUATING TECHNOLOGY-BASED SELF-MANAGEMENT INTERVENTIONS

Effective self-management in rehabilitation through technology-based interventions requires a rigorous development and evaluation process, guided by one or more well-established frameworks (Booth et al., 2019). The following paragraphs detail several commonly used frameworks that guide the design, implementation, and evaluation of these interventions.

Theoretical Models for Behavior Change

Health-related behavior and behavior change are central to self-management in rehabilitation, as individuals often need to adopt, maintain, or modify behaviors to support participation in daily activities. Health behavior theories help identify key factors to target when promoting behavior change (Byrne, 2020; Czajkowski et al., 2015). There is a broad consensus on the value of theory-driven approaches in designing, implementing, and evaluating health interventions (Glanz and Bishop, 2010). Evidence from prior reviews suggests that technology-based self-management programs that are grounded in theoretical frameworks tend to yield better outcomes across diverse populations (Lau et al., 2022; Lycett et al., 2018).

Many health behavior change theories have been developed to understand individual behaviors and have been used to support self-management interventions. These include the transtheoretical model (Prochaska and Velicer, 1997), self-determination theory (Deci and Ryan, 2012), Theory of Planned Behavior (Ajzen, 1991), health belief model (Janz and Becker, 1984), and social cognitive theory (Bandura, 1991). Among these, social cognitive theory is the most frequently cited conceptual framework in self-management research, particularly due to its emphasis on self-efficacy as a key driver of behavior change (Jones and Riazi, 2011).

Social cognitive theory (Bandura, 1991) emphasizes the role of self-efficacy – an individual's belief in their ability to perform specific behaviors – as a central driver of behavior change. Bandura identified four primary sources of self-efficacy: mastery experiences (successful past performances), vicarious experiences (observing others succeed), verbal persuasion (encouragement or feedback from others), and physiological and emotional states (internal responses during task performance) (Bandura, 1997). In practice, self-management programs grounded in Social Cognitive Theory often enhance stroke survivors' self-efficacy by fostering mastery experiences, supporting goal attainment, and strengthening problem-solving skills (Jones and Riazi, 2011). These interventions may also target other key constructs, such as social support, self-regulation, outcome expectations, and behavior capability. The strength of this theory lies in its consideration of both interpersonal and intrapersonal influences, making it particularly relevant to rehabilitation settings where success depends on interactions among clients, caregivers, and healthcare providers (Nieuwenhuijsen et al., 2006). The widespread influence of Social Cognitive Theory in self-management research is reflected in the frequent use of Stanford University's Chronic Disease Self-Management Program (Lorig et al., 1999), which has served as a foundation for numerous studies in chronic illness and rehabilitation (Lau et al., 2022).

User-Centered Design (UCD)

User-centered design (UCD) is an evidence-based method that emphasizes users' experiences to ensure that products or systems meet their needs, preferences, requirements, and contexts, ultimately helping translate evidence into practical application (Norman, 2013). According to the International Organization for Standardization (ISO), user experience refers to "a person's perceptions and responses resulting from the use or anticipated use of a product, system, or service" (ISO, 2010). UCD promotes the active involvement of target users throughout the design and evaluation processes (Gould and Lewis, 1985). It has become a cornerstone of mobile health development, playing a vital role in enhancing user satisfaction and ensuring that digital health technologies are both usable and effective (Van Velsen et al., 2022).

Gould and Lewis have outlined three key principles of UCD (Gould and Lewis, 1985). First, it is essential to develop a thorough understanding of users, their goals, and the contexts in which they will interact with the technology – this includes early exploration of user characteristics, needs, and environments. Second, a systematic and empirical evaluation is critical, involving representative users testing early versions of the product and providing feedback on their experiences and performance. Third, UCD relies on an iterative design process, with multiple rounds of prototyping, testing, and refinement to continuously improve usability and overall effectiveness.

UCD has been applied in developing digital self-management systems for rehabilitation. For example, a personalized self-management system for post-stroke rehabilitation was created using UCD principles (Mawson et al., 2014). The design process incorporated home visits, focus groups, in-depth interviews, cultural probes, and technology biographies, which were conducted iteratively to inform both the treatment content and the interactive interfaces of the system.

In addition, UCD has been increasingly influencing the development and assessment of eHealth technologies through several structured frameworks, such the Centre for eHealth and Wellbeing Research (CeHRes) Roadmap (Kip et al., 2025; Van Gemert-Pijnen et al., 2011), Intervention Mapping (IM) (Bartholomew et al., 1998), and the Integrate, Design, Assess, and Share (IDEAS) framework (Mummah et al., 2016). Among these, the CeHRes Roadmap is one of the most widely applied (Van Velsen et al., 2022), outlining five key phases where UCD principles are embedded: contextual inquiry, value specification, design, operationalization, and summative evaluation (Van Gemert-Pijnen et al., 2011). Each phase has distinct objectives and methodological guidelines. The CeHRes Roadmap is grounded in six overarching principles (Van Gemert-Pijnen et al., 2011): (1) eHealth development should be a participatory process; (2) it should involve continuous evaluation cycles; (3) it must be closely integrated with implementation; (4) it should account for organizational changes resulting from technology adoption; (5) it should incorporate persuasive design techniques; and (6) it requires advanced methods for assessing impact. For example, the CeHRes Roadmap was recently applied to adapt a digital monitoring system initially designed for home-based self-management among patients with COPD, tailoring it to the context of inpatient geriatric rehabilitation through a co-creation process with stakeholders (Debeij et al., 2025; Van Velsen et al., 2022).

Although IM is not explicitly designed for technology-based interventions, it provides a comprehensive and iterative framework for the systematic development of complex behavioral interventions (Bartholomew et al., 1998). The framework comprises six interconnected steps, beginning with problem identification and progressing through planning, implementation, and evaluation. Each step involves specific tasks that guide researchers and practitioners in integrating theoretical foundations, empirical evidence, and data gathered from target populations. IM also places strong emphasis on active stakeholder engagement throughout the development process to ensure that interventions are contextually appropriate and feasible. This framework has been effectively applied in the design of digital self-management interventions aimed at helping individuals manage chronic symptoms and enhance participation in daily life after stroke (Wong et al., 2023).

These frameworks differ in terminology and structure, but they share a common foundation grounded in the original philosophy of UCD. This foundation emphasizes systematic development, active engagement of end users and stakeholders, and continuous iterative refinement (Van Velsen et al., 2022).

Implementation Science

The Reach, Effectiveness, Adoption, Implementation, Maintenance (RE-AIM) framework was developed to evaluate both the success of implementation and the impact of translating research evidence into real-world settings (Glasgow et al., 1999). It encompasses five key dimensions that guide the evaluation of health interventions. *Reach* refers to the proportion of the target population that participates in the intervention. *Effectiveness (or efficacy)* measures both the immediate and long-term outcomes when the intervention is implemented as intended. *Adoption* assesses the extent to which relevant staff, organizations, or individuals choose to implement the program. *Implementation* examines whether the intervention is delivered as designed and adheres to established protocols in real-world settings. Finally, Maintenance evaluates the sustainability of the intervention over time and its integration into routine practice. Unlike traditional evaluation methods that often focus on short-term outcomes in controlled settings, the RE-AIM framework broadens the scope to emphasize long-term effectiveness and real-world applicability. It encourages researchers, developers, and stakeholders to prioritize external validity, ensuring that interventions are not only effective but also scalable and sustainable beyond research environments (Glasgow et al., 1999).

The RE-AIM framework has been widely applied in the design, evaluation, and reporting of self-management interventions, including those delivered through digital platforms such as web- or app-based programs (Yoshida et al., 2020). For example, RE-AIM was used to evaluate the PRIDE app, a self-management program developed to support individuals living with mild dementia (Lee, 2023). Specifically, this research team used RE-AIM to guide the evaluation of: (1) the program's reach within the target population, (2) its effectiveness in promoting self-management and user engagement, and (3) the potential for adoption in community and healthcare settings.

CURRENT LANDSCAPE OF TECHNOLOGY-BASED SELF-MANAGEMENT INTERVENTIONS

Traditional self-management interventions have primarily relied on educational approaches that teach individuals specific skills to manage chronic conditions. These methods assume that providing information in a didactic format will help patients adopt appropriate behavioral changes and better control their symptoms. However, research has shown that low adherence to self-management interventions is common in most patients (Lau et al., 2022; Newman et al., 2004). This challenge has underscored the need for targeted self-management interventions designed to enhance patient engagement and foster greater autonomy in managing health. One promising solution is harnessing technology to engage individuals in developing self-management skills. This section summarizes findings from several systematic reviews of technology-based self-management interventions for stroke and other chronic conditions, followed by tabulating a few illustrative examples that have demonstrated strong evidence in improving patient engagement, self-efficacy, and health outcomes.

Mobile Health (mHealth) Interventions

mHealth interventions refer to the use of wireless devices and wearable sensors that individuals can wear, carry, or access to monitor their health status or improve health outcomes (Kumar et al., 2013). Among these devices, smartphones have emerged as the most widely used due to their growing computational power and ubiquity. Notably, smartphones are equipped with motion-detecting sensors (e.g., accelerometers and gyroscopes), global positioning system (GPS), Bluetooth, and cloud storage capabilities, all of which can be leveraged to collect health-related data (Becker et al., 2014). In some instances, certain medical conditions require more specialized mobile technologies. For example, the Personalized Self-Managed Rehabilitation System, designed for stroke survivors, incorporates insole sensors into an "intelligent shoe" to gather data on pressure distribution during walking. The collected data can be used to provide real-time feedback to the user about their balance and heel strike, supporting home-based rehabilitation (Mawson et al., 2016).

In the context of stroke, a scoping review summarized mobile technology-based interventions for stroke self-management (Thompson et al., 2023). They showed that the interventions varied across the 26 studies reviewed: 10 (38%) focused on physical exercise (e.g., task-oriented training, balance, and strength), 5 (19%) on risk factor management (e.g., self-monitoring blood pressure, education on stroke risk factors and healthy lifestyle, and communication with health professionals), 3 (12%) on linguistic exercises (e.g., communication strategies and language rehabilitation exercises), 3 (12%) on activities of daily living training (e.g., self-care habit training, problem-solving, and goal setting), 2 (8%) on medication adherence (e.g., reminders), 2 (8%) on stroke education (e.g., emergency response for survival and rehabilitation skills), and 1 (4%) on weight management (e.g., culturally appropriate dietary counseling, goal setting, and calorie monitoring).

A systematic review summarized mHealth interventions to improve pain and functional disability in patients with chronic pain (Moreno-Ligero et al., 2023). Of the 22 studies included, self-management interventions consist of: 9 (41%) with home-based physical activity programs, 8 (36%) with educational sessions and materials, 5 (23%) with relaxation and mind-body interventions, and 4 (18%) with cognitive behavioral therapy. Another review analyzed 17 studies on mHealth self-management interventions for patients with hypertension (Li et al., 2020). They categorized the intervention into the following themes: 17 (100%) provided educational information about hypertension, 17 (100%) included self-monitoring of blood pressure, 15 (88%) offered educational content on a healthy lifestyle (e.g., low-salt diet and exercise), 10 (59%) included reminders for medication adherence, 4 (24%) provided motivational encouragement, 3 (18%) involved feedback from staff and social support, and 1 (6%) focused on stress management.

Telehealth and/or Telemedicine Interventions

Telehealth and/or telemedicine interventions refer to the delivery of healthcare services when patients and healthcare providers are separated by distance (World Health Organization, 2010). While telemedicine typically focuses on remote clinical services, telehealth is a broader term that encompasses both clinical and non-clinical services (The Center for Connected Health Policy). These interventions are commonly used for remote monitoring of physiological data, evaluating health symptoms, and facilitating communication with healthcare professionals through platforms such as telephone and videoconferencing. Importantly, the concept of "distance" in this context extends beyond geography to include temporal, economic, and cultural factors.

Another review summarized telehealth interventions of self-management in stroke survivors (Hwang et al., 2021). Out of the 10 reviewed studies, all (100%) provided education on general knowledge and self-management related to stroke. 9 (90%) offered psychological support focusing on goal setting, action planning, and problem-solving strategies. 7 (70%) implemented remote monitoring with feedback, while another 7 (70%) provided regular follow-up reviews. Additionally, 7 (70%) offered adherence support such as logbooks, reminder messages, and encouragement messages. 5 (50%) shared information on community resources, peer support, and adaptive equipment. 2 (20%) provided exercise training to improve physical function, and another two (20%) offered social support, including peer support, peer mentoring, and group socialization. Recently, a remote technology-support self-management intervention called interactive Stroke Management Augmented Rehabilitation Technologies (iSMART) has proven effective in increasing self-efficacy for managing post-stroke symptoms and applying strategies for active participation, as well as improving post-stroke functional outcomes and community reintegration (Lei et al., 2025; Li et al., 2024). Within this program, multicomponent intervention includes psychoeducation videoconferences, behavioral coaching sessions, and interactive text messages to enhance patient engagement and outcomes. Table 32.1 shows representative examples of some mHealth and telehealth self-management interventions for stroke survivors.

TABLE 32.1
Illustrative Examples of Mobile Health and Telehealth Interventions for Individuals after Stroke

Source and Sample Size	Intervention Goals & Devices	Intervention Structures	Intervention Contents	Key Findings
Mobile Health				
Kamal et al. (2020) (Pakistan) ***Sample size:*** 310	***Goal:*** To improve stroke risk factor control (e.g., blood pressure, blood sugar, and blood cholesterol) mortality, and functional outcomes ***Device:*** Tablet and mobile phone (Android, personally owned)	***Brief name:*** Movies4Stroke ***Number of sessions***: • Videos: 4 times (enrollment, discharge, first month after discharge, and third month after discharge) • SMS reminder messages: two times/ week ***Duration of each session:*** five mins for videos ***Program length:*** three months ***Supervision level:*** self-directed, professional-supported	***Content:*** Education on an introduction to stroke, emergency response for survival, rehabilitation skills, safe swallowing and speaking skills, medications, and stroke prevention	The intervention group demonstrated a significantly lower percentage of participants with high blood pressure, HbA1c levels, and low-density lipoprotein levels (Kamal et al., 2020).
Labovitz et al. (2017) (USA) ***Sample size:*** 28	***Goal:*** To improve medication adherence ***Device:*** Artificial intelligence application (app) via smartphones	***Brief name:*** AiCure ***Number of sessions:*** N.A. ***Duration of each session:*** N.A. ***Program length:*** 12 weeks ***Supervision level:*** self-directed, professional-supported	***Content:*** The provision of medication reminders, dose instructions, visual confirmation of medication ingestion through facial recognition, real-time data encryption and transmission, and connection to staff via SMS or email	Patients with limited experience using a smartphone showed improvements in medication adherence and successful application (Labovitz et al., 2017).

(Continued)

TABLE 32.1 ***(Continued)***
Illustrative Examples of Mobile Health and Telehealth Interventions for Individuals after Stroke

Source and Sample Size	Intervention Goals & Devices	Intervention Structures	Intervention Contents	Key Findings
Telehealth				
Chumbler et al. (2015) (USA) ***Sample size:*** 52	***Goal:*** To instruct patients in functionally based exercises and adaptive strategies ***Device:*** Telephone and messaging	***Brief name:*** STeleR ***Number and duration of sessions:*** • 3 1-hour home visits (tele-visits) • 5 telephone intervention calls • Daily message ***Program length***: three months ***Supervision level:*** Professional-directed	***Content:*** Telephone-delivered: • Exploration of potential barriers and identification solutions • Instructions for the exercises and adaptive strategies In-home messaging device • Self-report measurement • Instant feedback with positive encouragement for exercise adherence	The STeleR intervention significantly enhanced physical function, with benefits lasting up to three months (Chumbler et al., 2015).
Li et al. (2024) & Lei et al. (2025) (USA) ***Sample size***: 24	***Goal:*** To examine the feasibility and preliminary effects of the iSMART intervention on post-stroke function ***Device:*** Videoconferencing platform, SMS, and website-based, clinician-facing platform	***Brief name:*** iSMART ***Number and duration of sessions:*** • Skill-building training: 2.5-hour session/week • Human coaching: 0.5-hour/week • Interactive text messaging: up to three tips, daily check-in message to report mood states, and weekly motivational messages. ***Program length:*** 12 weeks ***Supervision level:*** Professional-directed	***Context:*** • ***Skill-building training***: Psychoeducation on self-management strategies (e.g., problem-solving, decision-making, communication, accommodation, and emotion and symptom management) • ***Human coaching***: Valued goal setting, activity scheduling, & action planning • ***Interactive text messaging:*** Goal reminders and monitoring, mood monitoring, self-management tips, ecological momentary assessment of needs, and motivational messages	iSMART participants showed improvements in self-efficacy and post-stroke functioning, including hand function, mobility, cognition, communication, social participation, and community re-integration (Lei et al., 2025; Li et al., 2024)

In addition, a systematic meta-review identified telehealth-mediated self-management interventions for six chronic conditions, including type 1 and type 2 diabetes, heart failure, asthma, COPD, and cancer (Hanlon et al., 2017). Interventions included in this meta-review can be grouped into (1) patient education and information provision, (2) remote monitoring with feedback, (3) facilitation of remote clinical review, (4) adherence support (e.g., medication and lifestyle intervention adherence), and (5) psychological support. Their findings indicate that, although telehealth-based self-management interventions are not always better than traditional in-person care, they are a safe alternative for delivering self-management support, especially in conditions like heart failure and Type 2 diabetes where the evidence is more robust.

TECHNOLOGIES UTILIZED IN SELF-MANAGEMENT INTERVENTIONS

Digital Technologies and Their Applications in Self-Management

The field of rehabilitation technology is rapidly evolving, with new innovations transforming how people manage their health independently and offering solutions for accessible, high-quality, and affordable healthcare services (World Health Organization, 2018). Supported by clinical supervision and assistance, rehabilitation technologies help individuals actively manage their recovery journey (Abedi et al., 2024; Pearce et al., 2024; Sands and Finn, 2025; World Health Organization, 2018). Technology-based interventions offer several advantages over traditional treatments for people with disabilities and chronic conditions. Unlike traditional rehabilitation approaches that focus primarily on face-to-face therapeutic sessions with clinicians, technology-based methods incorporate digital health tools into interventions that can be more easily monitored and tailored to individual needs. These technology-based solutions also increase user motivation (Strubbia et al., 2020) and provide particular benefits to people in rural areas who may have limited access to traditional healthcare services (Carswell and Rea, 2021). Staff shortages create barriers to patient education; however, technologies solve this challenge by delivering patient education outside the clinical setting (Ingram et al., 2025; Webb et al., 2020).

Rehabilitation professionals are increasingly integrating digital health technologies to support individuals with disabilities and chronic conditions in developing self-management strategies. These technologies offer personalized education, symptom monitoring (e.g., blood glucose, blood pressure, fall detection), behavioral prompts (e.g., goal-setting, reflective journaling), and interactive feedback (Ingram et al., 2025; Lee et al., 2018; Ramey et al., 2019; Tadas and Coyle, 2020). Common tools include video-based platforms, text-messaging, chatbots, mobile applications, and wearable sensors. These tools typically feature educational content, real-time symptom tracking, medication or exercise reminders, and motivational feedback, all of which enhance self-efficacy and promote sustained engagement in self-management behaviors (Cheung et al., 2023; Navarro et al., 2021; Tadas and Coyle, 2020). Many also provide condition-specific educational resources and incorporate a coach to support goal setting and action planning, thereby forming a closed-loop system aligned with core self-management principles (Lorig and Holman, 2003). This section will present several existing technologies that support self-management interventions in rehabilitation.

Video-Based Platforms

Video conferencing platforms such as Zoom and Microsoft Teams play a pivotal role in facilitating remote rehabilitation by enabling live consultations, virtual psychoeducation sessions, and supervised exercise sessions. These platforms allow clinicians to guide and monitor progress in real time, especially for individuals with disabilities and chronic conditions (Deshpande et al., 2023). Moreover, video conferencing fosters supportive learning environments by promoting meaningful interactions between clinicians and patients, as well as peer-to-peer engagement. This collaborative exchange of health-related information encourages problem-solving and helps individuals overcome barriers to applying self-management strategies in daily life (Morgado et al., 2024; Wong et al., 2023).

While some interventions incorporate pre-recorded educational videos, commonly delivered through study-specific websites or mobile applications, to demonstrate self-management strategies for home-based rehabilitation (Ingram et al., 2025). Research shows that these video modules can significantly enhance users' knowledge, self-efficacy, and health behaviors across a range of chronic conditions, including multiple sclerosis, diabetes, heart failure, and rheumatologic disorders (Deshpande et al., 2023; Van Denend et al., 2022; Xie et al., 2020). Moreover, interventions, asynchronous video formats allow users to engage with rehabilitation content at their convenience, offering flexibility that can improve adherence throughout the recovery process (Navarro et al., 2021).

Text Messaging and Chatbots

Text messaging (SMS) and chatbots are commonly used to send reminders, motivational notes, and brief educational content that enhance user motivation, engagement, and behavioral outcomes (Cheung et al., 2023). The goal of using text messages and chatbots is for quick understanding, personal accountability, and social connections, while also providing engagement support that does not overwhelm the target users (Cheung et al., 2023). Some text messaging- and chatbot-based interventions incorporate automated and interactive features to provide personalized feedback to support self-management behaviors in individuals with chronic conditions (Laymouna et al., 2024; Ramey et al., 2019; Tadas and Coyle, 2020). In stroke rehabilitation, Wong and colleagues have incorporated the SMS text messaging component into iSMART, along with psychoeducation and coaching, to support self-management behaviors among stroke survivors (Wong et al., 2023). Specifically, based on behavioral change techniques (Michie et al., 2013), this research team has developed different types of SMS text messages, including goal reminders, brief self-management education tips, general motivation, and check-in messages, to foster the practice of self-management strategies among stroke survivors.

Mobile Applications

Several studies have developed and tested mobile applications for self-management, such as SmartLossTM, iMHere, and SCI-Ex, in rehabilitation. These applications incorporate evidence-based education for people with disabilities and chronic conditions and provide multifunctional support to foster the recovery process (Ramey et al., 2019). Nowadays, most mobile self-management applications let users track symptoms, set and monitor goals, get medication or exercise reminders, detect and log falls, log workouts or activity targets, and view progress. Information gathered from these mobile applications can help healthcare providers modify treatment details and components (Maillart et al., 2020). Some applications also include features that enable sending personalized feedback and can adjust the treatment for different age groups and functional levels based on predefined rules. (Ingram et al., 2025; Ramey et al., 2019; Strubbia et al., 2020; Tadas and Coyle, 2020).

Wearable Sensors

Wearable sensors, such as commercially available activity trackers (e.g., Fitbit, Apple Watch, Garmin) and heart rate monitors, are widely used to measure step count, physical activity levels, and sleep quality (Carswell and Rea, 2021). These devices provide real-time, goal-oriented feedback to both users and healthcare providers, supporting self-directed rehabilitation and enabling effective progress monitoring. Their utility is particularly significant in home-based and rural settings, where access to therapeutic services may be limited (Carswell and Rea, 2021; Latif et al., 2024; Lee et al., 2021; Toh et al., 2023).

Furthermore, recent research has demonstrated the effectiveness of wearable sensors in supporting self-management in rehabilitation, especially for individuals with neurological conditions (Bonanno et al., 2025; Woelfle et al., 2023). A scoping review has highlighted how wearable sensors are utilized to track gait and mobility of individuals with multiple sclerosis in real-world environments (Woelfle et al., 2023). Data from wearable sensors help users recognize change in their condition, adjust activity levels, and engage in personalized rehabilitation strategies. Similarly, another review has examined the use of wearable sensors to assess risk fall in neurological disorders (Bonanno et al., 2025). This review emphasizes how these wearable sensors can detect early signs of mobility impairment and provide actionable feedback, empowering users to engage in proactive self-management and fall prevention strategies. These applications underscore the growing role of wearable technologies in enhancing autonomy and health outcomes for individuals managing long-term disabilities and chronic conditions.

Artificial Intelligence and Machine Learning

Artificial intelligence (AI) and machine learning (ML) are increasingly utilized across various medical domains, including rehabilitation medicine (Wei and Wu, 2023). AI-powered systems use predictive analytics to enable precise risk stratification and the development of tailored treatment plans, allowing individuals to receive personalized treatment recommendations based on their unique health profiles and recovery trajectories (Abedi et al., 2024; Ingram et al., 2025). Additionally, intelligent chatbots integrated with generative AI and large language models deliver natural, human-like text and voice interactions, providing continuous, personalized guidance and support without requiring constant clinician involvement (Cheng and Jiang, 2020; Kretzschmar et al., 2019; Laymouna et al., 2024).

Additionally, AI-enabled wearable sensors are emerging as powerful tools in rehabilitation, especially for individuals with motor impairments. A recent review demonstrates that AI algorithms embedded in wearable sensors can identify movement patterns, evaluate motor symptoms, and deliver personalized feedback to individuals with Parkinson's disease (Li et al., 2025). These innovative technologies empower individuals to actively manage their condition, track progress, and adjust activities based on real-time data. These results demonstrate the potential of AI and ML to improve self-management by enabling real-time monitoring and adaptive feedback in the rehabilitation process.

Other Emerging Technologies

Emerging and future technologies hold significant promise for advancing self-management and rehabilitation interventions. These include, but not limited to, computer vision for exercise form correction and assessment (Mennella et al., 2023), smart home devices for activity monitoring and fall detection (Pais et al., 2020), virtual and augmented reality for immersive therapy and training experiences (Berton et al., 2020; Gazzoni and Cerone, 2020; Muñoz-Tomás et al., 2023), and robotics for enhancing gait and mobility rehabilitation (Carpino et al., 2018; Rodríguez-Fernández et al., 2021). While these technologies offer considerable potential, future clinical trials are warranted to evaluate their effectiveness.

FUTURE DIRECTIONS

Opportunities for Innovation and Advancement

Integration of Multiple Technologies for Holistic Care

The future of rehabilitation technology depends on strategically combining various technological platforms to build comprehensive, holistic care systems that enable individuals to manage their health independently. This technological integration could help reduce disparities between countries and bring health benefits to nations with fewer resources, ultimately promoting more equitable access to rehabilitation services (Andrade et al., 2025).

The convergence of AI, wearable sensors, VR and AR, robotics, and digital therapeutics offers unprecedented opportunities to create seamless, interconnected systems that deliver continuous, personalized support for rehabilitation goals (Deshpande et al., 2023; Ingram et al., 2025). These integrated platforms can generate collaborative effects where data from multiple sources guides more advanced treatment recommendations, allowing individuals to receive coordinated care that addresses physical, cognitive, and psychosocial aspects of recovery (De La Torre et al., 2025).

Personalization and Adaptive Learning Algorithms

Personalization is a crucial cutting-edge area in developing rehabilitation technology, with adaptive learning algorithms expected to deliver truly personalized self-management experiences

(De La Torre et al., 2025). These intelligent systems can continuously learn from user behavior, physiological responses, and clinical outcomes to refine treatment recommendations in real-time (Kumar et al., 2023; Laymouna et al., 2024). By analyzing adherence patterns, progress markers, and user preferences, adaptive algorithms can modify exercise protocols, adjust difficulty levels, provide targeted motivational interventions, and predict potential setbacks before they occur (Gönül et al., 2021). This level of personalization guarantees that self-management tools remain engaging, relevant, and effective throughout the rehabilitation journey, adjusting to changing needs and circumstances as individuals work toward their goals.

Scalability and Cost-Effectiveness of Digital Health Technologies

The scalability and cost-effectiveness of digital interventions offer transformative opportunities to expand access to high-quality rehabilitation services (Bolinger and Tyl, 2024; Cheung et al., 2023). Unlike traditional in-person clinical models, digital self-management platforms can simultaneously serve an unlimited number of users across multiple stakeholder groups while maintaining consistent quality and evidence-based treatment protocol (Morimoto et al., 2022). Scalability is crucial for meeting rehabilitation needs in underserved areas, where conventional services are often inaccessible or too costly (Goldstein et al., 2023). Digital interventions can expand access to specialized rehabilitation expertise, providing evidence-based self-management tools to individuals regardless of their location or financial situation circumstances (Andrade et al., 2025).

Addressing Gaps and Challenges in Research

Need for More Rigorous Randomized Controlled Trials

Even though digital health technologies show great promise for self-management, significant research gaps still need to be filled to build a strong evidence base and improve their clinical use. Most current studies on digital technologies are small, short-term, and often carry a high risk of bias (e.g., poor data security and privacy measures, lack of healthcare professional engagement in technology development, insufficient validation from pilot studies (Cucciniello et al., 2021; Wang et al., 2017). These limitations lead to inconsistent findings with limited generalizability. This requires conducting more rigorous, large-sample, high-quality randomized controlled trials (RCTs) to establish conclusive evidence of efficacy and effectiveness (Fleming et al., 2019). However, traditional RCTs are structured and inflexible, while digital health technologies are adaptable and need frequent updates based on specific contexts. Therefore, there is an urgent need to develop more flexible evaluation strategies that can reflect the changing nature of digital technologies (Bolinger and Tyl, 2024; Mohr et al., 2015). These studies must employ appropriate control conditions, adequate sample sizes, and validated outcome measures to produce the high-quality evidence needed for clinical adoption and regulatory approval (Cucciniello et al., 2021; Kunkoski et al., 2025; Mäder et al., 2023).

Long-Term Efficacy and Sustainability Studies

Research on long-term efficacy and sustainability is another key priority, as existing studies mainly focus on short-term outcomes that might not accurately represent real-world implementation challenges (Isernia et al., 2019). When designing technology-based rehabilitation programs, adherence incentives must be carefully considered. Lower treatment adherence may result from the physical and cognitive fatigue that this population experiences both during treatment sessions and in daily life (Heesen et al., 2015; Isernia et al., 2019). Understanding the sustainability of technology-mediated behavior changes is essential for ensuring that initial improvements made during rehabilitation are maintained over the long term. Conversely, over-relying on digital technologies raises concerns, as electronic devices have been strongly linked to both physical and mental health issues

(De La Torre et al., 2025). Ensuring proper implementation of digital health technologies is essential to maximize their effectiveness.

Research on Equitable Access and Digital Inclusion

The evidence base for technologies varies greatly across populations: while these technologies show promise for rehabilitation in people with physical disabilities, their effectiveness for mental health conditions remains under-researched. For example, the comparative efficacy of new digital interventions (e.g., internet-delivered cognitive behavioral therapy, ecological momentary interventions delivered by smartphones or VR) versus traditional face-to-face treatment for depression and anxiety has not been definitively established (Hollis et al., 2018).

Many healthcare providers report receiving insufficient education on digital technologies and express a strong desire for additional training. Without proper training, the full potential of these technologies to improve health outcomes cannot be achieved. Effective training for healthcare providers is essential to deliver safe, efficient, and high-quality care, yet most medical schools do not include digital health technologies in their curriculum (Borges Do Nascimento et al., 2023; Jidkov et al., 2019). A comprehensive and actionable international digital health competencies framework should be adapted for health professional training and education globally (Borges Do Nascimento et al., 2023; Fleming et al., 2019; Rauzi et al., 2025). Research on equitable access and digital inclusion has become increasingly urgent as technology-based interventions grow more common in rehabilitation practice. Digital divides based on age, socioeconomic status (SES), education level, language barriers, geographic location, disability status, and technological literacy can worsen existing healthcare disparities if not properly addressed (Andrade et al., 2025).

Addressing digital health literacy is essential for the successful deployment of digital health interventions. Because low literacy can prevent individuals from participating effectively in research, it is important to examine how different populations interact with rehabilitation technologies, identify access and engagement barriers, and create inclusive design principles that ensure technology benefits are distributed equitably across diverse user groups (Bolinger and Tyl, 2024). Integrating digital health education into school curricula, vocational programs, and adult education platforms is essential for building generational digital fluency, especially given their low cost and potential significant impact (Andrade et al., 2025; Carter et al., 2021). Limited internet access has also sped up rural-urban disparities in health information sharing, since only 29% of the population in Africa has access to mobile Internet (Cariolle, 2021). Online health interventions through real-time consultations or video telehealth sessions are still hard to access for people in low- and middle-income countries who lack the necessary technology or internet access (Cariolle, 2021; Monlezun et al., 2024).

Ethical Considerations, Data Privacy, and Security

As rehabilitation technologies become more complex and data-driven, ethical issues, data privacy, and security challenges remain critical and require ongoing research attention (Andrade et al., 2025; Cordeiro, 2021). The collection of continuous physiological and behavioral data through self-management platforms raises complex questions about data ownership, consent, and privacy protection (Cordeiro, 2021). Research must address how to balance the benefits of comprehensive data collection with individual privacy rights, establish appropriate governance frameworks for sensitive health information, and ensure that vulnerable populations are protected from potential exploitation or discrimination based on rehabilitation technology data (Cordeiro, 2021; Maaß et al., 2024) Although many countries have enacted Data Protection Acts, LMICs often lack the enforcement mechanisms, technical infrastructure, and monitoring systems necessary for comprehensive data protection implementation (Andrade et al., 2025). Another significant issue is bias in machine learning models. Since datasets are mainly trained in high-income countries, they fail to include the genetic, behavioral, and socioenvironmental traits specific to low- and middle-income countries, leading to misclassification and misdiagnosis. (Weissglass, 2022). To ensure ethical digital health deployment, validating context and maintaining transparency in algorithm design are essential (Andrade et al., 2025; Benzinger et al., 2023; Cordeiro, 2021; Weissglass, 2022).

Potential for Widespread Implementation and Impact

Policy and Regulatory Considerations for Technology Adoption

The transition from research innovation to widespread clinical adoption requires careful attention to policy and regulatory considerations that may either help or hinder technology adoption. Policy initiatives must also address liability issues, scope of practice for professionals, and integration requirements with existing healthcare systems (Essén et al., 2022). Regulatory frameworks must continually adapt to the unique features of digital rehabilitation interventions while ensuring safety and effectiveness standards (Fleming et al., 2019). Such efforts involve developing and updating standards specifically designed for software-based interventions (De La Torre et al., 2025; Fleming et al., 2019); identify and serve areas' needs for broadband expansion (Goldstein et al., 2023); develop reimbursement systems that recognize the value of self-management technologies (Essén et al., 2022; Rauzi et al., 2025); and establishing quality standards to guarantee consistent performance across various platforms and providers (Andrade et al., 2025; Benzinger et al., 2023; Cordeiro, 2021; Weissglass, 2022).

Training Healthcare Professionals in Digital Health Competencies

Training healthcare professionals in digital health skills is an essential implementation need that extends far beyond basic technological literacy (Borges Do Nascimento et al., 2023). Clinicians must develop a thorough understanding of how to incorporate self-management technologies into comprehensive care plans, interpret data produced by digital platforms, and deliver appropriate support and oversight for technology-mediated interventions (Rauzi et al., 2025). This requires fundamental changes in rehabilitation education curricula (Borges Do Nascimento et al., 2023), continuing professional development programs, and clinical practice guidelines. Healthcare professionals should also develop competencies in digital health equity, ensuring they can identify and address barriers that may prevent specific populations from effectively utilizing self-management technologies and sustained adoption (Rauzi et al., 2025).

Global Health Implications and Access in Low-Resource Settings

Advances in rehabilitation technology have great potential to meet rehabilitation needs in resource-limited settings where traditional healthcare infrastructure might be lacking (Andrade et al., 2025). Self-management technologies are expected to surpass the limitations of traditional service models by offering evidence-based rehabilitation interventions in settings without specialized clinicians (Laymouna et al., 2024). However, successful implementation across diverse global settings requires careful attention to cultural adaptation, local infrastructure limitations, and sustainable financing models. Research and development efforts should focus on solutions that work effectively in resource-limited environments while ensuring cultural relevance, local appropriateness, and sustainability (Andrade et al., 2025; Cordeiro, 2021).

The convergence of these opportunities and challenges marks a critical turning point for rehabilitation technology. Achieving the transformative potential of self-management tools will rely on coordinated efforts across research, policy, education, and implementation sectors. By closing current gaps and leveraging emerging opportunities, the field can move toward a future where advanced, personalized, and accessible self-management solutions empower individuals to reach optimal rehabilitation outcomes, regardless of their health conditions or geographic locations.

REFERENCES

Abedi, A., Colella, T. J. F., Pakosh, M. & Khan, S. S. 2024. Artificial intelligence-driven virtual rehabilitation for people living in the community: A scoping review. *NPJ Digit Med*, 7, 201.

Ajzen, I. 1991. The theory of planned behavior. *Organ Behav Hum Decis Process*, 50, 179–211.

Allegrante, J. P., Wells, M. T. & Peterson, J. C. 2019. Interventions to support behavioral self-management of chronic diseases. *Annu Rev Public Health*, 40, 127–146.

Andrade, J. B. C., Fagundes, T. P., Katsuyama, E. & Silva, G. S. 2025. Digital health in low-resource settings: Comprehensive challenges and opportunities with a focus on stroke care. *Stroke*, 57(1), 245–253.

Arias López, M. D. P., Ong, B. A., Borrat Frigola, X., Fernández, A. L., Hicklent, R. S., Obeles, A. J. T., Rocimo, A. M. & Celi, L. A. 2023. Digital literacy as a new determinant of health: A scoping review. *PLOS Digit Health*, 2, e0000279.

Bandura, A. 1991. Social cognitive theory of self-regulation. *Organ Behav Hum Decis Process*, 50, 248–287.

Bandura, A. (1997). Sources of self-efficacy. In: *Self-Efficacy: The Exercise of Control*, Vol. 1, 79–113. New York, NY: Freeman & Company.

Bartholomew, L. K., Parcel, G. S. & Kok, G. 1998. Intervention mapping: A process for developing theory- and evidence-based health education programs. *Health Educ Behav*, 25, 545–563.

Becker, S., Miron-Shatz, T., Schumacher, N., Krocza, J., Diamantidis, C. & Albrecht, U. V. 2014. mHealth 2.0: Experiences, possibilities, and perspectives. *JMIR Mhealth Uhealth,*, 2, e24.

Benzinger, L., Ursin, F., Balke, W.-T., Kacprowski, T. & Salloch, S. 2023. Should artificial intelligence be used to support clinical ethical decision-making? A systematic review of reasons. *BMC Med Ethics*, 24, 48.

Berton, A., Longo, U. G., Candela, V., Fioravanti, S., Giannone, L., Arcangeli, V., Alciati, V., Berton, C., Facchinetti, G., Marchetti, A., Schena, E., De Marinis, M. G. & Denaro, V. 2020. Virtual reality, augmented reality, gamification, and telerehabilitation: Psychological impact on orthopedic Patients' rehabilitation. *J Clin Med*, 9, 2567.

Bolinger, E. & Tyl, B. 2024. Key considerations for designing clinical studies to evaluate digital health solutions. *J Med Internet Res*, 26, e54518.

Bonanno, M., Ielo, A., De Pasquale, P., Celesti, A., De Nunzio, A. M., Quartarone, A. & Calabrò, R. S. 2025. Use of wearable sensors to assess fall risk in neurological disorders: Systematic review. *JMIR Mhealth Uhealth*, 13, e67265.

Booth, V., Hood-Moore, V., Hancox, J. E., Logan, P. & Robinson, K. R. 2019. Systematic scoping review of frameworks used to develop rehabilitation interventions for older adults. *BMJ Open*, 9, e024185.

Borges Do Nascimento, I. J., Abdulazeem, H., Vasanthan, L. T., Martinez, E. Z., Zucoloto, M. L., Østengaard, L., Azzopardi-Muscat, N., Zapata, T. & Novillo-Ortiz, D. 2023. Barriers and facilitators to utilizing digital health technologies by healthcare professionals. *NPJ Digit Med*, 6, 161.

Boyle C. 2022. How do you meme?: Using memes for information literacy instruction. *Ref. Libr.*, 63(3), 82–101.

Byrne, M. 2020. Gaps and priorities in advancing methods for health behaviour change research. *Health Psychol. Rev.*, *14*(1), 165–175.

Cariolle, J. 2021. International connectivity and the digital divide in Sub-Saharan Africa. *Inf Econ Policy*, 55, 100901.

Carpino, G., Pezzola, A., Urbano, M. & Guglielmelli, E. 2018. Assessing effectiveness and costs in robot-mediated lower limbs rehabilitation: A meta-analysis and state of the art. *J Healthcare Eng*, 2018, 7492024.

Carswell, C. & Rea, P. M. 2021. What the tech? The management of neurological dysfunction through the use of digital technology. *Adv Exp Med Biol*, 1317, 131–145.

Carter, H., Araya, R., Anjur, K., Deng, D. & Naslund, J. A. 2021. The emergence of digital mental health in low-income and middle-income countries: A review of recent advances and implications for the treatment and prevention of mental disorders. *J Psychiatr Res*, 133, 223–246.

Cheng, Y. & Jiang, H. 2020. AI-Powered mental health chatbots: Examining users' motivations, active communicative action and engagement after mass-shooting disasters. *J Contingencies Crisis Manag*, 28, 339–354.

Cheung, N. W., Redfern, J., Thiagalingam, A., Hng, T.-M., Marschner, S., Haider, R., Faruquie, S., Von Huben, A., She, S., Mcintyre, D., Cho, J.-G. & Chow, C. K. 2023. Effect of Mobile phone text messaging self-management support for patients with diabetes or coronary heart disease in a chronic disease management program (SupportMe) on blood pressure: Pragmatic randomized controlled trial. *J Med Internet Res*, 25, e38275.

Chumbler, N. R., Li, X., Quigley, P., Morey, M. C., Rose, D., Griffiths, P., Sanford, J. & Hoenig, H. 2015. A randomized controlled trial on stroke telerehabilitation: The effects on falls self-efficacy and satisfaction with care. *J Telemed Telecare*, 21, 139–43.

Cordeiro, J. V. 2021. Digital technologies and data science as health enablers: An outline of appealing promises and compelling ethical, legal, and social challenges. *Front Med*, 8, 647897.

Cucciniello, M., Petracca, F., Ciani, O. & Tarricone, R. 2021. Development features and study characteristics of mobile health apps in the management of chronic conditions: A systematic review of randomised trials. *NPJ Digit Med*, 4, 144.

Czajkowski, S. M., Powell, L. H., Adler, N., Naar-King, S., Reynolds, K. D., Hunter, C. M., Laraia, B., Olster, D. H., Perna, F. M., Peterson J. C. & Epel, E. 2015. From ideas to efficacy: The ORBIT model for developing behavioral treatments for chronic diseases. *Health Psychol*. 34(10), 971.

Debeij, S. M., Van Dam Van Isselt, E. F., Kasteleyn, M. J., Krabben, H. V., Siemonsma, P., Achterberg, W. P. & Haaksma, M. L. 2025. Adapting a digital monitoring system for self-management to geriatric COPD rehabilitation: A participatory mixed method study. *Digit Health*, 11, 20552076251343782.

Deci, E. L. & Ryan, R. M. 2012. Self-determination theory. *In:* Handbook of Theories of Social Psychology, Vol. 1, 416–436. New York, NY: Sage Publications.

De La Torre, K., Min, S., Lee, H. & Kang, D. 2025. The application of preventive medicine in the future digital health era. *J Med Internet Res*, 27, e59165.

Deshpande, N., Wu, M., Kelly, C., Woodrick, N., Werner, D. A., Volerman, A. & Press, V. G. 2023. Video-based educational interventions for patients with chronic illnesses: Systematic review. *J Med Internet Res*, 25, e41092.

Egan, K. J. & Pot, A. M. 2016. Encouraging innovation for assistive health technologies in dementia: Barriers, enablers and next steps to be taken. *J Am Med Dir Assoc*, 17, 357–63.

Essén, A., Stern, A. D., Haase, C. B., Car, J., Greaves, F., Paparova, D., Vandeput, S., Wehrens, R. & Bates, D. W. 2022. Health app policy: International comparison of nine countries' approaches. *NPJ Digit Med*, 5, 31. https://doi.org/10.1038/s41746-022-00573-1

Fleming, G. A., Petrie, J. R., Bergenstal, R. M., Holl, R. W., Peters, A. L. & Heinemann, L. 2019. Diabetes digital app technology: Benefits, challenges, and recommendations. A consensus report by the European association for the study of diabetes (EASD) and the American diabetes association (ADA) diabetes technology working group. *Diabetes Care*, 43, 250–260.

Forducey, P. G., Glueckauf, R. L., Bergquist, T. F., Maheu, M. M. & Yutsis, M. 2012. Telehealth for persons with severe functional disabilities and their caregivers: Facilitating self-care management in the home setting. *Psychol Serv*, 9, 144–62.

Gazzoni, M. & Cerone, G. L. 2020. Augmented reality biofeedback for muscle activation monitoring: Proof of concept. In T. Jarm, A. Cvetkoska, S. Mahnič-Kalamiza, & D. Miklavcic (eds.), *8th European medical and biological engineering conference*. EMBEC 2020. IFMBE Proceedings. Springer, Cham, 143–150. https://doi.org/10.1007/978-3-030-64610-3_17

Glanz, K. & Bishop, D. B. 2010. The role of behavioral science theory in development and implementation of public health interventions. *Annu. Rev. Public Health*, 31(1), 399–418.

Glasgow, R. E., Vogt, T. M. & Boles, S. M. 1999. Evaluating the public health impact of health promotion interventions: The RE-AIM framework. *Am J Public Health*, 89, 1322–1327.

Glueckauf, R. L. & Lustria, M. L. A. 2008. E-health self-care interventions for persons with chronic illnesses: Review and future directions. *In:* Parker, J. & Thorson, E. (eds.) *Health communication in the new media landscape*. New York: Springer.

Goldstein, S. P., Tovar, A., Espel-Huynh, H. M. & Stowers, K. C. 2023. Applying a social determinants of health framework to guide digital innovations that reduce disparities in chronic disease. *Psychosom Med*, 85, 659–669.

Gönül, S., Namli, T., Coşar, A. & Toroslu I, H. 2021. A reinforcement learning based algorithm for personalization of digital, just-in-time, adaptive interventions. *Artif Intell Med*, 115, 102062.

Gould, J. D. & Lewis, C. 1985. Designing for usability: Key principles and what designers think. *Commun ACM*, 28, 300–311.

Grady, P. A. & Gough, L. L. 2014. Self-management: A comprehensive approach to management of chronic conditions. *Am J Public Health*, 104, e25-31.

Hanlon, P., Daines, L., Campbell, C., Mckinstry, B., Weller, D. & Pinnock, H. 2017. Telehealth interventions to support self-management of long-term conditions: A systematic metareview of diabetes, heart failure, asthma, chronic obstructive pulmonary disease, and cancer. *J Med Internet Res*, 19, e172.

Heesen, C., Bruce, J., Gearing, R., Moss-Morris, R., Weinmann, J., Hamalainen, P., Motl, R., Dalgas, U., Kos, D. & Visioli, F. 2015. Adherence to behavioural interventions in multiple sclerosis: Follow-up meeting report (AD@ MS-2). *Mult Scler J Exp Transl Clin*, 1, 2055217315585333.

Hollis, C., Sampson, S., Simons, L., Davies, E. B., Churchill, R., Betton, V., Butler, D., Chapman, K., Easton, K., Gronlund, T. A., Kabir, T., Rawsthorne, M., Rye, E. & Tomlin, A. 2018. Identifying research priorities for digital technology in mental health care: Results of the James Lind Alliance priority setting partnership. *Lancet Psychiatry*, 5, 845–854.

Hwang, N. K., Park, J. S. & Chang, M. Y. 2021. Telehealth interventions to support self-management in stroke survivors: A systematic review. *Healthcare (Basel)*, 9, 472. https://www.mdpi.com/2227-9032/9/4/472

Ingram, T. A., Barnett, R., Shakaib, N., Jones, S., Sengupta, R. & Rouse, P. C. 2025. Rehabilitation interventions delivered via telehealth to support self-management of rheumatic and musculoskeletal disease: A scoping review. *Arthritis Rheumatol.* https://www.iso.org/standard/77520.html

Isernia, S., Pagliari, C., Jonsdottir, J., Castiglioni, C., Gindri, P., Gramigna, C., Palumbo, G., Salza, M., Molteni, F. & Baglio, F. 2019. Efficiency and patient-reported outcome measures from clinic to home: The human empowerment aging and disability program for digital-health rehabilitation. *Front Neurol*, 10, 1206.

ISO. 2010. *9241–210, Ergonomics of human-system interaction – Part 210: Human-centred design for interactive systems* [Online]. Available: http://www.iso.org [Accessed].

Janz, N. K. & Becker, M. H. 1984. The health belief model: A decade later. *Health Educ Q*, 11, 1–47.

Jarvis, F., Clemson, L. M. & Mackenzie, L. 2017. Technology for dementia: Attitudes and practices of occupational therapists in providing assistive technology for way finding. *Disabil Rehabil Assist Technol*, 12, 373–377.

Jidkov, L., Alexander, M., Bark, P., Williams, J. G., Kay, J., Taylor, P., Hemingway, H. & Banerjee, A. 2019. Health informatics competencies in postgraduate medical education and training in the UK: A mixed methods study. *BMJ Open*, 9, e025460.

Jones, F. & Riazi, A. 2011. Self-efficacy and self-management after stroke: A systematic review. *Disabil Rehabil*, 33, 797–810.

Kamal, A., Khoja, A., Usmani, B., Magsi, S., Malani, A., Peera, Z., Sattar, S., Ahmed Akram, M., Shahnawaz, S., Zulfiqar, M., Muqeet, A., Zaidi, F., Sayani, S., Artani, A., Azam, I. & Saleem, S. 2020. Effect of 5-minute movies shown via a mobile phone app on risk factors and mortality after stroke in a low- to middle-income country: Randomized controlled trial for the stroke caregiver dyad education intervention (Movies4Stroke). *JMIR Mhealth Uhealth*, 8, e12113.

Kip, H., Beerlage-De Jong, N., Van Gemert-Pijnen, L. & Kelders, S. M. 2025. The CeHRes roadmap 2.0: Update of a holistic framework for development, implementation, and evaluation of eHealth technologies. *J Med Internet Res*, 27, e59601.

Kretzschmar, K., Tyroll, H., Pavarini, G., Manzini, A., Singh, I. & Group, N. Y. P. S. A. 2019. Can your phone be your therapist? Young people's ethical perspectives on the use of fully automated conversational agents (chatbots) in mental health support. *Biomed Inform Insights*, 11, 1178222619829083.

Kumar, S., Nilsen, W. J., Abernethy, A., Atienza, A., Patrick, K., Pavel, M., Riley, W. T., Shar, A., Spring, B., Spruijt-Metz, D., Hedeker, D., Honavar, V., Kravitz, R., Lefebvre, R. C., Mohr, D. C., Murphy, S. A., Quinn, C., Shusterman, V. & Swendeman, D. 2013. Mobile health technology evaluation: The mHealth evidence workshop. *Am J Prev Med*, 45, 228–236.

Kumar, Y., Koul, A., Singla, R. & Ijaz, M. F. 2023. Artificial intelligence in disease diagnosis: A systematic literature review, synthesizing framework and future research agenda. *J Ambient Intell Humaniz Comput*, 14, 8459–8486.

Kunkoski, E., Saha, A. & Kam, M. M. 2025. FDA perspective on the importance of digital health technologies in clinical trials. *JAMA Health Forum*, 6, e250165–e250165.

Labovitz, D. L., Shafner, L., Reyes Gil, M., Virmani, D. & Hanina, A. 2017. Using artificial intelligence to reduce the risk of nonadherence in patients on anticoagulation therapy. *Stroke*, 48, 1416–1419.

Latif, A., Al Janabi, H. F., Joshi, M., Fusari, G., Shepherd, L., Darzi, A. & Leff, D. R. 2024. Use of commercially available wearable devices for physical rehabilitation in healthcare: A systematic review. *BMJ Open*, 14, e084086.

Lau, S. C., Judycki, S., Mix, M., Depaul, O., Tomazin, R., Hardi, A., Wong, A. W. & Baum, C. 2022. Theory-based self-management interventions for community-dwelling stroke survivors: A systematic review and meta-analysis. *Am J Occup Ther*, 76, 7604205010.

Laymouna, M., Ma, Y., Lessard, D., Schuster, T., Engler, K. & Lebouché, B. 2024. Roles, users, benefits, and limitations of chatbots in health care: Rapid review. *J Med Internet Res*, 26, e56930.

Lee, A. R. 2023. *Promoting independence in dementia–changing lifestyles & improving outcomes: RE-AIM study of The PRIDE self-management app* [Doctoral dissertation, University of Nottingham (United Kingdom)].

Lee, J.-A., Choi, M., Lee, S. A. & Jiang, N. 2018. Effective behavioral intervention strategies using mobile health applications for chronic disease management: A systematic review. *BMC Med Inform Decis Mak,* 18(1), 12.

Lee, R., James, C., Edwards, S., Skinner, G., Young, J. L. & Snodgrass, S. J. 2021. Evidence for the effectiveness of feedback from wearable inertial sensors during work-related activities: A scoping review. *Sensors*, 21, 6377.

Lei, Y., Li, Z., Bui, Q., Depaul, O., Nicol, G. E., Mohr, D. C., Fong, M. W. M., Metts, C. L., Lee, S. I., Tomazin, S. E. & Wong, A. W. K. 2025. Satisfaction, user experiences, and initial efficacy of a technology-supported self-management intervention (iSMART) to improve post-stroke functioning: A remoted randomized controlled trial. *Top Stroke Rehabil*, 32, 677–691.

Li, R., Liang, N., Bu, F. & Hesketh, T. 2020. The effectiveness of self-management of hypertension in adults using mobile health: Systematic review and meta-analysis. *JMIR mHealth and uHealth*, 8, e17776.

Li, S., Chen, S., Yu, X., Shang, H., Tu, T. & Quan, M. 2025. Advances in AI-enabled wearable technologies for rehabilitation interventions and functional assessment in Parkinson's disease: A scoping review and evidence map. *J Med Internet Res*, 28, e85596.

Li, Z., Lei, Y., Bui, Q., Depaul, O., Nicol, G. E., Mohr, D. C., Lee, S. I., Fong, M. W. M., Metts, C. L., Tomazin, S. E. & Wong, A. W. K. 2024. A digital intervention to promote self-management self-efficacy among community-dwelling individuals with stroke: Pilot randomized controlled trial. *JMIR Rehabil Assist Technol*, 11, e50863.

Lorig, K., Ritter, P. L., Moreland, C. & Laurent, D. D. 2015. Can a box of mailed materials achieve the triple aims of health care? The mailed chronic disease self-management tool kit study. *Health Promot Pract*, 16, 765–774.

Lorig, K. R. & Holman, H. 2003. Self-management education: History, definition, outcomes, and mechanisms. *Ann Behav Med*, 26, 1–7.

Lorig, K. R., Sobel, D. S., Stewart, A. L., Brown, B. W., JR, Bandura, A., Ritter, P., Gonzalez, V. M., Laurent, D. D. & Holman, H. R. 1999. Evidence suggesting that a chronic disease self-management program can improve health status while reducing hospitalization: A randomized trial. *Med Care*, 37, 5–14.

Lycett, H. J., Raebel, E. M., Wildman, E. K., Guitart, J., Kenny, T., Sherlock, J. P. & Cooper, V. Theory-based digital interventions to improve asthma self-management outcomes: systematic review. *J. Med. Internet Res.*, *20*(12), e293.

Maaß, L., Hrynyschyn, R., Lange, M., Löwe, A., Burdenski, K., Butten, K., Vorberg, S., Hachem, M., Gorga, A., Grieco, V., Restivo, V., Vella, G., Varnfield, M. & Holl, F. 2024. Challenges and alternatives to evaluation methods and regulation approaches for medical apps as Mobile medical devices: International and multidisciplinary focus group discussion. *J Med Internet Res*, 26, e54814.

Mäder, M., Timpel, P., Schönfelder, T., Militzer-Horstmann, C., Scheibe, S., Heinrich, R. & Häckl, D. 2023. Evidence requirements of permanently listed digital health applications (DiGA) and their implementation in the German DiGA directory: An analysis. *BMC Health Serv Res,* 23, 369.

Maillart, E., Labauge, P., Cohen, M., Maarouf, A., Vukusic, S., Donzé, C., Gallien, P., De Seze, J., Bourre, B. & Moreau, T. 2020. MSCopilot, a new multiple sclerosis self-assessment digital solution: Results of a comparative study versus standard tests. *Eur J Neurol*, 27, 429–436.

Mawson, S., Nasr, N., Parker, J., Zheng, H., Davies, R. & Mountain, G. 2014. Developing a personalised self-management system for post stroke rehabilitation; Utilising a user-centred design methodology. *Disabil Rehabil Assist Technol*, 9, 521–528.

Mawson, S., Nasr, N., Parker, J., Davies, R., Zheng, H. & Mountain, G. 2016. A personalized self-management rehabilitation system with an intelligent shoe for stroke survivors: A realist evaluation. *JMIR Rehabil Assist Technol*, 3, e1.

Mennella, C., Maniscalco, U., Pietro, G. & Esposito, M. 2023. A deep learning system to monitor and assess rehabilitation exercises in home-based remote and unsupervised conditions. *Comput Biol Med*, 166, 107485.

Michie, S., Richardson, M., Johnston, M., Abraham, C., Francis, J., Hardeman, W., Eccles, M. P., Cane, J. & Wood, C. E. 2013. The behavior change technique taxonomy (v1) of 93 hierarchically clustered techniques: Building an international consensus for the reporting of behavior change interventions. *Ann Behav Med*, 46, 81–95.

Mohr, D. C., Schueller, S. M., Riley, W. T., Brown, C. H., Cuijpers, P., Duan, N., Kwasny, M. J., Stiles-Shields, C. & Cheung, K. 2015. Trials of intervention principles: Evaluation methods for evolving behavioral intervention technologies. *J Med Internet Res*, 17, e166.

Monlezun, D. J., Omutoko, L., Oduor, P., Kokonya, D., Rayel, J., Sotomayor, C., Girault, M. I., De Los Ríos Uriarte, M. E., Sinyavskiy, O. & Aksamit, T. 2024. Digitalization of health care in low-and middle-income countries. *Bull World Health Organ*, 103, 148.

Moody, L., Wood, E., Needham, A., Booth, A., Jimenez-Aranda, A. & Tindale, W. 2022. Identifying individual enablers and barriers to the use of digital technology for the self-management of long-term conditions by older adults. *J Med Eng Technol*, 46, 448–461.

Moreno-Ligero, M., Moral-Munoz, J. A., Salazar, A. & Failde, I. 2023. mHealth intervention for improving pain, quality of life, and functional disability in patients with chronic pain: Systematic review. *JMIR Mhealth Uhealth*, 11, e40844.

Morgado, M., Botelho, J., Machado, V., Mendes, J. J., Adesope, O. & Proença, L. 2024. Full title: Video-based approaches in health education: A systematic review and meta-analysis. *Sci Rep*, 14, 23651.

Morimoto, Y., Takahashi, T., Sawa, R., Saitoh, M., Morisawa, T., Kagiyama, N., Kasai, T., Dinesen, B., Hollingdal, M., Refsgaard, J. & Daida, H. 2022. Web portals for patients with chronic diseases: Scoping review of the functional features and theoretical frameworks of telerehabilitation platforms. *J Med Internet Res*, 24, e27759.

Mummah, S. A., Robinson, T. N., King, A. C., Gardner, C. D. & Sutton, S. 2016. IDEAS (integrate, design, assess, and share): A framework and toolkit of strategies for the development of more effective digital interventions to change health behavior. *J Med Internet Res*, 18, e317.

Muñoz-Tomás, M. T., Burillo-Lafuente, M., Vicente-Parra, A., Sanz-Rubio, M. C., Suarez-Serrano, C., Marcén-Román, Y. & Franco-Sierra, M. 2023. Telerehabilitation as a therapeutic exercise tool versus face-to-face physiotherapy: A systematic review. *Int J Environ Res Public Health,* 20(5), 4358.

Navarro, O., Escrivá, M., Faubel, R. & Traver, V. 2021. Empowering patients living with chronic conditions using video as an educational tool: Scoping review. *J Med Internet Res*, 23, e26427.

Newman, S., Steed, L. & Mulligan, K. 2004. Self-management interventions for chronic illness. *Lancet*, 364, 1523–1537.

Nieuwenhuijsen, E. R., Zemper, E., Miner, K. R. & Epstein, M. 2006. Health behavior change models and theories: Contributions to rehabilitation. *Disabil Rehabil*, 28, 245–256.

Norman, D. 2013. *The design of everyday things: Revised and expanded edition*. New York, NY: Basic Books.

Oldenburg, B., Taylor, C. B., O'neil, A., Cocker, F. & Cameron, L. D. 2015. Using new technologies to improve the prevention and management of chronic conditions in populations. *Annu Rev Public Health*, 36, 483–505.

Pais, B., Buluschek, P., Dupasquier, G., Nef, T., Schütz, N., Saner, H., Gatica-Perez, D. & Santschi, V. 2020. Evaluation of 1-year in-home monitoring technology by home-dwelling older adults, family caregivers, and nurses. *Front Public Health*, 8, 518957.

Pangrazio, L., Godhe, A.-L. & Ledesma, A. G. L. 2020. What is digital literacy? A comparative review of publications across three language contexts. *E-Learn Digit Media*, 17, 442–459.

Papastergiou, M. 2009. Exploring the potential of computer and video games for health and physical education: A literature review. *Comput Educ*, 53, 603–622.

Pearce, L. M. N., Pryor, J., Redhead, J., Sherrington, C. & Hassett, L. 2024. Advanced technology in a real-world rehabilitation setting: Longitudinal observational study on clinician adoption and implementation. *J Med Internet Res*, 26, e60374.

Prochaska, J. O. & Velicer, W. F. 1997. The transtheoretical model of health behavior change. *Am J Health Promot*, 12, 38–48.

Ramey, L., Osborne, C., Kasitinon, D. & Juengst, S. 2019. Apps and Mobile health technology in rehabilitation: The good, the bad, and the unknown. *Phys Med Rehabil Clin N Am*, 30, 485–497.

Rauzi, M. R., Balakrishnan, S., Flynn, S. M., Keysor, J. J. & Hoenig, H. M. 2025. Guiding technology adoption in rehabilitation: A framework from the rehabilitation technology implementation for promising solutions (Rehab TIPS) workgroup. *Arch Phys Med Rehabil*, 107(1), 123–133.

Rodríguez-Fernández, A., Lobo-Prat, J. & Font-Llagunes, J. M. 2021. Systematic review on wearable lower-limb exoskeletons for gait training in neuromuscular impairments. *J NeuroEng Rehabil*, 18(1), 22.

Sands, D. Z. & Finn, N. B. 2025. From internet to artificial intelligence (AI) bots: Symbiotic evolutions of digital technologies and e-patients. *J Particip Med*, 17, e68911.

Sauerzopf, L., Luft, A., Maeusli, V., Klamroth-Marganska, V., Sy, M. & Spiess, M. R. 2024. Technology use for home-based stroke rehabilitation in Switzerland from the perspectives of persons living with stroke, informal caregivers, and therapists: Qualitative interview and focus group study. *JMIR Rehabil Assist Technol*, 11, e59781.

Strubbia, C., Levack, W. M. M., Grainger, R., Takahashi, K. & Tomori, K. 2020. Use of technology in supporting goal setting in rehabilitation for adults: A scoping review. *BMJ Open*, 10, e041730.

Su, Z., Li, X., Mcdonnell, D., Fernandez, A. A., Flores, B. E. & Wang, J. 2021. Technology-based interventions for cancer caregivers: Concept analysis. *JMIR Cancer*, 7, e22140.

Tadas, S. & Coyle, D. 2020. Barriers to and facilitators of technology in cardiac rehabilitation and self-management: Systematic qualitative grounded theory review. *J Med Internet Res*, 22, e18025.

Thompson, A. N., Dawson, D. R., Legasto-Mulvale, J. M., Chandran, N., Tanchip, C., Niemczyk, V., Rashkovan, J., Jeyakumar, S., Wang, R. H., Cameron, J. I. & Nalder, E. 2023. Mobile Technology-based interventions for stroke self-management support: Scoping review. *JMIR Mhealth Uhealth*, 11, e46558.

Toh, S. F. M., Fong, K. N. K., Gonzalez, P. C. & Tang, Y. M. 2023. Application of home-based wearable technologies in physical rehabilitation for stroke: A scoping review. *IEEE Trans Neural Syst Rehabil Eng*, 31, 1614–1623.

Van Denend, T., Peterson, E. W., Mcarthur, A. R., Yarnot, R., Kish, J., Steinkellner, S., Sandhu, A. & Rice, L. A. 2022. A process evaluation of an on-line fall prevention and management program for individuals who use wheelchairs or scooters living with multiple sclerosis. *Front Public Health*, 10, 1042668.

Van Gemert-Pijnen, J. E., Nijland, N., Van Limburg, M., Ossebaard, H. C., Kelders, S. M., Eysenbach, G. & Seydel, E. R. 2011. A holistic framework to improve the uptake and impact of eHealth technologies. *J Med Internet Res*, 13, e111.

Van Kessel, R., Wong, B.L., Clemens, T. Brand, H. 2022. Digital health literacy as a super determinant of health: more than simply the sum of its parts. *Internet Interv.*, 27, 100500.

Van Velsen, L., Ludden, G. & Grünloh, C. 2022. The limitations of user-and human-centered design in an eHealth context and how to move beyond them. *J Med Internet Res*, 24, e37341.

Wang, Y., Xue, H., Huang, Y., Huang, L. & Zhang, D. 2017. A systematic review of application and effectiveness of mHealth interventions for obesity and diabetes treatment and self-management. *Adv Nutr*, 8, 449–462.

Webb, J., Peerbux, S., Smittenaar, P., Siddiqui, S., Sherwani, Y., Ahmed, M., Macrae, H., Puri, H., Bhalla, S. & Majeed, A. 2020. Preliminary outcomes of a digital therapeutic intervention for smoking cessation in adult smokers: Randomized controlled trial. *JMIR Mental Health*, 7, e22833.

Wei, S. & Wu, Z. 2023. The application of wearable sensors and machine learning algorithms in rehabilitation training: A systematic review. *Sensors*, 23, 7667.

Weissglass, D. E. 2022. Contextual bias, the democratization of healthcare, and medical artificial intelligence in low-and middle-income countries. *Bioethics*, 36, 201–209.

Woelfle, T., Bourguignon, L., Lorscheider, J., Kappos, L., Naegelin, Y. & Jutzeler, C. R. 2023. Wearable sensor technologies to assess motor functions in people with multiple sclerosis: Systematic scoping review and perspective. *J Med Internet Res*, 25, e44428.

Wong, A. W. K., Fong, M. W. P. S. P. M., Munsell, E. G. S., Metts, C. L., Lee, S. I., Nicol, G. E., Depaul, O., Tomazin, S. E., Kaufman, K. J. & Mohr, D. C. 2023. Using intervention mapping and behavior change techniques to develop a digital intervention for self-management in stroke: development study. *JMIR Hum Factors*, 10, e45099.

World Health Organization. 2010. *Telemedicine: opportunities and developments in member states: report on the Second Global Survey on eHealth* [Online]. Available: https://www.afro.who.int/publications/telemedicine-opportunities-and-developments-member-state [Accessed October 07 2025].

World Health Organization. 2018. Seventy-first world health assembly. *Agenda Item*, 12. https://www.who.int/about/governance/world-health-assembly/seventy-first

Xie, L. F., Itzkovitz, A., Roy-Fleming, A., Da Costa, D. & Brazeau, A.-S. 2020. Understanding self-guided web-based educational interventions for patients with chronic health conditions: Systematic review of intervention features and adherence. *J Med Internet Res*, 22, e18355.

Yoshida, Y., Patil, S. J., Brownson, R. C., Boren, S. A., Kim, M., Dobson, R., Waki, K., Greenwood, D. A., Torbjørnsen, A., Ramachandran, A. & Masi, C. 2020. Using the RE-AIM framework to evaluate internal and external validity of mobile phone–based interventions in diabetes self-management education and support. *J. Am. Med. Inform. Assoc.*, 27(6), 946–956.

33 New Technologies in Self-Management of Rheumatoid Arthritis

Pablo Rodríguez-Sánchez-Laulhé, Alberto Marcos Heredia-Rizo, Hermann Fricke-Comellas, and Jesús Salas-González

INTRODUCTION TO RHEUMATOID ARTHRITIS AND SELF-MANAGEMENT

Rheumatoid arthritis is a chronic, systemic autoimmune disease characterized by synovial inflammation, persistent pain, and progressive joint damage that frequently leads to disability (Damgaard et al., 2023). The worldwide prevalence ranges between 0.5% and 1% (Ma et al., 2025; Zhang et al., 2025), with women being affected up to three times more often than men (Zhang et al., 2025). The inflammatory process alters joint metabolism, promoting bone resorption, cartilage erosion, and fibroblast proliferation, resulting in deformity, structural damage, and loss of function (Scherer et al., 2020). Rheumatoid arthritis imposes a substantial psychosocial burden, including fatigue, sleep disturbances, emotional distress, and work limitations (Damgaard et al., 2023; de Thurah et al., 2022). Extra-articular complications such as pericarditis, vasculitis, anemia, or infection may also occur, making this condition a major public health concern (Ma et al., 2025).

The clinical course is highly variable (Scherer et al., 2020), requiring a sustained, individualized, and multidisciplinary approach to control flare-ups and minimize their impact (Sardana et al., 2023). Although advances in pharmacological therapy and integrated care have reduced rheumatoid arthritis-related mortality, the global burden of disability attributable to the disease has substantially increased in the past decades (Ma et al., 2025).

Effective management extends beyond medical treatment and relies on patients' ability to develop self-management skills (Damgaard et al., 2023). Self-management, closely linked to self-efficacy, refers to an individual's capacity to cope with symptoms, treatment demands, psychosocial challenges, and lifestyle adaptations when living with a chronic condition (Barlow et al., 2002). Interventions designed to enhance self-management in rheumatoid arthritis improve psychosocial well-being, functional capacity, and reduce healthcare utilization (Bounabe et al., 2024; Fu et al., 2025; Hinch and Sirois, 2024; Walrabenstein et al., 2023). Accordingly, the European Alliance of Associations for Rheumatology underscores structured strategies to strengthen self-management among people with rheumatoid arthritis (Nikiphorou et al., 2021).

Digital health technologies have become key resources to improve accessibility, efficiency, and continuity of care. The World Health Organization identifies them as strategic for achieving universal health coverage (WHO, 2016). By enabling real-time communication and remote access, digital tools facilitate the delivery and uptake of self-management programs (Hartman and Duttine, 2022; Mollard and Michaud, 2020). However, barriers such as limited educational resources, overburdened healthcare systems, and transportation difficulties persist (Chaleshgar-Kordasiabi et al., 2018; Kleinert et al., 2021). Only one in three patients living with rheumatoid arthritis engage with digital health, and just one in ten uses disease-specific apps (Magnol et al., 2021), despite a general willingness to adopt such tools (Becker et al., 2022).

DOI: 10.1201/9781003599074-36

Self-management encompasses education, lifestyle modification, adherence, and coping skills (Combe et al., 2017; Nikiphorou et al., 2021), shifting patients from passive recipients to proactive participants in their own care (Kongsted et al., 2021). Exercise and joint protection programs are also essential to preserve physical function and reduce pain. Collectively, these strategies foster patient autonomy, disease control, and quality of life.

Education is a cornerstone of self-management, providing practical guidance on living with rheumatoid arthritis (Bounabe et al., 2024; NICE, 2018). Effective programs cover disease mechanisms, benefits of physical activity, and strategies to limit functional decline (Peter et al., 2021), improving psychosocial and functional domains (Bounabe et al., 2024; Wu et al., 2022), as well as adherence (Najm et al., 2019). Yet, many patients report insufficient guidance on exercise, medication adherence, joint protection, and coping (Becker et al., 2022; Bobos et al., 2021a), which may contribute to treatment discontinuation and suboptimal outcomes (van den Bemt et al., 2012). Education also supports positive health behaviors such as smoking cessation, balanced diet, and stress management (Gioia et al., 2020; Nikiphorou et al., 2021). Addressing these educational gaps is therefore a priority in routine care.

Joint protection strategies, involving strengthening and stretching exercises and assistive devices, reduce inflammation, pain, and risk of deformities. Despite their recognized benefits, particularly for hand function, patient awareness remains limited (Bobos et al., 2021b).

Exercise programs are considered first-line therapy in the management of rheumatoid arthritis (Combe et al., 2017; Fu et al., 2025; NICE, 2018) and should be individually tailored to disease activity and function (Fu et al., 2025; Rodríguez-Sánchez-Laulhé et al., 2024). Exercise diaries and regular assessment of patient-reported outcomes can enhance communication (Roddy et al., 2005), self-monitoring, and engagement (Zhao et al., 2019), strengthening the patient's role within the multidisciplinary healthcare team (Wu et al., 2022).

Coping strategies, defined as cognitive and behavioral efforts to deal with stress (Lazarus and Folkman, 1984), are central to self-management (Nikiphorou et al., 2021). Adaptive coping, including acceptance, positive reframing, and active problem-solving, promotes psychological well-being, while maladaptive strategies such as rumination and emotional avoidance, increase distress and difficulty to adapt to the disease (Janiszewska et al., 2020; Peres and Lucchetti, 2010; Thompson et al., 2010; Wu et al., 2022). Avoidance-oriented strategies can delay proper management (Hinch and Sirois, 2024), while patients with better disease knowledge are less likely to adopt harmful behaviors (Janiszewska et al., 2020). All this underscores the strong link between education, adaptative coping, and self-management.

Integrating multiple self-management strategies and digital technologies represents a promising pathway to personalized, patient-centered care. Digital tools, e.g., apps, wearables, videoconferencing, and artificial intelligence, can enhance engagement, adherence, and remote monitoring. Despite existing challenges, these approaches offer opportunities for improved symptom tracking, disease control, communication, and patient autonomy. The next sections will address specific digital tools for rheumatoid arthritis, their effectiveness, and current challenges and limitations.

CONTEXT OF NEW TECHNOLOGIES IN RHEUMATOID ARTHRITIS MANAGEMENT

New Technologies in Rheumatology

The rising incidence and global burden of rheumatology disorders demand a re-evaluation of conventional clinical models where challenges remain to achieve sustained, equitable, and patient-centered care.

New technologies offer a wide range of clinical applications, from diagnosis and monitoring to patient education and remote treatment (Volkmar et al., 2025), thereby optimizing efficiency, time, and resources (Molina-Garcia et al., 2024). By providing accessible, interactive, intuitive, engaging, and evidence-based platforms, digital tools can help overcome logistical barriers while enhancing patient engagement (Molina-Garcia et al., 2024).

Integrating technology into rehabilitation settings enhances clinical efficiency and resource allocation (Seron et al., 2021), often yielding similar or even superior results to in-person rehabilitation (Aily et al., 2023), as well as greater confidence and autonomy in managing exercise routines (Eriksson et al., 2011). A recent large-scale survey in Germany showed that nearly half of respondents adopted at least one form of digital health technology and expressed positive perceptions (May et al., 2025).

Digital interventions are feasible, accessible, and cost-effective (Darlow et al., 2022; Safari et al., 2020), enabling individualized exercise programs (Krauss et al., 2017) and continuous monitoring of patient progress. They also strengthen the therapeutic alliance through ongoing feedback (Kolasinski et al., 2020; Ritschl et al., 2021). Although the current quality of evidence on the use of digital health in arthritis remains low to moderate (Safari et al., 2020), emerging research indicates promising trends and suggests a two-fold benefit: reducing direct costs, by lowering in-person consultations, follow-up visits (de Thurah et al., 2018; Molina-Garcia et al., 2024), patient travel, and work absenteeism (Seppen et al., 2020), and improving overall quality of care (Niknejad et al., 2021; Seron et al., 2021).

However, the effectiveness of these interventions depends on user-related factors, such as readiness, motivation, and digital literacy (Niknejad et al., 2021; Seron et al., 2021). Psychological (Nelligan et al., 2021), racial, and ethnic variables (Scheer et al., 2022) can also influence engagement and outcomes. In addition, exercise dose and adherence (completion rates) can act as moderators of changes in pain and physical function following exercise-based tele-rehabilitation (Rodríguez-Sánchez-Laulhé et al., 2024).

New technologies support the delivery of evidence-based treatments (Baroni et al., 2023) and allow personalized adaptation to individual needs (Mahmood et al., 2023; Thompson et al., 2023) through everyday devices, e.g., smartphones, tablets, or computers (Molina-Garcia et al., 2024). Digital tools facilitate tracking patient progress and adherence (Kataria and Ravindran, 2019; Rodríguez Sánchez-Laulhé et al., 2022; Safari et al., 2020), as well as remote multidisciplinary treatment for patients with limited access to healthcare services (Rodríguez-Sánchez-Laulhé et al., 2024) or cognitive behavioral therapy and goal-setting interventions (MacIver et al., 2021).

Overall, technology-supported rehabilitation represents a promising approach to strengthen self-management by promoting empowerment, education, and autonomy (Baroni et al., 2023). Within this framework, the concept of the *digitally engaged patient* has emerged, referring to individuals who actively incorporate digital resources into their daily routines. These tools enable access to interdisciplinary interventions along with direct communication with clinicians (Lupton, 2013).

Definitions

Following the increasing incorporation of digital tools into rheumatology and rehabilitation practice, it is important to clarify the terminology commonly used in technology-enabled healthcare. This section outlines the most frequently cited terms and their hierarchical relationships (Figure 33.1).

At the top of this conceptual framework lies *Digital Health*, a broad term referring to the use of digital, mobile, and wireless technologies to achieve health-related goals. It represents an overarching concept that integrates various information and communication technologies, applied to healthcare. Within this umbrella are several subdomains, including eHealth, Telehealth, and mHealth (Baroni et al., 2023).

According to the World Health Organization (WHO, 2016), *eHealth* denotes the secure and cost-effective use of information and communication technologies across multiple health-domains such as clinical services, education, research, and surveillance. Beyond direct patient care, eHealth includes digital infrastructures, e.g., electronic health records, clinical decision-support systems,

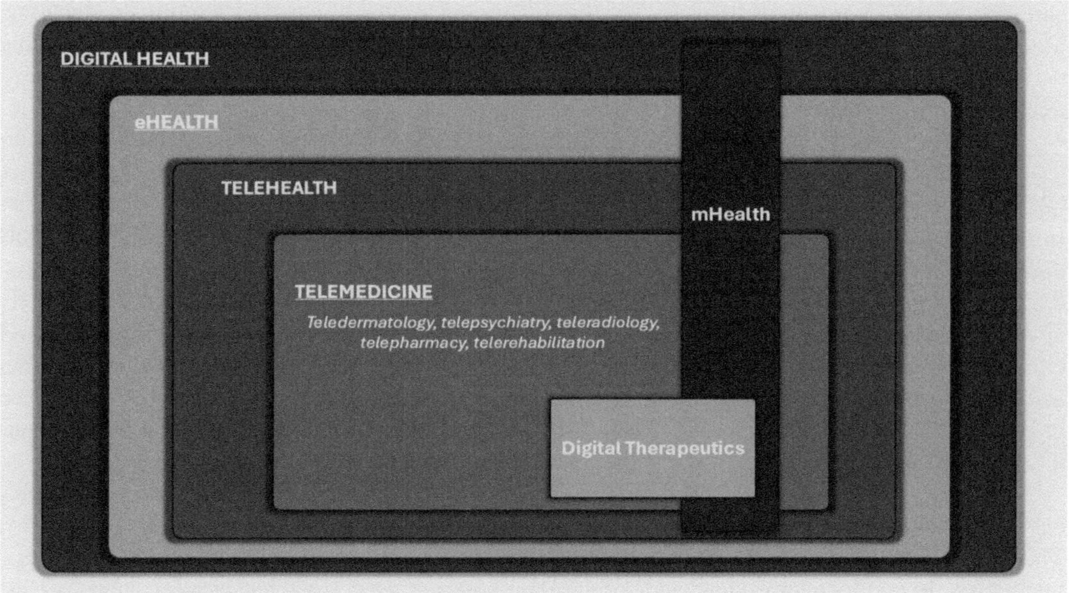

FIGURE 33.1 Terminology of new technologies in medicine.

and management platforms (WHO, 2016). Nested within eHealth is *Telehealth*, which refers to the remote delivery of healthcare services, including prevention, education, health promotion, and treatment through information and communication technology-based systems (Bashshur et al., 2011; van Dyk, 2014). Telehealth reduces geographical and logistical barriers, expanding access to care for vulnerable or remote populations, while offering cost-effective and efficient treatments (WHO, 2016). A specific subset of telehealth is *Telemedicine*, which focuses on the exchange of medical information for diagnostic and therapeutic purposes at a distance. It includes modalities such as telepsychiatry, teleradiology, and teledermatology (Baroni et al., 2023) and has been adapted to rehabilitation under the terms telerehabilitation or telephysiotherapy (Baroni et al., 2023; Cottrell et al., 2017). These interventions may be delivered synchronously (in real-time), through mobile technologies, videoconferencing, or virtual reality, or asynchronously, via apps and web-based platforms that provide therapeutic content, exercise guidance, or educational materials without simultaneous interaction (Fan et al., 2024).

Finally, *Mobile Health* (mHealth) refers to the implementation of eHealth principles via mobile and wireless devices. mHealth encompasses the practice of medicine and public health by using smartphones, wearable sensors, personal digital assistants, and monitoring systems (WHO, 2011). mHealth is a cross-cutting category that overlaps with eHealth, Telehealth, and Telemedicine, emphasizing the technological medium (mobile connectivity) rather than the clinical purpose (healthcare delivery) (van Dyk, 2014).

In the following sections, we will examine the main evidence-based approaches associated with each of these concepts, highlighting their implications for rheumatology practice.

TELEMEDICINE AND VIDEO CONSULTATION

Telemedicine interventions offer significant potential to enhance clinical management and expand healthcare coverage by reducing unnecessary in-person consultations, facilitating timely care, and improving access for underserved population. Within rheumatology, telemedicine has comparable effectiveness to face-to-face treatment (Kennedy et al., 2017). When carefully designed to address individual needs and preferences, these tools improve accessibility, self-management, continuity of care, fostering closer connections between patients and professionals (de Thurah et al., 2022; MacIver et al., 2021). However, limited training and experience in remote management remain key barriers, contributing to clinicians' skepticism and reluctance to incorporate telemedicine into routine practice (Lawford et al., 2018).

Modalities of Telemedicine in Rheumatology

In rheumatology, telemedicine is typically structured into three complementary modalities: *real-time* (synchronous), *store-and-forward* (asynchronous) and *remote monitoring*, each serving distinct clinical purposes (de Thurah et al., 2022).

Real-Time modalities such as video consultation enables live interaction between patients and clinicians for assessment, education, and follow-up. This format supports shared decision-making and is particularly useful for evaluating disease activity, functional status, and treatment adherence in rheumatoid arthritis (Latifi et al., 2021). Depending on the clinical goal, sessions may be conducted by different professionals, reinforcing an interdisciplinary approach to care.

Store-and-forward technology refers to asynchronous approaches in which pre-recorded clinical information, e.g., imaging, laboratory results, is transmitted for later review by a specialist. This system facilitates expert consultation and diagnostic support without requiring simultaneous interaction. In rheumatology, store-and-forward methods are used to exchange ultrasound images, joint photographs, or health records between primary and tertiary care providers (Latifi et al., 2021).

Remote monitoring involves the continuous or periodic collection and transmission of clinical or patient-reported data from the individual's home or community environment. Typical parameters include pain intensity, joint stiffness, fatigue, and physical activity levels. This modality enables longitudinal follow-up between in-person visits or teleconsultations and supports early detection of disease flares. Remote monitoring can be implemented via wearable devices, digital platforms, or mobile apps, often integrated within broader mHealth ecosystems (Latifi et al., 2021). These tools will be discussed in other sections.

Preparation and Setup of Teleconsultation

Before a teleconsultation, clinicians must ensure that all legal, safety, privacy, technical, and clinical requirements are met. This involves both the clinician's setup and the patient's readiness to engage effectively (Davies et al., 2021; Yedlinsky and Peebles, 2021). Clinicians' competence in adapting their professional practice to the digital environment is essential for safe and effective care (Davies et al., 2021).

From a legal and regulatory perspective, clinicians should verify patient eligibility for telehealth according to national or institutional frameworks, including reimbursement policies. They are responsible for holding appropriate licensure and ensuring that professional indemnity insurance covers teleconsultation practice. Informed consent must be obtained, and all actions should comply with institutional protocols and data protection laws to guarantee confidentiality and professional accountability. Teleconsultations should take place in a quiet, neutral, and private environment to preserve the dignity of the encounter. Platforms must comply with recognized data security standards (e.g., General Data Protection Regulation in the European Union, Health Insurance Portability and Accountability Act in the United States of America) and patients should be informed about how recordings, photos, videos, or data will be used, granting explicit consent when needed.

Safety is critical, as the clinician is not physically present. Before beginning, they must assess whether the patient's health status and environment allow for safe participation, confirm the patient's location in case of emergency, and have a protocol for managing incidents. Involving a caregiver or family member may improve safety and reduce mobility concerns. Patients should also be advised to arrange adequate lighting, space, and visibility for exercises or movement assessments.

Technological readiness underpins teleconsultation quality. Clinicians should evaluate the patient's digital literacy and access to reliable hardware, software, and internet connection. Platforms should meet privacy, encryption, and interoperability standards while remaining user-friendly. Clinicians must also master core features, such as audio, video, and screen-sharing, and provide patients with clear, step-by-step guidance beforehand. Keeping a backup communication channel ensures continuity if technical issues arise.

Finally, practitioners should adapt communication, assessment, and management strategies to the virtual context, using camera angles, lighting, verbal cues and gestures to compensate for the lack of physical interaction. Healthcare professionals should recognize the limits of remote assessment, adjust "hands-on" procedures accordingly and identify when in-person assessment is required. Effective teleconsultation integrates all these competencies to ensure safe, evidence-based, and patient-centered care (Davies et al., 2021).

Clinical Interview and Assessment in Teleconsultation

Physical examination and diagnosis via telemedicine can yield very good results, with acceptable levels of satisfaction reported by both patients and clinicians (Lee et al., 2024; Tong et al., 2024). However, the success of this approach depends on clinicians' competence and confidence in using and adapting to the virtual context (Tong et al., 2024; Ziade et al., 2022).

A well-prepared environment is essential for safe and effective communication and accurate clinical observation (Davies et al., 2021; Laskowski et al., 2020). Again, clinicians should ensure adequate lighting, audio, and a neutral background, maintaining professionalism. The camera should capture the head and shoulders during dialogue and a wider frame when demonstrating posture or movement-related tasks. Maintaining visual contact fosters rapport, whereas disabling notifications and minimizing interruptions help preserve privacy and focus. Adopting a structured approach to history taking and physical examination mirrors traditional clinical workflows. When necessary, clinicians can demonstrate or guide examination or movement tasks to facilitate understanding and accuracy.

Patient preparation is equally important. Patients should receive clear instructions on camera positioning, lighting, and sound quality. Adequate space must be ensured for mobility tasks, and involving a caregiver can be recommended to assist with camera positioning or technical issues and ensure safety during movement. Completing standardized questionnaires or patient-reported measures (e.g., pain, fatigue) beforehand supports a more efficient and comprehensive evaluation (Ahmed et al., 2022; Ziade et al., 2022). Teleconsultation requires deliberate communication strategies to overcome the absence of physical presence. Clinicians should use slower speech, plain language, visual cues, and active listening, ensuring that patients' concerns and expectations are addressed (Davies et al., 2021).

Visual inspection is crucial when assessing disease activity. The evaluation should begin by identifying the primary area of complaint and observing for swelling, erythema, deformities, or asymmetry (Wainberg et al., 2020). Guided self-palpation can complement inspection when appropriate (Ziade et al., 2022).

Functional assessment conducted remotely has shown high interrater reliability when compared with in-person evaluations, with minor differences in timing, although standardized procedures are still needed to maintain consistency and accuracy (Bird et al., 2022). Guided active range of motion testing is both feasible and clinically valuable in the context of a remote consultation (Lee et al., 2024). Patients should position the joint for full visibility, and clinicians may capture still images or use on-screen tools to estimate joint angles (Mo, 2025; Sahu et al., 2022). Reliable tests when administered during teleconsultation, include the Five-Times Sit-to-Stand, 3-Meter, and 4-Meter Walk, Timed Up-and-Go (Bird et al., 2022; Lawford et al., 2024), grip strength, functional reach, static balance (Bird et al., 2022), 30-Second Chair Stand, and stair climb, among others (Lawford et al., 2024). These measures provide valuable insights into postural control, mobility, and physical performance, informing clinical decision-making and monitoring over time.

Therapeutic Interventions and Telehealth

Interventions delivered through teleconsultation should follow the same evidence-based principles as in-person care (Ahmed et al., 2022; de Thurah et al., 2022; Ziade et al., 2022). Before treatment, clinicians can provide clear written or digital materials and reinforce a positive attitude toward telehealth (Davies et al., 2021). Establishing shared goals supports motivation and ensures a common direction throughout the entire process. Core components of telehealth-based interventions include patient education, focusing on disease understanding, adherence, pacing, and stress-management, pharmacological review, ensuring adherence and monitoring adverse effects, and non-pharmacological management, particularly individualized exercise programs adapted for remote delivery. Exercise-based interventions can be conducted synchronously (live supervision) or asynchronously (pre-recorded sessions), promoting accessibility and continuity of care without compromising quality.

Follow-up and Continuity of Care

Follow-up frequency should be determined by clinical status and disease activity, considering that not all patients are suitable for remote monitoring (de Thurah et al., 2022). In individuals with rheumatoid arthritis with low disease activity or clinical remission, follow-up based on patient-reported outcomes through telemedicine is equally effective as in-person visits to maintain disease control (de Thurah et al., 2018). Exclusive telemedicine follow-up should not exceed 12 months at a time, as disease activity may fluctuate (Ahmed et al., 2022). A hybrid model, alternating between remote and face-to-face consultations, provides flexibility, safety, and clinical accuracy.

Contraindications and Limitations

Some conditions may require in-person assessment or intensive medical management. Similarly, different barriers such as technological, environmental, or cognitive, may limit feasibility of telehealth (Lee et al., 2024; Ziade et al., 2022). Although conservative interventions such as exercise programs are generally safe and well-tolerated, mild adverse events have been reported in about 19% of cases (Niemeijer et al., 2019). Patients experiencing severe inflammatory flare-ups, acute pain crises, or signs of systemic complications should be promptly referred for in-person evaluation. Teleconsultation is also unsuitable when cognitive, sensory, or communication impairments hinder effective interaction, or when privacy, space, or connectivity issues arise. In such cases, face-to-face care remains the preferred and most effective therapeutic option.

MOBILE HEALTH APPS

Mobile Health or mHealth has gained relevance as an effective means of promoting self-management among adults with musculoskeletal pain (Marcuzzi et al., 2023). Evidence indicates that mobile app-based interventions are among the most effective digital modalities to reduce pain interference in chronic pain conditions (Slattery et al., 2019). Their portability and flexibility make them well suited to support long-term self-management behaviors, while gamification features enhance adherence and engagement through motivational and interactive elements (Giansanti, 2024).

In rheumatology, mHealth solutions contribute to lowering rheumatoid arthritis *disease* activity and facilitate clinicians' responses during symptoms exacerbations (Nikiphorou et al., 2021). Mobile apps have demonstrated growing potential for both therapeutic delivery and patient empowerment. For individuals with rheumatic hand disorders, home-based mHealth exercise programs with video demonstrations and tailored dosage have been proposed as a solution to bridge gaps during rehabilitation (Volkmar et al., 2025), especially for exercise prescription and self-management (Hammond and Prior, 2016). Previous literature supports the efficacy and safety of mHealth interventions in improving hand function (Rodríguez Sánchez-Laulhé et al., 2022), promoting self-monitoring (Seppen et al., 2020), and reinforcing self-management (Mollard and Michaud, 2020) among patients with RA. Comparable results have been observed in symptomatic hand osteoarthritis (Rodríguez Sánchez-Laulhé et al., 2023). Across broader arthritis populations, digital strategies have been associated with better clinical results (Safari et al., 2020) and adherence rates (Patten et al., 2022). To fully realize their potential, mHealth technologies should incorporate personalized management and adherence-support features, although evidence regarding their optimal design remains limited (Rodríguez-Sánchez-Laulhé et al., 2024).

A notable example is the *CareHand app*, a rigorously developed mHealth solution combining exercise video demonstrations with self-monitoring and educational components. Designed for patients with rheumatoid arthritis or osteoarthritis in the hands, CareHand records symptoms and exercise progression to constantly tailor therapeutic programs. Developed under the supervision of different professionals (physicians, physiotherapists, and occupational therapists), CareHand adheres to evidence-based guidelines and has proven effective in improving hand function, work performance, and pain intensity (Rodríguez Sánchez-Laulhé et al., 2022). The incorporation of such valid and user-friendly digital tools offers a cost-effective and scalable strategy to sustain self-management and compliance with treatment (Hammond and Prior, 2016; Mahmood et al., 2023), while complementing traditional care pathways.

However, implementing exercise regimens through mHealth presents certain challenges, particularly regarding functional status assessment and direct supervision of exercise technique, both essential for individualized prescription. However, these limitations can be partially mitigated using smartphone apps with visual guidance (Rodríguez Sánchez-Laulhé et al., 2022), computer vision-guided exercise systems (Zhu et al., 2025), and wearables capturing movement parameters (Chen et al., 2020).

Digital Therapeutics

The rapid growth of health technologies, especially after the COVID-19 pandemic, has increased the demand for simple, user-friendly, and scalable therapeutic options (Giansanti, 2024; Volkmar et al., 2025). Initially conceived as wellness-oriented devices, these technologies have evolved into software-based medical products that deliver therapeutic or preventive care (Wang et al., 2023), giving rise to the concept of digital therapeutics.

According to the Digital Therapeutics Alliance, digital therapeutics are *"health software intended to treat or alleviate a disease, disorder, condition, or injury by generating and delivering a medical intervention that has a demonstrable positive therapeutic impact on a patient's health"* (Digital Therapeutics Alliance, 2025). Accordingly, digital therapeutics must meet clinical and regulatory standards, including International Organization for Standardization norms, scientific validation through clinical trials, and a clearly defined intended purpose (Zovi et al., 2025). An illustrative example is ***ReHand*** (Figure 33.2), a telerehabilitation system designed for musculoskeletal, orthopedic, and neurological disorders affecting the wrist, hand, and fingers. Through an interactive touchscreen tablet interface, ReHand delivers tailored and guided therapeutic exercises with instant feedback. Several clinical trials have demonstrated its clinical

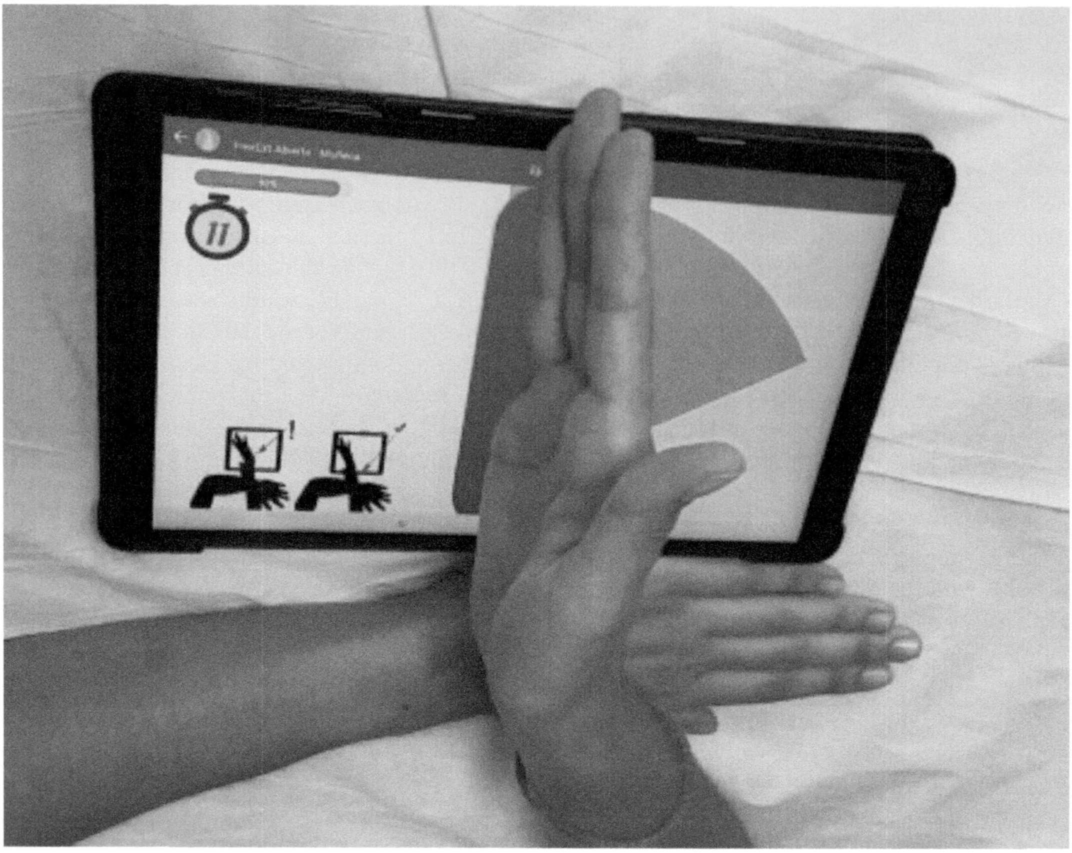

FIGURE 33.2 A mHealth telerehabilitation system for wrist, hand, and fingers disorders.

effectiveness and its capacity to reduce hospital-based healthcare resource utilization (Blanquero et al., 2020; Suero-Pineda et al., 2023).

Public Health Coverage of Digital Therapeutics: The Case of Germany

Germany has been a global pioneer in the regulatory integration of digital therapeutics. Through the Federal Institute for Drugs and Medical Devices, it became the first country to establish a "fast-track" evaluation system for digital health applications (Liang et al., 2025). The Digital Healthcare Act, enacted in November 2019, allows physicians and psychotherapists to prescribe digital health tools which may then be reimbursed by health insurance funds (Lantzsch et al., 2022).

This framework defines quality, safety, and data protection requirements for digital health applications, all subject to scientific evaluation. These must be listed in the official statutory health insurance directory to qualify for reimbursement, following one of two fast-track pathways: (1) permanent inclusion, granted when robust evidence of clinical benefit is already available; or (2) conditional inclusion, permitted for up to 12–24 months, when a plausible rationale for the contribution of digital health applications to positive outcomes can be provided, along with a scientific evaluation plan from an independent institution.

This pioneering system ensures that individuals have access to rigorously tested digital therapeutics with demonstrated value. Similar initiatives are being explored in France, while in the United States, the Food and Drug Administration has maintained an active digital therapeutics precertification program since 2017 (Lantzsch et al., 2022).

ARTIFICIAL INTELLIGENCE

Artificial Intelligence is defined as computer systems capable of performing tasks that normally require human cognition, such as pattern recognition, learning, reasoning, and decision-making (Momtazmanesh et al., 2022). The goal of artificial intelligence is to emulate the human brain function, enabling autonomous systems that can think, learn, and act based on data (Chandwar and Misra, 2024; Momtazmanesh et al., 2022). Main artificial intelligence applications include chatbots, which interpret and generate human-like conversations through text or voice (Rossettini et al., 2023); deep learning, based on multilayered neural networks that extract complex features from large datasets, with applications for voice recognition, medical imaging, and translation (Momtazmanesh et al., 2022); and computer vision, which analyzes images or videos to identify patterns or clinically relevant information (Olveres et al., 2021).

In medicine, and particularly in rheumatology, artificial intelligence has demonstrated great potential to analyze extensive clinical, imaging, and movement data. These systems can assist in clinical decision-making, enhance diagnostic precision, and guide individualized and evidence-based treatment. Furthermore, artificial intelligence enables continuous monitoring and prediction of disease flares or progression, thereby contributing to proactive and personalized patient management (Chandwar and Misra, 2024; Eriksen et al., 2024; Marcuzzi et al., 2023; Vlad et al., 2025).

Monitoring and Tailored Self-Management Interventions

Modern rehabilitation platforms can now collect real-time clinical data and integrate artificial intelligence-based algorithms that provide adaptive feedback to clinicians and patients (Chandwar and Misra, 2024; Marcuzzi et al., 2023; Vlad et al., 2025). By identifying individuals' patterns of disease activity, artificial intelligence can predict flares and trigger timely therapeutic or self-management strategies, including rest, tailored exercise programs, medication adjustments, or medical consultations (Chandwar and Misra, 2024; Marcuzzi et al., 2023). Gossec et al. (2019) demonstrated the feasibility of this approach: machine learning models analyzing daily physical activity and flare frequency in patients with rheumatoid arthritis and spondyloarthritis achieved excellent diagnostic accuracy, with 96% sensitivity, 95% specificity, 91% positive predictive value, and 99% negative predictive value. Similarly, artificial intelligence-based models have outperformed traditional screening tools to predict cardiovascular comorbidities in rheumatic diseases (Chandwar and Misra, 2024).

Patient Education and Communication

Artificial Intelligence chatbots and large language models, such as ChatGPT (OpenAI) or Gemini (Google), can serve as valuable tools for therapeutic education and communication. These systems can synthesize knowledge, translate complex terminology into accessible language, and even answer questions about disease, medication, or self-care. This fosters engagement, understanding, continuity of care, and treatment adherence (Rossettini et al., 2023).

Ayers et al. (2023) found that chatbot-generated responses to patient inquiries were perceived as more empathetic and clearer than those provided by human professionals in public online forums. Other studies evaluating ChatGPT's accuracy against official rheumatology guidelines (e.g., American College of Rheumatology, European Alliance of Associations for Rheumatology) mostly found accurate and reliable outputs, though occasional inconsistencies with evidence-based recommendations were reported. Therefore, artificial intelligence-generated content should always be supervised by qualified clinicians before use in clinical or educational settings (Uz and Umay, 2023).

Diagnosis Support and Clinical Decision-Making

Recent evidence suggests that large language models can assist in diagnosis and clinical decision-making with accuracy (Eriksen et al., 2024; Kremer et al., 2025). For example, ChatGPT-4 correctly identified the primary diagnosis in 57% of clinical cases, significantly outperforming clinicians (Eriksen et al., 2024). Artificial intelligence systems have also proven useful in diagnosing rare rheumatic diseases (Kremer et al., 2025). Despite these promising findings, limitations persist, primarily due to discrepancies between theoretical training data and real-world variability (Chandwar and Misra, 2024). Computer vision systems have also shown notable results in identifying signs of active arthritis. In artificial intelligence models trained with smartphone-captured images, Phatak et al. (2023) reported diagnostic accuracies ranging from 62% to 83% for different hand and wrist joints. Similarly, ARTHUR, an automated ultrasound analysis system, has shown accuracy in detecting synovitis and structural damage in patients with arthritis, with excellent acceptability and no additional risks (Frederiksen et al., 2022).

Artificial intelligence is also advancing precision medicine through machine learning analysis and integration of multi-omics datasets, including genomics, proteomics, and metagenomics, together with traditional biomarkers such as rheumatoid factor, erythrocyte sedimentation rate, and C-reactive protein. This combined multidimensional analysis facilitates a more precise patient stratification, earlier disease detection, and more personalized therapeutic approaches (Momtazmanesh et al., 2022).

Exercise Feedback and Self-Management

Artificial Intelligence combined with mobile device cameras and computer vision is capable of real-time analysis of exercise execution, monitoring movements and posture, and offering corrective feedback (Biebl et al., 2020; Luna et al., 2021; Zhu et al., 2025) comparable to that of an experienced physiotherapist (Biebl et al., 2020; Luna et al., 2021). Consequently, artificial intelligence enhances safety and self-management, allowing patients to perform exercises autonomously at home while maintaining proper technique, without in-person supervision (Luna et al., 2021).

Artificial intelligence and mHealth technologies have become integral components of multidisciplinary management of musculoskeletal disorders (Marcuzzi et al., 2023; Toelle et al., 2019). Toelle et al. (2019) demonstrated that an artificial intelligence-powered mHealth tool combining personalized and guided exercises, education, monitoring, and psychological support achieved better outcomes compared to conventional physiotherapy. Other adaptive artificial intelligence systems providing self-management strategies adapted to patient responses have also proven similar effectiveness to standard interventions, while improving accessibility and adherence (Marcuzzi et al., 2023).

LIMITATIONS OF NEW TECHNOLOGIES

As discussed throughout the different sections of this chapter, emerging technologies are reshaping the management of rheumatoid arthritis, primarily by strengthening individual self-management. However, technical, clinical, regulatory, economic, and socio-cultural limitations persist, all intersecting with a persistent concern for equity. Central among these challenges is the *digital divide*, which reflects unequal access to technological resources, as well as disparities in digital literacy and the ability to translate technological use into meaningful health benefits (Lyles et al., 2023). Additionally, willingness to engage in digital health interventions may differ among patients, shaping both adoption and adherence (Tang et al., 2024). Understanding these interrelated dimensions is essential for identifying the barriers that will be addressed below.

Technical and Practical Barriers

Technology-based interventions depend on access to appropriate digital infrastructure, sufficient processing power, reliable broadband connectivity, and compatible operating systems (Lee et al., 2024). The rapid advance of hardware and software updates often leaves certain users with obsolete or incompatible devices, creating barriers to participation and continuity.

Usability issues further constrain both end users and healthcare providers (Keel et al., 2023). Complex interfaces, unintuitive design, or difficulties during installation and configuration may discourage engagement, particularly for those with lower digital literacy or with visual, cognitive, or motor impairments (Lee et al., 2024). Likewise, language barriers and the lack of plain-language explanations can hinder comprehension and accessibility in multicultural contexts (Lee et al., 2024; Tang et al., 2024).

Local infrastructure reliability remains another major barrier. Poor connectivity can cause frequent call drops and disruptions during video consultations, limiting a proper evaluation or intervention. Lack of integration with electronic health records can also fragment care delivery (Barksdale et al., 2023; Lee et al., 2024; Vasconez-Gonzalez et al., 2025). Addressing these technical limitations is a prerequisite for ensuring that eHealth interventions are functional and inclusive.

Clinical Practice

The integration of digital technologies has transformed the patient-clinician relationship, expanding interactions beyond clinical settings and in-person contact. Yet, this paradigm shift introduces new complexities. For instance, differences in expectations and acceptance often determine the success of telehealth approaches (Keel et al., 2023). Clinicians may face additional workload and the need for new training while patients, especially older adults, may perceive a diminished therapeutic alliance due to reduced direct human contact or hands-on exercise guidance (Lumma et al., 2025; Zhang et al., 2024). Overall, achieving a proper balance between in-person and telehealth care appears crucial to sustain engagement and treatment efficiency (Lindberg et al., 2021).

Clinical assessment via telehealth presents specific concerns. The absence of direct physical examination limits palpation and manual testing, while reduced nonverbal communication can affect diagnostic accuracy. Technical issues, such as poor lighting or limited visualization of the affected body regions, can further compromise remote evaluations (Lee et al., 2024).

Most telehealth systems are designed for single-disease management, overlooking the complex multimorbidity profiles commonly seen in patients with rheumatoid arthritis (Volkmar et al., 2025). This may fragment care and increase the burden of using different digital tools, while recommendations from disease-specific algorithms can be conflicting and not account for interactions among overlapping comorbidities or treatments.

Age has often been cited as a potential barrier to digital health adoption. Yet, evidence suggests that digital engagement among older adults is more strongly influenced by sociodemographic and contextual factors (Jacob et al., 2022). This widespread misconception among clinicians reflects the underlying *ageism* in healthcare, which can unintentionally exclude older people from innovative approaches. Recent calls have emphasized the need to promote equitable digital inclusion across all age groups (Mace et al., 2022).

Artificial Intelligence

Artificial intelligence has introduced new opportunities into rheumatology for clinical decision support, patient education, and research, with distinct challenges to be considered. Artificial Intelligence-driven systems, particularly chatbots and large language models, generate responses based on large datasets, open access web sources, or user inputs (Uz and Umay, 2023). This process, while powerful, carries risks of reproducing protected copyrighted material or misusing third-party content, raising concerns regarding authorship, traceability, originality, and intellectual property (Rossettini et al., 2023).

A particularly relevant phenomenon is *artificial intelligence hallucination*, as the generation of inaccurate or entirely fabricated information presented as factual. In clinical and educational contexts, such misinformation can lead to incorrect self-management strategies, improper exercise routines, or medication misuse, thus artificial intelligence-generated content must be carefully reviewed (Tangsrivimol et al., 2025). Large language models, such as ChatGPT, currently rely on training datasets that do not include the most recent evidence and are unable to verify the information sources, which introduces further risk of bias (Uz et al., 2023). Artificial intelligence outputs also tend to exhibit redundancy and excessive verbosity, which may obscure key information, and reduce clarity and conciseness (Rossettini et al., 2023). For all these reasons, artificial intelligence-generated content should be consulted under professional guidance before use with education or clinical purposes.

Regulatory, Legal, and Privacy

A clear and comprehensive legal framework is a prerequisite for adopting new digital health practices within national healthcare systems. One of the main challenges for digital health developers is the absence or heterogeneity of legal regulations across countries, which hinders the development of products that can be safely deployed internationally (Keel et al., 2023).

In Europe, medical device regulation 2017/745 provides the legislative foundation governing the marketing, clinical evaluation, and commercialization of software-based health technologies (European Parliament and Council, 2017). This regulation aims to guarantee the safety, quality and efficacy of medical devices within the European market, by strengthening transparency and accountability oversight throughout their life cycle. Key elements include classification and certification procedures, clinical evaluation standards, market and post-market surveillance, and clearly defined responsibilities for manufacturers, importers and distributors.

Despite this framework, the absence of standardized and disease-specific guidance, particularly for rheumatic conditions such as rheumatoid arthritis, remains a significant gap. The absence of institutional guidelines addressing quality, safety, and data protection requirements, makes implementation of these digital practices difficult. This uncertainty discourages clinicians from adopting such tools and decreases the likelihood of integration into routine practice (Van Tilburg et al., 2024). Moreover, the rapid emergence of artificial intelligence-driven technologies introduces further complexity. Chatbots, clinical decision-support systems, and large language models process sensitive health data that may fall under strict privacy regulations, such as the European Union's General Data Protection Regulation. Ensuring robust informed-consent procedures, end-to-end encryption, and transparent data governance (Tangsrivimol et al., 2025), as well as adherence to region-specific regulatory frameworks is critical. The European Union Artificial Intelligence Act represents an important step toward regulating the development, deployment, and monitoring of Artificial Intelligence systems, including those used as medical devices (European Parliament & Council of the European Union, 2024). It is imperative that regulation evolves dynamically to keep pace with technological advances.

Economic and Organizational

Public investment in telehealth infrastructure remains insufficient, largely due to the substantial initial costs required for hardware acquisition, software development, and staff training (Barnett et al., 2025; Vasconez-Gonzalez et al., 2025). While countries like China have demonstrated successful implementation driven by robust technological infrastructure and centralized strategies (Ye et al., 2023), most health systems face persistent economic and logistical challenges.

In private healthcare models, adoption is not necessarily easier as financial constraints may be equally significant. Insurance reimbursement policies often limit coverage to in-person services, excluding or undervaluing telehealth interventions, thereby discouraging healthcare providers from adopting them (Keel et al., 2023).

Equity and Access Concerns

Certain population groups show lower levels of readiness and willingness to engage with digital health interventions. However, these traits are not inherently determined by demographic aspects, but rather reflect the interaction of social, educational, and contextual factors (Tang et al., 2024; Zhang et al., 2024). Gender inequities persist in some low- and middle-income countries, where women's digital access remains limited due to cultural and structural constraints (Tang et al., 2024). Although language, sex, cultural background, and immigration status have been cited as potential barriers, evidence indicates that these effects are largely mediated by socioeconomic disparities and digital literacy (Duggal et al., 2023; Tang et al., 2024). Promoting regular use of technology reinforces engagement and competence, creating a positive feedback loop and supporting trust and positive beliefs (Badr et al., 2024; Tan and Wong, 2025).

As healthcare systems continue to integrate digital strategies, some individuals may still experience delayed access to diagnosis and suboptimal disease management, conditioning their clinical progress.

Clinical Evidence

Despite the proliferation of technological tools for rheumatic diseases, the overall quality of available systems remains limited. Many interventions lack a solid scientific foundation, rigorous validation, or adequate professional supervision (Dantas et al., 2021; Knitza et al., 2019). Key challenges include ensuring clinical reliability, sustaining long-term patient engagement and integrating these solutions effectively into existing care pathways.

In primary care, deficits are particularly evident in the clinical management of individuals with hand rheumatic conditions (Kloppenburg, 2007), in which most of the commonly used interventions are not aligned with current guidelines or supported by robust evidence (Seppen et al., 2020). In rheumatoid arthritis, this gap between recommended practice and actual clinical management contributes to patient dissatisfaction (Porcheret et al., 2007) and underuse of primary care services, even among patients experiencing severe functional impairment (Dziedzic et al., 2007).

Thus, while technological advances hold enormous promise, these limitations spanning technical, clinical, ethical, economic, and equity dimensions must be systematically addressed. Only by closing these gaps can digital tools enhance self-management and quality of care in rheumatoid arthritis.

IMPLICATIONS AND FUTURE DIRECTIONS

Digital health has emerged as a valid, scalable, and cost-effective approach to deliver evidence-based treatments while promoting proactive self-management and patient empowerment in chronic health conditions (Dixon and Michaud, 2018). As highlighted in this chapter, the rising global burden of rheumatic diseases (Ma et al., 2025) underscores a pressing need for efficient and innovative care models.

A growing body of evidence reported clinical improvements and enhanced treatment adherence in patients with rheumatic conditions using digital interventions (Patten et al., 2022). Beyond direct clinical benefits, these technologies generate new opportunities for research (Thompson et al., 2023) and for strengthening routine clinical practice (Agnew et al., 2022). For instance, mobile applications facilitate continuous data collection, enabling the creation of accessible databases suitable for secondary analyses (Beukenhorst et al., 2022). Moreover, artificial intelligence algorithms can efficiently analyze such datasets to identify meaningful patterns and outcome clusters, potentially supporting more precise diagnosis, prognosis, and treatment optimization (Momtazmanesh et al., 2022).

The versatility of digital health technologies enables the integration of multidisciplinary interventions and the delivery of personalized treatment plans (Moman et al., 2019; Rodríguez Sánchez-Laulhé et al., 2022, 2023). For this purpose, these modalities should be coordinated through interoperable platforms connecting primary, secondary, and tertiary care, fostering continuity, avoiding redundancy, and enhancing efficiency in treatment. Similarly, it facilitates the adaptation of interventions to prognostic factors or patient preferences, promoting a more flexible and patient-centered medical care. These advantages are further amplified when artificial intelligence algorithms are incorporated to refine therapeutic recommendations based on biological and clinical data patterns (Momtazmanesh et al., 2022). Telerehabilitation, whether synchronous or asynchronous, also represents a promising complement to traditional treatments. When appropriately monitored by professionals, it can improve access to care, reduce in-person consultations, and improve efficiency in rheumatologic rehabilitation (de la Fuente Ballesteros et al., 2018).

Common challenges such as loss of motivation and poor adherence continue to compromise the effectiveness of interventions (Jones et al., 2025; Yang et al., 2022). In this context, digital self-management programs offering individualized feedback have shown potential to enhance patient engagement (Lindberg et al., 2021). However, these benefits may not be equitably distributed, as limited digital literacy, particularly among older adults, who represent the population most affected by rheumatoid arthritis (Ma et al., 2025), can hinder participation and adherence (Rodríguez-Sánchez-Laulhé et al., 2024).

A decisive factor for successful implementation lies in the digital competence and education of clinicians. Adequate training promotes acceptance, prevents inefficiencies, and empowers them to deliver technological high-quality and individualized interventions (Baroni et al., 2023; Le et al., 2023). Moreover, developing awareness of digital inequalities makes it possible to identify and support patients facing barriers to participation (Neter et al., 2025). Actively involving end users in the design and testing of digital health technologies is also key to improving usability, adherence, and perceived value (Yang et al., 2022).

Low- and middle-income countries exhibit lower levels of implementation and opportunities for professional training. Therefore, economic disparities, telecommunication infrastructure, and contextual adaptation must be considered when designing digital strategies (World Health Organization, 2016). Ensuring universal access to stable internet connections, suitable devices, and digital literacy programs is essential to prevent widening existing health disparities (Neter et al., 2025; Ye et al., 2023). Public policies promoting broadband expansion, subsidized connectivity, and inclusive design should be prioritized. From a research standpoint, equity considerations must be considered from the earliest stages of design, including recruitment, eligibility, and data analysis, so that digital health evidence truly reflects diverse populations (Badr et al., 2024). Hand function impairments should also be accounted for when designing user interfaces (World Health Organization & International Telecommunication Union, 2024).

As digital health continues to evolve, regulatory and policy frameworks must advance in parallel (Ziade et al., 2022). International guidelines and the experience of pioneering countries provide critical reference for defining appropriate clinical indications and safety and quality standards in technology implementation (Badr et al., 2024; Lee et al., 2024b). Aligning reimbursement and insurance systems with the clinical use of digital modalities is crucial to ensure their integration into healthcare provision. Additionally, secure systems for electronic prescriptions and medication monitoring remain equally important (Ziade et al., 2022). Digital health interventions also carry a responsibility to ensure the accuracy and scientific integrity of disseminated information (Najm et al., 2019).

Finally, future research in digital interventions should aim to improve replicability, methodological transparency, and the cumulative evidence base (Rodríguez-Sánchez-Laulhé et al., 2024). Standardized frameworks, such as the Template for Intervention Description and Replication checklist (Hoffmann et al., 2014) and the mHealth evidence reporting and assessment checklist (Agarwal et al., 2016) should therefore be systematically adopted in clinical studies to improve reporting quality and ensure reproducibility.

Looking ahead, the convergence of different digital health technologies, such as mobile health, telehealth, and artificial intelligence, heralds a new paradigm in rheumatologic care. By integrating patient-reported outcomes, predictive analytics, and personalized interventions, these innovations have the potential to transform self-management in rheumatoid arthritis, enhancing patient autonomy, optimizing clinical decisions, improving clinical results and ultimately promoting better disease control. To translate this progress into meaningful and equitable benefits, it is essential to address ethical, social and accessibility challenges through rigorous evaluation, inclusive design, and close collaboration between clinicians, researchers, and patients. Furthermore, high-quality clinical research is urgently needed to evaluate how the integration of these emerging technologies into self-management care may influence disease progression, patient engagement, and long-term outcomes in rheumatoid arthritis.

REFERENCES

Agarwal, S., Lefevre, A.E., Lee, J., L'engle, K., Mehl, G., Sinha, C., Labrique, A., Vasudevan, L., Tamrat, T., Kallander, K., Mitchell, M., Aziz, M.A., Froen, F., Ormel, H., Muniz, M., & Asangansi, I. (2016). Guidelines for reporting of Health interventions using mobile phones: Mobile Health (mHealth) evidence reporting and assessment (mERA) checklist. BMJ, 352, i1174. https://doi.org/10.1136/bmj.i1174.

Agnew, J.M.R., Hanratty, C.E., McVeigh, J.G., Nugent, C., & Kerr, D.P. (2022). An investigation into the use of mHealth in musculoskeletal physiotherapy: Scoping review. JMIR Rehabilitation and Assistive Technologies, 9(1), 1–20.

Ahmed, S., Grainger, R., Santosa, A., Adnan, A., Alnaqbi, K.A., Chen, Y., Kavadichanda, C., Kaw, N.S.K., Kelly, A., Khan, S.E.A., Masri, B., Nakarmi, S., Parlindungan, F., Rahman, N., So, H., Soroush, M.G., Thilakarathne, A.S., & Traboco, L. (2022). APLAR recommendations on the practice of telemedicine in rheumatology. International Journal of Rheumatic Diseases, 25(3), 247–258. https://doi.org/10.1111/1756-185X.14286

Aily, J.B., de Noronha, M., Approbato Selistre, L.F., Ferrari, R.J., White, D.K., & Mattiello, S.M. (2023). Face-to-face and telerehabilitation delivery of circuit training have similar benefits and acceptability in patients with knee osteoarthritis: A randomised trial. Journal of Physiotherapy, 69(4), 232–239.

Ayers, J.W., Poliak, A., Dredze, M., Leas, E.C., Zhu, Z., Kelley, J.B., Faix, D.J., Goodman, A.M., Longhurst, C.A., Hogarth, M., & Smith, D.M. (2023). Comparing physician and artificial intelligence chatbot responses to patient questions posted to a public social media forum. JAMA Internal Medicine, 183(6), 589–596. https://doi.org/10.1001/jamainternmed.2023.1838

Badr, J., Motulsky, A., & Denis, J.-L. (2024). Digital health technologies and inequalities: A scoping review of potential impacts and policy recommendations. Health Policy, 146, 105122. https://doi.org/10.1016/j.healthpol.2024.105122

Barksdale, S., Stark Taylor, S., Criss, S., Kemper, K., Friedman, D.B., Thompson, W., Donelle, L., MacGilvray, P., & Natafgi, N. (2023). Improving patient health literacy during telehealth visits through remote teach-back methods training for family medicine residents: Pilot 2-arm cluster, nonrandomized controlled trial. JMIR Formative Research, 7, e51541. https://doi.org/10.2196/51541

Barlow, J., et al. (2002). Self-management approaches for people with chronic conditions: A review. Patient Education and Counseling, 48(2), 177–187. https://doi.org/10.1016/S0738-3991(02)00032-0

Barnett, A., Kelly, J.T., & Scuffham, P. (2025). Funding of digital health care for the management of chronic conditions in Australia. Australian Health Review, 49(2), AH24310. https://doi.org/10.1071/AH24310

Baroni, M.P., Jacob, M.F.A., Rios, W.R., Fandim, J.V., Fernandes, L.G., Chaves, P.I., Fioratti, I., & Saragiotto, B.T. (2023). The state of the art in telerehabilitation for musculoskeletal conditions. Archives of Physiotherapy, 13(1), 1–14.

Bashshur, R., Shannon, G., Krupinski, E., & Grigsby, J. (2011). The taxonomy of telemedicine. Telemedicine and e-Health, 17(6), 484–494.

Becker, C., et al. (2022). Unmet information needs of patients with rheumatic diseases: Results of a cross-sectional online survey study in Germany. International Journal of Environmental Research and Public Health, 19(12), 7071. https://doi.org/10.3390/ijerph19127071

Beukenhorst, A.L., Druce, K.L., & De Cock, D. (2022). Smartphones for musculoskeletal research – Hype or Hope? Lessons from a decennium of mHealth studies. BMC Musculoskeletal Disorders, 23(1), 1–13.

Biebl, J.T., Marzena, R., Strobel, M., Kaur Bollinger, P., Ulm, B., Kraft, E., Huber, S., & Lorenz, A. (2020). Comparison of app-based correction feedback to exercise correction by physiotherapists in patients with osteoarthritis of the knee and/or hip: A prospective cohort study (preprint). Journal of Medical Internet Research, 23, 1–13. https://doi.org/10.2196/26658

Bird, M.-L., Peel, F., Schmidt, M., Fini, N.A., Ramage, E., Sakakibara, B.M., Simpson, D.B., Mather, C., Cadilhac, D.A., Ahuja, K.D.K., Bridgman, H., & English, C. (2022). Mobility-focused physical outcome measures over telecommunication technology (Zoom): Intra and interrater reliability trial. JMIR Rehabilitation and Assistive Technologies, 9(3), e38101. https://doi.org/10.2196/38101

Blanquero, J., Cortés-Vega, M.D., Rodríguez-sánchez-laulhé, P., Corrales-Serra, B.P., Gómez-Patricio, E., Díaz-Matas, N., & Suero-Pineda, A. (2020). Feedback-guided exercises performed on A tablet touchscreen improve return to work, function, strength and healthcare usage more than an exercise program prescribed on paper for people with wrist, hand or finger injuries: A randomised trial. Journal of Physiotherapy, 66(4), 236–242. https://doi.org/10.1016/j.jphys.2020.09.012

Bobos, P., MacDermid, J., et al. (2021a). Barriers, facilitators, preferences and expectations of joint protection programmes for patients with hand arthritis: A cross-sectional survey. BMJ Open, 11(1), e041935. https://doi.org/10.1136/bmjopen-2020-041935

Bobos, P., MacDermid, J.C., et al. (2021b). Joint protection programmes for people with osteoarthritis and rheumatoid arthritis of the hand: An overview of systematic reviews. Physiotherapy Canada, 73(1), 56–65. https://doi.org/10.3138/ptc-2019-0037

Bounabe, A., et al. (2024). Effectiveness of patient education on the quality of life of patients with rheumatoid arthritis: A systematic review and meta-analysis. Seminars in Arthritis and Rheumatism, 69, 152569. https://doi.org/10.1016/j.semarthrit.2024.152569

Chaleshgar-Kordasiabi, M., et al. (2018). Barriers and reinforcing factors to self-management behaviour in rheumatoid arthritis patients: A qualitative study. Musculoskeletal Care, 16(2), 241–250. https://doi.org/10.1002/msc.1221

Chandwar, K., & Misra, D.P. (2024). What does artificial intelligence mean in rheumatology? Archives of Rheumatology, 39(1), 1–9. https://doi.org/10.46497/ArchRheumatol.2024.10664

Chen, Y.-P., et al. (2020). Wearable motion sensor device to facilitate rehabilitation in patients with shoulder adhesive capsulitis: Pilot study to assess Feasibility. Journal of Medical Internet Research, 22(7), e17032. https://doi.org/10.2196/17032

Combe, B., et al. (2017). 2016 update of the EULAR recommendations for the management of early arthritis. Annals of the Rheumatic Diseases, 76(6), 948–959. https://doi.org/10.1136/annrheumdis-2016-210602

Cottrell, M.A., Galea, O.A., O'Leary, S.P., Hill, A.J., & Russell, T.G. (2017). Real-time telerehabilitation for the treatment of musculoskeletal conditions is effective and comparable to standard practice: A systematic review and meta-analysis. Clinical Rehabilitation, 31(5), 625–638.

Damgaard, A.J., et al. (2023). Self-management support needs of patients with inflammatory arthritis and the content of self-management interventions: A scoping review. Seminars in Arthritis and Rheumatism, 60, 152203. https://doi.org/10.1016/j.semarthrit.2023.152203

Dantas, L. O., Carvalho, C., Prando, B. C., McAlindon, T. E., & da Silva Serrão, P. R. M. (2021). Mobile health technologies for the management of rheumatic diseases: a systematic review of online stores in Brazil. Clinical Rheumatology, 40(7), 2601–2609. https://doi.org/10.1007/s10067-020-05561-y

Darlow, B., Brown, M., Hudson, B., Frew, G., Clark, J., Vincent, L., Abbott, J.H., Briggs, A.M., Grainger, R., Marra, C., McKinlay, E., & Stanley, J. (2022). Feasibility of a randomised controlled trial of two types of written information for people with knee osteoarthritis. Osteoarthritis and Cartilage Open, 4(2), 100254.

Davies, L., Hinman, R.S., Russell, T., Lawford, B., Bennell, K., Billings, M., Cooper-Oguz, C., Finnan, K., Gallagher, S., Gilbertson, D.K., Holdsworth, L., Holland, A., McAlister, J., Miles, D., & Roots, R. (2021). An international core capability framework for physiotherapists to deliver quality care via videoconferencing: A Delphi study. Journal of Physiotherapy, 67(4), 291–297. https://doi.org/10.1016/j.jphys.2021.09.001

Dixon, W. G., & Michaud, K. (2018). Using technology to support clinical care and research in rheumatoid arthritis. Current Opinion in Rheumatology, 30(3), 276–281. https://doi.org/10.1097/BOR.0000000000000485

de la Fuente Ballesteros, S.L., García Granja, N., Hernández Carrasco, M., Hidalgo Benito, A., García Álvarez, I., & García Ramón, E. (2018). Tele-medicine consultation as a tool to improve the demand for consultation in primary care. Semergen, 44(7), 458–462.

de Thurah, A., Bosch, P., Marques, A., Meissner, Y., Mukhtyar, C.B., et al. (2022). 2022 EULAR points to consider for remote care in rheumatic and musculoskeletal diseases. Annals of the Rheumatic Diseases, 81(8), 1065–1071. https://doi.org/10.1136/annrheumdis-2022-222341

de Thurah, A., Stengaard-Pedersen, K., Axelsen, M., Fredberg, U., Schougaard, L.M.V., Hjollund, N.H.I., Pfeiffer-Jensen, M., Laurberg, T.B., Tarp, U., Lomborg, K., & Maribo, T. (2018). Tele-health followup strategy for tight control of disease activity in rheumatoid arthritis: Results of a randomized controlled trial. Arthritis Care and Research, 70(3), 353–360. https://acrjournals.onlinelibrary.wiley.com/doi/abs/10.1002/acr.23280

Digital Therapeutics Alliance. (2025). Understanding DTx. What is a DTx? Retrieved October 24, 2025, from https://dtxalliance.org/understanding-dtx/what-is-a-dtx/

Duggal, M., El Ayadi, A., Duggal, B., Reynolds, N., & Bascaran, C. (2023). Editorial: Challenges in implementing digital health in public health settings in low and middle income countries. Frontiers in Public Health, 10, 1090303. https://doi.org/10.3389/fpubh.2022.1090303

Dziedzic, K., Thomas, E., Hill, S., Wilkie, R., Peat, G., & Croft, P. R. (2007). The impact of musculoskeletal hand problems in older adults: findings from the North Staffordshire Osteoarthritis Project (NorStOP). Rheumatology (Oxford, England*)*, *46*(6), 963–967. https://doi.org/10.1093/rheumatology/kem005

Eriksen, A.V., Sören, M., & Jesper, R. (2024). Use of GPT-4 to diagnose complex clinical cases. NEJM AI, 1(1), AIp2300031. https://doi.org/10.1056/AIp2300031

Eriksson, L., Lindström, B., & Ekenberg, L. (2011). Patients' experiences of telerehabilitation at home after shoulder joint replacement. Journal of Telemedicine and Telecare, 17(1), 25–30.

European Parliament & Council of the European Union. (2024). Regulation (EU) 2024/1689 of the European Parliament and of the Council of 13 June 2024 laying down harmonised rules on artificial intelligence and amending Regulations (EC) No 300/2008, (EU) No 167/2013, (EU) No 168/2013, (EU) 2018/858, (EU) 2018/1139 and (EU) 2019/2144 and Directives 2014/90/EU, (EU) 2016/797 and (EU) 2020/1828 (Artificial Intelligence Act). OJ L 1689. http://data.europa.eu/eli/reg/2024/1689/oj

European Parliament and Council. (2017). Regulation (EU) 2017/745 of the European Parliament on medical devices, amending directive 2001/83, regulation 178/2002 and regulation 1223/2009 and repealing council directives 90/385 and 93/42.

Fan, I., Govil, D., King, M.G., Scholes, M.J., & Semciw, A.I. (2024). How effective are exercises delivered digitally (requiring internet), amongst patients with hip or knee osteoarthritis? A systematic review and meta-analysis. Osteoarthritis and Cartilage, 32(3), 254–265.

Frederiksen, B.A., Schousboe, M., Terslev, L., Iversen, N., Lindegaard, H., Savarimuthu, T.R., & Just, S.A. (2022). Ultrasound joint examination by an automated system versus by a rheumatologist: From a patient perspective. Advances in Rheumatology, 62(1), 30. https://doi.org/10.1186/s42358-022-00263-2

Fu, X., et al. (2025). The effect of exercise therapy on pain, fatigue, bone function and inflammatory biomarkers individuals with rheumatoid arthritis and knee osteoarthritis: A meta-research review of randomized controlled trials. Frontiers in Physiology, 16, 1558214. https://doi.org/10.3389/fphys.2025.1558214

Giansanti, D. (2024). Joint expedition: Exploring telehealth and the digital healthcare landscape as a team integration. Healthcare (Switzerland), 12(5), 585. https://doi.org/10.3390/healthcare12050585

Gioia, C., et al. (2020). Dietary habits and nutrition in rheumatoid arthritis: Can diet influence disease development and clinical manifestations? Nutrients, 12(5), 1456. https://doi.org/10.3390/nu12051456

Gossec, L., Guyard, F., Leroy, D., Lafargue, T., Seiler, M., Jacquemin, C., Molto, A., Sellam, J., Foltz, V., Gandjbakhch, F., Hudry, C., Mitrovic, S., Fautrel, B., & Servy, H. (2019). Detection of flares by decrease in physical activity, collected using wearable activity trackers in rheumatoid arthritis or axial spondyloarthritis: An application of machine learning analyses in rheumatology. Arthritis Care & Research, 71(10), 1336–1343. https://doi.org/10.1002/acr.23768

Hammond, A., & Prior, Y. (2016). The effectiveness of home hand exercise programmes in rheumatoid arthritis: A systematic review. British Medical Bulletin, 119(1), 49–62. https://doi.org/10.1093/bmb/ldw024

Hartman, J., & Duttine, A. (2022). Rehabilitation 2030: A collective call that requires individual action. Brazilian Journal of Physical Therapy, 26(2), 100360. https://doi.org/10.1016/j.bjpt.2021.06.004

Hinch, R., & Sirois, F.M. (2024). A meta-analysis of coping strategies and psychological distress in rheumatoid arthritis. British Journal of Health Psychology, 29(3), 771–787. https://doi.org/10.1111/bjhp.12726

Hoffmann, T.C., Glasziou, P.P., Boutron, I., Milne, R., Perera, R., Moher, D., Altman, D.G., Barbour, V., Macdonald, H., Johnston, M., Kadoorie, S.E.L., Dixon-Woods, M., McCulloch, P., Wyatt, J.C., Phelan, A.W.C., & Michie, S. (2014). Better reporting of interventions: Template for intervention description and replication (TIDieR) checklist and guide. BMJ (Online), 348(March), g1687-g1687. https://doi.org/10.1136/bmj.g1687

Jacob, C., Sezgin, E., Sanchez-Vazquez, A., & Ivory, C. (2022). Socio-technical factors impacting Patients' adoption of Mobile health tools: Systematic literature review and narrative synthesis. JMIR mHealth and uHealth, 10(5), 1–27.

Janiszewska, M., et al. (2020). Coping strategies observed in women with rheumatoid arthritis. Annals of Agricultural and Environmental Medicine: AAEM, 27(3), 401–406. https://doi.org/10.26444/aaem/110958

Jones, M.D., Hansford, H.J., Bastianon, A., Gibbs, M.T., Gilanyi, Y.L., Foster, N.E., Dean, S.G., Ogilvie, R., Hayden, J.A., & Wood, L. (2025). Exercise adherence is associated with improvements in pain intensity and functional limitations in adults with chronic non-specific low back pain: A secondary analysis of A cochrane review. Journal of Physiotherapy, 71(2), 91–99.

Kataria, S., & Ravindran, V. (2019). Emerging role of eHealth in the identification of very early inflammatory rheumatic diseases. Best Practice & Research Clinical Rheumatology, 33(4), 101429. https://doi.org/10.1016/j.berh.2019.101429

Keel, S., Schmid, A., Keller, F., & Schoeb, V. (2023). Investigating the use of digital health tools in physiotherapy: Facilitators and barriers. Physiotherapy Theory and Practice, 39(7), 1449–1468. https://doi.org/10.1080/09593985.2022.2042439

Kennedy, C.A., Warmington, K., Flewelling, C., Shupak, R., Papachristos, A., Jones, C., Linton, D., Beaton, D.E., Lineker, S., & Hogg-Johnson, S. (2017). A prospective comparison of telemedicine versus in-person delivery of an interprofessional education program for adults with inflammatory arthritis. Journal of Telemedicine and Telecare, 23(2), 197–206. https://doi.org/10.1177/1357633X16635342

Kleinert, S., et al. (2021). A real-world rheumatology registry and research consortium: The German RheumaDatenRhePort (RHADAR) Registry. Journal of Medical Internet Research, 23(5), e28164. https://doi.org/10.2196/28164

Kloppenburg, M. (2007). Hand osteoarthritis--an increasing need for treatment and rehabilitation. Current Opinion in Rheumatology, 19(2), 179–183. https://doi.org/10.1097/BOR.0b013e32802106a8

Knitza, J., Tascilar, K., Messner, E. M., Meyer, M., Vossen, D., Pulla, A., Bosch, P., Kittler, J., Kleyer, A., Sewerin, P., Mucke, J., Haase, I., Simon, D., & Krusche, M. (2019). German Mobile Apps in rheumatology: Review and analysis using the Mobile Application Rating Scale (MARS). JMIR mHealth and uHealth, 7(8), e14991. https://doi.org/10.2196/14991

Kolasinski, S.L., Neogi, T., Hochberg, M.C., Oatis, C., Guyatt, G., Block, J., Callahan, L., Copenhaver, C., Dodge, C., Felson, D., Gellar, K., Harvey, W.F., Hawker, G., Herzig, E., Kwoh, C.K., Nelson, A.E., Samuels, J., Scanzello, C., White, D., & Wise, B. (2020). 2019 American college of Rheumatology/Arthritis foundation guideline for the management of osteoarthritis of the hand, hip, and knee. Arthritis Care & Research, 72(2), 149–162. https://doi.org/10.1002/acr.24131

Kongsted, A., et al. (2021). Self-management at the core of back pain care: 10 key points for clinicians. Brazilian Journal of Physical Therapy, 25(4), 396–406. https://doi.org/10.1016/j.bjpt.2021.05.002

Krauss, I., Katzmarek, U., Rieger, M.A., & Sudeck, G. (2017). Motives for physical exercise participation as A basis for the development of patient-oriented exercise interventions in osteoarthritis: A cross-sectional study. European Journal of Physical and Rehabilitation Medicine, 53(4), 590–602.

Kremer, P., Schiebisch, H., Lechner, F., Haase, I., Cirkel, L., Kötter, I., Kuhn, S., Krusche, M., & Knitza, J. (2025). Comparative analysis of large language models and traditional diagnostic decision support systems for rare rheumatic disease identification. EULAR Rheumatology Open, 1(2), 51–59. https://doi.org/10.1016/j.ero.2025.04.007

Lantzsch, H., Eckhardt, H., Campione, A., Busse, R., & Henschke, C. (2022). Digital health applications and the fast-track pathway to public health coverage in Germany: challenges and opportunities based on first results. *BMC Health Services Research*, 22(1). https://doi.org/10.1186/s12913-022-08500-6

Laskowski, E.R., Johnson, S.E., Shelerud, R.A., Lee, J.A., Rabatin, A.E., Driscoll, S.W., Moore, B.J., Wainberg, M.C., & Terzic, C.M. (2020). The telemedicine musculoskeletal examination. Mayo Clinic Proceedings, 95 (8), 1715–1731. https://doi.org/10.1016/j.mayocp.2020.05.026

Latifi, R., Doarn, C.R., & Merrell, R.C. (eds) (2021). Telemedicine, Telehealth and Telepresence: Principles, Strategies, Applications, and New Directions. Springer.

Lawford, B.J., Bennell, K.L., Kasza, J., & Hinman, R.S. (2018). Physical Therapists' perceptions of telephone- and internet Video–Mediated service models for exercise management of people with osteoarthritis. Arthritis Care and Research, 70(3), 398–408. https://doi.org/10.1002/acr.23260

Lawford, B. J., Dobson, F., Bennell, K. L., Merolli, M., Graham, B., Haber, T., Teo, P. L., Mackenzie, D., McManus, F., Lamb, K. E., & Hinman, R. S. (2024). Clinician-administered performance-based tests via telehealth in people with chronic lower limb musculoskeletal disorders: Test-retest reliability and agreement with in-person assessment. Journal of Telemedicine and Telecare, 30(8), 1300–1319. https://doi.org/10.1177/1357633X221137387

Lazarus, R., & Folkman, S. (1984). Stress, Appraisal, and Coping. Springer Publishing Company.

Le, T.V., Galperin, H., & Traube, D. (2023). The impact of digital competence on telehealth utilization. Health Policy and Technology, 12(1), 100724. https://doi.org/10.1016/j.hlpt.2023.100724

Lee, A.C., Deutsch, J.E., Holdsworth, L., Kaplan, S.L., Kosakowski, H., Latz, R., McNeary, L.L., O'Neil, J., Ronzio, O., Sanders, K., Sigmund-Gaines, M., Wiley, M., & Russell, T. (2024a). Telerehabilitation in physical therapist practice: A clinical practice guideline from the American physical therapy association. Physical Therapy, 104(5), pzae045. https://doi.org/10.1093/ptj/pzae045

Lee, H.-Y., Ju, M., Kang, M., Lee, H., Choi, J., & Oh, J. (2024b). Preparedness, challenges, and opportunities for digital intervention for chronic disease management: A qualitative study in rural areas of South Korea. Health Systems & Reform, 10(2), 2378503. https://doi.org/10.1080/23288604.2024.2378503

Liang, J., Fang, Q., Jiao, X., Xiang, P., Ma, J., Zhang, Z., Liu, Y., He, Y., Li, Y., He, Z., & Lei, J. (2025). Approved trends and product characteristics of digital therapeutics in four countries. NPJ Digital Medicine, 8(1), 308. https://doi.org/10.1038/s41746-025-01660-9

Lindberg, J., Bhatt, R., & Ferm, A. (2021). Older people and rural eHealth: Perceptions of caring relations and their effects on engagement in digital primary health care. Scandinavian Journal of Caring Sciences, 35(4), 1322–1331.

Lumma, F., Knitza, J., & Mühlensiepen, F. (2025). Potentials and barriers of digital patient education in rheumatic disease management: An exploratory qualitative interview study. Rheumatology International, 45(6), 148. https://doi.org/10.1007/s00296-025-05893-5

Luna, A., Casertano, L., Timmerberg, J., O'Neil, M., Machowsky, J., Leu, C.S., Lin, J., Fang, Z., Douglas, W., & Agrawal, S. (2021). Artificial intelligence application versus physical therapist for squat evaluation: A randomized controlled trial. Scientific Reports, 11(1), 1–8. https://doi.org/10.1038/s41598-021-97343-y

Lupton, D. (2013). The digitally engaged patient: Self-monitoring and self-care in the digital health era. Social Theory and Health, 11(3), 256–270.

Lyles, C.R., Nguyen, O.K., Khoong, E.C., Aguilera, A., & Sarkar, U. (2023). Multilevel determinants of digital health equity: A literature synthesis to advance the field. Annual Review of Public Health, 44(1), 383–405. https://doi.org/10.1146/annurev-publhealth-071521-023913

Ma, Y., et al. (2025). Global, regional and national burden of rheumatoid arthritis from 1990 to 2021, with projections of incidence to 2050: A systematic and comprehensive analysis of the global burden of disease study 2021. Biomarker Research, 13, 47. https://doi.org/10.1186/s40364-025-00760-8

Mace, R.A., Mattos, M.K., & Vranceanu, A.M. (2022). Older adults can use technology: Why healthcare professionals must overcome ageism in digital health. Translational Behavioral Medicine, 12(12), 1102–1105.

MacIver, A., Hollinger, H., & Carolan, C. (2021). Tele-health interventions to support self-management in adults with rheumatoid arthritis: A systematic review. Rheumatology International, 41(8), 1399–1418. https://doi.org/10.1007/s00296-021-04907-2

Magnol, M., et al. (2021). Use of eHealth by patients with rheumatoid arthritis: Observational, cross-sectional, multicenter study. Journal of Medical Internet Research, 23(1), e19998. https://doi.org/10.2196/19998

Mahmood, A., Nayak, P., Deshmukh, A., English, C., Manikandan, N., Solomon M, J., & Unnikrishnan, B. (2023). Measurement, determinants, barriers, and interventions for exercise adherence: A scoping review. Journal of Bodywork and Movement Therapies, 33, 95–105.

Marcuzzi, A., Nordstoga, A.L., Bach, K., Aasdahl, L., Ivar, T., Nilsen, L., & Bardal, E.M. (2023). Effect of an artificial intelligence – Based self-management app on musculoskeletal health in patients with neck and/or low back pain referred to specialist care a randomized clinical trial. JAMA Network Open, 6(6), 1–13. https://doi.org/10.1001/jamanetworkopen.2023.20400

May, S., Darkow, R., Knitza, J., Boy, K., Klemm, P., Heinze, M., Vuillerme, N., Petit, P., Steffens-Korbanka, P., Kladny, H., Hornig, J., Aries, P., Welcker, M., & Muehlensiepen, F. (2025). Digital transformation of rheumatology care in Germany: Cross-sectional national survey. Journal of Medical Internet Research, 27, 1–10.

Mo, R. (2025). Goniometer Chrome extension. https://chromewebstore.google.com/detail/goniometer/bgohdobpmnajfkhonaimnelpglcplhei

Molina-Garcia, P., Mora-Traverso, M., Prieto-Moreno, R., Díaz-Vásquez, A., Antony, B., & Ariza-Vega, P. (2024). Effectiveness and cost-effectiveness of telerehabilitation for musculoskeletal disorders: A systematic review and meta-analysis. Annals of Physical and Rehabilitation Medicine, 67(1), 101791.

Mollard, E., & Michaud, K. (2020). Self-management of rheumatoid arthritis: Mobile Applications. Current Rheumatology Reports, 23(1), 2. https://doi.org/10.1007/s11926-020-00968-7

Moman, R.N., Dvorkin, J., Pollard, E.M., Wanderman, R., Murad, M.H., Warner, D.O., & Hooten, W.M. (2019). A systematic review and meta-analysis of unguided electronic and mobile health technologies for chronic pain - is it time to start prescribing electronic health applications? Pain Medicine (United States), 20(11), 2238–2255.

Momtazmanesh, S., Nowroozi, A., & Rezaei, N. (2022). Artificial intelligence in rheumatoid arthritis: Current status and future perspectives: A state-of-the-art review. Rheumatology and Therapy, 9(5), 1249–1304. https://doi.org/10.1007/s40744-022-00475-4

Najm, A., et al. (2019). EULAR points to consider for the development, evaluation and implementation of mobile health applications aiding self-management in people living with rheumatic and musculoskeletal diseases. RMD Open, 5(2), e001014. https://doi.org/10.1136/rmdopen-2019-001014

Nelligan, R.K., Hinman, R.S., McManus, F., Lamb, K.E., & Bennell, K.L. (2021). Moderators of the effect of a self-directed digitally delivered exercise program for people with knee osteoarthritis: Exploratory analysis of a randomized controlled trial. Journal of Medical Internet Research, 23(10), e30768.

Neter, E., Western, M.J., Cooper, R., Silva, A.M., & König, L.M. (2025). Towards bridging the digital divide: Training healthcare professionals for digitally inclusive healthcare systems. Global Health Research and Policy, 10(1), 31. https://doi.org/10.1186/s41256-025-00433-x

Niemeijer, A., Lund, H., Stafne, S.N., Ipsen, T., Goldschmidt, C.L., Jørgensen, C.T., & Juhl, C.B. (2019). Adverse events of exercise therapy in randomised controlled trials: A systematic review and meta-analysis. British Journal of Sports Medicine, 54(18), 1073–1080. https://doi.org/10.1136/bjsports-2018-100461

Nikiphorou, E., et al. (2021). 2021 EULAR recommendations for the implementation of self-management strategies in patients with inflammatory arthritis. Annals of the Rheumatic Diseases, 80(10), 1278–1285. https://doi.org/10.1136/annrheumdis-2021-220249

Niknejad, N., Ismail, W., Bahari, M., & Nazari, B. (2021). Understanding telerehabilitation technology to evaluate Stakeholders' adoption of telerehabilitation services: A systematic literature review and directions for further research. Archives of Physical Medicine and Rehabilitation, 102(7):1390–1403. https://doi.org/10.1016/j.apmr.2020.12.014

Olveres, J., González, G., Torres, F., Moreno-Tagle, J.C., Carbajal-Degante, E., Valencia-Rodríguez, A., Méndez-Sánchez, N., & Escalante- Ramírez, B. (2021). What is new in computer vision and artificial intelligence in medical image analysis applications. Quantitative Imaging in Medicine and Surgery, 11(8), 3830–3853. https://doi.org/10.21037/qims-20-1151

Overview | Rheumatoid arthritis in adults: management | Guidance | NICE. (2018). NICE. Available at: https://www.nice.org.uk/guidance/ng100 (Accessed: 31 August 2025).

Patten, R.K., Tacey, A., Pile, R., Parker, A., De Gori, M., Tran, P., McKenna, M.J., Lane, R., Apostolopoulos, V., Said, C.M., Levinger, I., & Woessner, M.N. (2022). Digital self-management interventions for osteoarthritis: A systematic scoping review of intervention characteristics, adherence and attrition. Archives of Public Health, 80(1), 1–13. https://doi.org/10.1186/s13690-022-00854-x

Peres, M.F.P., & Lucchetti, G. (2010). Coping strategies in chronic pain. Current Pain and Headache Reports, 14(5), 331–338. https://doi.org/10.1007/s11916-010-0137-3

Peter, W.F., et al. (2021). Clinical practice guideline for physical therapist management of people with rheumatoid Arthritis. Physical Therapy, 101(8), pzab127. https://doi.org/10.1093/ptj/pzab127

Phatak, S., Chakraborty, S., & Goel, P. (2023). Computer vision detects inflammatory arthritis in standardized smartphone photographs in an Indian patient cohort. Frontiers in Medicine, 10, 1280462. https://doi.org/10.3389/fmed.2023.1280462

Porcheret, M., Jordan, K., Jinks, C., Croft, P., & Primary Care Rheumatology Society (2007). Primary care treatment of knee pain—A survey in older adults. Rheumatology (Oxford, England), 46(11), 1694–1700. https://doi.org/10.1093/rheumatology/kem232

Ritschl, V., Stamm, T., Aletaha, D., Bijlsma, J.W., Boehm, P., Dragoi, R., Dures, E., Estévez-López, F., Gossec, L., Iagnocco, A., Nudel, M., Marques, A., Moholt, E., Van Den Bemt, B., Viktil, K., Voshaar, M., De Thurah, A., & Carmona, L. (2021). 2020 EULAR points to consider for the detection, assessment and management of non-adherence in people with rheumatic and musculoskeletal diseases. Annals of the Rheumatic Diseases, 80, 707–713.

Roddy, E., et al. (2005). Evidence-based recommendations for the role of exercise in the management of osteoarthritis of the hip or knee—the MOVE consensus. Rheumatology, 44(1), 67–73. https://doi.org/10.1093/rheumatology/keh399

Rodríguez Sánchez-Laulhé, P., et al. (2022). An exercise and educational and self-management program delivered with a smartphone app (CareHand) in Adults With Rheumatoid Arthritis of the Hands: Randomized Controlled Trial. JMIR mHealth and uHealth, 10(4), e35462. https://doi.org/10.2196/35462

Rodríguez Sánchez-Laulhé, P., et al. (2023). The effects of a mobile app-delivered intervention in people with symptomatic hand osteoarthritis: A pragmatic randomized controlled trial. European Journal of Physical and Rehabilitation Medicine, 59(1), 54–64. https://doi.org/10.23736/S1973-9087.22.07744-9

Rodríguez-Sánchez-Laulhé, P., et al. (2024). Exploring factors associated with changes in pain and function following mHealth-based exercise therapy for chronic musculoskeletal pain: A systematic review with meta-analysis and meta-Regression. Applied Sciences, 14(15), 6632. https://doi.org/10.3390/app14156632

Rossettini, G., Cook, C., Palese, A., Pillastrini, P., & Turolla, A. (2023). Pros and cons of using artificial intelligence chatbots for musculoskeletal rehabilitation management. Journal of Orthopaedic and Sports Physical Therapy, 53(12), 728–734. https://doi.org/10.2519/jospt.2023.12000

Safari, R., Jackson, J., & Sheffield, D. (2020). Digital self-management interventions for people with osteoarthritis: Systematic review with meta-analysis. Journal of Medical Internet Research, 22(7), e15365.

Sahu, D., Shah, D., Joshi, M., Shaikh, S., Gaikwad, P., & Shyam, A. (2022). Validation of an on-screen application-based measurement of shoulder range of motion over telehealth medium. Journal of Shoulder and Elbow Surgery, 31(1), 201–208. https://doi.org/10.1016/j.jse.2021.06.017

Sardana, Y., et al. (2023). Progression of pre-rheumatoid arthritis to clinical disease of joints: Potential role of mesenchymal stem cells. Life Sciences, 321, 121641. https://doi.org/10.1016/j.lfs.2023.121641

Scheer, J., Costa, F., Molinos, M., Areias, A., Janela, D., Moulder, R.G., Lains, J., Bento, V., Yanamadala, V., Cohen, S.P., & Correia, F.D. (2022). Racial and ethnic differences in outcomes of a 12-week digital rehabilitation program for musculoskeletal pain: Prospective longitudinal cohort study. Journal of Medical Internet Research, 24(10), e41306. https://doi.org/10.2196/41306

Scherer, H.U., Häupl, T., & Burmester, G.R. (2020). The etiology of rheumatoid arthritis. Journal of Autoimmunity, 110, 102400. https://doi.org/10.1016/j.jaut.2019.102400

Seppen, B.F., L'ami, M.J., Duarte Dos Santos Rico, S., Ter Wee, M.M., Turkstra, F., Roorda, L.D., Catarinella, F.S., van Schaardenburg, D., Nurmohamed, M.T., Boers, M., & Bos, W.H. (2020). A smartphone app for self-monitoring of rheumatoid arthritis disease activity to assist patient-initiated care: Protocol for a randomized controlled trial. JMIR Research Protocols, 9(2), e15105. https://doi.org/10.2196/15105

Seron, P., Oliveros, M.-J., Gutierrez-Arias, R., Fuentes-Aspe, R., Torres-Castro, R.C., Merino-Osorio, C., Nahuelhual, P., Inostroza, J., Jalil, Y., Solano, R., Marzuca-Nassr, G.N., Aguilera-Eguía, R., Lavados-Romo, P., Soto-Rodríguez, F.J., Sabelle, C., Villarroel-Silva, G., Gomolán, P., Huaiquilaf, S., & Sanchez, P. (2021). Effectiveness of telerehabilitation in physical therapy: A rapid overview. Physical Therapy, 101(6), pzab053. https://doi.org/10.1093/ptj/pzab053

Slattery, B.W., Haugh, S., O'Connor, L., Francis, K., Dwyer, C.P., O'Higgins, S., Egan, J., & McGuire, B.E. (2019). An evaluation of the effectiveness of the modalities used to deliver electronic health interventions for chronic pain: Systematic review with network meta-analysis. Journal of Medical Internet Research, 21(7), e11086. https://doi.org/10.2196/11086

Suero-Pineda, A., Oliva-Pascual-Vaca, Á, Durán, M.R.P., Sánchez-Laulhé, P.R., García-Frasquet, M., & Blanquero, J. (2023). Effectiveness of a telerehabilitation evidence-based tablet app for rehabilitation in traumatic bone and soft tissue injuries of the hand, wrist, and fingers. Archives of Physical Medicine and Rehabilitation, 104(6), 932–941. https://doi.org/10.1016/j.apmr.2023.01.016

Tan, M.M.T., & Wong, R.S.H. (2025). Facilitators and barriers for use of digital technology in chronic disease management. Scientific Reports, 10(15), 1. https://doi.org/10.1038/s41598-025-15549-w

Tang, C. Y., Bastani, A., Sidhu, B., Saberi, G., & Baker, E. (2024). Access, readiness and willingness to engage in allied health telerehabilitation services for adults: Does cultural and linguistic diversity make a difference?. Healthcare (Basel, Switzerland), 12(11), 1141. https://doi.org/10.3390/healthcare12111141

Tangsrivimol, J.A., Darzidehkalani, E., Virk, H.U.H., Wang, Z., Egger, J., Wang, M., Hacking, S., Glicksberg, B.S., Strauss, M., & Krittanawong, C. (2025). Benefits, limits, and risks of ChatGPT in medicine. Frontiers in Artificial Intelligence, 8, 1518049.

Thompson, D., Rattu, S., Tower, J., Egerton, T., Francis, J., & Merolli, M. (2023). Mobile app use to support therapeutic exercise for musculoskeletal pain conditions may help improve pain intensity and self-reported physical function: A systematic review. Journal of Physiotherapy, 69(1), 23–34.

Thompson, R.J., et al. (2010). Maladaptive coping, adaptive coping, and depressive symptoms: Variations across age and depressive State. Behaviour Research and Therapy, 48(6), 459–466.

Toelle, T.R., Utpadel-Fischler, D.A., Haas, K.-K., & Priebe, J.A. (2019). App-based multidisciplinary back pain treatment versus combined physiotherapy plus online education: A randomized controlled trial. NPJ Digital Medicine, 2(1), 1–9. https://doi.org/10.1038/s41746-019-0109-x

Tong, S.Y.K., Jackson, T.M., & Lau, A.Y.S. (2024). Virtual physical examination in teleconsultation: A scoping review. International Journal of Medical Informatics, 191, 105561. https://doi.org/10.1016/j.ijmedinf.2024.105561

Uz, C., & Umay, E. (2023). "Dr ChatGPT": Is it a reliable and useful source for common rheumatic diseases? International Journal of Rheumatic Diseases, 26(7), 1343–1349. https://doi.org/10.1111/1756-185X.14749

van den Bemt, B.J.F., Zwikker, H.E., & van den Ende, C.H.M. (2012). Medication adherence in patients with rheumatoid arthritis: A critical appraisal of the existing literature. Expert Review of Clinical Immunology, 8(4), 337–351. https://doi.org/10.1586/eci.12.23

van Dyk, L. (2014). A review of telehealth service implementation frameworks. International Journal of Environmental Research and Public Health, 11(2), 1279–1298.

Van Tilburg, M.L., Spin, I., Pisters, M.F., Staal, J.B., Ostelo, R.W., Van Der Velde, M., Veenhof, C., & Kloek, C.J. (2024). Barriers and facilitators to the implementation of digital health services for people with musculoskeletal conditions in the primary health care setting: Systematic review. Journal of Medical Internet Research, 26, e49868. https://doi.org/10.2196/49868

Vasconez-Gonzalez, J., Alexander-León, H., & Ortiz-Prado, E. (2025). Digital health transformation in Ecuador: Progress, barriers, and future directions. Journal of Medical Systems, 49(1), 41. https://doi.org/10.1007/s10916-025-02174-3

Vlad, A.L., Popazu, C., Lescai, A.-M., Voinescu, D.C., & Balta, A. (2025). The role of artificial intelligence in the diagnosis and management of rheumatoid arthritis. Medicina, 61(689), 1–26. https://doi.org/10.3390/medicina61040689

Volkmar, A., Kleinert, S., Karberg, K., Gauler, G., Klennert, M., Klennert, J., Aries, P.M., Froschauer, S., Wildenhain, S., Späthling-mestekemper, S., Kuhn, C., Welcker, M., Bartz-bazzanella, P., & Englbrecht, M. (2025). Potential of digital applications for self-management and other outcomes in inflammatory rheumatic diseases: A systematic literature review. Frontiers in Medicine, 12, 1617151.

Wainberg, M.C., Jurisson, M.L., Johnson, S.E., & Brault, J.S. (2020). The telemedicine hand examination. American Journal of Physical Medicine & Rehabilitation, 99 (10), 883–883. https://doi.org/10.1097/PHM.0000000000001555

Walrabenstein, W., et al. (2023). A multidisciplinary lifestyle program for rheumatoid arthritis: The "Plants for Joints" randomized controlled trial. Rheumatology, 62(8), 2683–2691. https://doi.org/10.1093/rheumatology/keac693

Wang, C., Lee, C., & Shin, H. (2023). Digital therapeutics from bench to bedside. NPJ Digital Medicine, 6(1), 1–10. https://doi.org/10.1038/s41746-023-00777-z

WHO. (2011). mHealth: New horizons for health through mobile technologies. Observatory, 3(June), 66–71.

WHO. (2016). Global Diffusion of eHealth: Making Universal Health Coverage Achievable. Report of the Third Global Survey on eHealth. https://www.who.int/publications/i/item/9789241511780

World Health Organization & International Telecommunication Union. (2024). *Implementation toolkit for accessible telehealth services*. Geneva: World Health Organization. https://iris.who.int/handle/10665/378483

Wu, Z., et al. (2022). The effects of patient education on psychological status and clinical outcomes in rheumatoid arthritis: A systematic review and meta-Analysis. Frontiers in Psychiatry, 13, 848427. https://doi.org/10.3389/fpsyt.2022.848427

Yang, Y., Boulton, E., & Todd, C. (2022). Measurement of adherence to mHealth physical activity interventions and exploration of the factors that affect the adherence: Scoping review and proposed framework. Journal of Medical Internet Research, 24(6), e30817.

Ye, J., He, L., & Beestrum, M. (2023). Implications for implementation and adoption of telehealth in developing countries: A systematic review of China's practices and experiences. NPJ Digital Medicine, 6(1), 174. https://doi.org/10.1038/s41746-023-00908-6

Yedlinsky, N.T., & Peebles, R.L. (2021). Telemedicine management of musculoskeletal issues. American Family Physician, 103(3), 147–154.

Zhang, W., Ji, H., Wu, Y., Xu, Z., Li, J., Sun, Q., Wang, C., & Zhao, F. (2024). Patients' needs and experiences of telerehabilitation after total hip and knee arthroplasty: A qualitative systematic review and meta-synthesis. DIGITAL HEALTH, 10, 20552076241256756. https://doi.org/10.1177/20552076241256756

Zhang, Z., et al. (2025). Global, regional, and national epidemiology of rheumatoid arthritis among people aged 20–54 years from 1990 to 2021. Scientific Reports, 15(1), 10736. https://doi.org/10.1038/s41598-025-92150-1

Zhao, P., et al. (2019). Mobile applications for pain management: An app analysis for clinical usage. BMC Medical Informatics and Decision Making, 19(1), 106. https://doi.org/10.1186/s12911-019-0827-7

Zhu, D., et al. (2025). Effects of a computer vision-based exercise application for people with knee osteoarthritis: Randomized controlled Trial. JMIR mHealth and uHealth, 13, e63022. https://doi.org/10.2196/63022

Ziade, N., Hmamouchi, I., El Kibbi, L., Daou, M., Abdulateef, N., et al. (2022). Telehealth in rheumatology: The 2021 Arab league of rheumatology Best practice guidelines. Rheumatology International, 42(3), 379–390. https://doi.org/10.1007/s00296-021-05078-w

Zovi, A., Ferrara, F., Gelmi, M., Messina, N., Pagani, A.A.M., Patti, T., Zanetti Lorenzetti, E., Torri, T., & Langella, R. (2025). Digital therapeutics as a new weapon against diseases: Focus on the current European legislation and possible therapeutic strategies. Expert Review of Medical Devices, 22(2), 141–148. https://doi.org/10.1080/17434440.2025.2457468

Index

For Product Safety Concerns and Information please contact our
EU representative GPSR@taylorandfrancis.com Taylor & Francis
Verlag GmbH, Kaufingerstraße 24, 80331 München, Germany